Ophthalmic
LENSES AND
DISPENSING

For Elsevier:

Commissioning Editor: Robert Edwards
Development Editor: Rebecca Gleave
Project Manager: Frances Affleck
Designer: George Ajayi
Illustrator: Precision Illustration
Illustration Buyer: Merlyn Harvey

THIRD EDITION

Ophthalmic LENSES AND DISPENSING

Mo Jalie SMSA, FBDO(Hons), *Hon*FCGI, *Hon*FCOptom, MCMI

Visiting Professor in Optometry, School of Biomedical Sciences, University of Ulster, Coleraine, Northern Ireland

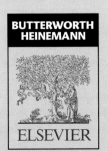

BUTTERWORTH
HEINEMANN

ELSEVIER

Edinburgh London New York Oxford Philadelphia St Louis Sydney Toronto 2008

ELSEVIER

BUTTERWORTH
HEINEMANN

First edition 1999
Second edition 2003
Third edition 2008
  Reprinted 2008

ISBN 9780750688949

British Library Cataloguing in Publication Data
A catalogue record for this book is available from the British Library

Library of Congress Cataloging in Publication Data
A catalog record for this book is available from the Library of Congress

Knowledge and best practice in this field are constantly changing. As new research and experience broaden our knowledge, changes in practice, treatment and drug therapy may become necessary or appropriate. Readers are advised to check the most current information provided (i) on procedures featured or (ii) by the manufacturer of each product to be administered, to verify the recommended dose or formula, the method and duration of administration, and contraindications. It is the responsibility of the practitioner, relying on their own experience and knowledge of the patient, to make diagnoses, to determine dosages and the best treatment for each individual patient, and to take all appropriate safety precautions. To the fullest extent of the law, neither the publisher nor the editors assumes any liability for any injury and/or damage.

The Publisher

The
publisher's
policy is to use
**paper manufactured
from sustainable forests**

Printed in China

Contents

Preface to the third edition

The proliferation of new spectacle lens designs over the last few years has necessitated a third edition of this work on the background to the selection and fitting of modern ophthalmic lenses. New aspheric, atoric and progressive power lens designs have appeared in the last four years, together with recommendations from the lens manufacturers upon how to measure, fit and verify their new lenses. The principles behind these methods are explained in the additions to the text. In addition to a new chapter devoted to lenses for sport, the section on tinted lenses has been enlarged to include the requirements of recent BS EN ISO standards. Advances in manufacturing methods and the implications of freeform technology are described.

Reports from readers have indicated that the explanations on the CD have proved to be particularly helpful in enabling them to obtain a better understanding of the topics presented and it is hoped that the new section on the CD relating to the theory, production and an overview of the different generations of progressive designs will be found equally useful.

Mo Jalie
2007, Balcombe, Sussex

Foreword to the second edition

A name that is renowned and revered in ophthalmic dispensing, Mo Jalie's reputation grows year by year and rightly so when he excels in a field where so few people have made any impact over the years. Mo represents many 'firsts': he was the first dispensing optician to lead a major academic department in his role as the Head of Department of Applied Optics at the former City and Islington College, the first dispensing optician to be awarded honorary Fellowship of The College of Optometrists and the first Professor in Ophthalmic Dispensing, having been invited to take up this visiting post in the Optometry department at the University of Ulster, Coleraine.

On a personal note, one of his most difficult tasks must surely have been to teach me in the first 'block release' courses in the final year of my correspondence course and, believe me, his reputation went before him, even then! He is the only person I have ever known who could recall logarithmic tables off by heart. His mind was just so quick and so clever he left many of us open-mouthed.

Over the years and since those experiences, I have come to know, like and respect the man. The love of his profession is always at the forefront and he has never stopped working and developing new ideas. The respect he engenders in all circles of optics is, I think, quite unique.

The first book written by Mo was published in 1967 and it soon became the 'bible' for students of dispensing. It has now become the standard text on the theory of spectacle lenses for the entire English-speaking world, being used in optometry courses from Canada to New Zealand. Unfortunately for me, the book appeared soon after I had finished my training, but I have been associated with many students who extol its virtues each time it is used. Ophthalmic Lenses and Dispensing, as shown by the publication of its Second Edition, is following suit. This new form of text book actually, and I think uniquely, brings together the theory and practice of Ophthalmic Dispensing. There are already numerous books on the refraction of light, the properties of lenses and their effects. However, to actually have such a comprehensive text that will be used by everyone who is dispensing in practice, dispensing opticians and optometrists alike, must be of enormous value to us all.

A very useful aspect of the text is that the use of the lenses is linked to the appropriate patient, so not only does the book talk about the best type of lenses for the individual, but it then discusses the treatments applicable to those types of lenses. The way in which the contents of the book has been structured, with the major points being repeated for convenience when dealing with each category, is so logical it is remarkable that a similar format has not appeared before. However, it is the measure of the author that it has at last been published.

Students in particular will gain enormously from the CD-ROM included with the book. This method of presenting quite difficult concepts in ophthalmic lens theory in such a visual form brings a far quicker understanding of the theory of ophthalmic lenses. The wide range of topics included on the CD-ROM vary from taking simple measurements for lens fitting to off-axis lens performance and the principles of best-form lenses.

As well as this book becoming essential reading for us all, I am quite sure it will not be long before it becomes a necessary reference book on every optician's bookshelf in every practice.

Colin Lee
President (1996–1998)
Association of British Dispensing Opticians

Preface to the first edition

Successful dispensing of modern ophthalmic lenses requires both knowledge of the different lens forms that are in use in current practice and an understanding of the performance and effects of these lenses. This topic is usually included in the curriculum for optometry and dispensing students under the heading, Dispensing. It presupposes some knowledge of the geometrical optics of ophthalmic lenses and the physiology of vision.

The information presented in this book is designed to provide a comprehensive introduction to the subject, ophthalmic dispensing. It first appeared in this form as a series of articles in Optician magazine, which the author was invited to produce as editor for a continuing education series in ophthalmic lenses and dispensing. Most of the material was written by myself and is the result of 30 years teaching experience of the subject, mainly to dispensing students at City and Islington College. Some of the material was contributed to the series by other authors, each of whom are expert in their own fields.

The section on anti-reflection coatings contained in Chapter 5 and most of the material in Chapter 6 was contributed by Dr Peter Wilkinson, who, as a technical director in the ophthalmic industry for many years, was responsible for the development of coatings and machinery for the treatment of ophthalmic lenses.

The chapter on tinted lenses was contributed largely by Trevor White who is Senior Lecturer in Ophthalmic Dispensing at City and Islington College, and the chapter on safety lenses by Richard Earlam, Lecturer in the Department of Optometry and Vision Science at the University of Wales, College Cardiff. I am very

grateful to these fellow contributors for allowing their original articles to reappear in the book, edited only slightly to follow the style of the rest of the material.

The original series in Optician was deliberately written as a non-mathematical treatment of the subject material. Rigorous proof of the theory is to be found in many other optometry textbooks. However, for the sake of completeness, it was felt that the book should include some information on the theory of geometrical optics and it is hoped that Chapter 1, Introduction to the theory of ophthalmic lenses, will be helpful to students as a résumé of the optics of spectacle lenses.

The CD-ROM included with the book enables much of the information to be presented in visual form designed to provide the reader with a better understanding of the theory of dispensing. Animations of the effects of prisms and lenses upon a crossline chart, how to use the focimeter, ray diagrams to explain the correction of ametropia and the effect of lenses in near vision, field diagrams showing the off-axis performance of lenses and how to take measurements for lens fitting, are just some of the topics included on the CD-ROM. This method of instruction is sure to become commonplace in teaching institutions and it is hoped that the presentation methods used will help not only students, but also give teachers some ideas when developing presentations for their own students.

Mo Jalie
1999, Balcombe, Sussex

Introduction to the theory of ophthalmic lenses

Laws of reflection and refraction

Ophthalmic lens theory is based upon the laws of geometrical optics,[1,2] which in their basic form are encompassed by the laws of reflection and refraction. This chapter considers these fundamental laws and how they relate to the theory of spectacle lenses.

Light is considered to travel in straight lines until it meets a surface that separates two media. What then happens to the light depends upon the nature of the surface and the two media on either side. If the surface is polished so that it acts as a mirror surface, the light is reflected at the surface, back into the incident medium (Figure 1.1).

Depending upon the degree of polish, the light may be reflected specularly (Figure 1.1a), the surface acting as a true mirror, or, if the surface is incompletely polished, it reflects the light diffusely (Figure 1.1b), scattering it in all directions.

In the case of specular reflection, the reflected light obeys the *law of reflection*, which states that:

- the incident ray, the reflected ray and the normal to the surface at the point of incidence all lie in the same plane
- the angle of incidence, i, equals the angle of reflection, i'.

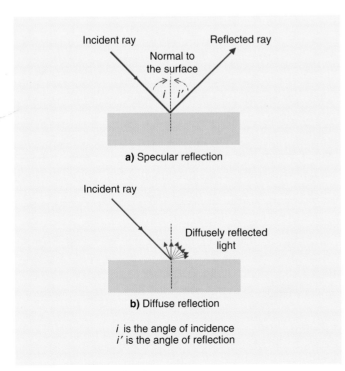

a) Specular reflection

b) Diffuse reflection

i is the angle of incidence
i' is the angle of reflection

Figure 1.1   Law of reflection

The normal lies at 90° to the surface. Note that the angles of incidence and reflection are measured from the rays to the normal to the surface at the point of incidence.

It follows from the laws of reflection that, when an object is placed in front of a plane mirror, the image formed by the mirror lies as far behind the mirror surface as the object lies in front. Also, the straight line that joins the object and its reflected image is normal to the mirror surface.

The laws of reflection are used to study reflection at plane and curved surfaces; they are met again in Chapter 5 (Reflections from spectacle lens surfaces.)

When light meets a polished surface at the boundary of two transparent media, some of the light is reflected, but most is refracted at the surface and passes into the new medium.

The refracted light undergoes a change in velocity. The ratio of the velocities of light in the first and second media is called the *relative refractive index* between the media.

The *absolute refractive index* of a medium, n, is defined as the ratio of the velocity of light in a vacuum to the velocity of the light in the medium:

$$\text{refractive index, } n = \frac{\text{velocity of light in vacuum}}{\text{velocity of light in the medium}}$$

When light is incident obliquely at the boundary between two media, the change in velocity in the refracted light as it enters the new medium causes a change in direction of the light.

Figure 1.2 illustrates a ray of light that is incident, in air, at point D on the surface of a plane-sided glass block. The refractive index of the first medium (air) is denoted by n and the refractive index of the second medium (the glass block) is denoted by n'.

The angle of incidence that the incident ray makes with the normal to the surface at D is denoted by i, and the angle of refraction is denoted by i'.

The *law of refraction* (Snell's Law) states that:

- the incident ray, the refracted ray and the normal to the surface at the point of incidence all lie in one plane
- the ratio of the sine of the angle of incidence, i, to the sine of the angle of refraction, i', is a constant for any two media.

The relationship between the angle of incidence and the angle of refraction is now usually quoted in the form:

$$n \sin i = n' \sin i'$$

By means of Snell's Law and the application of ordinary geometry to the light rays we can determine the effects of lenses and prisms.

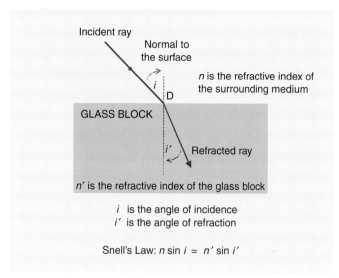

Figure 1.2   Law of refraction

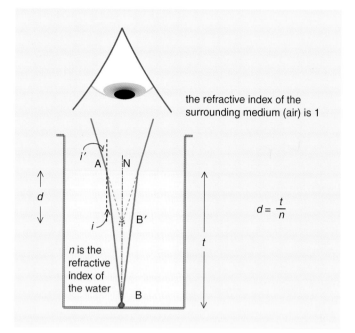

Figure 1.3   Equivalent air thickness

The most important application of Snell's Law of Refraction is to determine the effect of prisms and lenses on incident light, that is, to determine the change in direction and the change in vergence produced by a lens.

A very important application of the laws of refraction in geometrical optics is to determine the equivalent air thickness of a block of material of given refractive index, n.

Figure 1.3 illustrates a beaker of water, sitting on the bottom of which is a small stone B. To an eye looking down into the water, the stone appears to be at B′, closer to the surface than it really is. This illusion is familiar to everyone who has looked at the bottom of a swimming pool when the water in the pool is unruffled. The pool does not appear to be as deep as it really is.

The optics of the situation is illustrated in Figure 1.3. A ray of light, AB, emanates from B and meets the surface at A, where it makes an angle of incidence, i, with the normal to the surface at A. After refraction, the ray that travels in air makes an angle of refraction, $i′$, with the normal at point A. From Snell's Law, $n \sin i = \sin i′$ (since $n′ = 1$).

Now the beam of light that emanates from the water is very narrow. This is because the beam as it enters the pupil of the eye is only about 4 mm in diameter. Hence, the angles of incidence and refraction involved must be very small. For small angles we can replace the sines of the angles by their tangents and write:

$$n \tan i = \tan i′$$

From the geometry of the figure, $\tan i = AN/t$ and $\tan i′ = AN/d$. So:

$$n \times AN/t = AN/d$$

and:

$$d = t/n$$

Use is made of this expression when dealing with the back vertex power of spectacle lenses.

Prismatic power

A straightforward application of the law of refraction is found in the study of plano-prisms. Rotation of the eye is brought about by the action of the six extrinsic ocular muscles attached to the globe of the eye. Defects in these muscles, or defects to their innervation, are relieved by prisms.

An ophthalmic prism is illustrated in Figure 1.4a. It consists of two plane refracting surfaces inclined at an angle to one another.

The two surfaces meet at the *apex* of the prism and the point opposite the apex is the *base* of the prism. In the case of a flat circular prism, such as a trial case prism, the apex is the thinnest point on the edge of the prism and the base is the thickest point on the edge.

An imaginary line that joins the apex to the base represents the base setting of the prism. The angle between the two refracting surfaces is the apical angle, which in ophthalmic work rarely exceeds 10°.

When light meets a prism, it is always refracted towards the prism base. This is shown in Figure 1.4b, which has a ray of light incident normally upon the front surface. Since the angle of incidence at the front surface is zero, the angle of refraction, given by Snell's Law, must also be zero, and we can conclude that at the first surface the light ray does not change its direction.

When the ray meets the second face of the prism, it now makes an angle of incidence, i, with the normal to the second face at the point of incidence. From the geometry of Figure 1.4b, it is clear that angle i must equal the apical angle of the prism, a.

Upon refraction at the second face, the angle of refraction, $i′$, can be found by means of Snell's Law. Note from the refraction at the second face that the angle of refraction, $i′$, is equal to $i + d$, or, since $a = i$, angle $i′ = a + d$.

If the refractive index of the prism material is denoted by n and the prism is supposed to be in air, so that $n′ = 1$, we have from Snell's Law:

$$n \sin i = n′ \sin i′$$

and substituting a for i, $(a + d)$ for $i′$ and 1 for $n′$, we can write:

$$n \sin a = \sin(a + d)$$

In the case of an ophthalmic prism, the apical angle of the prism rarely exceeds about 10°; when the angles are small, we

Figure 1.4   Ophthalmic prism

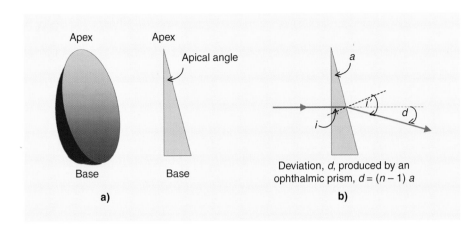

a)

b)

Deviation, *d*, produced by an
ophthalmic prism, $d = (n-1)a$

Figure 1.5   Action of a prism

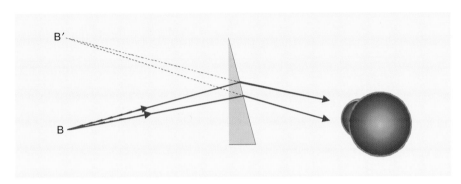

can replace the sine of the angle by the angle itself (expressed in radians), and so we can write:

$$na = (a + d)$$

from which we readily obtain:

$$d = (n-1)a$$

So the deviation produced by an ophthalmic prism is directly proportional to its apical angle.

To an eye that views through the prism, objects always appear displaced towards the prism apex. This is shown in Figure 1.5, in which light from an object point, B, is deviated by the prism and, to the eye viewing through the prism, the image, B′, appears to be displaced towards the prism apex.

If an eye views a crossline chart through a prism, held with its base down before the eye, that part of the chart viewed through the prism is displaced towards the apex and the crosslines appear to be broken, as illustrated in Figure 1.6a.

If the prism is now rotated clockwise, the limbs of the crosslines also appear to rotate clockwise, and the centre of the crosslines always remains displaced towards the prism apex (Figure 1.6b).

When the base–apex direction is horizontal, the appearance obtained is shown in Figure 1.6c, in which now only the vertical limb appears to be displaced.

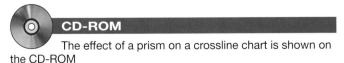

CD-ROM

The effect of a prism on a crossline chart is shown on the CD-ROM

The rotation test is a sensitive method for detecting both the presence of a prism in an optical element and locating and marking the direction of the base–apex line.

To locate the base–apex direction, the prism should be rotated in front of a crossline chart until the vertical limb of the chart appears unbroken, as depicted in Figure 1.6a. The base–apex direction then lies in the vertical meridian with the base downwards, and this direction may be marked on the prism, as shown in Figure 1.6a, in which the short horizontal red line depicts the base edge of the prism and the red arrow the prism apex.

The power of an unknown prism may be determined by means of the rotation test using a process of neutralization. A set of test prisms of known powers with their base–apex directions marked upon them is required, such as those found in a trial case. The base–apex direction of the unknown prism should be marked and the prism held in contact with prisms of known strength, with base–apex lines parallel and bases in opposition. When no displacement of the crosslines can be detected upon rotation of the pair, the unknown prism is neutralized and is of the same power as that of the test prism.

Prism units

Figure 1.7 depicts the path of a ray of light through a prism, the light being incident normally upon the first face of the prism. The apical angle of the prism is denoted by *a* and the deviation that the prism produces by *d*. If the refractive index of the prism material is denoted by *n*, the relationship between *a* and *d* for prisms of small refracting angle, which are usually employed in ophthalmic work, is shown above to be:

$$d = (n-1)a$$

In practice, it is difficult to measure angular values, so C. F. Prentice (1890) suggested that a far easier method for expressing prism power is to measure the displacement produced by the prism at a known distance. Prentice proposed that the distance should be 100 units from the prism and called the unit the prism dioptre, denoted by the Greek letter Δ. Today, the prism dioptre

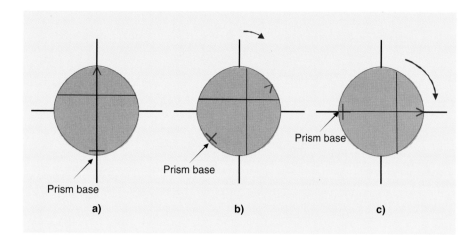

Figure 1.6   Appearance of crossline chart viewed through a prism held with its base DOWN before the chart

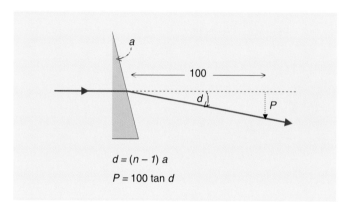

$$d = (n - 1)\, a$$
$$P = 100 \tan d$$

Figure 1.7   Prism units

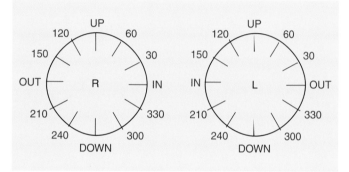

Figure 1.8   Prism base setting

is widely used and sometimes denoted by the suffix cm/m, since it expresses the displacement produced in centimetres at a distance of 1 metre from the prism. The prism dioptre is a unit of angular measure, being the angle with a tangent of 1/100 or 0.01. Degrees of deviation are converted to prism dioptres simply by multiplying the tangent of the angle by 100, that is:

$$P = 100 \ \tan d$$

The ophthalmic workshop method for measuring prism power is to use the thickness difference of the prism, g, at a given diameter. Denoting the semi-diameter of the prism by y, the thickness difference can be found from:

$$g = Py / \left[50 (n - 1) \right]$$

or, if g is given:

$$P = 50 (n - 1) g / y$$

Base setting of prisms

Images viewed through a prism appear displaced towards the prism apex, but in practice the orientation of a prism is always specified by stating the position of the prism base. The notation for the base setting is illustrated in Figure 1.8. Vertical prism is specified as base up or base down and horizontal prism is specified as base in or base out. Note that the vertical specification means the same thing for each eye whereas, in the case of the horizontal specification, base in means towards the nose and base out means towards the temple. Oblique prisms are specified simply by stating the desired position of the prism base using a 360° protractor.

Thus, base 30 means base up along 30, whereas base 210 means base down along the 30 meridian (210 = 180 + 30).

Summation of prisms

The process of adding prism powers together is known as *compounding prism powers*. If the base settings of the prisms are parallel with one another they can be added by simple arithmetic. Thus, the result of combining 2Δ base up and 3Δ base down is simply 1Δ base down.

When measuring heterophoria, the usual procedure is to test for deviation in the vertical and horizontal meridians separately. This may result in both a vertical and a horizontal prismatic correction being necessary.

A pair of prisms to be combined at right angles can be compounded into a single resultant prism, either graphically or by means of Pythagoras' theorem. In the graphical solution, the deviation that each prism produces is drawn to scale as a vector and, on completing the parallelogram, the resultant prism is represented by the magnitude and direction of the diagonal side of the parallelogram.

For example, Figure 1.9 illustrates how 3Δ base up and 4Δ base in is compounded into a single resultant prism, 5Δ base 37, for the right eye.

This result could be found by applying Pythagoras' theorem, to obtain the resultant prism, P_R, from:

$$P_R = \sqrt{\left(P_V^2 + P_H^2 \right)}$$

and the base-setting, θ, from:

$$\tan \theta = P_V / P_H$$

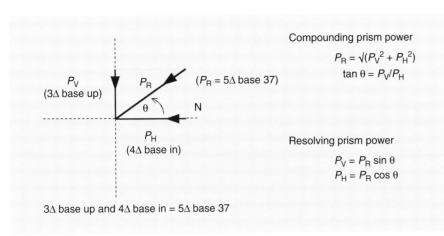

Compounding prism power

$$P_R = \sqrt{(P_V^2 + P_H^2)}$$
$$\tan \theta = P_V/P_H$$

Resolving prism power

$$P_V = P_R \sin \theta$$
$$P_H = P_R \cos \theta$$

3Δ base up and 4Δ base in = 5Δ base 37

Figure 1.9   Compounding and resolving prism powers

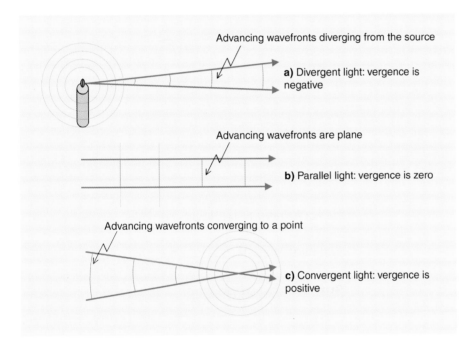

Figure 1.10   Concept of vergence

The reverse problem of finding the vertical and horizontal components equivalent to a given single oblique prism, P_R base θ, can also be carried out using a scale diagram (Figure 1.9), or from:

$$P_V = P_R \sin \theta$$

and

$$P_H = P_R \cos \theta$$

Obliquely combined prisms can be compounded, either by means of the cosine rule or, more simply, by first resolving each oblique prism into vertical and horizontal components, which can then be added mentally and finally compounded into a single oblique prism.

Vergence

The concept of vergence can be deduced from Figure 1.10. Light diverges from a source, such as the candle flame illustrated in Figure 1.10a. The curvature of the wavefront (see the next section for a mathematical treatment of *curvature*) at any moment is expressed as the reciprocal of the radius of the wavefront, assumed to be travelling in air (or, strictly, *in vacuo*).

Thus, at a distance *l* from the source, the curvature of the wavefront, L, is 1/*l*. The curvature is expressed in reciprocal metres or *dioptres*.

The curvature of a divergent wavefront is given a negative sign. Hence, 1 metre from the source, the divergence in the wavefront, or, we say, in the divergent pencils of light, is –1.00D.

At 1/2 metre from the source, or 50cm, the divergence is –2.00D, at 1/3 metre from the source, or 33.33cm, the divergence is –3.00D and so on.

The further the light travels from the source, the less becomes the curvature of the wavefront, until a long way from the source the curvature of the wavefront is zero. Parallel light arriving from a distant source of light, such as the sun, has zero vergence, L = 0.00D.

When an optical element is imposed in the path of divergent or parallel light it may cause the light to converge to a point. Converging light is given a positive sign, so that if we are considering the curvature of the wavefront at a point 1 metre from the point of convergence, the vergence in the pencil is said to be +1.00D. The vergence in the pencil 20cm from the point of convergence is said to be +5.00D and so on.

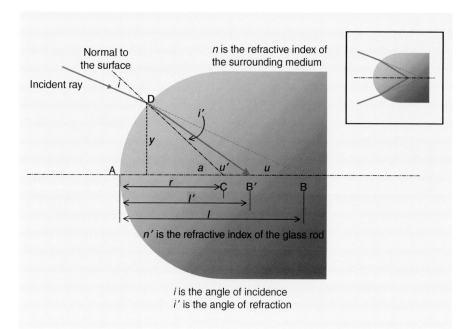

Figure 1.11   Conjugate foci relationship

Normal to the surface

Incident ray

D

i

i'

y

A

a u' u

r C   B'   B

l'

l

n is the refractive index of the surrounding medium

n' is the refractive index of the glass rod

i is the angle of incidence
i' is the angle of refraction

Figure 1.11 is used here to derive the *fundamental paraxial relationship*, which is used to study the effect that lenses have on light (although the proof is given in full for the sake of completeness, it is not necessary to know it to be able to apply the relationship). The inset to Figure 1.11 illustrates the situation. A beam of light is converging towards a point, B, on the axis of symmetry of the surface and the beam is intercepted by the convex spherical surface, ground onto the end of a rod of glass.

The centre of curvature of the surface lies at C and the distances AC and DC are equal to the radius of curvature of the surface.

The convex surface causes an increase in the convergence of the light, the reason for which is seen, from the main diagram, to be because the light is refracted towards the normal at the points of incidence. The light converging within the glass rod reunites at the point B′ on the axis. Points B and B′ are said to be *conjugate points* and, if we are given the position of the object point, B, and the details of the surface, the fundamental paraxial equation is used to locate the conjugate image point, B′.

The relationship can be deduced as follows.

From Figure 1.11 the angle DCA, denoted by a, is equal to $u + i$ and also $a = u' + i'$. So $i = u - a$ and $i' = u' - a$. In Figure 1.11, the distance AB, which is the distance of the object point, B, from the vertex of the surface, A, is denoted by l and the conjugate image distance, AB′, is denoted by l'.

If we now restrict the discussion to the paraxial region of the surface, that is to the narrow area around the vertex, A, it is clear that as the point of incidence, D, approaches A, the intercept height, y, becomes equal in length to the arc AD.

Expressing the angles in radians, we can then write:

$$a = y/\text{AC} = y/r$$
$$u = y/\text{AB} = y/l$$
$$u' = y/\text{AB}' = y/l'$$

Since the discussion has been restricted to very small angles, so that the angles of incidence and refraction, i and i', must also be very small, Snell's Law can be written in the form:

$$ni = n'i'$$

so that:

$$n(u - a) = n'(u' - a)$$

Now substituting the paraxial equivalents for the angles u, u' and a, we have:

$$n(y/l - y/r) = n'(y/l' - y/r)$$

from which:

$$\frac{n'}{l'} = \frac{n}{l} + \frac{n' - n}{r}$$

This is usually expressed in the form:

$$L' = L + F$$

where

$$L' = n'/l', \ L = n/l \text{ and } F = (n' - n)/r.$$

In the fundamental paraxial equation, L' represents the vergence leaving the surface, L represents the incident vergence arriving from the object and F represents the optical power of the surface.

In words, the fundamental paraxial equation, or the *conjugate foci relationship*, as it is often called, states that the vergence leaving the surface is the sum of the incident vergence and the power of the surface. The power of the surface can be looked upon as the vergence that the surface impresses upon the incident light, that is, how the surface changes the vergence of the light.

The use of these expressions to deal with the effects of lenses is considered shortly.

Curvature of surfaces

The ophthalmic prisms considered earlier in this chapter had flat, or plane, surfaces. Most optical elements have curved surfaces, the surface being described as convex if it bulges out of the material (as in the case of the glass rod in the previous section) and concave if it is depressed into the material. Figure 1.12 illustrates a cross-sectional view of a curved-form, or meniscus, lens with a convex surface on the left and a concave surface on the right. The

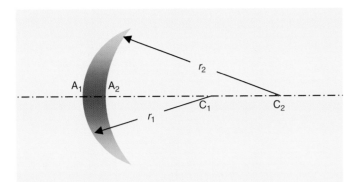

Figure 1.12   Optical axis and vertices of the surfaces of a curved form lens

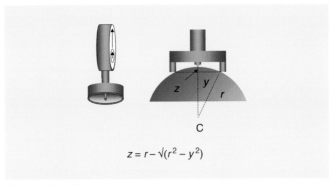

Figure 1.13   The simple sagometer

measure of the shape of a curved surface is known as *curvature*. In the case of a simple spherical surface, the curvature expresses the reciprocal of the radius of curvature of the surface in metres. The symbol for curvature is R, so we can write $R = 1/r$, where r is the radius of curvature of the surface in metres.

Thus, if two spheres have radii of curvature of 200mm and 100mm, respectively, the curvature of the first sphere is 5.0 reciprocal metres and the curvature of the second sphere is 10.0 reciprocal metres. The smaller sphere has a greater curvature than the larger. The unit, reciprocal metre, written as m^{-1}, is identical to the dioptre, but the term reciprocal metre is preferred to describe surface curvature, since surface *powers* are expressed in dioptres.

In Figure 1.12 the convex front spherical surface has radius r_1 and centre of curvature C_1, and the concave back surface has radius r_2 and centre of curvature C_2. The line that joins the two centres of curvature is called the *optical axis* of the lens and the intersection of the axis with the front surface, A_1, is the *front vertex* of the surface. The optical axis intersects the back surface of the lens at the *back vertex*, A_2.

The optical power of a surface is the product of the surface curvature and the refractivity of the material, $n' - n$, where n and n' are the refractive indices of the media to the left and right of the surface, respectively.

Since $R = 1/r$, we can write the surface power relationship in terms of its curvature in the form:

$$F = (n' - n)R$$

For surfaces other than spherical, the curvature varies in different zones and from one meridian to another. If the equation to the surface is known, then the curvature in the tangential meridian of the surface is given by the general mathematical expression:

$$R = d^2y/dx^2 / \left[1 + (dy/dx)^2\right]^{3/2}$$

where dy/dx and d^2y/dx^2 are the first and second differential coefficients of the equation to the curve.

The sagittal curvature at the point in question is the reciprocal of the distance from the surface to the point on the axis of revolution where the normal to the surface at the point meets the axis. This definition can be used at any instantaneous point on the surface, such as that on aspherical and progressive power surfaces.

In the case of a conicoidal surface the sagittal curvature at a point can be found directly from the expression:

$$R_S = 1 / \left[r_0^2 + (1 - p)y^2\right]^{1/2}$$

and the tangential curvature from:

$$R_T = R_S^{\ 3}/R_0^{\ 2}$$

The curvature of a spherical surface can be read with a simple instrument called a *spherometer*, which measures the height of the vertex of the curve above a fixed chord. If the height of the curve is denoted by z and the semi-chord length by y, then the curvature is given by:

$$R = 2000z / \left(y^2 + z^2\right)$$

where z and y are substituted in millimetres.

The common form of spherometer normally met with in practice is the optician's *lens measure*, which is calibrated for a refractive index in the region of 1.50 and gives the dioptric power of the surface directly. More accurate versions of the simple lens measure are used in surfacing laboratories and are known as *sagometers* (Figure 1.13).

Focal power

One of the most important applications of the fundamental paraxial equation is its use in the study of the effects of spectacle lenses and how they correct the eyes. We begin by looking again at the simple convex surface ground on the end of a glass rod, as depicted in Figure 1.11.

Suppose that the rod has a radius of curvature of 50.0mm, is made from a material of refractive index 1.5 and is set up in air, facing a distant object so the object distance, which we denote by l, is infinitely great. The vergence of the light arriving at the surface, L, is zero.

From above, the optical power of the surface, F, is found from:

$$F = 1000(n' - n)/r$$

when r is substituted in millimetres, so:

$$F = 1000(1.5 - 1)/50$$
$$= +10.00D$$

The vergence of the light leaving the surface is simply the sum of the incident vergence and the power of the surface, so the vergence leaving the surface, L', is the same as the power of the surface, F, which is +10.00D.

This can be deduced from the relationship:

$$L' = L + F$$
$$= F$$

when $L = 0$.

The convex surface on the end of the rod causes the light to converge to a focus at point B′ in Figure 1.11, which lies at the distance, l', from the vertex, A, of the rod. The image distance, l', is found from:

$$l' = n'/L'$$

where $n' = 1.5$ and $L' = +10.00$, so:

$$l' = 1.5/10 \text{ metres}$$
$$= 150\text{mm}$$

This situation is illustrated in Figure 1.14a. When the object lies at infinity, the image point, B′, is called the second principal focus, F′. The focusing distance for a distant object, AF′, is known as the second principal focal length, f', of the surface, where:

$$f' = n'/F$$

If an object is placed in front of the surface in such a position that $L' = 0$, then, from the fundamental paraxial relationship,

$L + F = 0$, and so, $L = -F$. This situation is illustrated in Figure 1.14b. The object lies at the first principal focus, F, and the distance AF is the first principal focal length of the surface, f.

Note that:

$$f = -n/F$$

In the case of a concave surface, the second principal focus of the surface lies in front of the surface. This is illustrated in Figure 1.15a, where it can be seen that, after refraction, the light appears to be diverging from a point to the left of the surface.

The first principal focus of a concave surface lies to the right of the surface; Figure 1.15b shows that, for the light to emerge with zero vergence from the surface (i.e. parallel to the axis), it must have been converging towards point F upon arrival at the surface.

We now consider the use of the fundamental paraxial equation to determine the power of an optical element with two surfaces, such as an ophthalmic lens. A spectacle lens has two surfaces, the front surface, F_1, which is taken to be the surface facing away from the eye, and the back surface, F_2, which is taken to be the surface next to the eye. In general, in ophthalmic optical diagrams the front surface is shown on the left (e.g. Figures 1.16, 1.17).

To begin with, we assume that the two surfaces are in close contact, so that the thickness of the lens can be ignored. Then the vergence leaving the first surface, L'_1, is the same as the vergence arriving at the second surface, L_2.

The vergence leaving the lens:

$$L'_2 = L_2 + F_2$$

but since:

$$L_2 = L'_1 = L_1 + F_1$$

we can write:

$$L'_2 = L_1 + F_1 + F_2$$

Now, $F_1 + F_2$ is the sum of the individual surface powers and is known as the *thin lens power* of the lens, F.

The thin lens power, F, can be looked upon as the power of a surface that has air on either side, and the fundamental paraxial equation for the thin lens is simply:

$$L' = L + F$$

where $L' = 1/l'$, $L = 1/l$ and the power, F, is the sum of the surface powers of the lens.

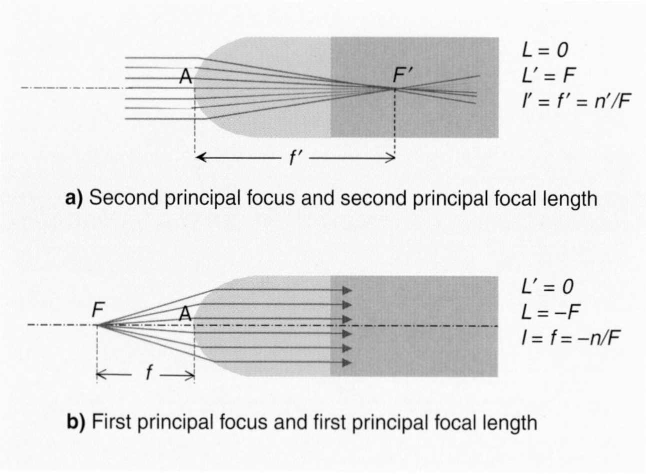

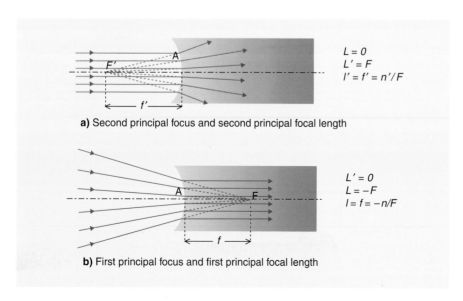

a) Second principal focus and second principal focal length

$$L = 0$$
$$L' = F$$
$$l' = f' = n'/F$$

b) First principal focus and first principal focal length

$$L' = 0$$
$$L = -F$$
$$l = f = -n/F$$

Figure 1.14   Principal foci and principal focal lengths of a convex surface

a) Second principal focus and second principal focal length

$$L = 0$$
$$L' = F$$
$$l' = f' = n'/F$$

b) First principal focus and first principal focal length

$$L' = 0$$
$$L = -F$$
$$l = f = -n/F$$

Figure 1.15   Principal foci and principal focal lengths of a concave surface

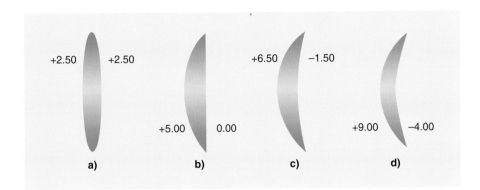

Figure 1.16 Various forms in which a +5.00D lens might be made

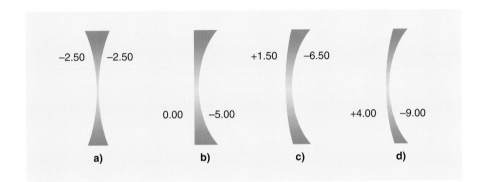

Figure 1.17 Various forms in which a −5.00D lens might be made

Thin lens power

We have just seen that when the thickness of a lens is ignored, the total thin-lens power of the lens is the sum of its surface powers. Thus, if a lens has a front surface power of +9.00D and a back surface power of −4.00D, then its thin lens power is +5.00D.

In theory, we could make a +5.00D lens in any form, such as those depicted in Figure 1.16, in which the first form has a pair of convex surfaces and is known as a *biconvex* lens form. When the surface powers are equal, as is the case with the lens shown in Figure 1.16a, the form is referred to as an *equi-convex* form. The second form (Figure 1.16b), which has one plane surface, is known as a *plano-convex* lens form. These lens forms are known as *flat-form* lenses. The remaining forms in Figure 1.16 each have one convex surface and one concave surface and are known as *curved* or *meniscus* lenses. In practice, modern lenses are curved in form, the reasons for which are given in Chapter 2.

Figure 1.17 illustrates various forms in which a −5.00D lens might be made. The first two forms are flat-form designs and the remainder are of curved form. The two flat-form designs are described as *biconcave* (*equi-concave* in the case illustrated in Figure 1.17a) and *plano-concave* forms.

The lower numerical surface power of a curved lens is known as the *base curve* and the curved forms illustrated in Figures 1.16d and 1.17d that have one surface of power 4.00D are described as *4.00 base meniscus* lens forms.

The relationship between the surface powers, F_1 and F_2, and the total thin-lens power of the lens, F, is simply:

$$F = F_1 + F_2$$

If the refractive index of the lens is denoted by n, and the radii of curvature of the front and back surfaces as r_1 and r_2, respectively, then the individual surface powers are given by:

$$F_1 = (n-1)/r_1$$

and

$$F_2 = (1-n)/r_2$$

These two expressions can be combined into the *lensmaker's equation*:

$$F = (n-1)(1/r_1 - 1/r_2)$$

The transverse test

When a plus lens is held in front of the eye and slowly moved from side to side, a vertical line viewed through the lens appears to move in the opposite direction to the movement of the lens. This transverse movement is known as *against movement* and is exhibited by all plus lenses, provided they are held closer to the eye than their own focal length.

When the transverse test is applied to a minus lens, the lens produces *with movement* under the test.

The movements are most easily seen if a crossline chart is employed; this consists, simply, of two black lines at right-angles to one another drawn on white card.

The power of an unknown lens can be determined by analysis of the movements produced during the transverse test by the process known as neutralization, details of which are given later.

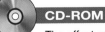

CD-ROM

The effect of spherical lenses under the transverse test is shown on the CD-ROM

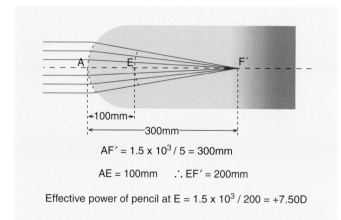

$$AF' = 1.5 \times 10^3 / 5 = 300\text{mm}$$

$$AE = 100\text{mm} \quad \therefore EF' = 200\text{mm}$$

Effective power of pencil at E = $1.5 \times 10^3 / 200 = +7.50\text{D}$

Figure 1.18   Effective power. The effective power of the pencil at E

Influence of thickness on lens power

The lensmaker's equation ignores the contribution played by the lens thickness in arriving at the power of the lens. When the thickness is taken into account, the actual power of a lens cannot be found from the simple sum of the surface powers, but it can be found by considering the change in vergence that the light undergoes after refraction at one surface.

Consider the pencil of light refracted by the surface illustrated in Figure 1.18, which has a radius of curvature of 100mm and separates air on the left from a material of refractive index 1.5. The optical power of the surface is +5.00D [from $F = (n-1)/r$].

If the incident vergence on the surface is zero ($L_1 = 0$), then the vergence after refraction, L'_1, is +5.00D. The light will converge to a focus l'_1 metres to the right of the surface, where $l'_1 = n'/L'_1$. So the light converges to a point 1.5/5 metres = 300mm to the right of the surface (Figure 1.18, in which AF' = 300mm).

Now consider the vergence in the converging pencil at point E, 100mm to the right of the vertex, A. Point E lies 200mm to the left of the second principal focus, F', and the vergence at E must be:

$$L'_E = n'/l'_E = 1.5 \times 1000/200 = +7.50\text{D}$$

In general, if the vergence, L, is known in one position, then the vergence at a distance, d, from the first position, L_E, is given by:

$$L_E = 1/(l - d)$$
$$= L/(1 - dL)$$

This quantity is called the *effective power* of the pencil at the new position.

Recall from Figure 1.3 that when light travels in some media other than air, the real thickness of material, t, through which the light travels can be replaced by an equivalent thickness of air, d, where $d = t/n$, the refractive index of the material being denoted by n.

In the example given in Figure 1.18, the distance, AE, within the material is 100mm. We can replace this 100mm distance in the material of refractive index 1.5 by 100/1.5 = 66.67mm of air. The effective power of the pencil at E can now be evaluated from $1/l_E$, since the refractive index of our supposed medium is now that of air.

It may have occurred to the reader that essentially we have said:

$$L_E = n/l_E = 1/l_E/n$$

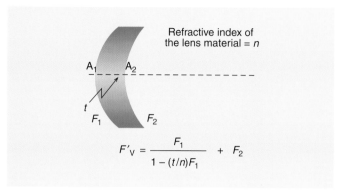

$$F'_V = \frac{F_1}{1 - (t/n)F_1} + F_2$$

Figure 1.19   Derivation of the back vertex power of a lens

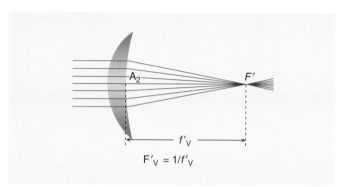

$$F'_V = 1/f'_V$$

Figure 1.20   Back vertex focal length of a plus lens

The concept of effective power enables us to determine the effect of thickness in the power of a spectacle lens.

Consider now the lens illustrated in Figure 1.19. The front surface power is denoted by F_1, the back surface by F_2, and the axial thickness, A_1A_2, is denoted by t. The power of the lens reckoned at the back vertex, A_2, is called the *back vertex power* of the lens, F'_V.

Spectacle lenses are numbered in terms of their back vertex powers. The back vertex power can be found from the sum of the effective power of the front surface at the back vertex and the back surface power. The effective power of the front surface at the back vertex is $F_1/[1 - (t/n)F_1]$, so the back vertex power is given by:

$$F'_V = F_1/\left[1 - (t/n)F_1\right] + F_2$$

which can be written in the form:

$$F'_V = \left[F_1 + F_2 - (t/n)F_1F_2\right]/\left[1 - (t/n)F_1\right]$$

Light from a distant object is focused by a lens at its second principal focus, F'. The distance from the back vertex of the lens to its second principal focus, A_2F', is called the *back vertex focal length* of the lens (Figure 1.20).

Accurate transposition

If the thickness and one surface power are known, then to make a lens of a given back vertex power, the other surface power that has to be compensated for the thickness of the lens is given by:

$$F_1 = F_{1N}/\left[1 + (t/n)F_{1N}\right]$$

where F_{1N} represents the nominal or uncompensated front curve, found by simple thin-lens transposition, $F_{1N} = (F'_V - F_2)$.

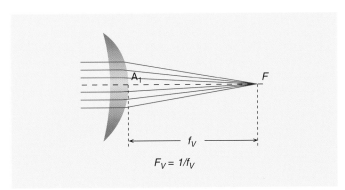

$$F_V = 1/f_V$$

Figure 1.21   Front vertex focal length of a plus lens

The compensated front curve is sometimes known as the reduced front curve, since the nominal surface power has to be made weaker to compensate for the thickness of the lens. The difference between the compensated and uncompensated surface powers is known as the *vertex power allowance* for the curve.

When the front surface power and the thickness are known, the compensated back curve is given by:

$$F_2 = F'_V - F_1 / \left[1 - (t/n) F_1 \right]$$

These expressions are used in the surfacing laboratory where, when the thickness of the lens has been calculated, they may be employed to compute the second surface of the lens.

When the lens is turned back-to-front so that light from a distant object meets the back surface of the lens, the light is focused at the first principal focus, F, of the lens (Figure 1.21). The distance from the front vertex of the lens to its first principal focus, A_1F, is called the *front vertex focal length* of the lens. The reciprocal of the front vertex focal length of a lens is called the *front vertex power*, F_V, of the lens. The front vertex power is given by the relationship:

$$F_V = \left[F_1 + F_2 - (t/n) F_1 F_2 \right] / \left[1 - (t/n) F_2 \right]$$

The reading given when a lens is placed in a focimeter with its back vertex in contact with the lens rest is the back vertex power. If the lens is reversed in the focimeter, the instrument reads the front vertex power of the lens.

Front vertex readings need to be taken when the lens is a bifocal or multifocal design with the segment on the convex surface, since the reading addition is defined as the difference between the vertex powers, measured from the surface that incorporates the segment.

Further details on the measurement of the reading addition are given in Chapter 10.

Swaine's step-along procedure for paraxial ray-tracing

Although formulae to determine the vertex powers and the positions of images formed by spectacle lenses are given above, the results can also be obtained, very simply, by successive application of the fundamental paraxial equation, $L' = L + F$, to each surface of the lens in turn.

The procedure is very straightforward and was first described by William Swaine[3] in the 1920s. The method is described below.

The effect of the first surface of the lens is given by:

$$L'_1 = L_1 + F_1$$

L_1 is the incident vergence, $= 1000/l_1$ when the object distance is expressed in millimetres (which is a suitable unit for spectacle lens work), and F_1 is the power of the surface. When L'_1 is known, the image distance, reckoned from the first surface, l'_1 is given by $1000/L'_1$. The object distance for the second surface, l_2, is given by $l'_1 - t/n$, where the actual thickness of the lens is replaced by its equivalent air thickness, found by dividing the real thickness by the refractive index of the lens material.

This procedure is now repeated for the second surface of the lens. The effect of the second surface is given by:

$$L'_2 = L_2 + F_2$$

L_2 is the incident vergence, $= 1000/l_2$, and F_2 is now the power of the second surface. The final image vergence is given by the value, L'_2, and might represent, say, the vertex power of the lens or the vergence that leaves the lens in near vision, depending upon the problem in hand. The work can be set out in columns with vergences on the left and distances on the right and, with a little practice and a simple calculator, the computing scheme takes just a few seconds to work through. The arrows signify that the next result is obtained by dividing the last result into 1000.

Computing scheme

	Vergences	Equivalent air distances
Line 1	L_1	← l_1
Line 2	L'_1	→ l'_1
Line 3		$-t/n$
Line 4	L_2	← l_2
Line 5	L'_2	→ l'_2

The following examples have been chosen both to demonstrate the use of the sequence and to indicate its application in typical problems that recur in ophthalmic lens work. Note that, in these examples, the computing template is always written in the order given above so that the suffix 1 relates to the front surface and 2 relates to the back surface. However, the computing sequence may start at Line 1 or Line 5 depending upon the unknown quantity in the problem.

Example i

Find the back vertex power of a lens made in glass of refractive index 1.60, with an axial thickness of 5.1mm and surface powers of +8.75 (front) and −4.00 (back).

Computing scheme

	Vergences	Equivalent air distances
Line 1	0.00	← infinity
Line 2	+8.75	→ +114.29
Line 3		−5.1/1.6
Line 4	+9.00	← +111.1
Line 5	+5.00	→ +200

Commentary

In this example the calculation starts at Line 1. Back vertex power is the vergence leaving the back surface when the vergence at the front surface is zero. The back vertex power of the lens (F'_V) is +5.00 and $f'_V = +200$mm.

Example ii

Find the front vertex power of the lens whose details are given in Example i.

Computing scheme

	Vergences		Equivalent air distances
Line 1	+4.80	→	−208.32
Line 2	−3.95	←	−253.19
Line 3			−5.1/1.6
Line 4	−4.00	→	−250.00
Line 5	0.00	←	infinity

Commentary

In this example the calculation starts at Line 5. Front vertex power is the vergence leaving the front surface when the vergence at the back surface is zero. Note the use of signs in Example ii; it is important to adhere rigidly to the correct sign. The front vertex focal length, $f_v = -1000/F_v$. The front vertex power of the lens (F_v) is +4.80 and $f_v = -208.32$ mm.

Example iii

Find the front surface power of a +8.00D lens made in glass of refractive index 1.50, with an axial thickness of 6.0mm and a back surface power of −3.00D.

Computing scheme

	Vergences		Equivalent air distances
Line 1	0.00	→	infinity
Line 2	+10.54	←	+94.91
Line 3			−6.0/1.5
Line 4	+11.00	→	+90.91
Line 5	+8.00		

Commentary

In this example the calculation starts at Line 5. The front surface power $F_1 = L'_1 - L_1$, where $L_1 = 0$, and so $F_1 = L'_1$. The back vertex power of the lens (F'_v) is given as +8.00D.

Example iv

A +10.00D lens is used for near vision at −333.33mm from the front surface of the lens. The lens is made in a plastic material of refractive index 1.50 with an axial thickness of 7.5mm, and has a +15.00D front curve. What is the vergence of the light leaving the back surface of the lens?

In this example, we must trace a ray of light from the near point through the lens, with a starting value $L_1 = -3.00$D. However, before undertaking this ray trace we must begin by finding the back surface power, F_2, of the lens.

Computing scheme to find F_2

	Vergences		Equivalent air distances
Line 1	0.00	←	infinity
Line 2	+15.00	→	+66.67
Line 3			−7.5/1.5
Line 4	+16.22	←	+61.67
Line 5	+10.00		

Commentary

Here, the calculation starts with the information known for both Line 1 and Line 5. The front surface power $F_1 = +15.00$. Since we now know L_2 and L'_2, $F_2 = -6.22$. The back vertex power of the lens (F'_v) is given as +10.00. So the back surface power of the lens is −6.22D.

Computing scheme to find L'_2

	Vergences		Equivalent air distances
Line 1	−3.00	←	−333.33
Line 2	+12.00	→	+83.33
Line 3			−7.5/1.5
Line 4	+12.77	←	+78.33
Line 5	+6.55		

Commentary

Here, the calculation starts with the information known for Line 1 and the surface powers are now known. The vergence leaving the lens is +6.55D.

Correction of ametropia

The correction of the two chief subdivisions of spherical ametropia, hypermetropia (long sight) and myopia (short sight), are depicted in Figures 1.22 and 1.23. Consider first the condition of hypermetropia (Figure 1.22).

In hypermetropia (meaning over-measure of the eye) the refracting surfaces are too weak for the length of the eye. This is usually because of faulty correlation of the optical components of the eye, but could be axial in origin if the eye is too short. In the case of the unaccommodated eye, incident parallel light is brought to a focus behind the macula, M′ (Figure 1.22a). The macula is the area on the retina that provides optimum vision. Instead of there being a sharp focus on the macula, the image consists of blur circles, the diameters of which depend upon the diameter of the pupil.

Since the eye is able to increase its dioptric power by the act of accommodation, it is possible for the young hypermetrope to exert sufficient accommodation to obtain a sharp focus of a distant object at the macula, on the retina, without any artificial aid such as a spectacle lens. Provided that the subject has sufficient accommodation, this is usually the case and as a result low degrees of hypermetropia often remain uncorrected.

Although the unaccommodated eye cannot bring light to a sharp focus at the macula, there is a point that is conjugate with the macula. This point is called the far point, M_R, of the eye, and is seen in Figure 1.22b to lie behind the macula.

The degree of hypermetropia is governed by the distance of the far point from the eye. If this distance (k) is measured in metres, then the ocular ametropia, K, is given by $K = 1/k$. Thus, if the far point lies 1 metre behind the eye, the ocular ametropia is +1.00D. If the far point lies 1/2 metre (or 50cm) behind the eye, the ocular ametropia is +2.00D and so on.

The far point of the hypermetropic eye lies behind the eye, that is, the far point is virtual. Unless the hypermetrope can exert accommodation it is not possible to focus a real object without an artificial aid such as a spectacle lens.

The correction of hypermetropia is illustrated in Figures 1.22c and 1.22d. A plus lens produces an image of a distant object at its second principal focus, which lies behind the lens (Figure 1.22c). If the second principal focus of the lens is made to coincide with

Figure 1.22   Correction of hypermetropia

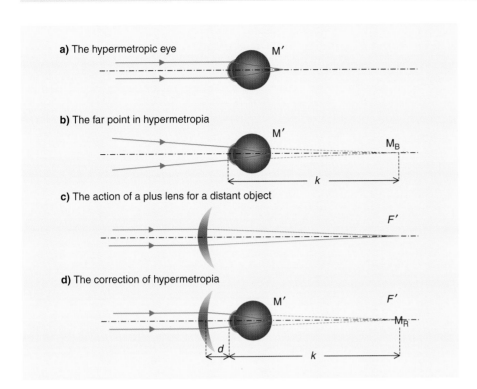

a) The hypermetropic eye

b) The far point in hypermetropia

c) The action of a plus lens for a distant object

d) The correction of hypermetropia

Figure 1.23   Correction of myopia

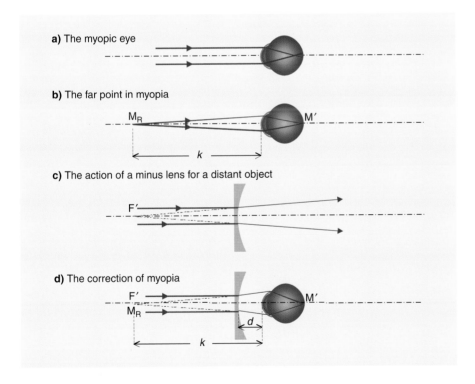

a) The myopic eye

b) The far point in myopia

c) The action of a minus lens for a distant object

d) The correction of myopia

the eye's far point, M_R, then the eye's own optical system can produce a sharp image of a distant object at the macula (Figure 1.22d). Effectively, the spectacle lens increases the power of the eye's optical system.

Plus lenses magnify the retinal image and, to minimize the spectacle magnification, the lens should be fitted as close to the eye as possible.

Figure 1.23 illustrates the condition of myopia. The refracting media are too strong when compared with the length of the eye. Again, this is usually because of faulty correlation of the optical

components of the eye, but in cases of high myopia it results from an increase in the axial length of the eye. In theory, it could also occur for an eye of normal length if the power of the cornea and/ or crystalline lens is too great, a condition known as refractive myopia.

In myopia, light from a distant object is focused in front of the macula (Figure 1.23a). Instead of there being a sharp focus on the macula, the image consists of blur circles the diameters of which, again, depend upon the diameter of the pupil. The smaller the pupil diameter, the smaller become the blur circle diameters, and if they can be made small enough, say, by the subject closing the lids, the image may become sharp enough to be recognizable. Myopia comes from the Greek '*muōps*', meaning '*I close the eye*'.

Although in uncorrected myopia images of a distant object are blurred, there is a point in front of the eye at which an object can be placed so that a sharp image is formed on the macula. This is the far point of the myopic eye (Figure 1.23b).

The degree of myopia is governed by the distance of the far point from the eye (k). The ocular ametropia, K, is given, as before, by $K = 1/k$. Thus, if the far point lies 1 metre in front of the eye, the ocular ametropia is −1.00D. If the far point lies 1/2 metre (or 50cm) in front of the eye, the ocular ametropia is −2.00D and so on.

Myopia is corrected by placing a minus lens in front of the eye. The action of the minus lens is to produce an image of a distant object at its second principal focus, which lies in front of the lens (Figure 1.23c). If the second principal focus of the lens coincides with the eye's far point then the image produced by the lens will be in sharp focus on the retina (Figure 1.23d). Effectively, the spectacle lens reduces the power of the eye's optical system.

An ancillary effect of the lens is to cause the image to appear smaller. The spectacle magnification of the lens is reduced by fitting the lens as close to the eye as possible. If contact lenses are used to correct the eye, the image is virtually the same size as in the uncorrected eye.

CD-ROM

The correction of ametropia by spectacle lenses is demonstrated on the CD-ROM

Astigmatic lenses

Eyes that suffer from astigmatism need a correcting lens for which the power differs along the principal meridians of the lens. The variation in power of an astigmatic lens is such that it has a minimum power along one meridian and a maximum power at right angles to the minimum meridian. These maximum and minimum meridians are known as the principal meridians of the lens. If no correction is required along one meridian, a cylindrical lens may be used. The cylindrical surface is illustrated in Figure 1.24a. It

can be seen that the surface curvature is plane along a meridian parallel with the axis of revolution of the cylinder, but circular at right angles to the axis meridian. The meridian at right angles to the axis meridian is known as the power meridian.

Cylindrical lenses are illustrated in Figure 1.24b. It can be seen that the surface curvature along a meridian parallel with the axis is plane. If a plano-cylindrical lens is moved along its axis meridian it has no effect upon the limbs of the crossline chart viewed through the lens.

If the lens is moved from side to side, along its power meridian, it produces the same effect as a spherical lens of the same power. When the lens is rotated in front of the crossline chart, it produces a characteristic scissors movement (Figure 1.25).

In Figure 1.25a, a plus plano-cylindrical lens has been placed in front of the crossline chart with its axis meridian held parallel with the vertical limb of the chart. There is no displacement of the crosslines.

In Figure 1.25b the lens has been rotated clockwise before the chart and the vertical limb appears to have rotated anti-clockwise, against the rotation of the lens, but the horizontal limb has rotated clockwise, with the rotation of the lens. This characteristic scissors movement is exhibited by all astigmatic lenses under the rotation test.

In Figure 1.25c a minus plano-cylindrical lens, held initially with its axis parallel with the vertical limb of the chart, has been rotated clockwise before the chart and the vertical limb appears to have rotated clockwise, with the rotation of the lens, but the horizontal limb has rotated anti-clockwise, against the rotation of the lens. This rotation test can be used both to verify whether a lens contains a cylindrical component for the correction of astigmatism and to locate its axis meridian.

CD-ROM

The effect of a cylinder on a crossline chart is demonstrated on the CD-ROM

Sphero-cylindrical lenses

A lens that has one spherical surface and one plano-cylindrical surface is called a sphero-cylindrical lens. The optical properties of such a lens can be deduced by imagining that a sphero-cylinder is constructed from a spherical lens that has been placed in contact

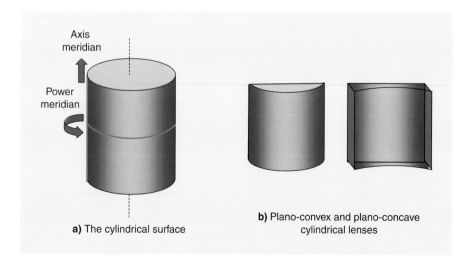

Figure 1.24 The cylindrical surface and plano-cylindrical lenses

Axis meridian

Power meridian

a) The cylindrical surface

b) Plano-convex and plano-concave cylindrical lenses

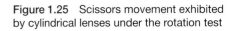

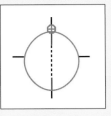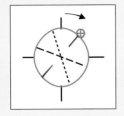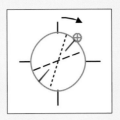

Figure 1.25   Scissors movement exhibited by cylindrical lenses under the rotation test

a) Axis meridian parallel with vertical limb of chart	**b)** Plus cylinder rotated clockwise causes vertical limb to rotate anti-clockwise	**c)** Minus cylinder rotated clockwise causes vertical limb to rotate clockwise

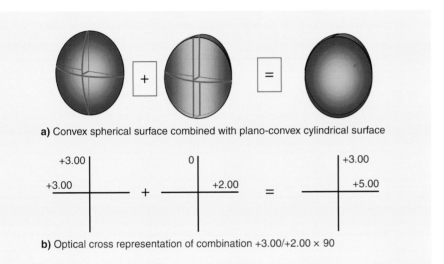

Figure 1.26   Sphero-cylindrical lenses

a) Convex spherical surface combined with plano-convex cylindrical surface

b) Optical cross representation of combination +3.00/+2.00 × 90

with a plano-cylinder (Figure 1.26a). Since a plano-cylinder has no power along its axis meridian, the power along the axis meridian of the combination must result from the spherical element alone. The power along the other principal meridian of the lens, at right angles to the axis meridian of the cylindrical surface, is the sum of the sphere and the cylinder.

Under the transverse test, a sphero-cylindrical lens exhibits movement along each of its principal meridians and under the rotation test it exhibits scissors movement in the same way as a plano-cylindrical lens.

The power of a sphero-cylindrical lens is expressed by stating the power of the spherical component first, followed by the power of the cylindrical component and, finally, the direction of the cylinder axis.

Thus the specification:

+3.00/ + 2.00 × 90

signifies that the spherical component of the lens is +3.00D, the cylindrical component is +2.00D and the axis of the cylindrical surface lies in the vertical, that is, along the 90° meridian.

It is convenient to represent the powers of a sphero-cylindrical lens by means of optical crosses, the limbs of which are marked with the principal powers of each component (Figure 1.26b). It is then an easy matter to sum the principal powers to determine the effect of the lens. Figure 1.26b illustrates the effect of a sphero-cylindrical lens made with a +3.00D spherical surface and a +2.00D cylindrical surface and with an axis that lies in the vertical meridian. It can be seen that the principal

powers are +3.00D in the vertical meridian and +5.00D in the horizontal meridian.

It may occur to the reader that another combination of spherical surface and plano-cylindrical surface produces a sphero-cylindrical lens with principal powers of +3.00D in the vertical meridian and +5.00D in the horizontal meridian (Figure 1.27). This second combination is a convex spherical surface of power +5.00D combined with a plano-concave cylindrical surface of power –2.00D, but this time the axis of the cylinder must lie in the horizontal meridian. This combination can be confirmed by the optical cross representation of the principal powers illustrated in Figure 1.27.

The pencil of light that results from refraction at an astigmatic lens is depicted in Figure 1.28. It is sometimes known as Sturm's Conoid, after the mathematician C. F. Sturm who wrote extensively[4] about the optics of cylindrical lenses. The cross-sectional shape of the astigmatic pencil can be seen to correspond with the shape of the aperture immediately after refraction, but then to narrow down to two focal lines at right angles to one another. The distance between the two line foci $(l'_2 - l'_1)$ in Figure 1.28, is known as the *interval of Sturm*. The lengths of these line foci are dependent upon their positions, the diameter of the aperture and the interval of Sturm.

At the dioptric mean of the pencil $(L'_1 + L'_2)/2$, the pencil has its narrowest cross-section, a position described as the position of the disc of least confusion in the astigmatic pencil. The shape of the pencil at the position of the disc of least confusion corresponds, once more, with that of the aperture, at least in the case of a single surface. In the general case, the shape of the pencil at

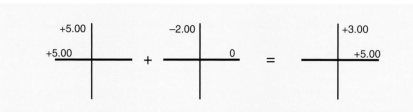

Figure 1.27 Optical cross representation of combination +5.00/−2.00 × 180

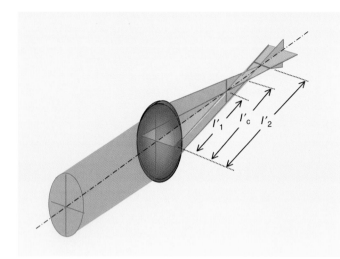

Figure 1.28 The astigmatic pencil

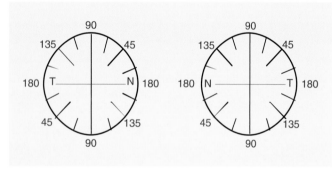

Figure 1.29 Standard axis notation

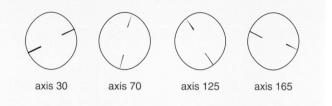

axis 30 axis 70 axis 125 axis 165

Figure 1.30 Axis direction of astigmatic lenses

usual mathematical convention, round to 180 on the left. The notation then re-numbers below the horizontal meridian, again beginning with 0 and passes back to the origin where it becomes 180. The origin lies at the nasal side of the right eye (marked N in Figure 1.29), but at the temporal side of the left eye (marked T in Figure 1.29).

The horizontal meridian is always referred to as the 180 meridian (never the 0 meridian) and the vertical meridian as the 90 meridian. The notation is usually expressed in 5° steps, but occasionally 2.5° or 1° steps may be stipulated. The degree sign itself is always omitted, to safeguard against a carelessly written 5° being mistaken for 50, etc. Most optical protractors used in practice are numbered in standard notation.

Reversed protractors are met with in surfacing workshops, where the semi-finished blank is blocked with its finished convex surface downwards.

Older methods for specifying the axis direction of astigmatic lenses,[6] such as *binasal notation* (in which the axis direction commences on the nasal side of each lens) and *bitemporal notation* (in which the axis direction commences on the temporal side of each lens), are no longer used, except in some mathematical treatments (e.g. formulae for finding prismatic effects at any point on a lens) in which these systems have the advantage of symmetry between the eyes.

Some examples of cylinder axis direction are shown in Figure 1.30, for which it should be remembered that the lenses are being viewed from the front.

In the case of lenses that are mounted in a spectacle frame, the open sides of the frame prevent the lenses from being laid down with their concave surfaces in contact with an optical protractor, in which case it may be necessary to lay the frame with its front surface in contact with the protractor. Great care should be taken in these circumstances, since it must be remembered that the supplement of the true axis direction is being read on the protractor.

When prescriptions need to be transposed from one form to another, the axis direction must be changed by 90. The rule for this transposition is that if the axis direction is greater than 90, then 90 must be subtracted from the value given. In all other cases, 90 must be added to the given axis direction. For example, the axes directions given in Figure 1.30 would transpose to 120, 160, 35 and 75, from left to right.

the position of the disc of least confusion is more complicated and its shape must be derived from the geometry of the pencil. For example, in the case of a circular aperture, the cross-sectional shape of the disk of least confusion can be said to be elliptical which, under some circumstances, may reduce to a circle.

Cylinder axis direction

The axis direction of astigmatic lenses is specified in *Standard Notation* (sometimes called TABO Notation after the technical committee[5] that first proposed its universal use), which has superseded all the earlier methods used to specify axis direction.

Standard notation is illustrated in Figure 1.29 and assumes that the spectacle lenses are being viewed from the front, for instance, as they would be seen when worn on a subject's face. The subject's right eye is on the observer's left and the left eye is on the observer's right. A horizontal line drawn through the wearer's eyes represents the zero meridian for the notation. The axis direction is specified in degrees, starting on the right side of each eye and numbering anti-clockwise in the same way as the

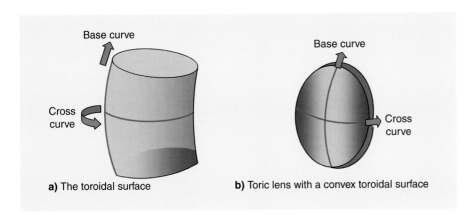

Figure 1.31   The toroidal surface and toric lens

a) The toroidal surface

b) Toric lens with a convex toroidal surface

Figure 1.31   The toroidal surface and toric lens

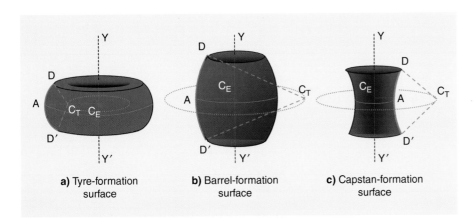

a) Tyre-formation surface

b) Barrel-formation surface

c) Capstan-formation surface

Figure 1.32   Types of toroidal surfaces

Transposition of lens powers

A prescription that incorporates a correction for astigmatism, such as $+2.00/-0.50 \times 45$, may be written either in minus cylinder form, as here, or in its plus cylinder transposition, $+1.50/+0.50 \times 135$. Usually, the prescription that is provided at the end of the sight test is written in its minus-cylinder transposition, but it is often necessary to order the lenses in their plus-cylinder transposition, for example for pricing purposes. A written prescription may be transposed from one form to another in the following way:

Given original sphere/cylinder $\times$ axis:

New sphere = algebraic sum of old sphere and cylinder

New cylinder = old cylinder with sign changed

New axis = old axis plus or minus 90

If the old axis is less than 90, add 90 to it to obtain the new axis. If the old axis is greater than 90, subtract 90 from it to obtain the new axis.

Toric lenses

In practice, sphero-cylindrical lenses are dispensed in curved form for the same reasons as spherical lenses. Curved lenses result in better quality images when the eye views through off-axis portions of the lens (see Chapter 2).

Figure 1.31 illustrates a cylinder that has been bent so that the original plane axis meridian is now curved. Such a surface is called a toroidal surface. A toroidal surface has two different principal powers, neither of which is zero. The lower power is usually referred to as the base curve of the surface and the higher power as the cross curve. In the simple cylindrical surface shown in Figure 1.24, the 'base-curve' power along the axis is zero and

the 'cross-curve' power is simply the power of the cylindrical surface. In the case of the toroidal surface (Figure 1.31), the 'axis meridian' is curved and the cylindrical power of the surface is the difference between the cross curve and the base curve.

A toroidal surface is formed by the rotation of an arc of a circle about an axis in the plane of the circle, but lying outside it. Toroidal surfaces now exist for which the generator is not a circular arc, and these *atoroidal* surfaces are described in Chapter 4.

Three quite distinct forms of the surface are used in ophthalmic work, illustrated in Figure 1.32. They take their names from their obvious similarity to a car tyre's inner tube, a barrel and a capstan. Figure 1.32 shows that each form of the surface has two principal radii of curvature that correspond to its two principal meridians. The generator in each figure is the arc DD' and the centre of curvature of the generating arc is C_T, the locus of which around the axis of revolution YY' is indicated in the figures. The axis of revolution meets the axis of symmetry passing through the vertex of the surface, A, at C_E, which represents the equatorial centre of curvature of the surface.

C_T represents the transverse centre of curvature of the surface and the distance AC_T represents the transverse radius of curvature, r_T. The distance AC_E is the equatorial radius of the surface, r_E.

In the tyre-formation toroidal surface illustrated in Figure 1.32a, which is the most common form of the surface in practice, r_E is the base-curve radius and r_T is the cross-curve radius. The tyre-form surface results when the centre of curvature of the generating arc, C_T, lies between the pole of the surface, A, and the axis of revolution, YY'.

In the case of the barrel-formation toroidal surface illustrated in Figure 1.32b, r_E is the cross-curve radius and r_T is the base-curve radius. The barrel-form of the surface results when the centre of curvature of the generating arc, C_T, lies on the other side of the axis of revolution, YY′, from the pole of the surface, A.

The rarely encountered capstan formation surface illustrated in Figure 1.32c is concave in one meridian and convex in the other. In this form, the surface lies between the centre of curvature of the generating arc, C_T, and the axis of revolution, YY′. It is conventional in this form of surface to describe the convex curve as the base curve, whatever the numerical value of the concave curve happens to be.

The tyre-formation toroidal surface is the usual form of surface to be found on stock-range toric lenses, since it lends itself well to mass production. The barrel-form surface is hardly ever used for mass production, since fewer lenses can be produced from a single toric block. From an optical point of view, the barrel-form surface does possess certain advantages, in that it improves the off-axis performance of the usual range of low-power toric lenses. Some toric generators are able to cut a toroidal surface in either tyre or barrel form.

Toric lenses are described by the power of their base curve; a +6.00 base toric signifies that the toroidal surface is convex and that the power of the base curve of the surface is +6.00D. The spherical surface of the lens is known as the sphere curve. To differentiate between spherical and astigmatic surfaces, the suffices DS and DC are used to signify either spherical or cylindrical surfaces.

The prescription $-4.00/+1.00 \times 30$, made in a toric form with +5.00D base curve, would have surface powers:

$$\frac{(+5.00DC \times 120 + 6.00DC \times 30)}{-9.00DS}$$

If the same prescription is made with a –7.50D base curve it would have surface powers:

$$+4.50DS/(-7.50DC \times 30 - 8.50DC \times 120)$$

If the prescription is considered in the sphere–cylinder transposition that has its cylinder with the same sign as the base curve, the sum of the base curve and the sphere curve gives the spherical element of the prescription. The difference between the cross curve and the base curve gives the cylindrical component of the prescription and the axis direction of the cylinder corresponds with the axis of the cross curve.

Effective power of a lens in distance vision

If a correcting lens is moved closer to or further away from the eye, its second principal focus no longer coincides with the far point and the effective power of the lens is no longer correct. The distance from the back vertex of the spectacle lens to the cornea is known as the *vertex distance*; it is important that the vertex distance employed during the sight test procedure be maintained for the final correcting lens, certainly for lens powers over ±5.00D. The vertex distance is indicated by the distance *d* in Figures 1.22d and 1.23d, where it can be seen that the back vertex focal length, f'_v, is made up from the sum of the far point distance, *k*, and the vertex distance, *d*, that is:

$$f'_v = k + d$$

The vertex distance is included in the prescription specification, simply by writing **at** followed by the number of millimetres.

Thus $+8.00/+2.00 \times 90$ **at 12** means that the vertex distance at which the prescription is effective is 12mm. If the final lens cannot be fitted at 12mm the power must be recalculated for the new vertex distance.

In distance vision, when a plus lens is moved away from the eye the effective power of the lens at the eye increases. A minus lens moved away from the eye, on the other hand, causes a decrease in effective power, that is, the lens becomes weaker. The reverse is true when lenses are moved towards the eye. Plus lenses become weaker and minus lenses become stronger. It follows that when a plus lens is to be fitted further from the eye than the testing distance, the back vertex power of the final lens must be decreased, whereas when a minus lens is to be fitted further from the eye than the testing distance, the back vertex power of the final lens must be increased.

The calculation for the final lens power is very simple, as it is only necessary to adjust the focal length of the lens by the change in vertex distance. Thus, if the prescription $+8.00/+4.00 \times 90$ at 12 is to be dispensed at 14mm, a forward shift of 2mm, the focal lengths of each principal power meridian of the lens must be increased by 2mm. The calculation is set out below. It is assumed that when a forward shift of the lens occurs the change in vertex distance is given a minus sign.

+8.00

focal length = 1000/8 = +125mm

add 2mm

gives +127mm

+12.00

focal length = 1000/12 = +83.33mm

add 2mm

gives +85.33mm

The final powers at 14mm are:

1000/+127 = +7.87

and

1000/+85.33 = +11.75

So the final prescription is $+7.87/+3.87 \times 90$ at 14.

In a similar way, the prescription $-10.00/-4.00 \times 180$ at 12 is equivalent to $-10.37/-4.25 \times 180$ at 15, which can be deduced as follows:

−10.00

focal length = 1000/−10 = −100mm

add 3mm

gives −97mm

−14.00

focal length = 1000/−14 = −71.43mm

add 3mm

gives −68.43mm

The final powers at 15mm are:

1000/−97 = −10.31

and

1000/−68.43 = −14.61

So the final prescription is −10.37/−4.25 × 180 at 15, when rounded to the nearest 0.12D.

Table 1.1 gives changes in effective power for distance vision when the vertex distance is altered.

CD-ROM

Further explanation of effective power is to be found on the CD-ROM

Effects of lenses in near vision

The back vertex power of a lens represents the vergence that leaves the lens when the light originates from a distant object. In near vision the light originates from a point that lies at a finite distance in front of the lens, so the vergence leaving the back surface depends not just upon the back vertex power, but also upon the form and thickness of the lens. Vertex power notation gives only an approximate indication of the performance of the lens in near vision.

The vergence leaving the back surface of the lens, L'_2, which has arrived from a near object lying at L_1 dioptres in front of the lens, is given by:

$$L'_2 = (L_1 + F_1) / \left[1 - (t/n)(L_1 + F_1) \right] + F_2$$

As expected, when L_1 is zero, this expression reduces to the expression already given for the back vertex power of the lens.

The difference between the vergence leaving a lens when the light originates from a near object, L'_2, and the anticipated vergence obtained from the sum of the incident vergence and the back vertex power, $L_1 + F'_V$, is called the near vision effectivity error (NVEE) of the lens.

It can be shown that the NVEE is given by the approximate relationship:

$$\text{NVEE} = (t/n) L_1 (L_1 + 2F_1)$$

NVEE is usually only a problem when the thickness of the lens becomes appreciable, which occurs with plus lenses of moderate-to-high power. Its significance is that lenses of the same back vertex power but of different forms are not interchangeable in near vision. Typically, for a lens of power +10.00 to be employed for near vision, the power of the final curved-form lens that the subject is dispensed needs to be increased by about +0.50D from that of the flat-form trial lens. The use of the above expression is illustrated in the next but one section (which deals with the theory of trial case lenses).

CD-ROM

Further explanation of NVEE is given on the CD-ROM

Effective power of a lens in near vision

In distance vision, whenever a plus lens is moved further from the eye, its effective power at the eye increases. This is not necessarily the case for near vision, when the change in effective power depends upon the power of the lens and also upon whether the object remains stationary or itself moves with the lens.

This can be deduced from Figure 1.33, which illustrates the situation for a subject who is wearing a +3.00D lens for near vision at −33.3cm in front of the lens. Assuming an emmetropic eye, no accommodation is required to see the near object. Moving the lens away from the eye, towards the object, which is assumed to remain in the same position, causes an increase in divergence of the light arriving at the lens. It is assumed that the lens has been moved forward from the eye to the point where the vergence of the light arriving at the lens is −3.25D. The vergence leaving the lens is now −0.25D, ignoring the lens thickness, and the eye needs to accommodate by +0.25D to produce a sharp image of the near object on the fovea.

If the near object, B, had moved away from the eye at the same rate as the lens, there would be no change in effective power since the lens is simply collimating the light (Figure 1.34).

The change in effective power, δF, for a lens of power F when moved through a distance x used for near vision at a dioptral distance L_1 from the lens, is given by the approximate relationship:

object remains stationary: $\delta F = -xF\left(2L_1 + F\right)$

object moves with lens: $\delta F = -x\left(L_1 + F\right)^2$

The graph in Figure 1.35 shows the results of plotting these expressions for lens powers in the range −10.00D to +10.00D, where the lens has been moved forwards by 5mm ($x = -0.005$ metres in the expression), the near point being assumed to lie at a dioptral distance −3.00D from the lens (object lies 33.3cm in front of the lens).

It can be seen that, when the object remains stationary, lens powers in the range 0.00D to +6.00D moved away from the eye cause the eye to accommodate more to see a near object. If the object is assumed to move away from the eye at the same rate as the lens, the action of moving the lens away from the eye causes a decrease in accommodation in all cases except that of a +3.00D lens, for which there is no change in effective power, since the lens collimates the light.

CD-ROM

Further details on the effective power of lenses in near vision is given on the CD-ROM

Trial case lenses

Various standards are laid down for ophthalmic trial case lenses. In addition to tolerances on lens powers, cylinder axis directions, prism powers and orientation and centration of the lenses, lens diameters and thicknesses are also recommended. Among the recommendations concerning power and diameter, the Standards specify that the marked power of a lens should be in terms of its back vertex power and that, if the front vertex power differs significantly from the back vertex power, a table should be provided by the manufacturer to show the front vertex powers of the lenses. The overall diameters of the lenses should be 38mm and the optical centres of the lenses should coincide with their geometric centres.

In most of the earliest trial cases, the spheres were equi-convex or equi-concave, and the cylinders plano-cylindrical in form with

Table 1.1 Compensation for changes in vertex distance

Plus lens fitted further from eye, or minus lens fitted closer to eye						Original power	Plus lens fitted closer to eye, or minus lens fitted further from eye					
Change in vertex distance (mm)						↓	Change in vertex distance (mm)					
6	5	4	3	2	1		1	2	3	4	5	6
4.38	4.40	4.42	4.44	4.46	4.48	4.50	4.52	4.54	4.56	4.58	4.60	4.62
4.85	4.88	4.90	4.93	4.95	4.98	5.00	5.03	5.05	5.08	5.10	5.13	5.15
5.32	5.35	5.38	5.41	5.44	5.47	5.50	5.53	5.56	5.59	5.62	5.66	5.69
5.79	5.83	5.86	5.89	5.93	5.96	6.00	6.04	6.07	6.11	6.15	6.19	6.22
6.26	6.30	6.34	6.38	6.42	6.46	6.50	6.54	6.59	6.63	6.67	6.72	6.76
6.72	6.76	6.81	6.86	6.90	6.95	7.00	7.05	7.10	7.15	7.20	7.25	7.31
7.18	7.23	7.28	7.33	7.39	7.44	7.50	7.56	7.61	7.67	7.73	7.79	7.85
7.63	7.69	7.75	7.81	7.87	7.94	8.00	8.06	8.13	8.20	8.26	8.33	8.40
8.09	8.15	8.22	8.29	8.36	8.43	8.50	8.57	8.65	8.72	8.80	8.88	8.96
8.54	8.61	8.69	8.76	8.84	8.92	9.00	9.08	9.17	9.25	9.34	9.42	9.51
8.99	9.07	9.15	9.24	9.32	9.41	9.50	9.59	9.68	9.78	9.88	9.97	10.07
9.43	9.52	9.62	9.71	9.80	9.90	10.00	10.10	10.20	10.31	10.42	10.53	10.64
9.88	9.98	10.08	10.18	10.28	10.39	10.50	10.61	10.73	10.84	10.96	11.08	11.21
10.32	10.43	10.54	10.65	10.76	10.88	11.00	11.12	11.25	11.38	11.51	11.64	11.78
10.76	10.87	10.99	11.12	11.24	11.37	11.50	11.63	11.77	11.91	12.05	12.20	12.35
11.19	11.32	11.45	11.58	11.72	11.86	12.00	12.15	12.30	12.45	12.61	12.77	12.93
11.63	11.76	11.90	12.05	12.20	12.35	12.50	12.66	12.82	12.99	13.16	13.33	13.51
12.06	12.21	12.36	12.51	12.67	12.83	13.00	13.17	13.35	13.53	13.71	13.90	14.10
12.49	12.65	12.81	12.97	13.15	13.32	13.50	13.68	13.87	14.07	14.27	14.48	14.69
12.92	13.08	13.26	13.44	13.62	13.81	14.00	14.20	14.40	14.61	14.83	15.05	15.28
13.34	13.52	13.71	13.90	14.09	14.29	14.50	14.71	14.93	15.16	15.39	15.63	15.88
13.76	13.95	14.15	14.35	14.56	14.78	15.00	15.23	15.46	15.71	15.96	16.22	16.48
14.18	14.39	14.60	14.81	15.03	15.26	15.50	15.74	16.00	16.26	16.52	16.80	17.09
14.60	14.81	15.04	15.27	15.50	15.75	16.00	16.26	16.53	16.81	17.09	17.39	17.70
15.01	15.24	15.48	15.72	15.97	16.23	16.50	16.78	17.06	17.36	17.67	17.98	18.31
15.43	15.67	15.92	16.18	16.44	16.72	17.00	17.29	17.60	17.91	18.24	18.58	18.93
15.84	16.09	16.36	16.63	16.91	17.20	17.50	17.81	18.13	18.47	18.82	19.18	19.55
16.25	16.51	16.79	17.08	17.37	17.68	18.00	18.33	18.67	19.03	19.40	19.78	20.18
16.65	16.93	17.23	17.53	17.84	18.16	18.50	18.85	19.21	19.59	19.98	20.39	20.81
17.06	17.35	17.66	17.98	18.30	18.65	19.00	19.37	19.75	20.15	20.56	20.99	21.44
17.46	17.77	18.09	18.42	18.77	19.13	19.50	19.89	20.29	20.71	21.15	21.61	22.08
17.86	18.18	18.52	18.87	19.23	19.61	20.00	20.41	20.83	21.28	21.74	22.22	22.73
18.25	18.59	18.95	19.31	19.69	20.09	20.50	20.93	21.38	21.84	22.33	22.84	23.38
18.65	19.00	19.37	19.76	20.15	20.57	21.00	21.45	21.92	22.41	22.93	23.46	24.03
19.04	19.41	19.80	20.20	20.61	21.05	21.50	21.97	22.47	22.98	23.52	24.09	24.68
19.43	19.82	20.22	20.64	21.07	21.53	22.00	22.49	23.01	23.55	24.12	24.72	25.35
20.21	20.63	21.06	21.52	21.99	22.48	23.00	23.54	24.11	24.70	25.33	25.99	26.68
20.98	21.43	21.90	22.39	22.90	23.44	24.00	24.59	25.21	25.86	26.55	27.27	28.04
21.74	22.22	22.73	23.26	23.81	24.39	25.00	25.64	26.32	27.03	27.78	28.57	29.41
22.49	23.01	23.55	24.12	24.71	25.34	26.00	26.69	27.43	28.20	29.02	29.89	30.81
23.24	23.79	24.37	24.98	25.62	26.29	27.00	27.75	28.54	29.38	30.27	31.21	32.22
23.97	24.56	25.18	25.83	26.52	27.24	28.00	28.81	29.66	30.57	31.53	32.56	33.65
24.70	25.33	25.99	26.68	27.41	28.18	29.00	29.87	30.79	31.76	32.81	33.92	35.11
25.42	26.09	26.79	27.52	28.30	29.12	30.00	30.93	31.92	32.97	34.09	35.29	36.59

full-apertures, 38mm round. Many modern trial case lenses are plano-convex or plano-concave with an effective aperture of just 20mm, these small diameter lenses being mounted in metal or plastics rims with an overall diameter of 38mm to enable them to be used in standard trial frames. It is also possible to obtain curved trial lenses with form that approximates that of the final lens that the subject will eventually wear.

In distance vision it is sufficient for the final lens to have the same back vertex power as the trial lens combination, provided that it is mounted at the same vertex distance with the same

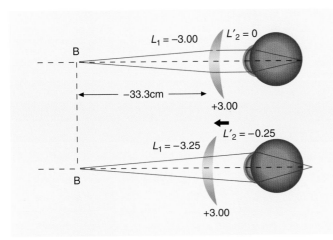

Figure 1.33 Effective power in near vision. Object remains stationary

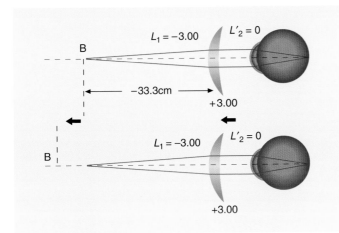

Figure 1.34 Effective power in near vision. Object moves with lens

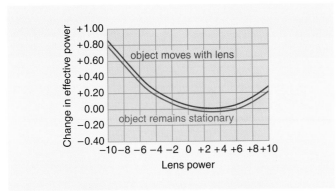

Figure 1.35 Effective power of lenses in near vision

centration and pantoscopic angle as the trial lens combination. In the case of strong lenses, the back vertex power of the trial lens system cannot be obtained simply by adding together the numbers marked on the lenses, but this problem can be overcome by recording the back vertex power of the trial lens system in position in the trial frame by means of a focimeter. An alternative solution is to use *additive vertex power* test lenses, in which the trial lenses occupy specific positions in the trial frame and the

lenses are numbered, not in terms of their back vertex powers, but, instead, with their effective powers at the back vertex of the combination. With these lenses, the problem of cylindrical effectivity in distance and near vision is overcome by placing all the cylinders in the rear cell of the trial frame with their cylindrical surfaces facing the eye. The spherical lenses can be numbered with their effective powers at the cylindrical surface and the back vertex power of the combination is then the sum of the powers marked on the two components.

To put this principle into practice it is necessary for all the cylinders to have the same thicknesses to maintain a constant separation between the front surface of the spherical component and the cylindrical surface. In cases where there is no cylindrical correction, a parallel plate of glass is inserted into the rear cell of the trial frame to maintain the same optical path length. The theory of these lenses is explained below. The modern refractor unit, or phoropter, which may, one day, replace the simple trial frame and separate lenses, employs additive vertex power test systems.

The theory of the various types of trial lenses in use today is summarized below.

An important consideration in the design of plus trial lenses of appreciable thickness is the amount of NVEE that the trial lenses exhibit. It is pointed out in the section on lens power that the vergence impressed by a lens in near vision depends not just upon the back vertex power of the lens, but also upon its form and thickness. Lenses of the same back vertex powers but of different forms are not interchangeable in near vision. The difference between the vergence that actually leaves a lens in near vision and the anticipated vergence found, simply from $L_1 + F'_V$, is defined as the near vision effectivity error, NVEE, and is given with good approximation by:

$$NVEE = (t/n)L_1(L_1 + 2F_1)$$

For instance, a +10.00D lens made in glass of refractive index 1.5 with a centre thickness of 9mm and a +12.00D front curve when used for near vision at one-third metre ($L_1 = -3.00$) would have:

$$NVEE = (t/n)L_1(L_1 + 2F_1)$$
$$= (0.009/1.5) \times -3 \times (-3 + 2 \times 12) = -0.4D$$

If the thickness of the lens had been ignored, we would expect the vergence leaving the lens to be $L_1 + F'_V$ or +7.00D. The actual vergence leaving the lens is the anticipated vergence plus the NVEE, which is +6.6D.

If the eye had been tested with an equi-convex trial lens of the same thickness, the individual surface powers would be +4.93D each and the NVEE exhibited by the trial lens would be:

$$NVEE = (t/n)L_1(L_1 + 2F_1)$$
$$= (0.009/1.5) \times -3 \times (-3 + 2 \times 4.93) = -0.1D$$

The vergence leaving the trial lens during the sight test would have been +6.9D and, ideally, the vergence leaving the final lens should also be +6.9D. For this to be the case, either the final lens should have exactly the same form and thickness as the trial lens, or the back vertex power of the final lens must be increased. The final lens would normally be dispensed in curved form to provide good off-axis performance, so unless the trial lenses are also curved, it is necessary to increase the power of the final lens for it to duplicate the effect of the trial lens.

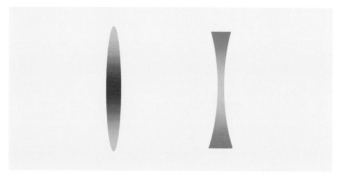

Figure 1.36   Symmetrical trial lenses

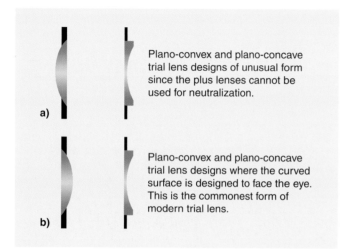

a)   Plano-convex and plano-concave trial lens designs of unusual form since the plus lenses cannot be used for neutralization.

b)   Plano-convex and plano-concave trial lens designs where the curved surface is designed to face the eye. This is the commonest form of modern trial lens.

Figure 1.37   Reduced aperture plano-convex and plano-concave trial lenses

It should be clear that in the choice of trial lens form, it is better for the lenses to have the same NVEEs as the final lenses that will be dispensed from the trial frame prescription.

Symmetrical trial case lenses

Symmetrical trial lenses (Figure 1.36) are full-aperture lenses for which the plus series are all equi-convex and the minus lenses all equi-concave in form. They have the advantage that, when *in situ* in the trial frame, the refractionist can still see the eye behind the lens. Also, they are reversible, an important consideration in the darkness of the examination room, so it does not matter which way round they are put into the trial frame.

Since the back vertex power of a symmetrical trial lens is almost the same as $2F_1$, the NVEE of these designs is given by:

$$(t/n)L_1(L_1+F_V')$$

We have just seen that in the case of an equi-convex +10.00D trial lens made with the parameters outlined above, the NVEE would be –0.1D compared with –0.4D for the final lens.

Reduced aperture plano-convex and plano-concave trial lenses

The series shown in Figure 1.37a is very unusual because the curved surface of the plus lenses is designed to face away from the eye. At first sight, this seems to be the natural way in which the trial lens should be used, but a moment's thought confirms that if the lens is used this way round, the power of the

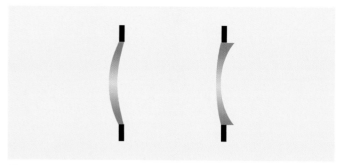

Figure 1.38   Reduced aperture curved-form trial lenses

front surface of the trial lens will not be equal and opposite in power to the minus lenses in the series, since it would be necessary to compensate this surface for the thickness of the lens. Thus, the plus lenses cannot be used for neutralization, which was always one requirement of trial case lenses, and, perhaps more important, the lenses in the series do not neutralize one another!

On the other hand, the plus lenses do have moderate errors of near vision effectivity like those of the final lenses that replace them.

For this series, the front surface power is almost the same as the back vertex power, so $2F_1=2F'_V$ and hence the NVEE is given by:

$$(t/n)L_1(L_1+2F_V')$$

For a +10.00D trial lens made in glass of refractive index 1.5 with thickness 4.5mm, the NVEE would be:

$$\text{NVEE} = (t/n)L_1(L_1+2F_V')$$
$$= (0.0045/1.5)\times-3\times(-3+2\times10) = -0.2\text{D}$$

The trial lenses illustrated in Figure 1.37b are plano-convex and plano-concave in form, with the curved surfaces designed to face the eye. In the case of the plus lenses, the final lens is effectively turned back to front from the trial lens. This design has the advantage that the power of the curved surface is the same as the back vertex power of the lens and so the design can be used for neutralization when this is necessary for high powered lenses. Furthermore, the convex surfaces of the plus lenses have identical curvature to the minus lenses in the series and, obviously, neutralize one another.

For this series, the front surface power is zero so the NVEE is simply $(t/n)L_1^2$. For a +10.00D trial lens made in glass of refractive index 1.5 with thickness 4.5mm, the NVEE would be:

$$\text{NVEE} = (t/n)L_1^2$$
$$= (0.0045/1.5)\times9 = +0.03\text{D}.$$

Curved-form trial lenses

In practice, these should be the best trial lenses of all to use for refraction, for they duplicate the form of the manufacturer's own best-form lens series (Figure 1.38). They do not violate the principle of direct substitution in that they exhibit the same errors of near vision effectivity as the final lenses. They also have the advantage that the off-axis performance of the trial lens matches that of the final lens, so that prescription translation should be easier in the case of high power prescriptions.

Additive vertex power test lenses

This series of trial lenses (Figure 1.39), together with its special trial frame, which holds the lenses in specific positions in the frame, has the spherical lenses numbered not in terms of their back vertex powers, but instead with their effective powers at the back vertex of the combination. In use, the spherical lenses are placed in the front cell of the frame and the cylinders in the rear cell, with their cylindrical surfaces facing the eye. A specially designed protractor enables the axis direction to be read despite the rear position of the cylinders. The spherical lenses are numbered with their effective powers at the cylindrical surface and the back vertex power of the combination is the sum of the powers marked on the two components.

The cylinders all have the same thicknesses to maintain a constant separation between the front surface of the spherical component and the cylindrical surface. In cases where there is no cylindrical correction, a parallel plate of glass is inserted into the rear cell of the trial frame to maintain the same optical path length.

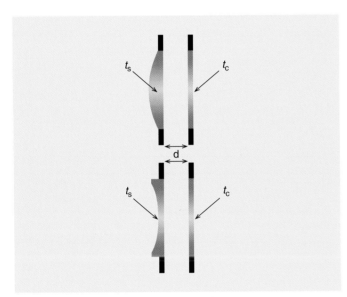

Figure 1.39   Additive vertex power test lenses

If the thicknesses of the spherical and cylindrical components are denoted by t_S and t_C, respectively, and the separation of the two lenses by d, then the front surface power of the spherical component is given by:

$$F_1 = F'_V/(1 + xF'_V)$$

where

$$x = (t_S + t_C + nd)/1000n$$

For example, for a series of test lenses made in glass of refractive index 1.5, with cylindrical components that are all 3mm thick, as is the separation between the two cells, in the case of the +10.00D lens, assuming this to be 4.5mm thick, the front surface power of the spherical component would be +9.26D.

Measurement of lens power

In practice, the back vertex power of spectacle lenses is found with the aid of a focimeter, which reads the dioptric power of the lens, the cylinder axis direction, any prismatic power and the base direction of the prism. Many modern instruments measure the lens powers and print out the prescription automatically, requiring no more skill from the user than the ability to insert the lens the right way round.

In the absence of a focimeter, the power of lenses of low power can be determined quite satisfactorily by hand neutralization. Here, ordinary trial case lenses of known power are placed in contact with the unknown lens until no more movement can be observed under the transverse test. The power of the unknown lens is equal and opposite to that of the lens required for neutralization.

The vergence leaving the back surface of a spectacle lens in near vision can be measured with the assistance of an auxiliary minus lens, which is placed in contact with the front surface of the lens under test when it is placed in the focimeter. For near vision at one-third of a metre, a −3.00D lens is employed for the auxiliary lens, or for near vision at 40cm a −2.50D lens is employed and so on. The auxiliary lens enables the focimeter, which normally is used to measure vertex power, to duplicate the ray path in near vision (see the section below on use of the focimeter).

Neutralization

One of the most significant influences in the design of trial lenses is the role they also play in the neutralization of an unknown lens to determine its power. It is the back vertex power that has to be determined and the trial lenses used should be numbered in terms of their back vertex powers.

The condition for neutralization is shown schematically in Figure 1.40. The second principal foci (i.e. the back vertex foci) of the two lenses should coincide and the back vertices of the unknown lens and the trial lens must be in contact. If the trial lenses are symmetrical in form it does not matter which way round the trial lens is placed in contact with the back surface of the lens under test. When the trial lenses are plano-convex or plano-concave in form, the powers marked on the trial lenses are usually those operative at the poles of the curved surfaces and so it is the curved surface that should be placed in contact with the back vertex of the unknown lens.

It will be appreciated that neutralization will apparently occur when the back vertices are not held in contact if the separation of the vertices is equal to the difference between the focal lengths

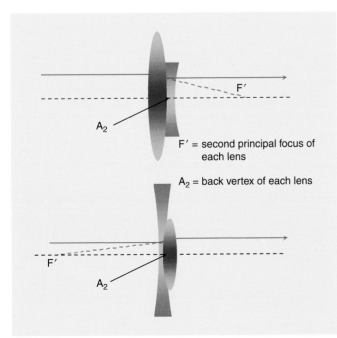

F′ = second principal focus of each lens

A₂ = back vertex of each lens

Figure 1.40   Condition for neutralization of plus and minus lenses

of the two lenses. Thus, a +5.00D lens and a –10.00D lens will apparently 'neutralize' if they are held 10cm apart. On a more practical scale, a +8.00D and a –8.12D lens will 'neutralize' if they are held 2mm apart.

Problems may occur when neutralization is attempted with a system of trial lenses that may be necessary when dealing with non-integer powers in the higher ranges. For example, it is unlikely that a trial lens of power –10.50D will be included in a trial set, so this power would need to be made up by adding two lenses together, such as –10.00D and –0.50D. Assuming the use of a symmetrical trial lens series, if this pair is placed in contact with a +10.50D lens with the –10.00D component in contact with the back vertex of the plus lens, then despite the air gap of some 2mm between the –10.00D lens and the –0.50D lens, the combination will appear to neutralize. If the –0.50D lens was inadvertently placed in contact with the plus lens under test, the combination would now exhibit an error of about +0.25D and it would not be difficult to conclude that the lens under test was actually +10.75D.

Further problems occur when neutralization is attempted upon a near object, because of the NVEE of the system. In particular, the values obtained are different when the plus lens faces the near object and when the minus lens faces the near object.

So far it has been assumed that it is possible to place the back vertices of the unknown lens and the test lens in contact. Perhaps the greatest difficulty found in practice concerns curved lenses when it proves to be impossible to place the pole of the trial lens

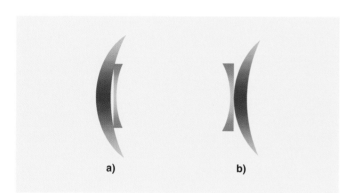

a)   b)

Figure 1.41   Neutralization of curved lenses showing the impossibility of placing the back vertices in close contact

in contact with the back vertex of the lens under test (Figure 1.41a). In such cases the trial lens may be held in contact with the front surface of the unknown lens, in which case the *front* vertex power of the lens under test is obtained (Figure 1.41b). In the case of negative lenses with negligible thickness, the front and back vertex powers are virtually the same and no error is made by adopting this procedure. However, in the case of positive lenses the front vertex power is invariably weaker than the back vertex power, so this procedure underestimates the power of the lens. The error is about –0.25D in the case of a +5.00D lens and –0.75D in the case of a +10.00D lens.

The focimeter

In view of the difficulties just outlined in the above section on neutralization, it is no small wonder that the vertex power measuring instrument, or focimeter, is so widely employed. The focimeter is an instrument that measures the vertex power of a lens, or of a system of lenses, such as the trial frame combination. In addition to giving the back vertex power of a spectacle lens, the instrument also finds the orientation of the cylinder axis of an astigmatic lens and may be used to locate the optical centre of a lens or to record the prismatic effect at a point on the lens.

The optical system of a simple focimeter is illustrated in Figure 1.42a, which shows the positions of the components in the system without a lens under test. The instrument is seen to consist, basically, of a collimator that issues parallel light and a telescope that focuses parallel light. A lens rest, at which the lens under test is placed, lies at the second principal focus of the collimating lens, F_O. A graticule on which is engraved the prism and axis scales lies at the common focus of the objective and eyepiece lenses that form the telescope. The prism scales are simply circular rings, each one representing 1Δ of prism.

In Figure 1.42b a plus lens is placed under test at the lens rest. The target T has to be refocused for it to be imaged at infinity by the telescope. To refocus the target, which is done manually in most instruments, the power dial is rotated, the action of which is to move the target, in the case of a plus lens under test, towards the standard lens, F_O, in the instrument. In the case of a minus lens under test, the target moves away from the standard lens.

Figure 1.42   The focimeter

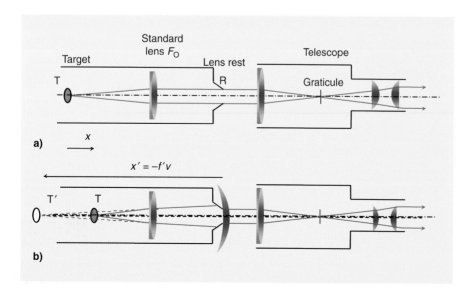

The movement of the target is denoted by x, and represents the position of the object with respect to the first principal focus of the system.

When an image of the target is seen clearly through the telescope, the light leaving the lens under test must, once more, be parallel, and appears to be coming from the point T', which is the image of T formed by the system comprising the standard lens and the lens under test. Since the back vertex of the lens under test lies upon the lens rest, which coincides with the second principal focus of the standard lens, the distance of the image T' from the lens rest, x', must also be the back vertex focal length of the lens under test, f'_V.

By means of Newton's Relationship, $xx' = -f'^2$, we find that $xf'_V = -f_O^2$, or the back vertex power of the lens under test, F'_V, is given by:

$$F'_V = xF_O{}^2$$

The movement of the target per dioptre of power of the lens under test is linear. If the standard lens of the instrument is +25.00D, the movement of the target would be 1.6mm per dioptre. To be able to measure lens powers in the range +20.00D to –20.00D the total travel of the target needs to be $40 \times 1.6\text{mm} = 64\text{mm}$.

The following instructions are intended for new users of manually operated focimeters.

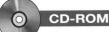

CD-ROM

Tips on how to use a manually operated focimeter are given on the CD-ROM

Setting up the instrument for use

To zero the instrument and ensure that instrument accommodation is not stimulated, the following procedure should be carried out.

Before switching on, rotate the power knob to one of its stop positions (highest plus or minus reading position) and rotate the eyepiece adjustment knob so that the eyepiece is withdrawn to its maximum setting.

Switch on the instrument and, viewing through the eyepiece, adjust the eyepiece by rotating it slowly inwards until the scales engraved on the graticule (e.g. the protractor scale) just come into

sharp focus. Cease the movement of the eyepiece as soon as the graticule comes into focus. (Further rotation of the eyepiece simply stimulates accommodation.)

Rotate the power knob to adjust the dioptre scale until the target is seen in sharp focus. The scale should now read zero. Keep both eyes open, if possible, during the setting up procedure to ensure that accommodation remains relaxed.

A first-time user will find it very helpful to determine first the powers of known lenses (such as trial case lenses). Start with spherical lenses.

There are usually two types of targets. Circular targets that comprise a circle of dots, each one of which defocuses when a lens is placed under test, and linear targets that comprise lines of dots at right angles to one another, usually two lines running in one direction and a single line in the other. Some targets are made up from a combination of these two types of target.

When the focimeter is used to measure the back vertex power of a spectacle lens, the ray path of the light through the instrument exactly simulates the ray path by which a spectacle lens corrects the eye for distance vision. This is illustrated in Figure 1.43, which compares the ray paths of a plus lens under test in the focimeter with the method by which a plus lens corrects an eye in hypermetropia. Clearly, the standard lens in the focimeter performs the same function as the eye's optical system. In the case of the focimeter, the standard lens produces an image of the target, T, at T', which coincides with the second principal focus of the lens under test. In the case of the eye, the macula, M', is conjugate with the far point, M_R, which coincides with the second principal focus of the lens.

Back vertex power is a measure of the vergence leaving the back surface of the lens when the incident vergence on the front surface is zero. The light is assumed to originate from a distant object.

In near vision, we are not dealing with a distant object and the back vertex system of numbering spectacle lenses only provides an approximate indication of the vergence impressed by a lens in near vision.

To measure the vergence leaving a spectacle lens when it is used in near vision, we can employ an auxiliary lens that is placed in contact with the front surface of the lens under test and is designed to simulate the ray path in near vision. For near vision at 33.3cm we would use a –3.00D auxiliary lens, whereas for near vision at 40cm we would use a –2.50D auxiliary lens and so on.

Trial lenses are ideal to use as auxiliary lenses. In theory, the minus auxiliary lens should be plano-concave in form and placed with its

Figure 1.43 Measurement of spectacle lenses for distance vision

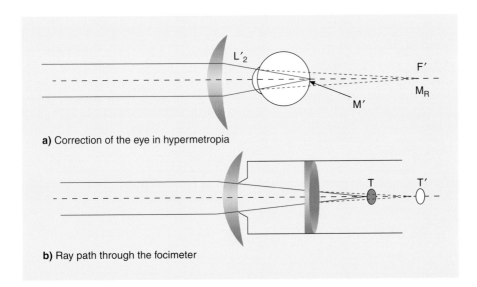

a) Correction of the eye in hypermetropia

b) Ray path through the focimeter

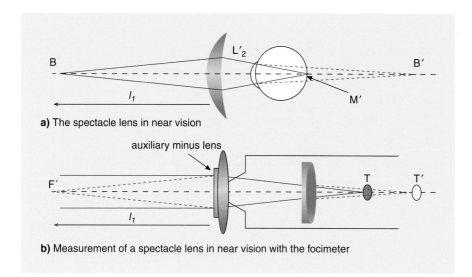

Figure 1.44   Measurement of spectacle lenses in near vision

a) The spectacle lens in near vision

b) Measurement of a spectacle lens in near vision with the focimeter

concave surface in contact with the front surface of the lens under test. However, since the auxiliary lens is of low power and likely to be thin, from a practical point of view its form is immaterial.

The optical principle is illustrated in Figure 1.44, which confirms that the action of the auxiliary lens is to enable the focimeter to simulate the ray path in near vision.

The action of the auxiliary lens is, effectively, to reduce the power of the front surface by the magnitude of the incident vergence from the near point. For example, if the front surface power is +10.00D and the auxiliary lens used is –3.00D, to simulate a near point distance of 33.3cm, the effect of the auxiliary lens is, in essence, to reduce the front surface power to +7.00D. This has exactly the same mathematical effect as would an incident vergence of –3.00D upon the front surface.

To duplicate the effect of a lens for near vision it is necessary to match not the back vertex power of the lens but, rather, the vergence that the lens impresses in near vision. Two lenses of different forms have the same effect in near vision when the vergence leaving the back surface of each lens, L'_2, is the same when measured by the focimeter with an auxiliary lens in contact with the front surface of the lens under test.

The scanning focimeter

The focimeter can be adapted to read the oblique vertex sphere powers of a spectacle lens by the following method. A lens holder must be made that enables the lens to pivot about a point, the assumed position of the eye's centre of rotation, measured back from the plane of the lens rest. An angular scale needs to be provided to indicate the rotation of the lens from the optical axis of the focimeter. A rotary prism device placed next to the objective lens of the telescope ensures that the light leaving the lens under test can be focused by the telescope. The principle is shown in Figure 1.45.

The optical axis of the instrument becomes the direction of the principal ray in the oblique ray path when the eye has rotated to view through off-axis portions of the lens.

Focimeter types

The focimeters described so far are essentially manually operated instruments with the collimator and telescope sharing a common optical axis. When a prismatic lens is under test the target remains

on the common optical axis, as does its image, at the position of the combined focal point for the rays which have passed through both the lens under test and the standard lens (Figure 1.46a). The image viewed through the eyepiece (or viewed on a screen in the case of projection focimeters) no longer lies on the optical axis of the telescope and its displacement must be judged on the graticule, or it can be restored to the telescope axis by means of a neutralizing prism.

Instruments of this type with which the focal point remains on the axis of the instrument are referred to as FOA (focal point on axis) focimeters.

In the case of modern automatic lens meters (automatic focimeters), some models are designed to read prismatic lenses with the collimated beam leaving the lens under test remaining on the optical axis, in which case the focal point of the system must have moved away from the axis (Figure 1.46b).

Instruments of this type with which the infinite conjugate remains on the axis of the instrument are referred to as IOA (infinite on axis) focimeters.

In the case of a non-prismatic lens under test, when the target is viewed without displacement, there is no practical difference between the readings given by the two types of instrument but in the case of strong prismatic lenses the readings obtained with one type of focimeter may differ slightly from those obtained with the other.

Summation of lenses

Thin lenses in contact, or the two surface powers of a spectacle lens, can be summed as follows.

Spherical lenses

Calling each component F_1 and F_2, the sum, $F, = F_1 + F_2$. Thus, the sum of –1.00 and –0.75 is –1.75. The sum of +2.50 and –2.50 is zero, which is the principle of neutralization.

In the case of optical components with thickness that cannot be ignored, or thin components that are separated by a given distance, the effective power of the first component at the second must be calculated. The effective power, F_E, of an optical component, F, at a distance, d, is given by:

$$F_E = F / (1 - dF)$$

Figure 1.45   The scanning focimeter

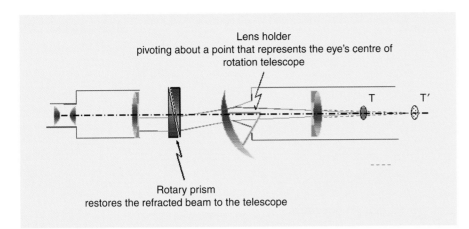

Lens holder
pivoting about a point that represents the eye's centre of rotation telescope

T   T'

Rotary prism
restores the refracted beam to the telescope

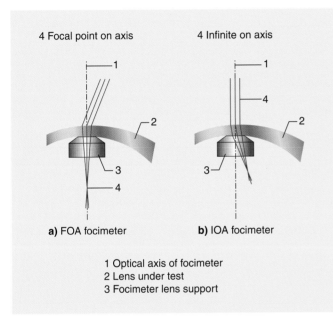

4 Focal point on axis   4 Infinite on axis

a) FOA focimeter   b) IOA focimeter

1 Optical axis of focimeter
2 Lens under test
3 Focimeter lens support

Figure 1.46   Measuring methods for different types of focimeter. (a) Measurement by classic manual and projection focimeters with focal point remaining on the optical axis (FOA design). (b) Method adopted by some automatic focimeters (auto lens meters) with the infinite conjugate remaining on the axis (IOA design).

In this relationship, d must be substituted in metres.

Alternatively, the step-along system described earlier can be employed.

Astigmatic lenses

If the axes of the two components are parallel to one another, the spheres and the cylinders can be added just as if they were spherical components. Thus, the sum of the two lenses: $+1.00/-0.50 \times 30$ and $-0.75/+1.25 \times 30$ is $+0.25/+0.75 \times 30$.

In the same way, if the two axes are at right angles to one another, the sum of the two lenses can be found by first transposing one component so that its axis is parallel with the axis of the other. Thus, the sum of the lenses: $-1.25/-0.75 \times 45$ and $+2.25/-0.50 \times 135$ can be found by first transposing the second component to its alternate sphero-cylindrical form, $+1.75/+0.50 \times 45$ and then adding the first, to obtain $+0.50/-0.25 \times 45$.

When the axes are not parallel with one another, addition of two astigmatic lenses can be undertaken by a process known as astigmatic decomposition, in which each astigmatic lens is broken down into three components that can be summed directly. These components are the mean refractive error (MRE) of the lens and two cylindrical components, one with an axis that lies along the 180 meridian, C_0, and one with an axis that lies along the 45 meridian, C_{45}. If the sphero-cylindrical prescription is represented by a sphere of power S, a cylinder of power C, with its axis along θ ($S/C \times \theta$), then:

$$MRE = S + C/2$$
$$C_0 = C \cos 2\theta$$
$$C_{45} = C \sin 2\theta$$

When each astigmatic lens has been reduced to these components, the MRE of the resultant is the sum of the MRE of each component, the C_0 of the resultant is the sum of all the C_0 components and the C_{45} of the resultant is the sum of all the C_{45} components.

To convert the sum back to its sphero-cylindrical form, the resultant cylinder, C_R, is first calculated from:

$$C_R = \sqrt{\left(C_0{}^2 + C_{45}{}^2\right)}$$

Either the plus or minus root can be taken to give the plus or minus cylinder axis direction, as required.

The axis of the resultant cylinder, θ_R, is given by:

$$\tan 2\theta_R = C_{45}/C_0$$

If the axis resulting from this expression turns out to be negative, simply add 180 to it to obtain the axis direction in standard notation.

The resultant sphere, S_R, is given by:

$$\text{total } MRE - C_R/2$$

As an example, the sum of the two lenses $+2.00/+2.00 \times 30$ and $-1.00/-2.00 \times 150$ yields the following:

Lens 1

$$MRE = S + C/2 = 2 + 2/2 = +3$$
$$C_0 = C \cos 2\theta = 2 \cos 60 = +1$$
$$C_{45} = C \sin 2\theta = 2 \sin 60 = +1.732$$

Lens 2

$$MRE = S + C/2 = -1 + -2/2 = -2$$
$$C_0 = C \cos 2\theta = -2 \cos 300 = -1$$
$$C_{45} = C \sin 2\theta = -2 \sin 300 = +1.732$$

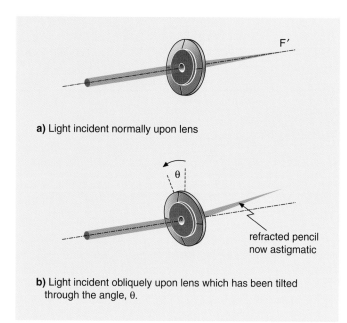

a) Light incident normally upon lens

b) Light incident obliquely upon lens which has been tilted through the angle, θ.

Figure 1.47   Oblique central refraction by a spherical lens. (a) The lens is stopped down so that only a narrow space around the optical centre is considered. (b) When the lens is tilted through an angle θ, the refracted pencil becomes astigmatic and its third-order effect can be calculated as shown in the accompanying text.

Adding the components separately gives:

	MRE	C_0	C_{45}
Lens 1	+3	+1	+1.732
Lens 2	−2	−1	+1.732
Sum	+1	0	+3.464

To convert back to sphero-cylindrical form, the resultant cylinder, C_R, is given by:

$$C_R = \sqrt{\left(C_0^2 + C_{45}^2\right)}$$
$$= \sqrt{\left(0^2 + 3.464^2\right)}$$
$$= +3.46$$

The resultant axis is found from:

$$\tan 2\theta_R = C_{45}/2C_0 = 3.464/0$$
$$\text{so } 2\theta_R = 90, \text{ and } \theta_R = 45.$$

The resultant sphere, S_R, is given by:

$$\text{total } MRE - C_R/2$$
$$= +1 - 3.464/2$$
$$= -0.73$$

The sum of the lenses is −0.73/+3.46×45.

The sum or difference of any two astigmatic prescriptions can be also found from a graphical construction developed by Stokes,[6] or from mathematical methods based on Stokes' Construction.

Tilted spherical lenses

When a narrow pencil of light from a distant object passes centrally through a spherical lens, which can be arranged by stopping down the lens so that just a small zone around the optical axis of the lens is in use as shown in Figure 1.47a, the pencil of light refracted

by the lens is focused at the second principal focus of the lens. If the spherical lens is then tilted so that the pencil is now incident obliquely on the lens, the refracted pencil becomes astigmatic. It is afflicted with aberrational astigmatism (Figure 1.47b).

It can be shown[6] that for a thin lens of power F, made in a material of refractive index, n, when the lens is tilted through an angle, θ, the spherical power of the lens, F_{SPH}, becomes:

$$F_{SPH} = F\left(1 + \sin^2\theta/2n\right)$$

and its cylindrical power,

$$F_{CYL} = F_{SPH}\tan^2\theta$$

with the axis of the cylinder parallel with the axis about which the lens is tilted.

Thus a +8.00D lens made in a material of refractive index 1.50 and tilted 10° about the horizontal axis (as shown in Figure 1.47b) would become:

$$F_{SPH} = +8.00\left(1 + \sin^2 10/3\right) = +8.08D$$
$$F_{CYL} = +8.08\tan^2 10 = +0.25D$$
$$\text{axis} = 180.$$

So tilting a +8.00D sphere through 10° about a horizontal axis would produce the effect +8.08/+0.25×180.

Tilting a −8.00D spherical lens through 10° about a horizontal axis would result in an effect of −8.08/−0.25×180.

The cylindrical component of spectacle prescriptions is usually quite small and if this component is ignored when tilting the spherical component it can be simply added to the tilted lens prescription. Hence, it follows that a lens of power +8.00/−0.25×180 tilted through 10° about a horizontal axis would become +8.08D sphere, the +0.25DC×180 introduced by tilting the lens has neutralized the prescription cylinder!

A lens of power +8.00/+0.25×60 tilted through 10° about a horizontal axis would become +8.20/+0.25×30 (summing +0.25DC×60 and +0.25DC×180 produces +0.12/+0.25×30) and it is seen that there is a change not only in the power but also the axis direction of the resultant cylinder.

These effects can be seen when spherical lenses are deliberately tilted in a focimeter, the small aperture of the focimeter lens support forming the narrow stop that restricts the zone of the lens which is being analysed. It will be seen in Chapter 2 that the real effect of a spectacle lens before the eye depends upon the form and position of the lens in addition to the zone of the lens which is in use at any time. However, the effect of lens tilt does have a bearing upon the power of a lens when it is read in a focimeter.

Mounted spectacle lenses may be tilted about the 180 meridian (pantoscopic angle) or about the 90 meridian (dihedral or wrap-round angle) or a combination of both. The significance of these changes in power due to lens tilt is considered in detail in Chapter 3.

References

1. Fincham W H A, Freeman M H 1980 Optics. Butterworth, London
2. Meyer-Arendt J R 1989 Introduction to classical and modern optics. Prentice-Hall, New Jersey
3. Swaine W 1922 Geometrical ophthalmic optics. Optician Hatton Press
4. Sturm C F 1861 Cours de mecanique de l'Ecole Polytechnique. Paris
5. Technischer Ausschuss für Brillenoptik 1917 German Committee named the notation TABO
6. Jalie M 1984 Principles of ophthalmic lenses. ABDO, London

Form and material of ophthalmic lenses

One of the first decisions to be made when dispensing a new prescription is the choice of lens form and material. Ophthalmic lenses may be made in flat or curved forms and from glass (inorganic or mineral) material or plastics (organic) material. Should a given prescription be dispensed in flat or curved form and should the lenses be made in a plastics material, with its inherent safety and lightness, or are there positive advantages to be gained by using one of the many types of ophthalmic glass? This chapter considers these fundamental questions.

Spectacle lenses are numbered in terms of back vertex power, which, when the thickness of a lens is ignored, is the same as the sum of its two surface powers. Thus, if the front surface power of a lens is +9.00D and the back surface power is –5.00D, then the total power of the lens is +4.00D. In theory, we could make a +4.00D lens in any of the forms shown in Figure 2.1a. The first two forms in the figure each have a pair of convex surfaces and are known as *flat-form* lenses. The third form, which has one plane surface, is also a flat-form lens and is known as a *plano-convex* lens form. The remaining forms in the figure each have one convex surface and one concave surface and are known as *curved* or *meniscus* lenses.

Figure 2.1b illustrates various forms in which a –4.00D lens might be made. Once more, the first three forms are flat-form designs and the remainder are of curved form. The lower numerical surface power of a curved lens is known as the *base curve* and the designs furthest right in Figures 2.1a and 2.1b are described as *5.00D base meniscus* lens forms.

When a spectacle lens is mounted in front of the eye in such a position that the optical axis of the lens coincides with the visual axis, the form of the lens does not matter. The eye is then viewing through the optical centre of the lens and the image formed by the lens is not afflicted with any defects or aberrations that might affect its sharpness or its shape. Figure 3.15 in Chapter 3 summarizes the correct centration of a spectacle lens for either distance or near vision. For distance vision, in the absence of any prescribed prism, the optical centres lie on a line that passes through the centre of the pupil, and in the vertical meridian the height has been adjusted to take into account the pantoscopic angle of the frame. Although the lens in Figure 3.15 has been centred correctly for one direction of gaze, in practice the eye turns behind the lens to view through off-axis visual points. It is under these circumstances that the form in which a lens is made assumes importance. Ideally, the off-axis performance of the lens should be the same as the optical performance of the lens at the optical centre. In general, the off-axis performance of the lens is not the same as its performance along the optical axis, the off-axis images being afflicted with various aberrations that spoil the quality of the images formed by the lens.[1]

The aberrations of significance to the spectacle wearer are:

- transverse chromatic aberration (TCA)
- oblique astigmatism
- curvature of field
- distortion.

The effect of these aberrations on image quality is best understood by viewing the targets shown in Figures 2.2 and 2.7 through a strong plus lens, such as a trial lens in the range +12.00 to +16.00D, made in plano-convex form. The appearance of the figures viewed through the lens is described below and demonstrates well the effects of the individual aberrations that might be reported by spectacle wearers.

Transverse chromatic aberration

Although transverse chromatic aberration (TCA) is caused by the material of the lens, it is convenient to deal with it here. The effect of TCA is to cause coloured fringes to be seen surrounding the image of a high-contrast target.

For example, when Figure 2.2 is viewed through a strong plus lens held close to the eye and the figure is focused by bringing the page slowly towards the lens with the centre of the target central in the lens aperture, coloured fringes are seen around the circular lines.

The order of colours and their positions should be noted. When light from a small white object is refracted by a prism, the light is dispersed into its monochromatic constituents, the blue wavelengths being deviated more than the red. To an eye that views through the prism the image of the object appears fringed with blue on the apex side of the prism. If the vertical line that forms the 90 meridian of the target in Figure 2.2 passes through the optical centre of the lens, no fringes are seen on either side of the vertical line. However, a yellow–red fringe can be seen on the outer edge of the circular lines and a blue–cyan one on the inner edge of the circular lines. Clearly, it is the white paper between the lines that acts as the source. The dispersion increases the further the rings are from the optical centre, and the fringes are most easily seen on the outermost ring.

Under conditions of low contrast, colour fringes may not be noticed. Instead, the effect of TCA is to cause a reduction in visual acuity. This effect is usually referred to as off-axis blur, and often gives rise to the complaint 'the lenses are fine when I look through the centres, but are blurred when I look through the edge'.

TCA results from the dispersive power of the lens, that is, the fact that the refractive index of the lens material varies with the wavelength of the incident light. It is usual to express the dispersive power by its reciprocal, the *constringence* of the material, denoted by the *V-value* or *Abbe number* for the material.

To a good approximation the magnitude of the TCA at any given point on a lens can be found by calculating the prismatic effect, P, at that point and dividing by the Abbe number of the material, that is, $TCA = P/V$. It is generally considered that the average

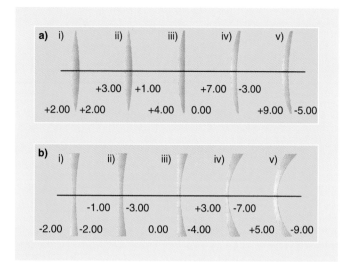

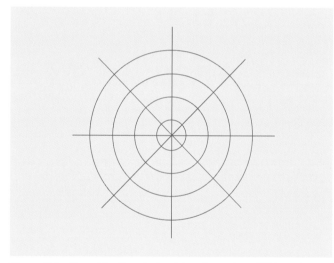

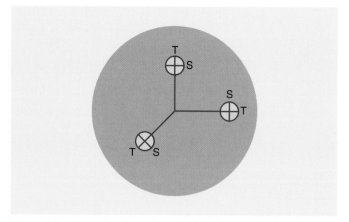

Figure 2.3   Tangential (T) and sagittal (S) planes of refraction

Figure 2.1   (a) Some forms in which a +4.00D lens might be made: (i) equi-convex; (ii) biconvex; (iii) plano-convex; (iv) –3.00D base meniscus; (v) –5.00D base meniscus. (b) Various forms in which a –4.00D lens might be made: (i) equi-concave; (ii) biconcave; (iii) plano-concave; (iv) +3.00D base meniscus; (v) +5.00D base meniscus

Figure 2.2   Target for the study of the aberrations, TCA, astigmatism and curvature

Oblique astigmatism

When a narrow pencil of rays is refracted obliquely by a spherical surface the refracted pencil becomes astigmatic. Instead of the rays re-uniting in a single image point, they form two separated line foci at right angles to one another with a disc of least confusion, where the refracted pencil has its least cross-sectional area somewhere between the two foci. The plane that contains the incident ray and the optical axis of the surface is referred to as the tangential plane and the plane at right angles to the tangential plane is referred to as the sagittal plane.

Figure 2.3 illustrates the tangential and sagittal meridians for three narrow pencils of rays incident at different points on the surface. The focal lines formed by the refracted pencil are at right angles to the meridian of corresponding power.

As a rule, the tangential power of a lens worn close to the eye, for a given oblique pencil, is in excess of the sagittal power and both are generally greater than the paraxial power. The effect of oblique astigmatism is to produce a blurring of the image as though an unwanted sphero-cylinder had been interposed between the lens and the eye.

Figure 2.4 shows the passage of a narrow pencil of oblique rays through a plus lens mounted before the eye. The refracted pencil is afflicted with aberrational astigmatism and the tangential focus, T′, lies closer to the lens than the sagittal focus, S′. Ideally, the lens should produce a point image of a distant point object on the eye's far point sphere. The terminology used for off-axis imagery is summarized in the caption to Figure 2.4. The vertex sphere is an imaginary reference surface concentric with the eye's centre of rotation from which the positions of the tangential and sagittal foci are measured. The far-point sphere is the imaginary surface, also concentric with the eye's centre of rotation, upon which we can assume the far point to remain as the eye rotates to view through off-axis zones of the lens. The distance between the vertex sphere and the far-point sphere measured through the eye's centre of rotation, Z, is constant and equal to the back vertex focal length of the lens, $A_2F′$.

A good idea of the effect of oblique astigmatism upon the eye can be obtained by studying the target depicted in Figure 2.2 through a strong plus lens. Lines in a radial direction correspond to tangential meridians and so are seen clearly when sagittal fans of rays are in focus on the retina. Similarly, the concentric circles form the sagittal meridians of the target and are seen clearly when tangential fans of rays are in focus.

Again, the target should be held well beyond the focusing distance and brought slowly towards the lens, which itself should

threshold value for TCA is 0.1Δ. TCA less than 0.1Δ is unlikely to give rise to complaints. The Abbe number for materials with a refractive index in the region of 1.5 (e.g. crown glass and CR39), is about 60 and the prismatic effect at the visual point needs to be about 6Δ before the typical threshold is reached. Using paraxial theory, this amount of prism would be encountered, for example, at a point 15mm from the optical centre of a +4.00D lens.

Materials with Abbe numbers in the region of 40 give rise to 0.1Δ of TCA at a point where the prismatic effect is 4Δ, that is 10mm away from the optical centre of a +4.00D lens. It is for this reason that it is wise to select a material with the highest possible Abbe number.

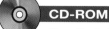
CD-ROM

The effect of dispersion in prisms and lenses is demonstrated on the CD-ROM

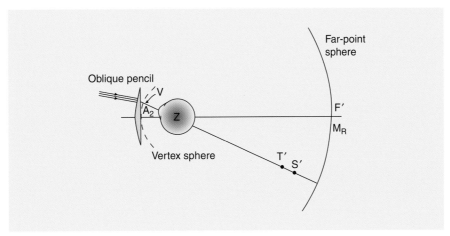

Figure 2.4 Terms used for discussing off-axis performance of spectacle lenses. Shown is a plano-convex lens, used for distance vision to correct a hypermetropic eye, that exhibits oblique astigmatism under these conditions. In the case of myopia, the far-point sphere and tangential and sagittal foci would lie in front of the lens. The following terms and expressions apply equally to plus and minus lenses:

A_2 is the back vertex of the lens
Z is the eye's centre of rotation
F' is the second principal focus of the lens
M_R is the eye's far point
T' is the tangential focus of the refracted pencil
S' is the sagittal focus of the refracted pencil
ZA_2 is the radius of the vertex sphere
ZM_R is the radius of the far-point sphere
V is the intersection of the principal ray of the refracted pencil with the vertex sphere
Back vertex power of lens, $F'_v = 1/A_2F'$
Tangential oblique vertex sphere power, $F'_T = 1/VT'$
Sagittal oblique vertex sphere power, $F'_S = 1/VS'$
Oblique astigmatic error (OAE) $= F'_T - F'_S$
Mean oblique power $= (F'_T + F'_S)/2$
Mean oblique error (MOE) $=$ Mean oblique power $- F'_v$

be held close to the eye. The first area of the target to come into focus is the central zone. This indicates that the power of the lens is weakest in the paraxial region. As the target is brought closer still to the eye, so each successive zone comes into and goes out of focus, which shows that the power of the lens increases gradually and continuously towards the periphery.

Also, for any given zone, the radial line in the neighbourhood of that zone comes into focus before the concentric circle, confirming that the tangential power is in excess of the sagittal power for the zone.

If the target is observed through a plano-convex lens, the difference in the clarity of the lines at each position is much greater (i.e. the astigmatism is much greater) when the curved surface of the lens is placed next to the eye, than when the plane surface is next to the eye.

The reduction of oblique astigmatism is very important in the design of spectacle lenses, and it may be achieved (see later) by a suitable choice of lens bending or by the use of an aspherical surface.

Curvature of field

Figure 2.2 can also be used to detect the presence of any curvature of field. In the above demonstration of the effects of oblique astigmatism, note that when the central zone of the target is in focus, the outer zones are not.

If the central zone is now brought into focus and attention turned to the horizontal radial line (along the 180 meridian of the target), the circular rings become progressively out of focus as the eye rotates away from the centre of the target.

If the page is now flexed, so that it presents a vertical concave cylindrical face to the eye (by bending the horizontal edges of the page towards the eye), all the rings along the 180 line are in focus at the same time. The curvature of the object field is being made to match, mechanically, the desired curvature for the image plane. As a rule, when the aberration oblique astigmatism is corrected, the effects of curvature of field are also reduced.

Field diagrams

A most useful guide to the effects of oblique astigmatism and curvature of field in a given spectacle lens is obtained by studying a field diagram for the lens form. A field diagram (Figure 2.5) is a plot of the tangential and sagittal oblique vertex sphere powers against the ocular rotation of the eye viewing through the lens. In the case of a perfect lens, such as the +4.00D design for which the ideal field diagram is illustrated in Figure 2.5a, the tangential and sagittal oblique vertex sphere powers remain +4.00D for all zones of the lens. Unfortunately, this performance is impossible to obtain in a single lens with just two surfaces, at least for this power.

The performance of the plano-convex +4.00D design, shown in Figure 2.4, is illustrated in Figure 2.5b. When the eye views along the optical axis of the lens the power of the lens is, indeed, +4.00D. When the eye rotates through 30° from the optical axis, however, the real effect of the lens is +4.25D in the sagittal meridian and +5.25D in the tangential meridian. We can express this effect as being equivalent to a power +4.25D sphere with a +1.00D cylinder. This is so different from the paraxial power that it cannot be ignored. Clearly, the choice of a plano-convex design for a lens of power +4.00D is a poor one.

In general, the surface powers chosen for any given lens are those that make the power obtained during oblique gaze as close as possible to the power obtained when the eye looks along the optical axis of the lens. Although we cannot make a +4.00D lens for which the power remains the same for all directions of gaze, we can certainly improve upon the performance given in Figure 2.5b (see later).

CD-ROM

The significance of field diagrams is considered in more detail on the CD-ROM

Distortion

The aberration distortion affects the shape of the image rather than its sharpness, and also occurs because the power of a spherical surface increases towards the periphery. Instead of remaining constant, the magnification increases more and more as the eye uses wider and wider zones of a spherical lens. Airy[2] showed at the beginning of the nineteenth century that distortion could be eliminated only by correcting spherical aberration between the entrance and exit pupils of a system, thereby satisfying his celebrated Tangent Condition.

Figure 2.6 shows the effects of distortion on a square grid target such as graph paper (Figure 2.6a) viewed through plus and minus lenses. Plus lenses produce *pincushion* distortion (Figure 2.6b), a type of distortion typically seen when a strong plus lens is used as a magnifier. Note that, in addition to obtaining the characteristic image in the shape of a pincushion, the impression is also obtained that the object being viewed is concave, the centre of the object being further from the eye than the edges.

Minus lenses produce *barrel* distortion (Figure 2.6c), which is often reported by myopes who view through peripheral zones of their lenses. Note the convex appearance of the target afflicted with barrel distortion; the centre of the target appears to be closer than the edges.

That distortion is very sensitive to lens form is immediately seen with a strong plano-convex lens. If the undistorted square grid object of Figure 2.6a is viewed with the lens held close to the eye, and with the plane surface nearer the eye, the amount of distortion is much less than when the lens is held with the curved surface closer to the eye. It can also be confirmed that when the plano-convex lens is used as a hand-held magnifier, close to the object being viewed, but now at some distance from the eye, the distortion is much less when the curved surface faces the eye than when the plane surface faces the eye. Clearly, the lens is now reversed from its usual position in front of the eye. When the form of a lens is changed, the amount of distortion that is exhibited by the lens also changes, which may be the chief cause of the perceptual problems that occur when a subject is given new lenses of different form. The sources of these effects are discussed later.

Best-form spectacle lenses

A *best-form* spectacle lens is one for which the surface powers have been specially computed to eliminate, or at least minimize, certain stated defects in its image-forming properties.

As already pointed out, transverse chromatism is a function of the Abbe number of the lens material and is minimized for a given power by selecting a material with the highest available Abbe number. Any further improvement in chromatism can only be made by constructing an achromatic doublet, that is, a pair of lenses bonded together, and in which the chromatism of one component is designed to neutralize the chromatism of the second. Such devices are too bulky to be considered seriously as spectacle lenses. For most people, the brain readily adapts to distortion and usually this aberration is an ongoing problem only for cases in which there has been a significant change in lens form or a significant change in prescription.

The aberrations that remain over which the designer can exert some influence are oblique astigmatism and curvature of field. The control that the designer can exercise over these two aberrations is illustrated in Figure 2.7, which shows how the off-axis

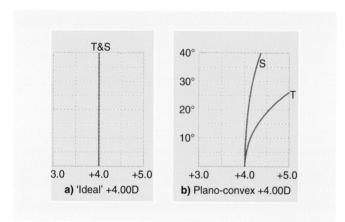

Figure 2.5 Field diagrams for spectacle lenses. (a) Field diagram for an ideal +4.00D lens. (b) Field diagram for +4.00D lens made in plano-convex form

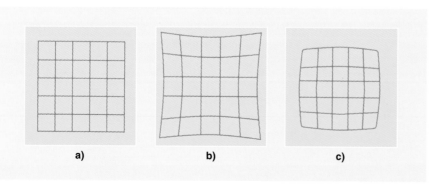

Figure 2.6 Distortion in spherical spectacle lenses. (a) Target for the study of distortion; (b) pincushion distortion; (c) barrel distortion

performance of +4.00D lenses varies for three meniscus forms with base curves –6.00D, –4.50D and –4.00D.

In Figure 2.7a, the lens has been bent into a form in which the oblique astigmatism has been eliminated entirely. Such a form is described as a *point-focal lens form*, from the German word *Punktal*, which means point-forming, and is, of course, the name still used by Carl Zeiss to describe their classic series of point-focal lenses.

At 35°, the power of the lens drops to +3.75D, that is, when the astigmatism is fully corrected, the mean oblique power of the lens changes by –0.25D. We say that the lens has a *mean oblique error at 35°* of –0.25D.

If the form of the lens is flattened from the point-focal bending, the tangential power increases and for the –4.50 bending depicted in Figure 2.7b, it is now the same as the back vertex power of the lens. Such a form is described as a *minimum tangential error* form and is seen to suffer from an ever-increasing amount of aberrational astigmatism, albeit small, as the eye rotates away from the optical axis. The oblique astigmatic error amounts to about +0.25D at 35° and the blurring effect of this small cylinder is certain to be less than the 0.25 sphere blur found in the point-focal form depicted in Figure 2.7a.

In Figure 2.7c the bending of the lens is reduced still further to a –4.00D base curve, and it can be seen in the field diagram that the tangential and sagittal oblique vertex sphere powers increase to just the point where the focal lines within the eye lie either side of, and equidistant from, the retina. At 35° the off-axis power of the lens is +3.85DS/+0.30DC, the tangential power is +0.15D too great and the sagittal power 0.15D too weak compared with the paraxial power. The mean oblique power of the lens is +4.00D. This form of lens is known as a *Percival lens* design and is free from mean oblique error for the zone in question.

Figure 2.8 illustrates field diagrams for –4.00D lenses made in point-focal form (+5.00D base curve), minimum tangential error form (+3.87D base curve) and Percival form (+3.25D base curve).

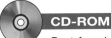

CD-ROM

Best-form lenses are considered in more detail on the CD-ROM

Tscherning's ellipses

Modern spectacle lens design is undertaken with the aid of a computer that can perform high-speed, exact trigonometric ray tracing through a lens and produce field diagrams, such as those depicted in Figures 2.7 and 2.8, in a matter of seconds, rather than days, as was the case when ray traces were performed by hand. In an attempt to speed up lens design in the days before the computer, it was customary to derive approximate equations for best-form lenses using so-called third-order theory, in which the trigonometric functions of the angles were replaced by a power series that gave reasonable results for angles up to about 15°. Such methods were applied to spectacle lens design during the nineteenth century, notably by Airy (1827)[2] and Tscherning (1904)[3]. Tscherning, in particular, pointed out that the relationship between the form and power of a spectacle lens, according to third-order calculations, was quadratic in nature. Whitwell[4] later showed that if the solutions to Tscherning's equations were plotted graphically they would form an ellipse, known

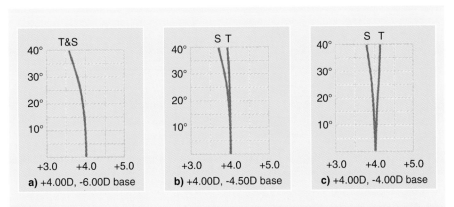

Figure 2.7　Field diagrams illustrating off-axis performance of +4.00D best-form lenses. (a) Point-focal lens, –6.00D base; (b) minimum tangential error form, –4.50D base; (c) Percival lens form, –4.00D base

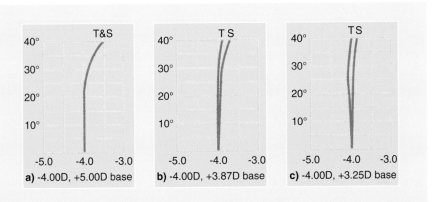

Figure 2.8　Field diagrams illustrating off-axis performance of –4.00D best-form lenses. (a) Point-focal lens, +5.00D base; (b) minimum tangential error form, +3.87D base; (c) Percival lens form, +3.25D base

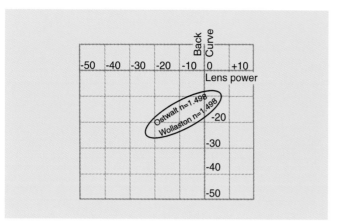

Figure 2.9   Tscherning's Ellipse for distance vision point-focal lenses. Constructed for $n = 1.498$, centre of rotation distance (CRD) = 27mm

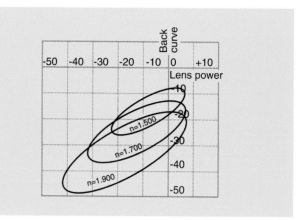

Figure 2.10   Tscherning's Ellipses for distance vision point-focal lenses. Constructed for $n = 1.50$, 1.70 and 1.90, CRD = 27mm

now as *Tscherning's Ellipse*. Such ellipses can be constructed for point-focal, Percival or minimum tangential error forms, and for both distance or near vision designs.

Figure 2.9 illustrates Tscherning's Ellipse constructed for point-focal forms, used for distance vision. The lenses are made from CR39 material of refractive index 1.498 and mounted 27mm in front of the eye's centres of rotation.

The ellipse shows very neatly that lenses can be made free from astigmatism only over a certain range of powers (+7.25D to –22.25D in the case of the ellipse illustrated in Figure 2.9), and that within this range there are two forms for each power. The shallower form, and the form usually supplied in practice, is known as the Ostwalt point-focal form, and the steeper form as the Wollaston point-focal form.

Lens powers outside the range depicted in Figure 2.9 cannot be made free from oblique astigmatism when restricted to the use of spherical surfaces. Later it is shown that powers outside the range of the ellipse can be made in point-focal form by the use of an aspherical surface that can be designed to neutralize the astigmatism of oblique incidence.

When Tscherning's Ellipses are constructed for media of higher refractive index, hardly any change in the upper limit is found for the plus range of powers, but the lower limit for minus lenses does increase, as shown in Figure 2.10, which compares ellipses constructed for materials of refractive index 1.50, 1.70 and 1.90.

It can also be seen from Figure 2.10 that, as a general rule, when the refractive index increases, the bending of the lens also needs to increase to eliminate astigmatism.

When the third-order results given by Tscherning's Ellipses are compared with those obtained by accurate trigonometric ray trac-ing, the third-order results are found to be somewhat too steep. The tendencies, however, which are so graphically depicted by the ellipses, are the same as those for lens forms determined by more accurate means. Generally, two forms of lens within a certain range of powers can be corrected for oblique astigmatism.

Dispensing problems that result from lens form

As a general rule, it is wise to dispense lenses in best-form cur-vatures, for then not only are off-axis errors minimized, but also different series do not differ much in form from one another and the distortion is about the same for a given power.

It is well-known that myopes, in particular, who become accus-tomed to a particular lens form are often dissatisfied when their lens form is changed and usually the only solution to their prob-lem is to provide a new pair of lenses in a similar form to their previous pair. Typically, a myope may have become accustomed to wearing flat-form lenses, and although, in theory, curved-form lenses provide better off-axis performance, many do not tolerate a change from their flat-form design. An idea of the difference in performance between flat-form and curved-form lenses can be obtained by comparing the differences in off-axis performance of the following pairs of lenses (Table 2.1).

Considering first the –4.00D lens forms, it can be seen that in the case of the +5.00D base form, as the eye rotates away from the optical axis of the lens, the off-axis power decreases as the mean oblique error becomes positive. The eye is undercorrected in oblique gaze and accommodation only worsens the situation.

For the plano-concave form, on the other hand, the off-axis power increases, the mean oblique error being negative and the eye is over-corrected in oblique gaze. If the eye accommodates, however, it can sharpen the image, especially if the eye views an object with principal features at right angles to the axis of the oblique astigmatism.

Also, the distortion, which is of the barrel variety, increases at a faster rate for the flat-form lens, and it is virtually double that of the best-form design.

Similar conclusions can be drawn from the data given for the –10.00D lens forms, but it is clear that, numerically, the changes are less dramatic than for the weaker power lens. Of course, this is because the change in form is less dramatic for the –10.00D lens. Nevertheless, the off-axis power becomes positive for the curved-form lens, whereas it becomes negative for the plano-concave form as the eye rotates away from the optical axis of the lenses.

The chief cause of the perceptual problems that these differ-ences in off-axis performance produce is not well-understood. An obvious explanation is the large difference in off-axis pow-ers of the two lens forms illustrated in Table 2.1. However, the symptoms usually described by subjects imply a change in retinal image shape. Certainly, they suffer a large change in distortion as evidenced by the values given in Table 2.1, and it could be that it is really the change in distortion that is the underlying source of complaint. In the absence of any history of problems associated with a change in lens form, when a subject is happily wearing an unexpected lens form, such as a –4.00D lens in plano-concave form, it is sensible, in the absence of any symptoms, not to change the form from that to which the subject has become accustomed.

Table 2.1   Comparison of optical performance of −4.00D and −10.00D lenses made in different forms

	−4.00D lens +5.00D base form			−4.00D lens plano-concave form		
	OAE	MOE	Distortion (%)	OAE	MOE	Distortion (%)
10°	0.00	+0.01	0.3	−0.08	−0.06	0.4
20°	+0.01	+0.02	1.4	−0.32	−0.24	2.3
30°	−0.01	+0.15	3.7	−0.77	−0.56	6.2
40°	−0.10	+0.36	7.8	−1.46	−1.01	14.4
	−10.00D lens +2.00D base form			−10.00D lens plano-concave form		
	OAE	MOE	Distortion (%)	OAE	MOE	Distortion (%)
10°	−0.01	+0.02	0.9	−0.07	−0.04	1.1
20°	−0.03	+0.09	4.3	−0.28	−0.15	5.0
30°	+0.01	+0.28	11.3	−0.61	−0.32	13.5
40°	+0.23	+0.70	25.2	−1.03	−0.51	32.2

Table 2.2   Form of higher-index lenses

Lens power (D)	Original front curve (1.498/1.523)	Required front curves when new refractive index is			
		1.600	1.700	1.800	1.900
−4.00	plano	+0.25	+0.50	+0.75	+1.00
−6.00	plano	+0.25	+0.75	+1.25	+1.62
−8.00	plano	+0.37	+0.87	+1.50	+2.00
−10.00	plano	+0.37	+1.00	+1.75	+2.25
−12.00	plano	+0.37	+1.00	+1.75	+2.50

Changes in form for materials of higher refractive index

Inspection of Figure 2.10 confirms that when the refractive index of the lens material changes, the lens form does need to change to provide the same off-axis powers. Table 2.2 indicates the form required for various lens powers that have approximately the same off-axis performance as plano-concave forms made in spectacle crown glass or CR39 material. Needless to say, the transverse chromatism exhibited by the lens is dependent upon the Abbe number of the material and only matches if the Abbe number of the new material matches that of crown glass or CR39.

Toric lens forms

Astigmatic lenses are normally supplied in curved form for the same reason as spherical lenses, to improve the off-axis performance of the lens. A *toroidal* surface can be imagined to be a cylindrical surface with an axis meridian that is also curved, and a *toric* lens is simply a curved lens with one toroidal surface (Figure 2.11). Three different types of toroidal surface are used in ophthalmic lens manufacture:

- the *tyre-formation* surface (Figure 2.11a), which lends itself well to mass-production techniques
- the *barrel-formation* surface (Figure 2.11b), which is better suited to individual surface working
- the rarer *capstan-formation* surface (Figure 2.11c).

The lower numerical curve on the toroidal surface is called the *base curve* and the steeper curve the *cross curve*. For example, the prescription +4.00/+2.00 × 90 could be supplied in either of the forms given below:

front curve + 8.00 × 180/+ 10.00 × 90, back curve − 4.00

or,

front curve + 9.00, back curve − 3.00 × 90/− 5.00 × 180

The first of these two forms is described as a +8.00 base toric lens and the second as a −3.00 base toric lens.

Stock glass single-vision uncut lenses are usually made in plus-base toric form employing a tyre-formation surface, since they are easier to mass-produce in this form. Stock plastics single-vision uncut lenses are usually made in minus-base toric form. Singly worked toric lenses could be surfaced in plus-base form, but today, in general, the preferred method of working by the surfacing workshop is to use a minus-base toric form. This method of working has several advantages from the workshop's point of view. Single-vision lenses can be processed using the same tools as those required for bifocal lenses in which the segment or progressive surface is on the front of the blank. Also, the cylinder power of the tool is the same as the cylinder power required for the lens. The cross curve does not need any compensation for the thickness of the lens, as it would for a plus-base toric design. Finally, if the blank manufacturer provides a reasonable compensation for lens thickness appropriate to the curve under consideration, the minus-base toric form permits the fewest number of surfacing tools to be maintained by the workshop.

From an optical point of view, plus-base toric lenses give slightly better performance for plus prescriptions and low-power minus prescriptions, whereas, in moderate and high myopia, the optical performance is better when the cylinder is incorporated

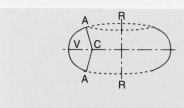

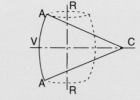

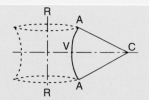

The axis of rotation RR and the vertex V of the generating arc AA are on the opposite sides of the latter's centre of curvature C.

a) Tyre formation

The axis of rotation RR lies between the vertex V of the generating arc AA and its centre of curvature C.

b) Barrel formation

The axis of rotation RR and the centre of curvature C of the generating arc AA are on opposite sides of the vertex V.

c) Capstan formation

Figure 2.11   Toroidal surfaces. Tyre, barrel and capstan formation surfaces

on the back surface, the lenses being supplied as minus-base toric designs. Ideally, the toroidal surface should be of barrel form, which is possible with singly worked lenses if toroidal tools are maintained by the surfacing house in barrel form. Minus-base toric construction also improves the appearance of the lens, since the variation in edge thickness that occurs along different power meridians can be hidden on the back of the lens. For very deep minus lenses it is easier for the manufacturer to incorporate the cylinder on the front surface of the lens in the form of a plano-convex cylindrical surface.

CD-ROM

Toric forms are considered in more detail on the CD-ROM

Lens materials

To make an informed assessment of a spectacle lens material several items of data need to be known about the material. Four of these are physical data provided by the material manufacturer and have a direct bearing on the performance of the material:

- refractive index
- density
- Abbe number (constringence or V-value)
- durability.

The remaining two concern availability and may be supplied by the blank manufacturer (or the lens supplier):

- availability of curves
- efficacy of surface treatments.

Table 2.3 gives a typical selection of lens materials and lists various physical properties pertinent to the choice of material. The significance of the physical data is discussed below.

Refractive index

Refractive index expresses the ratio of the velocity of light of a given wavelength in air to the velocity of light of the same wavelength in the refracting medium.

At present, in the UK and the USA, refractive index is measured on the helium d-line (wavelength 587.56nm) whereas in Continental Europe it is measured on the mercury e-line (wavelength 546.07nm). Both indices, n_d and n_e, are given in Table 2.3 to facilitate identification of the material. Note that the value for n_e is a little greater than that for n_d, so that when the value of

n_e is given the material appears to have a slightly higher refractive index. Curve variation factor (CVF), Abbe number and the reflectance, ρ, are quoted for n_d.

BS 7394 Part 2: *Specification for prescription spectacles*[5] classifies materials in terms of refractive index as follows:

- Normal index, $n \geq 1.48$ but < 1.54
- Mid index $n \geq 1.54$ but < 1.64
- High index $n \geq 1.64$ but < 1.74
- Very high index $n \geq 1.74$.

The curvature required to produce a given surface power is inversely proportional to the refractive index of the lens material. As the refractive index increases, the curvature decreases and so the sag of the surface for a given diameter also decreases. Hence, the higher the refractive index of the material, the thinner is the lens. Table 2.4 shows how the weight and edge thicknesses of a series of minus lenses varies at various diameters and it can be seen that, as a general rule, the higher the index the thinner the lens.

Study of the information given in Table 2.4 reveals some interesting facts about the variation in thickness and weight of finished spectacle lenses and provides several useful pointers to successful dispensing.

Consider spectacle crown glass (1.523/2.54), tabulated in the second row of Table 2.4, when the lens diameter is increased from 40 to 50mm the edge thickness increases by 40% and the weight of the lens doubles. Increasing the diameter again from 50mm to 60mm causes the edge thickness to increase by another 40% and, once again, the weight of the lens doubles. Compared with a lens diameter of 40mm, at 60mm diameter the edge thickness has virtually doubled and the weight has increased four times. Although the table considers only lenses of power −5.00D, these tendencies are true for all lens powers.

Refractive index is useful to inform of the likely change in thickness that will be obtained when the material is compared with a standard ordinary crown glass. The information is usually quoted in terms of the CVF, since this enables a direct comparison in thickness to be made. For example, a 1.700 index material has a CVF (see Table 2.1) of 0.75, which informs us that the reduction in thickness will be about 25% if this material is substituted for crown glass. One of the most practical uses for the CVF is to convert the power of the lens that is to be made into its crown glass equivalent. This is done simply by multiplying the power of the lens by the CVF for the material. For example, suppose it is necessary to dispense a −10.00D lens in 1.700 index material, the crown glass equivalent is 0.75 × −10 or −7.50. In other words, the use of a 1.700 index material results in a lens that has a power of −10.00D, but in all other respects looks like

Table 2.3 Physical data for typical lens materials

Medium	n_d	n_e	CVF	Density	Abbe number	ρ (%)
Glasses						
White crown	1.523	1.525	1.0	2.5	59	4.3
Light flint	1.600	1.604	0.87	2.6	42	5.3
1.7 glasses	1.700	1.705	0.75	3.2	35	6.7
	1.701	1.706	0.75	3.2	42	6.7
1.8 glasses	1.802	1.807	0.65	3.7	35	8.2
	1.830	1.838	0.63	3.6	32	8.6
1.9 glasses	1.885	1.893	0.59	4.0	31	9.4
Plastics						
PMMA	1.490	1.492	1.07	1.2	58	3.9
CR39	1.498	1.500	1.05	1.3	58	4.0
Trivex™ PPG	1.532	1.534	0.98	1.1	46	4.4
Sola Spectralite	1.537	1.540	0.97	1.2	47	4.5
PPG HIP	1.560	1.563	0.93	1.2	38	4.8
AO Alphalite 16XT	1.582	1.585	0.9	1.3	34	5.1
Polycarbonate	1.586	1.589	0.89	1.2	30	5.2
Hoya Eyas 1.6	1.600	1.603	0.87	1.3	42	5.3
Polyurethanes	1.600	1.603	0.87	1.3	36	5.3
	1.609	1.612	0.86	1.4	32	5.4
	1.660	1.664	0.79	1.4	32	6.2
	1.670	1.674	0.78	1.4	32	6.3
Hoya Teslalid	1.710	1.715	0.74	1.4	36	6.9
Nikon	1.740	1.745	0.71	1.4	32	7.3

The CVF is quoted in comparison with crown glass to enable lens thickness to be estimated by means of the sag factors given in Chapters 8 and 9.
The reflectance shown assumes that the surface is uncoated. In practice, many higher index lenses are automatically supplied with a multilayer anti-reflection coating.

Table 2.4 Comparison of edge thickness (et) and weight (wt) of −5.00D lenses at various diameters (ct, centre thickness)

n_d/D	ct	Diameter 40		Diameter 50		Diameter 60		Diameter 70	
		et	wt (g)	et	wt (g)	et	wt (g)	et	wt (g)
1.498/1.32*	2.0	4.1	5.1	5.4	9.5	7.2	16.7	9.5	27.8
1.523/2.54	1.0	3.0	6.4	4.2	12.9	5.9	23.9	8.0	41.8
1.600/2.63	1.0	2.7	6.1	3.8	12.2	5.1	22.2	6.8	38.2
1.600/1.34*	1.0	2.7	3.1	3.8	6.2	5.1	11.3	6.8	19.6
1.660/1.35*	1.0	2.6	3.0	3.5	5.9	4.7	10.6	6.1	18.1
1.700/3.21	1.0	2.5	7.0	3.3	13.5	4.1	22.8	5.8	41.0
1.740/1.40*	1.0	2.3	2.9	3.1	5.6	3.9	9.9	4.8	16.2
1.802/3.65	1.0	2.3	7.5	3.0	14.3	3.9	25.3	5.1	42.1
1.885/4.00	1.0	2.2	7.9	2.8	14.9	3.6	26.1	4.7	43.0

*Plastics material.
Note the reduction in weight of plastics lenses compared with their glass counterparts.

a −7.50D lens made in crown glass. A 1.600 index material has a CVF of 0.87, so that we may expect a 13% reduction in thickness and a −10.00D lens made in this material would look like a −8.75D lens made in crown glass. CVF is simply the ratio of the refractivity of crown glass to that of the material, $0.523/(n_d - 1)$, and compares the actual curves obtained on crown glass and the material in question for a given curvature of the surface.

Density

The density quoted in Table 2.3 tells us how heavy the material is and a comparison of densities can indicate the likely change in weight to be expected by using the material.

The value given is the mass per unit volume of the material. Many years ago, glass manufacturers would publish the relative density (or specific gravity) of the material, which is the ratio of the density of the material to the density of water. However, in recent years, glass types are expected to be used in, and indeed

survive, a wide variety of operating conditions and temperatures. For this reason, and for the sake of accuracy, Pilkington's optical glass division decided to quote density in g/cm^3 rather than the unitless specific gravity of the material. At normal temperature and pressure the two quantities are almost the same, so it is very convenient to look upon the figure quoted for the density as the weight in grams of one cubic centimetre of the material.

Densities of materials with high refractive index may be compared with that of crown glass, which is about 2.5, but to compare the weights of lenses made in different materials it is also necessary to take any saving in volume into account. For example, if the density of a material is quoted as 3.0, it means that the material is 20% heavier than crown glass. As a guide, provided that the saving in volume obtained (the saving as indicated by the CVF) is greater than the increase in density, the final lens should be no heavier in the new material than if it had been made in crown glass.

A good working rule is that if the density of a material is less than $5-2.5 \times CVF$, then the finished lens will be no heavier if made in a material of high refractive index than it would be if made in crown glass.

Until 1970, the few glass lenses of high refractive index that were dispensed were made from dense barium crown glasses ($n = 1.63$, CVF = 0.8, density = 3.7), or from extra dense flint glasses ($n = 1.700$, CVF = 0.75, density = 4.3). The barium or lead content of these glasses made them notoriously heavy.

Using the rule given above, the density for a glass with a CVF of 0.8 needs to be less than 3.0, whereas the density for a glass with a CVF of 0.75 needs to be less than 3.12. Neither of these two glass types obeyed the above rule and the wearer always paid the penalty of heavier, albeit thinner, lenses.

In 1973 a revolutionary new light-weight, high-index glass was introduced by Schott (USA), in which they replaced the heavier elements with titanium oxide and enabled, for the first time, thinner high-index lenses to be produced without an increase in weight.

This glass, obtainable from many sources and known by several different brand names, has a refractive index of about 1.700 (CVF = 0.75) and a density in the region of 3.0.

Abbe number

The Abbe number (constringence or *V*-value) of a material indicates the optical properties of the material rather than its mechanical characteristics. Constringence is the reciprocal of the dispersive power of the material and indicates the degree of TCA that the wearer will experience. The values quoted in Table 2.3 are the Abbe numbers for the helium d-line, V_d:

$$V_d = (n_d - 1)/(n_F - n_C)$$

where:

- n_C is the refractive index of the material for the wavelength of hydrogen C (656.27nm)
- n_F is the refractive index of the material for the wavelength of hydrogen F (486.13nm).

The effects of chromatic aberration are described above, where it is pointed out that when the target illustrated in Figure 2.2 is viewed through a strong plus lens held close to the eye, the figure being focused by bringing the page slowly towards the lens, with the centre of the target central in the lens aperture, coloured fringes are seen around the circular lines. The order of colours and their positions is noted. When light from a small white object is refracted by a prism, the light is dispersed into its monochromatic constituents, the blue wavelengths being deviated more than the red (Figure 2.12). To an eye that views through the prism, the image of the object appears fringed with blue on the apex side of the prism. If the vertical line that forms the 90 meridian of the target in Figure 2.2 passes through the optical centre of the lens, no fringes are seen on either side of the vertical line. However, a yellow–red fringe can be seen on the outer edge of the circular lines and a blue–cyan one on the inner edge of the circular lines. Clearly, it is the paper between the lines that acts as the source. The dispersion increases as the rings move further from the optical centre, with fringing most easily seen on the outermost ring.

Under conditions of low contrast, colour fringing may not be noticed. Instead, the effect of TCA is to cause a reduction in visual acuity. This effect is usually referred to as off-axis blur and often gives rise to the complaint 'these lenses are fine when I view through the centres, but are blurred when I view through the edge'.

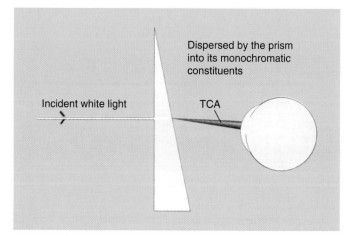

Figure 2.12   Dispersion by a prism

To a good approximation, the magnitude of the TCA at any given point on a lens can be found by calculating the prismatic effect, *P*, at that point and dividing by the Abbe number of the material,[1] that is, TCA = *P*/*V*. It is generally considered that the average threshold value for TCA is 0.1Δ. A TCA less than 0.1Δ is unlikely to give rise to complaints. The Abbe numbers for materials with a refractive index in the region of 1.5 (e.g. crown glass and CR39) are about 60 and the prismatic effect at the visual point would need to be about 6Δ before the typical threshold is reached. Using paraxial theory, this amount of prism would be encountered, for example, at a point 15mm from the optical centre of a +4.00D lens.

Materials for which the Abbe numbers are in the region of 40 give rise to 0.1Δ of TCA at a point where the prismatic effect is 4Δ, that is, 10mm away from the optical centre of a +4.00D lens. It is for this reason that it is wise to select a material with the highest possible Abbe number.

BS 7394: Part 2, *Specification for prescription spectacles*,[5] classifies materials in terms of their Abbe numbers as follows:

- Low dispersion, $V \geq 45$
- Medium dispersion, $V \geq 39$ but < 45
- High dispersion, $V < 39$.

Ordinary crown glass and plastics materials, such as CR39, have Abbe numbers in the region of 59. Experience has shown that these low dispersion materials almost never give rise to complaints of coloured fringes or off-axis blur.

Until the mid-1970s ophthalmic glasses with refractive indices in the region of 1.700 had Abbe numbers of about 30. These glasses exhibit twice as much chromatic aberration as crown glass lenses. The introduction in the early 1970s of the new glasses with high refractive index and low density caused an upsurge in the use of materials with high refractive index, especially for minus lenses where the benefit of thinner lenses was immediately apparent. Sadly, there were also many disappointed spectacle wearers who could not reconcile the poor off-axis performance with the improved appearance of their lenses. Glass manufacturers began to turn their attention to the problems of chromatic aberration, recognizing that it was important to produce glasses with as high an Abbe number as possible. Today, one would expect glasses of refractive index 1.700 to possess Abbe numbers of about 40.

Reflectance, ρ

Knowledge of the refractive index of a material also enables the reflectance of the lens surfaces to be calculated, that is, how much light is reflected away if the surface is not treated to either increase (by means of a vacuum deposited tint) or decrease (by means of an anti-reflection coating) the amount of reflected light. When light is incident normally on a lens surface in air, the percentage of light reflected at each surface is given by:[6]

$$\rho = (n-1)^2 / (n+1)^2 \times 100\%$$

Thus, a material of refractive index 1.5 has a reflectance of:

$$(0.5/2.5)^2 \times 100 = 4\% \text{ per surface}$$

The amount of light transmitted by a lens made in 1.5 index material can be deduced as follows. After a loss of 4% of the original light at the first surface, 96% of the original intensity arrives at the back surface. Here, a further 4% is lost by reflection, which amounts to a further 3.84% (0.04 × 96). So the light transmitted by the lens is 92.16%. (This value ignores further losses by multiple total internal reflections at the surfaces.)

A similar calculation for a lens material of refractive index 1.80 shows that the reflectance of each surface is 8.2% and the transmission of a lens that has negligible absorptance by the material itself would be 84.3%, over 15% of the light being lost by surface reflection. One purpose of an anti-reflection coating is to prevent this loss of light by reflection from the lens surfaces. It should be borne in mind that many modern lens series, notably the higher-index plastics lens series, are only available with multilayer, reflection-free coatings.

As a general guide, at 50mm diameter, 1.70 index glasses offer a thickness reduction of about 40% compared with CR39 lenses and 20% compared with normal crown glass lenses. Table 2.4 shows that these 1.70 index lenses are about the same weight as their crown glass counterparts. To obtain an even greater reduction in thickness, glasses with indices that exceed 1.80 are available. These glasses offer a thickness advantage of 45% over CR39 lenses and 30% over crown glass lenses. 1.90 index glasses offer a thickness advantage of almost 50% over CR39 lenses and 35% over crown glass lenses at 50mm diameter. These glasses of very high refractive index enable high-power lenses to be dispensed in larger eye sizes than would normally be considered possible and in some markets have proved to be highly acceptable to ametropes who previously were unable to choose large fashion frames.

The 1.80 and 1.90 index glasses possess quite remarkable densities and Abbe numbers for materials of such high refractive index (see Table 2.3). The highest refractive index material currently in use in Europe is the Corning 1.9 glass (n_d 1.885, Abbe number 30.5 and density 3.99), which is sure to be made available in several different lens series.

A further development in glass materials is the wide use of light flint glass of refractive index 1.60 for some specialist ranges of lenses, in particular glass low-power aspheric lens series from Zeiss and Rodenstock and 1.60 index photochromic glasses from Corning. It is shown in a later chapter that the combination of material of higher refractive index and aspheric technology leads to even thinner lens designs.

Plastics media of higher refractive index

Before 1970 the two principal plastics media for spectacle lenses were PMMA (*Igard* lenses from Combined Optical Industries Ltd) and CR39 (*Columbia Resin 39* – the monomer first produced by the Pittsburg Plate Glass Company of America, but now available from several sources).

The arrival of FDA safety legislation in the USA in 1972 brought about a great interest in the use of plastics lenses, which, naturally, are inherently safer in use than ordinary, untoughened glass lenses. The first alternative plastics material was polycarbonate, a plastics material capable of being injection moulded and vastly superior to CR39 in terms of impact resistance.

Polycarbonate has a refractive index of 1.586, but this does not necessarily mean that thinner lenses are obtained compared with CR39, since to ensure its superior qualities as a safety lens, the centre thickness of a polycarbonate lens must not fall below a minimum amount. With increasing use of this material, and in an attempt to take full advantage of its higher refractive index, some prescription laboratories are prepared to surface polycarbonate lenses to centre thicknesses as small as 1.0mm. At such a centre thickness it is absolutely essential not to overglaze these lenses to ensure that they do not flex in the mount.

For lenses of ordinary power, and with recommended thicknesses, polycarbonate provides safety and strength and there is no doubt that this material will be used increasingly in Europe. Already, polycarbonate lens series are available from several sources. The low Abbe number for the material suggests caution if its use is considered for medium- to high-power prescriptions. The processing of polycarbonate lenses differs somewhat from that for other plastics materials. In general, the front surface of the blank is produced by injection moulding techniques and dry machining processes are employed for satisfactory completion of the lens.

Pittsburg Plate Glass Industries, the original suppliers of CR39 monomer, have developed a mid refractive index plastics monomer (HIP), which has also been adopted by several lens manufacturers. The refractive index of this material is 1.56 and, unlike polycarbonate, it can be surfaced to provide a reasonable centre thickness comparable with CR39.

The newest material from Pittsburg Plate Glass Industries, generally known as Trivex™, was introduced to rival polycarbonate as a very safe, yet lightweight material for ophthalmic lenses. It is a normal index material, $n_d = 1.532$, with an Abbe number of about 46 and a density of just 1.1. It is claimed to be even stronger than polycarbonate, but more flexible to enhance even further its safety aspect. It offers 100% ultraviolet (UV) attenuation and is easily tinted by the usual surface-dyeing process. Minus lenses can be surfaced down to just 1.0mm centre thickness, without the lens losing its inherent safety features. Several lens manufacturers now produce lenses in Trivex™ material. For example, Younger Optics call its lenses *Trilogy*™ and Hoya calls its lenses *Phoenix*™ (*PNX*). Each company has modified the monomer to its own needs.

The Japanese chemical company, Toray Industries, has developed a 1.60 index HIP material that is employed by many major lens manufacturers both in Japan and in Europe for series of thin plastics lenses, some of which are aspheric in form. This material has excellent UVA absorption and, being more rigid than other plastics materials, it is possible to produce finished minus lenses with the same centre thickness as their glass counterparts.

Several manufacturers are offering lenses made in plastics materials with a high index refractive index of 1.66 or 1.67. The Mitsubishi Gas Chemical Corporation of Japan has developed a 1.71 refractive index plastics material with an Abbe number of 36, first utilized by Hoya in their Teslalid series of lenses. More recently, Nikon have introduced a 1.74, very high refractive index plastics material with an Abbe number of 32, which is being offered initially for their Nikon-Lite 5 HCC-AS aspheric lens series. The excellent mechanical qualities of these mid-to-high refractive index plastics materials can be deduced from the information on thickness and weight presented in Table 2.4.

Most of these lens series of high refractive index are produced with hard coatings that are hydrophobic and have superb broad-band anti-reflection properties.

Durability

An important requirement of any spectacle lens material is the ability to withstand either mechanical abuse or chemical attack. The durability of white ophthalmic crown is legendary. It is very hard and therefore difficult to scratch under ordinary circumstances. It is completely stable in normal atmospheric conditions and has excellent resistance to common chemical substances. Needless to say, it is not quite perfect as a spectacle lens material. It is brittle and, in common with all glass-like substances, when subjected to violent mechanical shock, ordinary untoughened crown glass easily fractures.

The rare earth content of glasses of high refractive index tends to make them less resistant to chemical attack, which may occur during the grinding and polishing operations, or under extreme atmospheric conditions. For this reason, glass lenses of high refractive index are normally dispensed with an anti-reflection coating that protects the surfaces from chemical attack as well as reducing surface reflections.

The ability of a glass to withstand chemical attack can be assessed reliably from an acid durability test. To quantify such chemical attack is extremely difficult and has been the subject of much international research.[6] A visually qualitative grading of durability has been developed based upon the exposure of polished samples to a constant pH reagent, namely 0.5N nitric acid. The nature and extent of surface corrosion is expressed by a code, the first digit of which indicates the exposure time before surface attack becomes apparent; the second indicates the severity of the attack and the third indicates the manner in which the surface is affected.[7] Glass catalogues include information on acid durability, but the major lens manufacturers also conduct their own tests on material and surface reaction to their individual processing regimes.

Plastics lenses emulate glass in their transparency and, being less brittle, are less likely to break. Furthermore, when plastics lenses do break, they are less dangerous than glass lenses since the fragments have relatively blunt edges. However, because they are less brittle, plastics lenses are generally softer when compared with glass and the lens surfaces are more prone to scratches. Modern hard coatings for plastics lenses greatly reduce the likelihood of surface damage, particularly in-mould hard coatings.

Tests for suitability of lens materials

An important new standard, BS EN ISO 14889:2003 Ophthalmic optics – Spectacle Lenses – Fundamental requirements for uncut finished lenses,[8] gives the following recommendations for lens materials.

Physiological compatibility

Lenses shall not be made from materials known to be physiologically incompatible or known to create allergic or toxic reactions amongst a significant proportion of wearers when the lenses are used as intended. In short, the lens material employed must not cause any irritation to the eyes or skin.

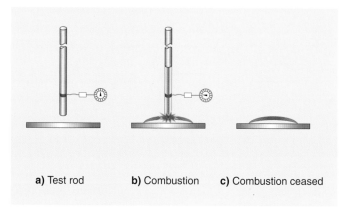

a) Test rod   **b)** Combustion   **c)** Combustion ceased

Figure 2.13   Test for inflammability of uncut lenses (BS EN ISO 14899:2003)

Inflammability

Lens material is tested for flammability using the method illustrated in Figure 2.13. A steel rod, 300mm in length and 6mm diameter, with a flat face and fitted with a thermocouple 20mm from the heated end of the rod, is heated over a length of 50mm to a temperature of 650°C and allowed to rest under its own weight on the surface of the test sample for a period of 5s. A visual inspection is then carried out to establish whether combustion continues after removal of the rod. The material is deemed to have passed the test if there is no continued combustion after withdrawal of the test rod.

Mechanical strength

Uncut spectacle lenses must be able to withstand the quasi-static loading type test illustrated in Figure 2.14.

The support system on which the lens is placed has a cylindrical cavity 1.5mm deep measured from its upper face into which is placed a disc of white paper with a disc of carbon paper on top. The support itself consists of a steel supporting plate and a pressure ring. The pressure ring weighs 250g and its purpose is to ensure that the silicone seating presses securely against the upper surface of the lens under test. The 3mm thick silicone support rings are attached to the lower face of the pressure ring and to the upper face of the support plate upon which the lens sits.

The loading mass, consisting of a steel ball of 22mm diameter fastened to the lower end of a tube, the length of which is 70mm, must be such that the force acting on the test specimen is 100N. The loading mass is lowered onto the lens at a speed not exceeding 400mm/min and a force of 100N is applied for 10s before being removed.

The test is carried out immediately after conditioning the lens at a temperature of 23°C and the test lens is deemed to have passed if there is no lens fracture or deformation as a result of the test.

The lens is considered to have fractured if it has cracked through its entire thickness into two or more pieces, or if more than 5mg of the lens material has become detached from the surface away from the surface in contact with the ball, or if the ball has passed right through the test specimen.

Deformation is considered to have taken place if a mark has appeared on the white paper beneath the lens.

This test for the mechanical strength of the lens material is intended for lenses for which no enhanced robustness is claimed. Chapter 14 gives details of the tests required for lenses which have increased robustness.

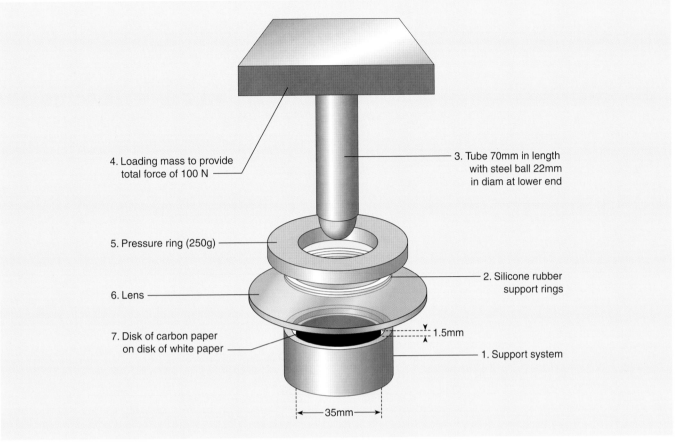

4. Loading mass to provide total force of 100 N

5. Pressure ring (250g)

6. Lens

7. Disk of carbon paper on disk of white paper

3. Tube 70mm in length with steel ball 22mm in diam at lower end

2. Silicone rubber support rings

1.5mm

1. Support system

35mm

Figure 2.14 Test for mechanical strength of uncut lenses (BS EN ISO 14899:2003)

Estimation of refractive index of lens material

With the plethora of available lens types, it is difficult in practice to identify precisely the material from which a given spectacle lens is made. It is fairly easy to establish if the material is glass or plastics and some lens series incorporate a trademark on the front surface, but it is possible with ordinary equipment to obtain an approximate value for the refractive index of the material by employing a focimeter to determine the back vertex power of the lens and a lens measure to obtain the thin-lens power from the sum of the surface powers. From thin-lens theory, the ratio of the thin-lens power to the true back-vertex power is the same value as the CVF for the material. For example, suppose the power of a finished lens is found by means of the focimeter to be −6.00D, but when a lens measure is applied to each surface the sum of the surface powers is found to be −4.50D. The ratio of the lens measure power to the back vertex power is 4.5/6 = 0.75. Inspection of Table 2.3 shows that a material with a refractive index of 1.700 has a CVF of 0.75 and the refractive index of the lens material must therefore lie in the region of 1.70.

In the absence of a table giving CVF, the refractive index, n_T, of the unknown material can be found from:

$$n_T = 1 + F_T (n_{LM} - 1)/F_{LM}$$

where F_T = the true power of lens given by a focimeter, F_{LM} = the sum of surface powers as given by lens measure and n_{LM} = the refractive index for which the lens measure has been scaled.

References and notes

1. Jalie M 1984 Principles of ophthalmic lenses. ABDO, London
2. Airy G B 1827 On a peculiar defect of the eye and a mode of correcting it. Trans Camb Phil Soc 2:267–271
3. Tscherning M 1904 Verres de lunettes. In: Lagrange F, Valude E (eds) Encyclopedie Française d'ophtalmologie, Vol 3. Octave Doin, Paris
4. Whitwell A 1913 On the best form of spectacle lenses. Ran in Optician from 1913 to 1926.
5. BS 7394: Part 2 Complete Spectacles. Specification for Prescription Spectacles. BSI, London, 1994
6. Reid A M, Parry R J, Blackburn J 1965 Jap J Appl Physiol 4(Suppl 1):330
7. Codes vary from **1.1.a** (best) to **7.5.c** (worst). Readers who would like a full explanation of the significance of the digits are referred to the article by Reid et al., reference 6.
8. BS EN ISO 14889:2003 Ophthalmic optics – Spectacle Lenses – Fundamental requirements for uncut finished lenses. BSI, London, 2003

Lens centration

Correct centration of spectacle lenses before the eyes is important for several reasons, all of which contribute towards the wearer obtaining the best and most comfortable visual performance from the lenses. Correct centration positions the zone of the lens where the paraxial prescription is most effective, in the optimum position as far as the visual field is concerned. It also minimizes problems that might arise from unwanted differential prismatic effects and reduces the possibility of ghost images formed by reflection at the lens surfaces.

When considering lens centration it is important to differentiate between face and frame measurements. Facial features and their dimensions remain constant for long periods of time, at least in adults, and the pupillary distance, for example, can be established and recorded as an absolute measurement. However, centration of the correcting lenses varies with the position and inclination of the spectacle frame that holds the lenses. Although consequential errors are often small, to achieve the optimum result from the correcting lenses it is important to understand the relationship between the facial measurement and the corresponding spectacle dimension. As it is useful, a review of the terminology that relates to lens centration is given in Table 3.1, the definitions in which are found in the relevant Standards on ophthalmic lenses.[1] Abbreviations suggested in the Standard are included and terms that appear in italics are themselves defined in the Standard.

Some of the terms and methods currently recommended for use when dealing with measurement and centration have been revised from those used in the past. In particular, the *datum system* is no longer recommended as a system for frame measurement and use of the term 'datum line' is now officially deprecated. The distance between the boxed centres of the frame is now known as the *distance between centres*. This new dimension replaces that formally known as the datum centre distance, which measurement should no longer be used. There can be no doubt that communication between the optician and the workshop will improve when the new terminology and definitions given above gain universal acceptance and become commonly employed.

Most of the dimensions described above are illustrated in Figures 3.1 to 3.4.

Horizontal centration of spectacle lenses

When an eye is directed to a point on an object the image of that point is produced on the fovea. The line that joins the object point and the fovea is the eye's visual axis. It is implicit in this statement that the eye's entrance and exit pupils also lie on the visual axis. If a spectacle lens is placed before the eye so that its optical axis coincides with the visual axis, there will be no prismatic effect and the object will not be displaced. In the following treatment it is assumed that the visual axis passes through the centre of the eye's pupil and the minor complications that arise from this assumption (such as the usual inclination of the eye's own optical axis to the visual axis, the so-called angle alpha), are ignored. Furthermore, it is assumed that the image produced by the anterior surface of the cornea of an illuminated source placed on the visual axis in front of the eye (the first Purkinje image) also lies on the visual axis and that this axis also passes through the assumed position of the eye's centre of rotation.

Figure 3.4 depicts a plan view of the eyes directed towards an object lying at infinity. The visual axes are parallel and, making use of the foregoing assumptions, the distance between the eyes' visual axes is the same as the distance between the eyes' centres of rotation, the pupil centres and the centration points (CPs) in the spectacle plane. The inter-pupillary distance, or PD, is a facial measurement, whereas the centration distance (CD) in the spectacle plane is a frame measurement. As will emerge shortly, it is strictly the CD in which we are interested.

In the circumstances depicted in Figure 3.4 we can measure the PD or CD in several ways. The traditional method using a simple millimetre rule works well in practised hands and is based upon the following procedure. The subject's and the fitter's eyes should be on the same level, which is easily achieved if the fitter uses a stool of adjustable height.

The fitter sitting in front of the subject closes his/her right eye and directs the subject to look at his/her open left eye. The situation is depicted in Figure 3.5a. The fitter can now line up the zero of the rule with the centre of the subject's right pupil. In practice, if the rule does not employ a hairline with which to locate the pupil centre, the zero may be aligned with the temporal junction of either the pupil margin and the iris, or, in the case of dark irides, the temporal junction of the iris and the sclera. Under normal circumstances, this latter reference point gives accurate results and obviates the uncertainty of unequal or decentred pupils.

Having zeroed the rule on the subject's right eye, the fitter asks the subject to look at the fitter's other (fitter's right) eye and notes the measurement to the nasal junction of the subject's left pupil/ iris or iris/sclera (Figure 3.5b). Having noted the reading, the fitter can check that the zero is still in its desired position by asking the subject to look once more at his/her left eye and, if necessary, repeating the sequence for the other eye. It may be helpful for the fitter to rest the fingers lightly on the subject's temples to steady the rule, and it is important that neither the subject nor the fitter moves their head during the measurement.

An economy of instructions to the subject simplifies the measurement and the following concise statements could be employed:

1. 'Please look straight into my open eye.'
2. 'Now, without moving your head, please look into my other eye.'

Table 3.1 Terminology of lens centration

Term	Definition
Vertex	Point of intersection of the optical axis with a surface of the lens.
Back	Relating to the surface of a lens nearer to the eye.
Optical centre, O	That point (real or virtual) on the optical axis of a lens that is, or appears to be, traversed by rays emerging parallel to their original direction. When applied to an ophthalmic lens the optical centre is regarded as coinciding with the front or back *vertex* of the lens.
Visual point	Point of intersection of the eye's visual axis with the *back* surface of the lens.
Distance visual point, DVP	An assumed position of the *visual point* on a lens that is used for distance vision under given conditions, normally when the eyes are in the primary position.
Near visual point, NVP	An assumed position of the *visual point* on a lens that is used for near vision under given conditions.
Lens shape	Outline of the lens periphery with the nasal side and the horizontal indicated.
Boxed lens size	Size of the rectangle that contains the *lens shape* and formed by the horizontal and vertical tangents to the *lens shape*.
Horizontal centre line, HCL	The line midway between and parallel to the horizontal tangents at the highest and lowest points of a lens.
Boxed centre	The midpoint of the rectangle that contains the *lens shape*.
Standard optical centre position	A reference point specific to each *lens shape* situated on the vertical line that passes through the *boxed centre* (or situated at the *boxed centre* if the manufacturer has published no contrary indication to its height).
Centration point, CP	Point at which the *optical centre* is to be located in the absence of prescribed prism or after any prescribed prism has been neutralized. NOTE: If the *centration point* is not specified it is located at the *standard optical centre position*.
Pantoscopic angle	The angle between the optical axis of a lens and the visual axis of the eye in the primary position, usually taken to be the horizontal.
Optical centre distance, OCD	The actual horizontal distance between the *optical centres* of a pair of mounted lenses.
Centration distance, CD	The specified horizontal distance between the right and left *centration points*. NOTE: If an inter-pupillary distance only is stated, this is taken to be the *centration distance*.
Decentration (dec)	Displacement, horizontal and/or vertical, of the *centration point* from the *standard optical centre position*.
Bodily decentration	(1) Of lenticular lenses. *Decentration* that is applicable to the lenticular aperture as well as to the *centration point*. (2) Of multifocal lenses. *Decentration* that is applicable to the segment as well as to the *centration point*.

Terms relating to optical centration of bifocals

Term	Definition
Segment top (segment extreme point)	The point of contact of the curve formed by the upper boundary of the segment with its horizontal tangent or, in the case of a straight-topped segment, with the midpoint of the straight line.
Segment top position	The vertical distance of the *segment top* above or below the *horizontal centre line*.
Segment drop	Vertical height of the *distance optical centre* above the segment top. NOTE: It is essential to specify the *segment drop* when ordering one lens of a pair to avoid introducing relative vertical prism.
Progression height	The vertical distance of the fitting cross above or below the *horizontal centre line*.
Distance optical centre	The *optical centre* of the distance portion.
Intermediate optical centre	The *optical centre* of the intermediate portion.
Near optical centre	The *optical centre* of the near portion.
Insetting	Displacing a bifocal segment towards the nose, usually without reference to the effect on the near optical centres, with the purpose generally of bringing the right and left reading fields into coincidence. NOTE: This term should not be used for an inward decentration of distance optical centres.
Geometrical inset (G in)	The distance between vertical lines through the *distance centration point* and the midpoint of the segment diameter. NOTE: For lenses with round segments the conventional method of *insetting* in workshop practice is by rotation about the *distance centration point* and is frequently based upon the *horizontal displacement* of an arbitrary point usually taken to lie 15mm below the distance centration point.
Fitting cross	A reference point (indicated by two intersecting lines) on a progressive power lens that is specified by the manufacturer. NOTE: The *fitting cross* is usually coincident with the start of the progression.
Prism reference point	The point, stipulated by the lens manufacturer, for checking the prescribed relative prism between a pair of progressive power lenses.

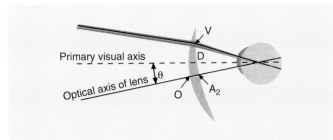

Figure 3.1   Terms used in discussing lens centration: V = visual point; D = distance visual point; O = optical centre; A₂ = back vertex of lens; θ = pantoscopic angle

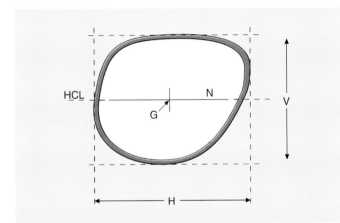

Figure 3.2   Lens shape: boxed lens size = H × V. G = boxed centre. HCL = horizontal centre line

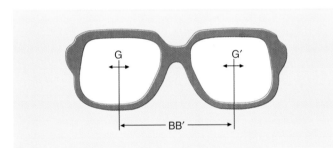

Figure 3.3   GG′ = distance between centres

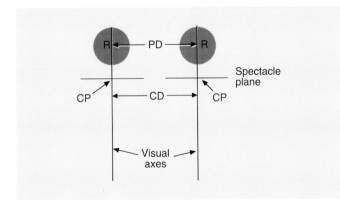

Figure 3.4   Inter-pupillary distance and centration distance: R = eye's centre of rotation; CP = centration point; CD = centration distance; PD = inter-pupillary distance

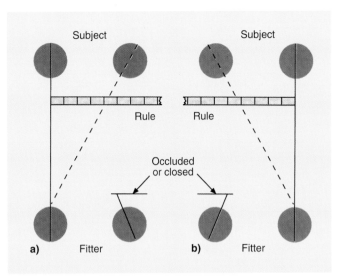

Figure 3.5   Measuring the inter-pupillary distance

The measurement that is obtained by this procedure is the binocular inter-pupillary distance or PD. This dimension is a facial measurement. If it is desired to separate the CPs of the correcting distance vision lenses by this value, the corresponding measurement in the spectacle plane is the centration distance.

The principle of the measurement is depicted in Figure 3.5 and, after a little practice, produces consistent results.

CD-ROM

Centration is also considered in detail on the CD-ROM

The sixteenth-of-a-millimetre rule

It is evident from Figure 3.5 that, from the theoretical point of view, the above procedure is only strictly valid when the PDs of the fitter and the subject are exactly the same. In practice, this is not always the case and some compensation must be made for the difference in the two measurements. The necessary compensation can be deduced from Figure 3.6, which assumes that the PD of the fitter is somewhat greater than the PD of the subject, who might be, for example, a small child.

It is evident from the geometry of Figure 3.6 that the true PD of the subject differs from the value measured by the fitter by δp where, by similar triangles:

$$\delta p = \delta P \times s/(s+l)$$

δP is the difference between the PD of the fitter and the subject.

If the distance of the eye's centre of rotation from the spectacle plane, s, is taken as 27mm and the distance of the fitter from the spectacle plane, l, is assumed to be 400mm, this reduces to

$$\delta p = \delta P/16$$

The sign convention is ignored in these statements.

In words, this helpful rule reminds us that for every 1mm difference between the PD of the fitter and the subject, the fitter will *over*-estimate the subject's PD by 1/16mm if the fitter's PD is *larger* than that of the subject. On the other hand, if the fitter's PD is *smaller* than the measured amount, the fitter will *under*-estimate the subject's PD.

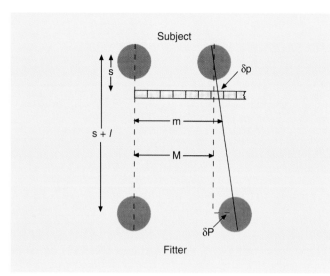

Figure 3.6   The 16th millimetre rule: m = measured PD; M = true PD; δp = error in measurement; δP = difference between PDs of fitter and subject

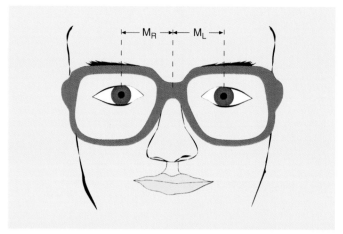

Figure 3.7   Monocular centration distance. Note that the midpoint of the bridge of the frame does not coincide with the point midway between the pupil centres. M_R = right monocular CD; M_L = left monocular CD

For example, suppose the PD of the fitter is 68mm and the measured PD of the subject is 60mm. The subject's true PD should be taken as 59.5mm. Alternatively, if the fitter's PD is 68mm and the measured PD of the subject is 76mm, the subject's true PD should be taken as 76.5mm. Clearly, the large differences in PD between the fitter and the subject suggested in these two examples are unusual and in most cases the theoretical drawback of the method can be ignored.

Precautions

If the pupil–iris margin is being used to take the measurement, this method produces the correct result only when the pupil diameters are equal. In the rare cases of unequal pupil diameters, the measurement should be repeated from the nasal edge of the subject's right pupil to the temporal edge of the left pupil and the mean of the two measurements recorded as the PD.

In the case of a squinting subject, the PD may be obtained with the aid of the cover-test technique. The rule should be held with one hand and the non-fixating eye covered with the free hand to ensure that each visual axis in turn moves into the primary position.

Monocular centration distances

In practice, it is necessary to centre the correcting lenses separately for each eye and, in these cases, to take the CD accurately it is necessary for the subject to wear the final spectacle frame (into which the lenses will be mounted) during the measurement. This is because the monocular CD is measured from the centre of the bridge of the frame to each CP, which may not coincide with the centre of the bridge of the subject's nose. This is demonstrated in Figure 3.7, which illustrates in somewhat exaggerated fashion how the bridge of the frame may be offset by gross asymmetry of the wearer's nose. Clearly, monocular PDs (or semi-PDs, as they are sometimes called) are of no use without reference to the final frame.

In many cases the spectacle frame is glazed with dummy plano lenses; this is certain to be the case if the frame is new. If the frame is empty, transparent adhesive tape may be attached to the eyes of the frame to enable the pupil centres to be marked on the tape. It is sensible to begin by measuring the binocular PD as described above, not just so that the adhesive tape can be attached in approximately the right place, but also as verification that the sum of the two monocular CDs does, indeed, equal the binocular PD.

To take the monocular CD, the procedure described above for ensuring that the visual axes are parallel can be employed during the measurement, but instead of using a ruler, the positions of the pupil centres can be marked with a fine ink pen.

The procedure can be summarized as follows:

- Using a grease pencil (or fine pen), mark the dead centre of the bridge on the front of the frame. If using ink, make sure it is of the type that will not stain or leave a permanent mark on the frame!
- Place the frame on the subject and, using the procedure outlined above, but without using a rule, direct the subject to look straight into your left eye.
- Using a fine pen, mark the position of the centre of the subject's right pupil on the dummy lens or transparent tape. A single dot should suffice.
- Direct the subject to look straight into your right eye and mark the position of the centre of the subject's left pupil on the dummy lens or tape.
- Verify that the dots are in front of the pupil centres by repeating the sequence, but now just look to ensure that the dots are in the correct position.
- Remove the frame and measure the horizontal distances between the centre of the bridge of the frame and the marks on the dummy lenses or tape. Record these as the two monocular CDs in the form 31/33, the first number representing the monocular CD for the right eye.

Naturally, the sum must equal the measured binocular PD. Any vertical asymmetry between the heights of the two dots should also be noted.

It will be recognized that this procedure is no different from that described below to determine the vertical centration of the lenses, nor from the usual procedure for determining progression heights when taking measurements for progressive power lenses.

PD gauges

Many different devices that simplify the taking of the PD measurement are available today, the most popular of which is the corneal reflection pupillometer. The instrument makes use of the

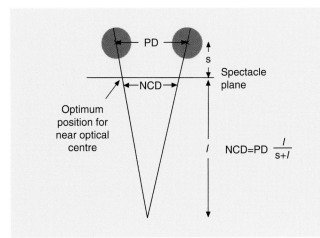

Figure 3.8   Near centration distance, NCD

Table 3.2   Relationship between PD and NCD for various working distances (s = 27)

PD (mm)	NCD for near vision at			
	25cm	33.3cm	35cm	40cm
74	67.0	68.5	68.5	69.5
72	65.0	66.5	67.0	67.5
70	63.0	65.0	65.0	65.5
68	61.5	63.0	63.0	63.5
66	59.5	61.0	61.5	62.0
64	58.0	59.0	59.5	60.0
62	56.0	57.5	57.5	58.0
60	54.0	55.5	55.5	56.0
58	52.5	53.5	54.0	54.5
56	50.5	52.0	52.0	52.5

telecentric principle, which is as follows. A small stop is placed at the first principal focus of a plus lens and the subject views an image formed at infinity of a small illuminated ring, which is concentric with the stop in the first focal plane. The anterior surface of the cornea produces an image of this source (Purkinje image I), and the observer moves a vertical hairline until it bisects the annular image of the source. The position of the hairline may be indicated on a scale, or its position may be read electronically by means of a digital readout. These instruments assume that the corneal reflection coincides with the visual axis, which would be the case if the angle between the optical axis and the visual axis (the angle alpha) is zero.

Some autorefractors also transmit the distance between the collimated binocular beams to a digital readout or, indeed, to the phoropter head itself, setting it up automatically for the user.

Near centration distance

When recording the PD, or CD, for distance vision, we measure the distance between the visual axes, which are supposed to be parallel and directed to infinity, and are assumed to pass through the centres of the pupils. In near vision, however, the separation of the centres of the converging pupils is not required. Instead, we are interested in the horizontal separation of the converging visual axes as they intersect the spectacle plane. This distance is known as the *near centration distance* (NCD) and is invariably less than the inter-pupillary distance in near vision, owing to the forward position of the spectacle plane (Figure 3.8).

If the PD is taken to be the distance between the eye's centres of rotation, it can be seen from Figure 3.8 that the NCD is a function of the PD, the working distance l and the position of the spectacle plane in relation to the eye's centres of rotation, s.

By means of similar triangles it is easy to show that:

$$NCD = PD \times l/(s + l)$$

Using the value of 27mm for s, this expression reduces to the following forms for various working distances, l:

Working distance			
	25cm NCD	=	0.903PD
	33.3cm NCD	=	0.925PD
	35cm NCD	=	0.928PD
	40cm NCD	=	0.937PD

Table 3.2 gives the NCD for various PDs obtained by means of this expression. The results have been rounded to the nearest 0.5mm.

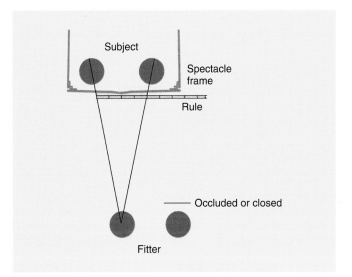

Figure 3.9   Measurement of near centration distance

Figure 3.9 shows how the NCD can be measured with a simple rule by placing the rule in contact with the front surface of an empty spectacle frame that is being worn by the subject. Without the frame, if the ruler was placed in contact with, say, the forehead, we would be trying to measure the near PD.

The fitter should place his/her left eye so that it lies centrally in front of the subject's nose at the subject's conventional reading distance. This would usually be some 300–400mm in front of the subject, but it will vary with height and posture, which should be noted before taking the measurement.

If the subject is now directed to look at the centrally placed eye of the fitter, the rule can be zeroed on the temporal edge of the pupil–iris or the iris margin–sclera, just as for distance vision. Keeping everything else still, the fitter should now direct the gaze to the subject's left eye and read the NCD from the rule by noting the position of the nasal edge of the subject's left pupil–iris or iris margin–sclera from the scale.

Decentration to provide the correct centration distance

In many cases, a spectacle frame is dispensed in which the *distance between centres* of the frame is larger than the subject's CD. To position the optical centres of the lenses directly in front of the subject's pupils, decentration must be ordered to shift the optical centres so that their horizontal separation corresponds with the subject's CD. For example, if the *distance between centres* for the frame is 70mm and the subject's CD is 64mm, then there is a discrepancy of 6mm and the lenses must be decentred inwards to compensate for this. If just a binocular CD of 64mm is given, then the decentration must be assumed to be divided equally between the eyes and the decentration is given simply by:

$$\text{decentration} = (\text{distance between centres} - CD)/2$$

In this example the decentration is given by $(70-64)/2 = 3mm$ each eye.

If monocular CDs are given, such as 33/31 (which sums to 64mm, as before), then the decentrations for each lens will differ. Again assuming the frame dimension to be 70mm, the decentration for each lens can be calculated from:

$$\text{decentration} = (\text{distance between centres}/2) - \text{monocular CD}$$

In the above example, the decentration for the right eye would be $35 - 33 = 2mm$ in, whereas the decentration for the left eye would be $35 - 31 = 4mm$ in. Needless to say, the sum of the monocular decentrations must be the same as the difference between the *distance between centres* and the binocular CD.

Centration distance and optical centre distance

In the absence of a prescribed prism, the optical centres of the spectacle lenses would be separated by the CD. Any prescribed prism, or unintentional prism, would remove the optical centres from the CPs.

The inter-relationship of the terms CD, optical centre distance (OCD) and *distance between centres* is best explained by means of an example. Consider a subject whose prescription is BE −5.00 combined with 2Δ base in. Suppose that the subject's PD is 66mm and that a frame has been chosen for which the *distance between centres* is 70mm. The glazed spectacles are illustrated in Figure 3.10.

Ignoring the prism for a moment, the optical centres need to be decentred inwards by 2mm for each eye to fulfil the CD requirement. However, to obtain the prismatic effect of 2Δ base in, the optical centres must be displaced outwards by 4mm (from Prentice's rule, $P = cF$; see below). In this example, it is likely that the prism will be obtained by decentration, but it could also be obtained by surfacing the lens.

Hence, as far as the finished spectacles are concerned, the OCD will be 74mm. This result is found by starting at the geometrical centre, decentring first 2mm inwards to fulfil the centration requirements and then 4mm outwards to obtain the prescribed prism. So if the *distance between centres* for the frame is 70mm, the optical centres will end up displaced outwards from the geometrical centres by 2mm for each eye, resulting in an OCD of 74mm. Since the full specification is known from the outset, we know that for this particular pair of spectacles, the CD is 66mm and the OCD is 74mm, and that the prismatic effect operative at the CPs is 2Δ base in.

No such certainty exists, however, when the original specification is unknown. Suppose that we were to examine the finished spectacles with no prior knowledge of their original specification. After reading the powers and dotting the optical centres by means of the focimeter, we could say with certainty that the power of each lens is −5.00D and that the OCD is 74mm. We might also give any of the following results as the true specification for the lenses:

- BE −5.00D with 1.0Δ base in, CD = 70mm
- BE −5.00D with 1.5Δ base in, CD = 68mm

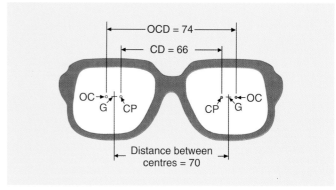

Figure 3.10 Centration distance, CD, and optical centre distance, OCD. OC = optical centre; G = boxed centre; CP = centration point

- BE −5.00D with 2.0Δ base in, CD = 66mm (which is the true specification)
- BE −5.00D with 2.5Δ base in, CD = 64mm

and so on.

Bifocal insetting

The purpose of insetting bifocal segments is to bring the near fields of view into coincidence. Contrary to popular belief, this is not achieved simply by insetting the segment by half the difference between the CD and the NCD. That so many bifocal wearers do not have problems with insetting deduced from the above rule is explained, quite simply, by the fact that current bifocal segments are relatively large. Large-diameter segments enable the individual monocular fields of view to overlap sufficiently to provide a large binocular field. If we were to attempt to dispense segments of only 10mm diameter, many more grief cases would arise from incorrect insetting.

The effect that insetting tries to achieve may be explained as follows. Imagine, first, that the segment is no more than a small aperture in an occluder placed close to the eye. The field of view through the aperture, of course, depends only on the size and shape of this aperture. If a subject wearing a pair of D-shaped apertures (like most modern bifocal segments) that have not been centred correctly on the converging visual axes looks at a sheet of paper, the fields of view projected onto the paper would appear as shown in Figure 3.11, in which it is assumed that the apertures have not been sufficiently inset. The shaded area represents the binocular field, whereas the areas that remain unshaded either side of the binocular field are seen in monocular vision. The areas seen only by the right and left eye are marked R and L, respectively. Ideally, of course, the areas should overlap exactly to provide a single D-shaped field.

It is an easy matter to bring the near fields depicted in Figure 3.11 into coincidence. The amount of inset necessary to do so is exactly the same as that given in Table 3.2, which also gives the geometrical insetting required when the distance portion of a bifocal lens has no power. Usually, however, the distance portion is not afocal and the main lens exerts horizontal prismatic effect at the near visual point (NVP). The influence that this has upon the geometrical inset can be deduced from Figure 3.12, which illustrates a plan view of a plus lens, centred for distance vision, in front of the right eye.

If the lens had no power, the visual axis would lie in the direction shown by the dashed line. Since the distance portion of the lens is positive and exerts a base-out prismatic effect in the region of the NVP, the direction that the visual axis must take up to view the near point B is indicated in Figure 3.12 by the direction RG. Clearly, the centre of the aperture that governs the near visual field, which is the bifocal segment itself, must be positioned at G, the distance OG being the geometrical inset.

The inset, g, that is required to bring the near fields into coincidence is given by the relationship:

$$g = pL/(L + F - S)$$

where p is the monocular CD, L the working distance in dioptres, F the power of the spectacle lens in the horizontal meridian and S the dioptral distance from the eye's centre of rotation to the spectacle plane.

If the spectacle plane is assumed to lie 27mm in front of the eye's centre of rotation, and the working distance is taken to be 33.3cm, this expression reduces to:

$$g = 3p/(40 - F)$$

Table 3.3 has been compiled from this relationship for various lens powers and a working distance of 33.3cm. Since the geometrical inset is a function of the monocular CD, it cannot properly be expressed in terms of the binocular CD and is listed in Table 3.3 for various monocular CDs that cover the same range of values as those considered in Table 3.2.

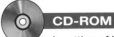

CD-ROM

Insetting of bifocal segments is also considered in detail on the CD-ROM

Vertical centration of lenses

Spectacle lenses are mounted before the eyes in a plane that is approximately parallel to the plane joining the supra-orbital ridge to the chin (Figure 3.13). This plane is usually inclined at an angle

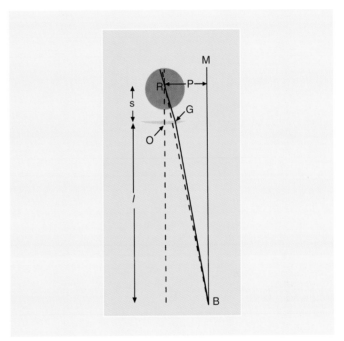

Figure 3.12 Geometrical inset. OG = g, the geometrical inset; B = near point; MB = midline measured from the geometric centre of the bridge of the frame; R = eye's centre of rotation; G = required position for the geometrical centre of the segment

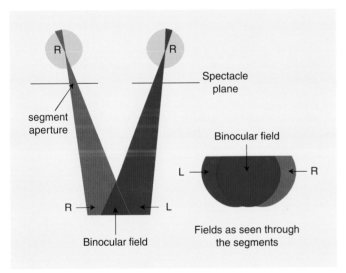

Figure 3.11 Non-coincident fields of view with D-shaped segments

Table 3.3	Geometrical insetting									
	Geometrical inset in mm for working distance of 33.3cm									
Lens power (D)	Monocular centration distances									
	28	29	30	31	32	33	34	35	36	37
+12.00	3.0	3.1	3.2	3.3	3.4	3.5	3.6	3.8	3.9	4.0
+10.00	2.8	2.9	3.0	3.1	3.2	3.3	3.4	3.5	3.6	3.7
+8.00	2.6	2.7	2.8	2.9	3.0	3.1	3.2	3.3	3.4	3.5
+6.00	2.5	2.6	2.6	2.7	2.8	2.9	3.0	3.1	3.2	3.3
+4.00	2.3	2.4	2.5	2.6	2.7	2.8	2.8	2.9	3.0	3.1
+2.00	2.2	2.3	2.4	2.4	2.5	2.6	2.7	2.8	2.8	2.9
0.00	2.1	2.2	2.3	2.3	2.4	2.5	2.6	2.6	2.7	2.8
−2.00	2.0	2.1	2.1	2.2	2.3	2.4	2.4	2.5	2.6	2.6
−4.00	1.9	2.0	2.0	2.1	2.2	2.3	2.3	2.4	2.5	2.5
−6.00	1.8	1.9	2.0	2.0	2.1	2.2	2.2	2.3	2.3	2.4
−8.00	1.8	1.8	1.9	1.9	2.0	2.1	2.1	2.2	2.3	2.3
−10.00	1.7	1.7	1.8	1.9	1.9	2.0	2.0	2.1	2.2	2.2
−12.00	1.6	1.7	1.7	1.8	1.8	1.9	2.0	2.0	2.1	2.1

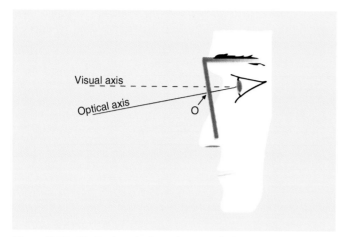

Figure 3.13 Vertical centration of spectacle lenses, the pantoscopic angle. O = optimum position for the optical centre

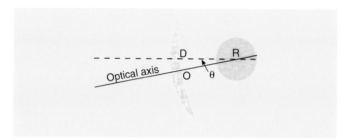

Figure 3.14 Vertical centration of spectacle lenses, the centre of rotation condition. R = eye's centre of rotation; D = distance visual point; O = optical centre of the lens; θ = pantoscopic angle; OR = s, the centre of rotation distance. From the geometry of the figure, AO = s tan θ

Table 3.4 Vertical centration of lenses and pantoscopic angle

Pantoscopic angle (°)	Lower optical centre (mm)
2.5	1.2
5.0	2.4
7.5	3.6
10.0	4.8
12.5	6.0
15.0	7.2

of between 5° and 15° to the normal to the primary direction of the eye and the angle is referred to as the *pantoscopic angle*. If the line of the side of the spectacle frame is horizontal, as it often is, the pantoscopic angle is the same as the *angle of side*. For the optical performance of the lens to match that which the designer intended it is necessary for the optical axis of the lens to pass through the eye's centre of rotation. This can be achieved by lowering the optical centre of the lens to compensate for the tilted spectacle plane.

The amount by which the optical centre should be lowered, DO, can be deduced from Figure 3.14. If the pantoscopic angle is denoted by θ, and the distance from the back vertex of the lens to the eye's centre of rotation by *s*, then the amount by which the optical centre should be lowered, DO, can be seen to be:

DO = *s* tan θ

Table 3.4 gives values of DO for various values of pantoscopic tilt, θ, when *s* is assumed to be 27mm. The dispensing rule, that the optical centre should be lowered by 0.5mm for every 1° angle of pantoscopic angle, has its origin here.

It can be deduced from Table 3.4 that, in general, the optical centre of a lens should not be placed directly in front of the centre of the eye's pupil, but on average some 4–5mm below the pupil centre. In practice, this position of the optical centre is often obtained with no specific instruction on the prescription order, simply because modern cosmetic dispensing dictates that the frame occupies a position such that the centre of the pupil lies 4–8mm above the *horizontal centre line* (HCL). If the optician does not give any instructions to the contrary, it is usual for the prescription house to place the optical centre at its own *standard*

optical centre position, which is either on the HCL or 1–3mm above it. This practice has the obvious advantage that the edge thicknesses at the top and bottom edges of the lens match more closely.

It is an easy matter to ensure that the optical centres occupy the correct position in the vertical meridian. The pupil centres can be dotted using exactly the same method described earlier for obtaining monocular CDs. Alternatively, for an empty frame, the height of the pupil centre can be measured up from the lower horizontal tangent to the lens periphery. To compensate for the pantoscopic angle, the optical centre of the lens must now be lowered from this position by the amount given in Table 3.4.

By way of example, suppose the pupil centres are found to lie at a height of 28mm above the lower horizontal tangents to the lens periphery and the pantoscopic angle is 10°. Using Table 3.4, the optical centres need to be 5mm lower than the measured pupil height and a height of 23mm should be ordered for the optical centres. If the height of the HCL is known to be 24mm, then the instruction to the glazing department might be: OC 1mm below HCL.

It must be pointed out that the advent of aspheric lenses for the normal power range emphasizes the importance of the correct vertical centration of spectacle lenses. Before 1985, aspheric lenses were reserved for the high-power plus range and in such cases the very nature of the prescription made the dispensing optician proceed with the centring of lenses with great care. The use of aspherical surfaces for low-power prescriptions demands the same attention to detail be paid in fitting the lenses. This is because the pole of the aspherical surface should also be made to coincide with the visual axis when it passes normally through the aspherical surface. This is achieved simply by obeying the rule for centration given above.

In cases of anisometropia, lowering the optical centres may give rise to discomfort since a vertical differential prismatic effect is introduced at the distance visual points (DVPs). In such cases it is usual to specify the vertical positions of the optical centres of the lenses. For distance vision these would normally be placed directly in front of the centres of the pupils when the eyes occupy the primary position. In such cases, unless the pantoscopic angle is zero, that is, the lens is not tilted at all, the wearer cannot benefit fully from the best-form principle of the lens. On the other hand, if the lens is mounted perpendicular to the primary direction of sight, the bottom edge of the lens appears to jut out from the cheek and the cosmetic appearance of the frame suffers.

Vertical centration in near vision

When the spectacle lens has been centred correctly for distance vision by lowering the optical centre to compensate for the pantoscopic angle, no further vertical decentration of the optical centre is necessary for near vision. This should be obvious from Figure 3.15, in which it can be seen that lowering the optical

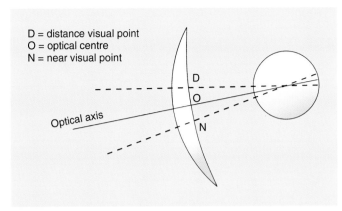

D = distance visual point
O = optical centre
N = near visual point

Figure 3.15   Vertical centration of lenses for near vision

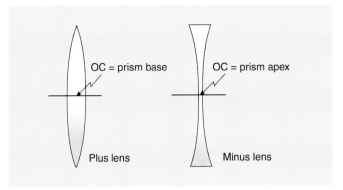

Figure 3.17   Direction of the prism base

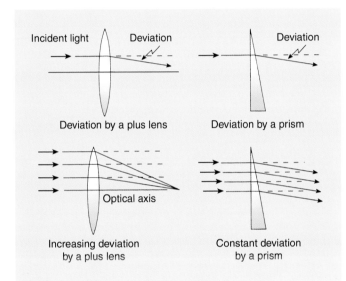

Figure 3.16   Similarity in the action of lenses and prisms

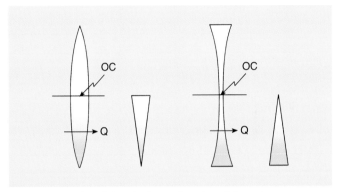

Figure 3.18   Visualizing the base direction of the prism

centre of the lens results in the centre of the distance visual zone lying as far above the optical centre as the centre of the near visual zone lies below the optical centre. In other words, centring the lenses correctly for distance vision in the vertical meridian also centres them correctly for near vision.

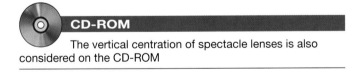

CD-ROM

The vertical centration of spectacle lenses is also considered on the CD-ROM

Prismatic effect of decentration

Figure 3.16 shows that when a single ray of light passes through a spectacle lens at any point other than its optical centre, it is deviated in much the same way as the ray would be deviated by a prism. In the case of a prism the deviation is constant when the angle of incidence is the same, whereas in the case of a lens, the deviation is such that all rays reunite at, or appear to diverge from, a single point (the effects of spherical aberration being ignored). If the rays of incident light emanate from an infinitely distant object, they reunite at the second principal focus of the lens. The deviating power of a lens increases from zero at the optical centre to a maximum at the lens periphery.

The deviating power of the lens at any point is called the *prismatic effect* of the lens at that point. It can be imagined that every lens is made up from a large number of plano-prisms of differing powers, the powers increasing at a steady rate as the light meets the lens further and further from its optical centre.

In the case of a plus lens the prism bases are all directed towards the optical centre of the lens. At the optical centre the prismatic effect is zero; the lens is parallel-sided here (Figure 3.17). In the case of a minus lens, the bases of the prisms are directed towards the lens periphery, away from the optical centre. The prismatic effect at any point on a lens is defined as the power of the plano-prism that would produce the same deviation as the lens at that point. It is expressed in prism dioptres (Δ), but in continental Europe the unit is sometimes known as cm/m, since the prism dioptre expresses the displacement of the ray in centimetres, measured at a distance of one metre from the prism.

The prismatic effect in prism dioptres, P, at a point c centimetres from the optical centre of a lens of power, F, is given by the decentration relationship (Prentice's rule):[2]

$$P = cF$$

Thus, the prismatic effect at a point that lies 6mm below the optical centre of a +5.00D lens is $0.6 \times 5.00 = 3\Delta$ base up. The prismatic effect at a point that lies 8mm below the optical centre of a −4.00D lens is $0.8 \times 4 = 3.2\Delta$ base down.

The base direction of the prismatic effect in these two instances can be found by visualizing where the thickest portion of the lens lies in relation to the point in question (Figure 3.18). In the case of the +5.00D lens, the thickest portion of the lens lies at the optical centre, which lies above the point at which the prismatic effect was found. Thus, the base direction is up. In the case of

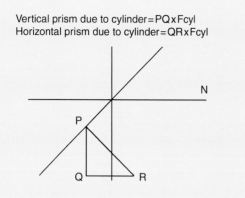

Figure 3.19 Author's construction for prismatic effect caused by a cylinder

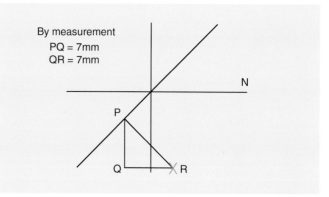

Figure 3.20 Construction for prismatic effect at a point 10mm down and 4mm in from the GC of the plano-cylinder +2.00DC × 45

the –4.00D lens, the optical centre is the thinnest point on the lens and represents the position of the prism apex. Since the optical centre lies directly above the point in question, the base direction at a point below the optical centre is base down.

In the case of astigmatic lenses for which the vertical and horizontal decentrations are known, the prismatic effect at any point on the lens can still be found by simple arithmetic provided that the cylinder axis lies at 90 or 180, that is when the powers of the lens coincide with the given decentration. For example, the prismatic effects at a point 8mm above and 4mm inwards from the optical centre of the lens, $L – 3.00/–2.00 \times 90$, can be determined simply since the power of the lens in the vertical meridian is known to be –3.00D and the power of the lens in the horizontal meridian is known to be –5.00D. Hence, the prismatic effects are $0.8 \times 3 = 2.4\Delta$ base up and $0.4 \times 5 = 2\Delta$ base in, the base directions being obtained by inspection as before.

When the cylinder axis is oblique, the prismatic effect can be determined by means of a graphical construction. The method described below treats an astigmatic lens as a sphere and a separate plano-cylinder and was first published by the author in 1965.[3] A ruler and a protractor are employed to obtain reasonable accuracy.

Begin by finding the prismatic effect caused by the spherical component of the prescription. To find the prism caused by the cylinder use the following method, illustrated in Figure 3.19:

- Construct 90 and 180 meridians to form an origin and indicate the nasal side of the lens.
- Draw the cylinder axis along its prescribed direction.
- Locate the position of the point (R in Figure 3.19) at which the prismatic effect is to be determined, choosing a suitably large scale (10× or 1cm representing 1mm should be sufficient for most purposes).
- Drop a perpendicular from R to the cylinder axis, meeting it at P.
- Determine the base direction of the prism caused by the cylinder by noting the position of P with respect to R and using the following rules:
  - If the cylinder power has a plus sign, P represents the position of the prism base.
  - If the cylinder power has a minus sign, P represents the position of the prism apex and the prism base lies in the opposite direction.
- Resolve PR into vertical and horizontal components (PQ and QR, respectively, in Figure 3.19) by making PR the hypotenuse

of a right-angled triangle. Measure PQ and QR and express their lengths in centimetres.
- Find the vertical prismatic effect at R caused by the cylinder by multiplying the distance PQ, expressed in centimetres, by the power of the cylinder.
- Find the horizontal prismatic effect at R caused by the cylinder by multiplying the distance QR, in centimetres, by the power of the cylinder.
- Add any prism from the spherical component of the prescription to the values just found for the cylinder to obtain the total vertical and horizontal prismatic effects at R.

The procedure is demonstrated by the following example.
Example. Find the vertical and horizontal prismatic effects encountered when the eye views through a point 10mm below and 4mm inwards from the optical centre of the right lens, $–4.00/+2.00 \times 45$.

1. The prism caused by the spherical component, –4.00, is $1 \times 4 = 4\Delta$ base down and $0.4 \times 4 = 1.6\Delta$ base in.
2. The construction for the prism caused by the cylinder is illustrated in Figure 3.20. By inspection, point P lies upwards and outwards from the point R at which the prism is to be found. The cylinder is positive in sign, so the base direction of the prism caused by the cylinder is base up and out.
3. By measurement, the distances PQ and QR are each 0.7cm in length, so the prism caused by the cylinder is $0.7 \times 2 = 1.4\Delta$ base up and $0.7 \times 2 = 1.4\Delta$ base out.
4. Adding the prism caused by the sphere, we obtain the total prismatic effect at the point:
   - vertically, 4Δ base down and 1.4Δ base up $= 2.6\Delta$ base down.
   - horizontally, 1.6Δ base in and 1.4Δ base out $= 0.2\Delta$ base in.

 CD-ROM

Prismatic effect at any point on a lens is considered in detail on the CD-ROM

Differential prismatic effect

When the prescription is the same for each eye, the prismatic effects encountered during version movements of the eyes, as they rotate away from the optical centres to view through extra-axial points on the lenses, are also the same and, normally, do not provide discomfort to the wearer. For example, in the case of the prescription BE –4.00DS, the prismatic effects encountered at the lenses by a pair of eyes that have rotated downwards and to the right to view through points 9mm below and 6mm to the right of the optical centres, are:

R, 3.6Δ base down and 2.4Δ base out

L, 3.6Δ base down and 2.4Δ base in

These prismatic effects cancel one another, since the base directions point in the same direction.

In near vision, the zone of the lens that is used to read lies below the distance visual zone. The centre of the near visual zone, the NVP, is normally taken to lie some 8–10mm below the DVP and 2.5mm inwards. As pointed out above, the optical centre of a spectacle lens is lowered from the position directly in front of the pupil by an amount that depends upon the pantoscopic angle of the lens. However, in cases of anisometropia, in which the prescription differs for each eye, it is likely that the pantoscopic angle has been reduced so that the optical centres are not far removed from the visual axes when the eyes are in their primary position, and the NVPs may well lie some 8mm below the optical centres of the lenses.

In these cases, the prismatic effects generally differ at the visual points. The difference in the prismatic effects between the eyes is called *differential prism* and requires the eyes to rotate by different amounts to maintain binocular single vision of the object of regard. It is well known that, normally, the eyes can cope with quite large amounts of horizontal differential prismatic effect, but that great discomfort arises if the eyes are called upon to overcome vertical differential prism. Supravergence movements of the eyes quickly produce diplopia. As a rule, the eyes can cope with only some 2Δ of vertical differential prismatic effect for long periods and 50% of this value, just 1Δ of vertical differential prism, was proposed many years ago by Emsley[4] as being the maximum amount that the eyes should be called upon to tolerate for prolonged periods.

Thus, in the case of the prescription R –3.00, L –6.00, and assuming reasonable visual acuities for each eye, the vertical prismatic effects that the subject encounters at points 8mm below the distance optical centres are R 2.4Δ base down and L 4.8Δ base down. The differential prismatic effect between the eyes is 2.4Δ base down in the left eye. This is certain to prevent comfortable binocular vision and some form of prism compensation may need to be provided for near vision.

More recent work by Henson and North[5] has shown that the eyes do adapt to vertical differential prism when worn permanently and that they re-adapt to their previous fusional state when the differential prism is removed. However, this is of no help to an anisometrope whose visual points roam about the lens as the eyes rotate, since they expect immediate binocular single vision at all times.

Anisometropes who are given simple single-vision spectacle lenses without any compensation for differential prism learn to restrict the area of the lens that they use to zones close to the optical centres of their lenses. For near vision, they lower their heads rather than just the eyes and, for example, at table, when eating a meal, adopt a characteristic chin-on-chest position when they are looking at the plate in front of them.

Needless to say, this expedient does not help when the subject becomes presbyopic and requires a bifocal correction, as the segment area that incorporates the near prescription requires the subject to view through extra-axial zones of the lenses. The

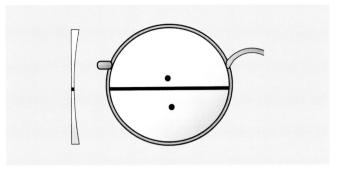

Figure 3.21 Split single-vision lens design

provision of prism control in bifocal lenses is considered in detail in Chapter 10.

Prism compensation in anisometropia

Compensation for vertical differential prism can be provided in several ways using lens designs in which the prismatic effects are controlled separately in the distance and reading areas of the lenses. Perhaps the simplest remedy is to provide the anisometrope with two separate pairs of spectacles, one centred for distance vision and a second pair centred for near vision.

Another method that provides separately centred distance and reading lenses, but this time in the form of a single pair of spectacles, is by means of a *split design* (Figure 3.21), similar to the split bifocal. Here, separate distance and reading lenses are cut in half and mounted together in a frame, each lens component being individually centred for distance or for near vision.

Alternatively, prism compensation can be provided in the form of a plano-prism segment bonded to the lower half of the lens (Figure 3.22). For example, in the case of the prescription R –3.00, L –6.00, considered above, a plano-prism of power 2.4Δ base down might be bonded to the right lens to increase the prismatic effect at the right NVP to 4.8Δ base down, which would now match that of the left eye. In this example, it might appear at first sight to be more sensible to provide prism compensation in the form of a segment for the left lens of 2.4Δ base up. However, this places the maximum depth of ridge in the worst position at the top of the reading segment, at just the point where the eye crosses from distance to near.

Perhaps the neatest method of providing prism control in the case of a single-vision design is in the form of a *bicentric lens*, in which the base-down prism is removed from the lower portion of the lens by means of a slab-off.

The slab-off technique can be performed by any surfacing workshop using ordinary machinery and results in a straight horizontal dividing line between the distance and reading areas of the lens (Figure 3.23a). Either the more minus lens of a pair should be worked (in the above example, the –6.00D lens would be selected for the slab-off), or both lenses could be slabbed off to provide a pair of bicentric lenses, with each portion separately centred for distance and near vision (Figure 3.23b).

Iso-V-differential prism zones

As pointed out above, it is *vertical* differential prismatic effect that is generally troublesome and may prevent comfortable binocular vision. Of course, vertical differential prismatic effects may

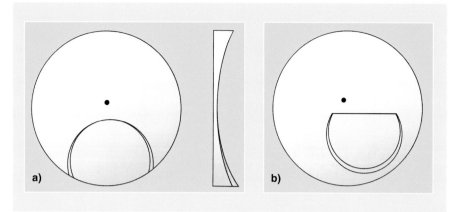

Figure 3.22 (a) Use of a bonded prism segment to compensate for vertical differential prism at the NVPs. (b) The segment can have any shape

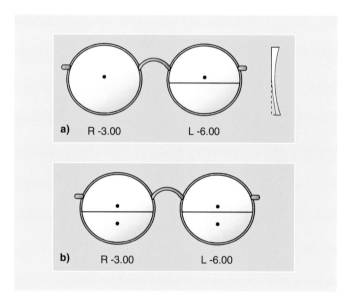

a) R -3.00   L -6.00

b) R -3.00   L -6.00

Figure 3.23 (a) The left lens has had 2.4Δ base down removed by slab-off from the lower portion of the lens to balance the prismatic effects at the NVPs. (b) Bicentric spectacles with separate optical centres for distance vision and near vision

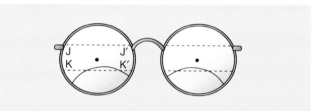

Figure 3.24 Iso-V-differential prism zones for the Rx: R −3.00, L −6.00. The zones are bands 13.3mm wide lying along 180°

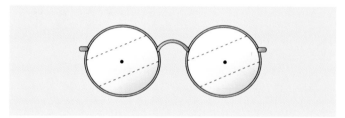

Figure 3.25 Iso-V-differential prism zones for the Rx: R +1.50/+2.00×135, L +3.50/+2.00×105. The zones are bands 32.3mm wide lying along 23.8°

result simply from poorly centred lenses, or may occur when the subject tries to use zones of the lenses in which differential prism exists because the powers of the lenses differ.

Perhaps the most helpful method of determining whether a subject is likely to be troubled by prismatic effects is to consider the areas on a pair of lenses within which the vertical differential prism does not exceed a stipulated amount – say 2Δ. In practice, these *iso-V-differential prism zones* can be generated instantly by computer and inform the dispensing optician whether, for example, prism control is necessary in a given case.

Figures 3.24 and 3.25 show how the zones are illustrated in a dispensing software package that calculates the sizes and orientations of the zones for any prescription and then indicates their positions and orientation on a pair of lenses on the VDU screen.

Figure 3.24 shows the areas on a pair of spectacles that have been glazed with the prescription considered earlier (R −3.00, L −6.00) within which the subject nowhere encounters more than 2Δ of vertical differential prismatic effect. Along the line JJ′ the base direction of the prismatic effect is up, whereas along KK′ the base direction is down.

It is very easy to show that the width of the band is 13.33mm, that is, the eyes can roam 6.67mm upwards or downwards from

the optical centres of the lenses before they encounter 2Δ of vertical differential prismatic effect. It is also obvious that if the lenses were a pair of bifocals with the segments positioned in the areas shown, the subject would not obtain comfortable near vision in the great majority of the near portion.

Figure 3.25 illustrates the 2Δ iso-V-differential prism zones for the prescription:

R +1.50/+2.00×30

L +3.50/+2.00×135

There is very little to indicate in the written prescription that there are large areas on the lenses within which comfortable reading vision would not be possible.

Construction of iso-V-differential prism zones

It can be shown that the iso-prism line that connects all points on a lens at which the *vertical* prismatic effect is the same is a straight line. Bennett[6] called these lines *iso-V-prism lines*. The area on a lens between the iso-V-prism line for which the vertical prismatic

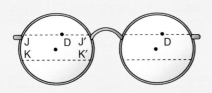

Figure 3.26　Iso-V-differential prism zones for the Rx: R +3.00, L +5.00. The zones are bands 20mm wide lying along 180°. At points D the vertical differential prism is 2Δ base down

effect is 1Δ base up and the iso-V-prism line for which the vertical prismatic effect is 1Δ base down is a band within which the vertical prismatic effect nowhere exceeds 1Δ. This band is the 1Δ iso-V-prism zone for the lens. It can be shown that, in the case of spherical lenses, iso-V-prism zones are horizontal bands, as is also the case with astigmatic lenses in which the cylinder axis lies at 90 or 180. However, in the case of sphero-cylindrical lenses with oblique axes, the bands lie along a meridian that does not coincide with the cylinder axis direction. When the iso-V-prism zones are constructed for the differential prescription, they show the areas on a pair of spectacle lenses within which the vertical differential prism nowhere exceeds the stipulated amount for the zone, known as iso-V-differential prism zones.

When the differential prescription has been determined, the dimensions of the zones can be calculated by the use of formulae or, more easily, they can be found by means of a graphical construction. Here, a graphical method is demonstrated.

Spherical lenses

In the case of a spherical prescription the iso-V-differential prism zones are horizontal bands centred on the optical centre of the lenses. Remember that all horizontal prismatic effect is ignored and we are only concerned with how far from the optical centres of the pair of lenses the eyes can roam before they encounter the stipulated vertical differential prismatic effect. Using the decentration relationship, the width of the band is given in millimetres by $20\delta P/\delta F$ where δP is the vertical differential prism and δF is the differential prescription.

Consider the prescription R +3.00, L +5.00. The differential prescription, δF is +2.00D, that is, the left lens is +2.00D stronger than the right.

Since the eyes can roam 10mm up or down from the optical centres of the differential lens before they encounter 2Δ of vertical prism, the 2Δ iso-V-differential prism zone is a horizontal band 20mm wide (Figure 3.26). To confirm this result, it is only necessary to show that at any point on the line JJ′ (or KK′), the vertical differential prismatic effect is 2Δ. When the eyes view through points D that lie 10mm above and 6mm to the left of the optical centres of the lenses, the prismatic effect encountered by the right eye is 3Δ base down and 1.8Δ base out. The prismatic effect encountered by the left eye is 5Δ base down and 3Δ base in. The vertical differential prismatic effect at D is 2Δ base down. The horizontal prismatic effects are simply ignored.

Plano-cylindrical lenses

In cases for which the differential prescription is a plano-cylinder, the iso-V-differential prism zone is again a band, but it now lies parallel with the cylinder axis. Since the power of a plano-cylinder lies at right angles to its axis, it is necessary to determine how far the eye can roam along the power meridian of the cylinder before it encounters the stipulated *vertical* differential prismatic effect.

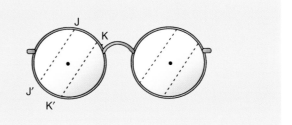

Figure 3.27　Iso-V-differential prism zones for the Rx: R +1.00/+2.00×150, L +3.00/+2.00×60. The differential Rx is +4.00DC×60. The zones are bands 20mm wide lying along 60°

Denoting the vertical differential prism by δP_V, the oblique prism, P, along the power meridian that gives rise to δP_V is given by:

$$P = \delta P_V/\cos\theta$$

where angle θ is the cylinder axis direction.

Consider the prescription: R +1.00/+2.00×150, L +3.00/+2.00×60. The differential prescription, which can be found by subtracting the weaker prescription from the greater (i.e. changing the sign of the right lens and adding the result to the left lens), is the plano-cylinder, +4.00DC×60.

The prism along 150 that gives rise to 2Δ of vertical prismatic effect is:

$$P = \delta P_V/\cos\theta$$
$$= 2/\cos 150$$
$$= 4\Delta \text{ base } 150$$

From the decentration relationship, the eye can roam $10P/F\text{mm} = 10\text{mm}$ along the 150 meridian before it encounters 4Δ of prism along 150, so the iso-V-differential prism zone is a band that is 20mm wide lying along the 60 meridian (Figure 3.27). Along JJ′ the vertical prism component is base down and along KK′ the base is up.

Sphero-cylindrical lenses

In the general case of a sphero-cylindrical lens, the iso-V-differential prism zone coincides with the axis meridian of the cylinder only when the principal powers of the differential prescription are vertical and horizontal. In all other cases the band lies along some other meridian. Since the edge of the band is a straight line, it is only necessary to plot two points to construct the band. These two points can be plotted, one on each principal meridian of the differential lens, using exactly the same method as is described above for a plano-cylinder.

It is essential to check the base direction along each principal meridian to ensure that the vertical prism components are both base up or both base down. Failure to do this results in the band being 90° off.

Consider the prescription that is illustrated in Figure 3.25:

R + 1.50/+ 2.00×135
L + 3.50/+ 2.00×105

The differential prescription is found, as before, by changing the sign of the minuend and adding the result to the stronger. Since the cylinder axes are not parallel, the powers must be summed by astigmatic decomposition or by means of Stokes' Construction.[2,6] The differential prescription is found to be +1.00/+2.00×75.

The graphical construction is illustrated in Figures 3.28 and 3.29.

The principal powers of the differential prescription lie along the 75 meridian (+1.00), and the 165 meridian (+3.00). Treating each of the principal meridians separately, the prism along the 75 meridian that gives rise to 2Δ of vertical prism is 2/cos 165 or 2.071Δ. If the eye is imagined to rotate up along the 75 meridian, the base direction of the prism is down along 75.

Since the power of the differential lens is +1.00 along 75, using the decentration relationship, the eye must roam 2.071/1cm, or 20.71mm up along 75 before it meets 2.071Δ base down along 75 (Figure 3.28). If a graphical solution is attempted, the prism along 75 is found by drawing a vertical line 2 units long from the 75 meridian to the 180 meridian (PN in Figure 3.28) and measuring OP, which represents the prism along 75. The point H, lying 20.71mm up along 75, can also be marked to scale on the construction (Figures 3.28 and 3.29).

Now turning our attention to the 165 meridian, the prism along this meridian, which gives rise to 2Δ of vertical prism, is 2/cos 75 or 7.727Δ. The eye needs to roam up along 165 to meet the prism base down along 165. The power of the differential

lens is +3.00D along 165, so the eye must roam 7.727/3cm or 25.758mm up along 165 before it meets 7.727Δ base down along 165. Once more, the prism along 165, which gives rise to 2Δ along 165, is found graphically by drawing a line 2 units long from the 165 meridian to the 180 meridian (QN′ in Figure 3.28). The point G, lying 25.758mm up along 165, can also be marked to scale on the construction (Figures 3.28 and 3.29).

Points G and H are the two points necessary to draw the 2Δ iso-V-prism line GH. Constructing a line parallel with GH that passes through the origin, AA′, and the line KK′, parallel with AA′ and the same distance from AA′ as GH, produces the iso-V-differential prism zone for the prescription. The position of the zone on the pair of lenses is illustrated in Figure 3.25.

As pointed out earlier, in practice it is much easier to generate the zones with a computer and the method described above forms an important part of comprehensive dispensing software packages.

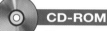

CD-ROM

The construction of iso-V-differential prism zones is demonstrated on the CD-ROM

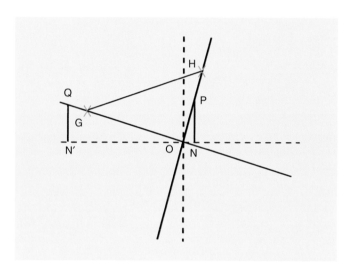

Figure 3.28   Graphical construction for iso-V-differential prism zone for the Rx: R +1.50/+2.00×30, L +3.50/+2.00×135. Determination of the prisms OP and OQ and the iso-V prism line GH

Prescription compensation for pantoscopic or dihedral tilt

The centre of rotation condition discussed earlier in this chapter under the heading, Vertical centration of lenses, states that when a lens is tilted before the eye (as when applying a pantoscopic tilt), it should be decentred to compensate for the tilt in order to ensure that the optical axis of the lens passes through the eye's centre of rotation. The same rule can also be applied to a lens tilt about a vertical axis in cases where the lens has a significant dihedral angle to provide a wrap-round effect to the spectacle front and the optical effects of this are discussed in detail in Chapter 16.

When a spherical lens is tilted before the eye, the refracted pencil is afflicted with aberrational astigmatism, which arises from the fact that the pencil passes obliquely through the lens. With their flagship designs, particularly progressive lens ranges, some manufacturers compensate the ordered prescription to take into account the induced astigmatism.

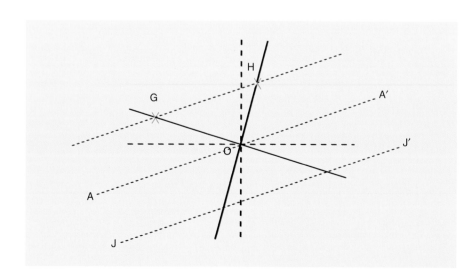

Figure 3.29   Graphical construction for iso-V-differential prism zone for the Rx: R +1.50/+2.00×30, L +3.50/+2.00×135. The zones are bands 32.3mm wide lying along 23.8°

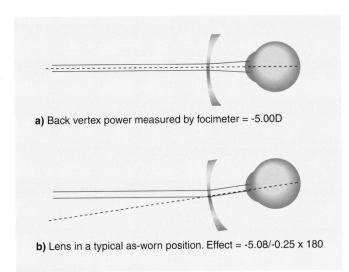

a) Back vertex power measured by focimeter = -5.00D

b) Lens in a typical as-worn position. Effect = -5.08/-0.25 x 180

Figure 3.30   Comparison of reading given by focimeter and the actual effect in wear. (a) Back vertex power of lens as read with the focimeter with no pantoscopic angle. (b) As-worn power – the effect obtained by the wearer when the lens is worn with a pantoscopic angle of 12.5°

Table 3.5 As-worn and compensated prescriptions	
As-worn prescription	**Compensated prescription**
–5.00	–4.92/+0.25 × 180
–5.00/–0.25 × 180	–4.92
–5.00/–0.25 × 90	–5.17/+0.50 × 180
–5.00/–0.25 × 30	–4.80/–0.25 × 60

Assuming that the third-order expressions given in Chapter 1 for the effects of tilting spherical lenses remain valid for tilts up to about 20°, the compensation required for a change in pantoscopic or dihedral angle can be obtained as follows.

Consider the prescription –5.00D which has been obtained with the trial frame (or phoropter head) fitted so that the subject's primary line passes normally through the lenses. This is the prescription which will be ordered from the lens manufacturer. When this lens is fitted with a pantoscopic angle of 12.5° it will no longer have an effect of –5.00D but instead (assuming it is made in CR 39 material):

$$F_{SPH} = F\left(1 + \sin^2 \theta / 2n\right) = -5\left(1 + \sin^2 12.5/3\right) = -5.08D.$$

$$F_{CYL} = F_{SPH}\ \tan^2 \theta = -5.08\ \tan^2 12.5 = -0.25D$$

$$\text{axis} = 180$$

so the as-worn power is –5.08/–0.25 × 180 (Figure 3.30).

The power of the lens which must be supplied so that the as-worn power is –5.00D can be found by changing the subject of the formula for the new spherical power, F_{SPH}, to find F and then neutralizing the induced cylinder. We have:

$$F_{RX} = 2nF/\left(2n + \sin^2 \theta\right) = 3 \times -5.00/\left(3 + \sin^2 12.5\right) = -4.92D$$

$$F_{CYL} = -F_{RX}\ \tan^2 \theta = +0.25 \times 180$$

and the power of the lens which must be supplied (the compensated prescription provided by the lens manufacturer to enable the lens to be checked) is –4.92/+0.25 × 180. When this lens is tilted before the eye to provide a pantoscopic angle of 12.5°, the –4.92D spherical component will increase its effect to –5.00D sphere and the astigmatism induced by the tilt, –0.25DC × 180, will be cancelled by the +0.25DC × 180 which the manufacturer has provided.

Table 3.5 lists some typical compensated prescriptions which will provide the given as-worn prescriptions (assuming CR 39 lenses) and mounted with a pantoscopic angle of 12.5°.

Note that in the case of the last example given in Table 3.5, there is a change in the axis direction of the cylinder. The required axis of 30 will only be obtained when the eye views straight ahead through the lens. As the direction of gaze changes (for example, in Figure 3.30, if the eye rotates downwards by 12.5°, it will be viewing normally through the lens and the effective cylinder axis will now be 60 instead of 30) the effective cylinder axis direction will change and for this reason, care must be undertaken when prescription compensation involves a change in cylinder axis direction!

References

1. BS 3521: Part 1: 1991, Terms Relating to Ophthalmic Lenses and Spectacle Frames. BSI, London
2. Jalie M 1984 Principles of ophthalmic lenses. ABDO, London
3. Jalie M 1965 An analysis of near prismatic effects – part 2. Optician 149
4. Emsley HH 1936 Visual optics. Hatton Press, London
5. Henson DB, North R 1980 Adaptation to prism induced heterophoria. Am J Optom Physiol Opt 57:129–137
6. Bennett AG 1968 Emsley & Swaine's ophthalmic lenses. Hatton Press, London

Aspheric lenses

The question of lens form is considered in Chapter 2, in which it is explained how the choice of bending influences the off-axis performance of the lens. In general, the ideal bending for any given power enables the wearer to obtain the same off-axis effect when viewing obliquely through the lens as obtained when viewing along the optical axis. When limited to the use of spherical surfaces, optimization of the off-axis performance can only be achieved by bending the lens. However, modern spectacle lens forms are no longer restricted to the simple spherical surface that can be produced by rotating machinery. Computer-assisted design and computer-controlled grinding methods have caused a revolution in modern spectacle lens forms and enabled surfaces of almost any shape to be produced, and reproduced, with accuracy. We now look in detail at lenses that employ an aspherical surface.

When a circle is rotated about its diameter, the solid of revolution that is obtained is called a sphere and the surface of a sphere is said to be spherical. Any surface that is not spherical can be termed *aspherical*, which means that the cylindrical surface, or the more widely used toroidal surface, might be described as an aspherical surface.

In lens design, the term 'aspherical surface' usually refers to a surface that is rotationally symmetrical, but at the same time not spherical, such as the ellipsoid illustrated in Figure 4.1, which would be generated by an ellipse that rotates about its major diameter.

The circle and the ellipse are two members of a series of curves known collectively as the *conic sections*, since they are the sections obtained when a plane intersects a right cone such as that depicted in Figure 4.2. If the plane intersects the cone exactly at right-angles to a vertical line that passes through the apex of the cone, the cut face of the cone is a *circle* (Figure 4.2a).

If the plane of intersection is slightly inclined to the plane that has a circular section, the section obtained is an *ellipse* (Figure 4.2b). Clearly, the eccentricity of the ellipse depends upon the angle that the plane makes with the circular section. If the plane of intersection is exactly parallel to one side of the cone, the section is a *parabola* (Figure 4.2c) and if inclined beyond this plane the cut section is a *hyperbola* (Figure 4.2d).

These conic sections are all described by the single equation:

$$y^2 = 2r_0x - px^2$$

where r_0 is the radius of curvature of the surface at the vertex, and the type of conic depends upon the value of p as indicated in Figure 4.3.

When the conic sections are rotated about their x-axes, the solid figures that they generate are known as the conicoids. A circle rotated about its x-axis produces the solid of revolution known as the sphere. The sphere is the best-known spectacle lens surface and has a great advantage over other members of the family in that it is easy to produce with simple rotating machinery.

An ellipse rotated about its x-axis produces an *ellipsoid*. If the major axis of the ellipse is horizontal, the solid is referred to as a prolate ellipsoid. If the minor axis is horizontal, the solid is referred to as an oblate ellipsoid. When a parabola is rotated about the x-axis it generates a *paraboloid* and a hyperbola generates a *hyperboloid*.

The advantages that these other conicoids confer when compared with a spherical surface are three-fold. Firstly, their tangential power changes as the point under consideration on the surface moves away from the vertex of the curve. This is most easily understood by imagining how the reading given by a lens measure would vary as the instrument slides over the surface. For example, it is easy to see, in the case of the prolate ellipsoidal surface, that the maximum curvature of the surface lies at the vertex and that the tangential surface power decreases as the curve departs from the vertex.

Secondly, at every point on the surface, except at the vertex, there is surface astigmatism that can be used to counteract the aberrational astigmatism of oblique incidence.

Thirdly, the sag of the curve is smaller than that of a spherical surface for the same diameter, which enables thinner lenses to be produced.

The sag, x, of a conicoid over a chord diameter $2y$ may be found from the expression:

$$x = y^2/[\,r_0 + \sqrt{(r_0{}^2 - py^2)}\,]$$

For example, a convex spherical curve of power +6.00D on CR39 material of refractive index 1.498 has a radius of curvature of $498/6 = 83.0$mm and a sag of 7.74mm over a 70mm diameter. This value can be found from the above expression, substituting the value of 1.0 for p, since the surface in this case is spherical.

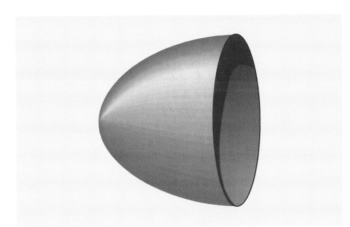

Figure 4.1   Aspherical surface – prolate ellipsoid

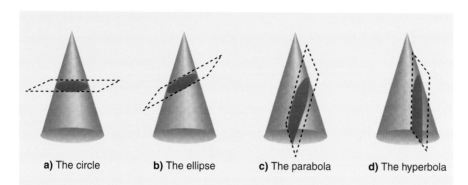

Figure 4.2   Conic sections

a) The circle   **b)** The ellipse   **c)** The parabola   **d)** The hyperbola

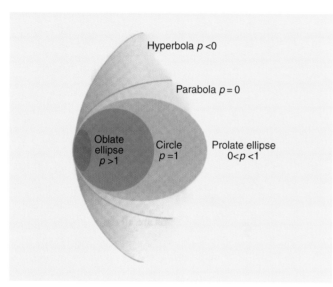

Figure 4.3   The conic sections. Significance of value of *p*:
p > 1, oblate ellipse
p = 1, circle
0 < *p* < 1, prolate ellipse
0 < *p* = 0, parabola
0 < *p* < 0, hyperbola

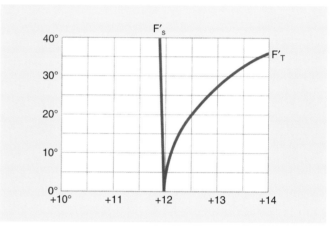

Figure 4.4   Field diagram for +12.00D lens made with spherical surfaces $n = 1.498$, $F_2 = -3.00$, $t = 10$mm, centre of rotation distance (CRD) = 25mm. Note that for a 20° rotation of the eye, the effective Rx is +12.00/+0.50 and at 30°, the effective Rx is +11.93/+1.37

If the spherical surface is replaced by a convex hyperboloid with a *p*-value of –2.0, but otherwise of the same power at the vertex, then the radius of curvature at the vertex remains 83.0mm and the sag reduces to 6.82mm over a diameter of 70mm.

In the design of spectacle lenses we are concerned with the aberrations that occur when the eye, rotating behind the lens, views through extra-axial points on the lens, that is, points removed from the optical centre. It is shown in Chapter 2 that the most significant aberration, in the case of spectacle lenses, is oblique astigmatism.

Aspheric lenses for the correction of aphakia

It is also pointed out in Chapter 2 that spectacle lens powers over about +7.00D cannot be made free from oblique astigmatism when confined to the use of spherical surfaces. This fact is demonstrated neatly by Tscherning's Ellipses for distance vision point-focal lenses, illustrated in Figures 2.9 and 2.10.

The field diagram illustrated in Figure 4.4 shows the off-axis performance of a +12.00D lens made in a form that employs spherical surfaces. The increase in tangential power of the lens and the large amount of aberrational astigmatism can be read from the diagram.

When the eye views through the optical centre, the vergence in the refracted pencil that leaves the lens is the prescribed value, +12.00D. When the eye begins to rotate through 10°, 20°, 30°, and so on, from the optical axis there is a dramatic change in the vergence of this refracted pencil. This is indicated by the curves shown as F'_T and F'_S in the field diagram, which represent the tangential and sagittal oblique vertex sphere powers of the lens, in other words, the real off-axis effect of the lens upon the eye.

The sagittal power remains about +12.00D, but the tangential power can be seen to increase, reaching about +14.00D at 35° from the optical axis. This ocular rotation corresponds to the eye viewing through a point about 17mm from the optical centre of the lens. At 35°, the real effect of this lens form with spherical surfaces is +11.91 with a +2.00 cylinder, and certainly not the +12.00 sphere intended. At this point, the lens exhibits 2.00D of unwanted astigmatism.

Ideally, the oblique vertex sphere powers should remain +12.00 for all zones of the lens. Clearly, if the subject's distance prescription is +12.00D, when wearing this spherical lens form the maximum visual acuity will be obtained only in a small zone around the optical axis. The aberrations impose a limit on the field in which the subject obtains optimum vision.

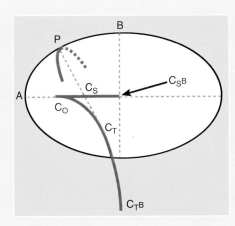

Figure 4.5 Evolutes for the section AB of an ellipsoidal surface: A is the vertex of the curve; C_0 is the centre of curvature of the surface at the vertex; and AC_0 is the radius of curvature of the surface at the vertex, r_0.
P is a point on the curve; PC_T is the radius of curvature of the surface at point P in the tangential meridian, which is the plane of the diagram; C_T lies on the evolute, C_0C_TB, which is the locus of the tangential centres of curvature of the surface between points A and B.
PC_S is the radius of curvature of the surface at point P in the sagittal meridian, which lies at right angles to the plane of the diagram. C_S lies on the evolute, C_0C_SB, which is the locus of the sagittal centres of curvature of the surface between points A and B

When the designer is not limited to the use of spherical surfaces, oblique astigmatism can be eliminated to provide a large increase in the field of useful vision. This is achieved by employing a surface that itself is astigmatic, the surface astigmatism varying in just the right way to counteract the astigmatism of oblique incidence.

One of the simplest surfaces to provide the correct variation in neutralizing astigmatism is the ellipsoid. It is easy to see how such a surface introduces neutralizing astigmatism by considering how the surface alters in shape as the eye rotates away from the pole of the curve. Figure 4.5 illustrates the instantaneous centres of curvature for the point P on the surface of a convex prolate ellipsoidal surface. The evolutes for the section AB are also shown and it can be seen that both the tangential and the sagittal radii of curvature for the surface increase, that is, the tangential and the sagittal surface powers decrease, with the tangential radius changing at a faster rate than the sagittal radius. Inspection of the field diagram in Figure 4.4 confirms that this is just what is required to combat the aberrational astigmatism for this form of lens – that is, a greater decrease in the tangential power of the lens.

By careful choice of eccentricity for the ellipsoid it is possible to eliminate oblique astigmatism for wide zones of the lens.

Aspheric lenses of the type needed to correct aphakia usually employ a convex prolate ellipsoidal surface to eliminate aberrational astigmatism in the post-cataract range of prescriptions.

The improvement in off-axis performance can be judged from the field diagram shown in Figure 4.6, which illustrates the zonal variation in oblique vertex sphere powers for a point-focal +12.00D lens made with a –3.00D back curve and a suitably chosen ellipsoidal front surface with a p-value of +0.65. It can be seen for this design that the tangential and sagittal oblique vertex sphere powers remain the same for all zones out to 40°, but

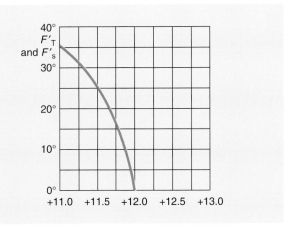

Figure 4.6 Field diagram for +12.00D lens made with convex prolate ellipsoidal surface: $p = +0.65$, $n = 1.498$, $F_2 = -3.00$, $t = 10$mm, CRD = 25mm.
Note that for a 20° rotation of the eye, the effective Rx is +11.68DS and at 30°, the effective Rx is +11.31DS

the lens performance is by no means perfect. The mean oblique power, which now is the same as the tangential and sagittal oblique vertex sphere powers, drops off rapidly as the eye rotates away from the optical axis of the lens.

This loss in power, the mean oblique error (MOE), amounts to almost 1.00D at 35° from the optical axis, but at least the error in off-axis performance is a spherical one. Ideally, the designer would like to be able to increase the marginal power of the aspheric design to provide a constant correction for all zones of the lens.

The large drop in tangential power does provide one advantage for lens powers in this range: there is a worthwhile reduction in distortion compared with the spherical design.

Most of the major lens manufacturers offer CR39 aspheric lenses with convex prolate ellipsoidal surfaces. These series are available in both full-aperture and lenticular form, usually with a 40mm aperture diameter. They can also be obtained in bifocal form with round or D-shape segments. However, the segment surface itself is normally not aspherical and, since it is cast on the ellipsoidal DP surface, the segment tends to be oval in shape rather than circular.

Needless to say, it is important when dispensing these high-power aspheric lenses that they are carefully centred both vertically and horizontally (see Chapter 3), since incorrect centration may well obviate the advantages of the ellipsoidal surface.

Also, note that when these lenses are prescribed for near vision, the loss in power caused by near vision effectivity errors (NVEEs) is exacerbated by the loss in mean oblique image vergence (MOIV) when the eye uses extra-axial zones of the lens. In the case of deep plus lenses with spherical surfaces, there is a gain in MOIV as the eye rotates away from the optical centre of the lens. In effect, the aberrations replace the loss in power caused by NVEE. However, in the case of the aspheric lens, the loss through NVEE is increased by the drop in MOIV. About 1.00D would be lost in the case of an aspheric design that employs a convex prolate ellipsoidal surface.

Needless to say, the aphakic eye has no mechanism to compensate for this loss in power in near vision and it would be to the subject's advantage to increase the prescribed reading addition, by an amount that depends, like the change in NVEE, upon the form of the trial lens used during refraction.

The first aspheric lenses were made in glass by hand-figuring the aspherical surface, such as the Zeiss *Katral* lens (1909), which employed a concave figured surface akin to an oblate ellipsoid, to provide the neutralizing surface astigmatism required to eliminate the positive aberrational astigmatism of oblique incidence. These lenses were individually made to prescription and were, therefore, expensive. Aspheric lenses for the correction of aphakia that employ a convex prolate ellipsoidal surface were really made feasible by the advent of CR39 during the 1950s. Using this plastics material, one glass mould could be used to cast several finished surfaces, greatly reducing the cost of production.

At the end of the 1960s, in the ophthalmic world, the term *aspherical surface* was taken to mean a conicoidal surface of one form or another. In addition to the ellipsoidal surface described above for the post-cataract range of powers, paraboloidal and hyperboloidal surfaces were being used to provide low-distortion magnifiers and better quality subnormal vision aids. Aspheric designs from Combined Optical Industries Ltd are particularly well known in the low vision field and have been in production since the 1950s (Chapter 15).

The equations to conicoidal surfaces are well known and it is not difficult to calculate and assess the performance of a lens that incorporates such a surface.

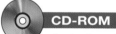

CD-ROM

Aspheric surfaces are considered in more detail on the CD-ROM

Blended lenticulars

During the 1970s several new aspheric lens series appeared with optical performances deliberately compromised towards the edge of the field to produce lenses with improved mechanical characteristics. The mechanical advantages and optical disadvantages of these *blended lenticular* designs are understood most easily by considering the principles of ordinary lenticular lenses. The usual lenticular lens for the correction of aphakia has a central aperture that incorporates the optical correction, surrounded by a carrier or margin of lower power, or even afocal.

Naturally, sharp foveal vision is only possible when the wearer views through the aperture and, in the case of a deep plus lens that has a spherical aperture surface, when the visual axis is close to the optical axis of the lens. Off-axis, the useful field of view is limited by the severe aberrations obtained if spherical surfaces are used.

The carrier, however, which may be afocal, does permit some awareness of objects and movement provided these lie outside the ring scotoma that occurs at the dividing line. Obviously, peripheral vision is important and an essential part of the normal visual function.

During the 1970s, 'aspheric' lenses were introduced in which the dividing line between the aperture and the margin was blended to make it invisible. Removal of the dividing line both improved the appearance of the lens and also increased the field of vision by removing the ring scotoma associated with the abrupt change in power at the edge of the aperture.

The performance of these designs can be understood by considering the female glass mould, shown in Figure 4.7, which is used to mould the convex aperture side of a plastics lenticular.

It can be seen that a concave annulus with its centre of curvature at C_B would blend the aperture curve and marginal curve to produce a continuous surface on the mould. The blending tool must be arranged so that its centre of curvature rotates about Q through a circle of radius QC_B that is concentric with the aperture.

Smoothing and polishing of the blended annulus can be achieved with a floating pad system in which the pads follow the generated curve. The necessary radius of curvature of the blending curve depends upon the width of the blended zone $(y_M - y_A)$ and the radii of curvature of the aperture and marginal curves.[1]

If the width of the blended zone is made too narrow, then the blending curve on the mould becomes convex and the corresponding curve on the cast lens becomes concave, which is undesirable.

The blended zone is of the same form as a barrel-form toroidal surface and as such is, indeed, highly astigmatic. In general, the blended region of the lens cannot provide good vision, which is restricted to the central zone of the design – just as in the case of a normal lenticular lens.

These blended lenticular designs have been described as *zonal aspherics*, and are simply lenticular lenses without a visible dividing line. They have a central power some 3.00 to 6.00D greater than their marginal power. For example, a +10.00D blended lenticular may have a marginal power of just +6.00D, so the design has a power of +10.00D, but the centre thickness, t_c is of a lens of power +6.00D. The field of view is also the same as a +6.00D lens, without the ring scotoma that occurs at the normal lenticular dividing line. Furthermore, at the edge of the lens, where the ring scotoma does occur, it is smaller than would be the case if the central power was maintained to the edge of the lens.

Against these undoubted merits must be offset the obvious disadvantage that the wearer obtains the optimum correction only in the central zone of the lens and must learn to turn the head to view laterally placed objects.

The first zonal aspheric, or blended lenticular, design was introduced in the early 1970s by Dr Robert Welsh, who was one of the first people to recognize the advantages of a thinner full-aperture lens for the correction of aphakia. Known originally as the *Welsh 4-drop Aspheric*, since the zones dropped in power by 4.00D from centre to edge, it was made available in several forms, such as the Signet *Hyperaspheric*, the Sola *Hi-drop* and the *Thi-Aspheric* in high-refractive index glass from Hoya.

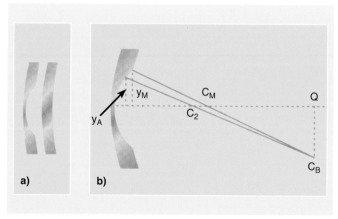

Figure 4.7   Blending the dividing line of a mould for a convex lenticular

Aspheric lenses with polynomial surfaces

Although the optical performance of these designs is a compromise, there can be no reservations about their superior mechanical characteristics. It is not surprising that they attracted the attention of other lens manufacturers.

With the advent of computer-assisted design and computer numerically controlled grinding techniques, it became possible to design and manufacture surfaces of almost any complexity. Surfaces of higher order than the conicoids could be reproduced at a cost that made them viable in ophthalmic lens terms.

By the end of the 1970s, designs with convex polynomial surfaces made an appearance (Figure 4.8). The term *polynomial* is used because the equation to the convex surface is of polynomial form, involving powers of y up to the 10th or 12th degree, for example:

$$x = Ay^2 + By^4 + Cy^6 + Dy^8 + Ey^{10} + \dots$$

(see Chapter 17 for a more detailed discussion of the mathematics of polynomial surfaces).

If the zone AA´ in Figure 4.8 is indistinguishable from, say, a convex prolate ellipsoid, then this zone of the lens would enjoy the same optical properties as a traditional aspheric lens that employs an ellipsoidal surface. Zone AA´ could be free from aberrational astigmatism. It also exhibits less distortion since the tangential surface power within this zone decreases as the eye rotates away from the optical axis.

Zone A´M is seen to be concave in its tangential section. The surface flexes backwards in this region. Since the surface is continuous, however, there is no annular scotoma between the central ellipsoidal zone and the margin.

Zone MM´ has the same purpose as the margin of a lenticular design. It supports the central aperture. If the polynomial surface becomes parallel with the back surface in this region, then the margin is virtually afocal.

The polynomial surface acts in much the same way as the blending process described earlier – but with two very important differences. Firstly, the aspheric zone has excellent optical properties. It does not have the aberrational astigmatism associated with spherical surfaces. Secondly, the blending is concave. It can be imagined that the region between the aspheric aperture and spherical margin of a traditional lenticular has been filled with material to eliminate the dividing line. The result of this is to eliminate the ring scotoma that exists at the edge of every plus lens and the accompanying *jack-in-the-box* effect, which is so annoying to wearers of deep plus lenses.

The optical performance of a post-cataract lens that employs a convex polynomial surface can be judged from the field diagram in Figure 4.9, which shows the variation in tangential and sagittal oblique vertex sphere powers for a +12.00D lens used for distance vision. The lens has been designed to provide an optical zone of 40mm diameter within which the tangential error is negligible out to 25° and the aberrational astigmatism very well corrected out to 30°, which is about 20mm from the optical axis. Beyond the optical zone the tangential power falls off rapidly as the surface begins to change direction.

The first ophthalmic lens design to be introduced that employed this type of convex polynomial surface was the *Ful-Vue Aspheric* cataract lens produced by the American Optical Corporation in 1978. It was available in both single-vision and bifocal form, the bifocal version incorporating a 22mm diameter segment on the convex surface.

Other manufacturers were to follow suit in the next few years, such as Essilor with their *Omega Aspheric* design in 1981. The convex surface of the Omega is a figured ellipsoid that has an optical zone of 43mm diameter (zone AA´ in Figure 4.8) and is indistinguishable from the ellipsoidal surface used for their traditional aspheric lenticular. Such a surface could be produced by blending the ellipsoidal aperture curve with a spherical margin. The *blending* zone, A´M, is about 10mm in width and is designed to blend the aperture curve with the peripheral zone MM´, which

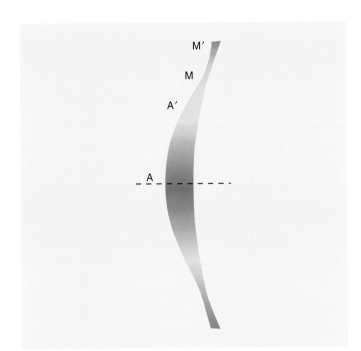

Figure 4.8 A post-cataract lens design with a convex polynomial surface

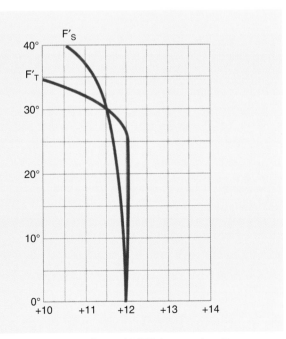

Figure 4.9 Field diagram for a +12.00D lens made with a convex polynomial surface. Note that for a 20° rotation of the eye, the effective Rx is +11.75/+0.25 and at 30°, the effective Rx is +11.50DS

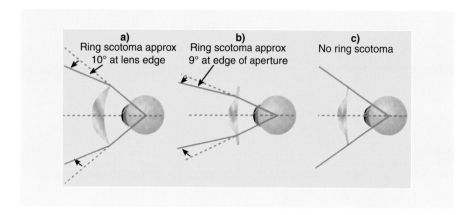

Figure 4.10 Comparison of aspheric post-cataract design lenses of power +12.00: (a) Full-aperture aspheric lens with a convex prolate ellipsoidal surface; (b) aspheric lenticular with 40mm aperture and convex ellipsoidal aperture curve; (c) aspheric lens with convex polynomial surface

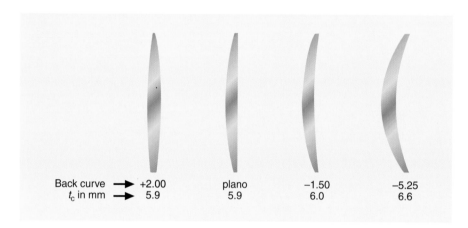

Figure 4.11 Comparison of centre thickness, t_c, of +4.00D lenses made in CR39, 70mm in diameter, with edge thickness 1.0mm, in various forms

forms the margin of the design. A bifocal version is also available with a 22mm diameter segment incorporated on the polynomial surface.

Similar designs are available from Zeiss, the *Clarlet Aphal*, and Rodenstock, the *Perfastar*.

Polynomial lens designs combine the advantages of both lenticular lenses and full-aperture lens designs (Figure 4.10). The lenses are thinner and lighter than full-aperture designs for just the same reasons as a lenticular lens, but there is no visible dividing line between the aperture and the margin. This is of particular benefit when strong plus lenses need to be dispensed in frames with large eye sizes. The wearer obtains a wide central field within which the aberrations, which are normally severe in the case of post-cataract lenses, are exceptionally well corrected, together with a useful peripheral field with no ring scotoma between them.

Aspheric lenses for the normal power range

So far, we have considered the use of aspherical surfaces for high-power plus lenses beyond the range of powers that can be corrected for aberrational astigmatism with spherical surfaces. In recent years, aspherical surfaces have been employed on lenses of low power, as are required for the usual range of prescriptions.

In 1980, the author obtained patents[2] for lenses in the power range +7.00 to –20.00D for a series of spectacle lenses that incorporate a hyperboloidal curve for the major surface of the lens, the major surface being the convex surface for plus powers and the concave surface for minus lenses. The use of aspheric forms for the low- to medium-power range allows the production of thinner and lighter lenses for the normal range of prescriptions.

The reduction in thickness is the result of a two-stage process. First, the lens is made much flatter in form by employing a shallower base curve. For example, the centre thicknesses of a series of +4.00D lenses made in CR39 material at 70mm diameter and with edge thicknesses of 1.0mm in the forms indicated have the centre thicknesses shown in Figure 4.11.

It can be seen that, simply by flattening the lens form, we obtain a saving in centre thickness. The flatter the lens, the thinner it becomes. If the lens is made with a –1.50 base curve instead of the usual –5.25 inside curve necessary to make the lens point-focal, a saving in centre thickness of 0.6mm is obtained.

Needless to say, this flatter form does not have good optical properties. It is afflicted with positive aberrational astigmatism when the eye rotates to view through off-axis portions of the lens.

Just how poor the off-axis performance becomes through flattening the lens form is shown in Figure 4.12. Figure 4.12a illustrates a field diagram for a +4.00D lens made with a –5.25 back curve and it can be seen that the tangential and sagittal oblique vertex sphere powers are the same for all directions of gaze. This form is free from oblique astigmatism and represents a point-focal form for this power. Figure 4.12b illustrates the off-axis performance of a +4.00D lens made with a –1.50 back surface power using spherical surfaces and it is seen that the real effect of the lens when the eye has rotated 35° from the optical axis is +4.05/+0.87. Clearly, there is almost 1.00D of aberrational astigmatism 35° from the optical axis for this very shallow bending. However, to eliminate the aberrational astigmatism an aspherical surface can be employed with a form such that it introduces negative surface

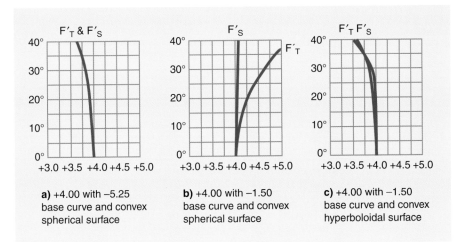

Figure 4.12   Comparison of off-axis performance of +4.00D lenses made in different forms

a) +4.00 with −5.25 base curve and convex spherical surface

b) +4.00 with −1.50 base curve and convex spherical surface

c) +4.00 with −1.50 base curve and convex hyperboloidal surface

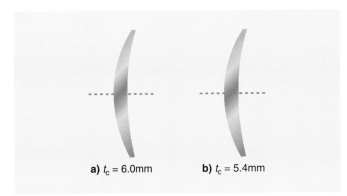

a) t_c = 6.0mm   b) t_c = 5.4mm

Figure 4.13   Comparison of centre thickness, t_c, of +4.00D lenses made in spherical and hyperbolic forms

astigmatism to neutralize the astigmatism of oblique incidence. A correctly chosen aspherical surface completely neutralizes the aberrational astigmatism that arises from oblique incidence.

Figure 4.12c illustrates the off-axis performance of the +4.00D lens made with a −1.50 back surface power and a convex aspherical surface with a p-value chosen to neutralize the astigmatism of oblique incidence. This form has the same oblique vertex sphere powers as the point-focal form with spherical surfaces that has the performance depicted in Figure 4.12a. The surface is a convex hyperboloid with a p-value of −1.8 and it can be seen that the field diagram is almost identical to that shown in Figure 4.12a for the design with spherical surfaces.

The second stage of the thinning process occurs since, for a given diameter, the required aspherical surface has a smaller sag than a spherical surface of the same vertex radius. The smaller front surface sag causes a further reduction in the centre thickness of the lens.

The original patent proposed that a hyperboloid should be employed for the major surface of the lens, since the rate of flattening of a hyperboloid is just what is required to neutralize aberrational astigmatism. Figure 4.13 shows just what additional saving in centre thickness is achieved when the convex spherical surface is replaced by a suitable convex hyperboloidal surface with its asphericity chosen to restore the off-axis performance of the lens. A further saving of 0.6mm is achieved for a 70mm diameter when the spherical surface is made aspherical to eliminate the aberrational astigmatism that arises from oblique incidence.

The aspheric lens form has a total saving in centre thickness of 1.2mm when compared with the traditional spherical form.

Needless to say, any higher order aspherical surface could be used but, in practice, it would not depart significantly from a hyperboloid since this curve regulates the astigmatism at the correct rate.

The optical performance of an aspheric design can be made to match any design philosophy. The lens may be made point-focal, just like the designs illustrated in Figure 4.12, or it may be made in Percival form or, more typically, a compromise bending between these two forms to provide a reasonable performance over a wide range of fitting distances, as discussed in Chapter 2.

An even greater saving in thickness is obtained when a higher refractive index material is used. If the same power base curve is used the saving is two-fold. Firstly, there is the obvious reduction in the sags of the curves, since longer radii of curvature are employed. Secondly, since the use of the same power base curve on a higher refractive index material requires a longer radius of curvature at the vertex, r_0, effectively, the lens is flatter still and requires greater asphericity on the convex surface to restore the off-axis performance.

This is illustrated in Figure 4.14, which shows how the centre thickness of a 70mm diameter +4.00D lens reduces when made in 1.60 and 1.70 index materials. The asphericity of the convex surfaces indicated in Figure 4.14 is chosen to provide the same off-axis performance for each lens.

Another important advantage of these low-power aspheric designs for hypermetropia can be gleaned from Figure 4.14. The original best-form +4.00D design with spherical surfaces required a centre thickness of 6.6mm to obtain an edge thickness of 1.0mm at 70mm diameter. If this uncut lens is edged down to a finished diameter of 50mm, it will have an edge thickness of 4.1mm, which is not acceptable for a lens of this power.

The aspheric design made in 1.60 index material, on the other hand, has a centre thickness of 4.5mm and would have an edge thickness of 2.6mm when edged down to a finished diameter of 50mm. The aspheric design lends itself far better to a system of supply of large-diameter plus uncut lenses that need to be edged to smaller diameters, depending upon the choice of shape and size of the lens.

Aspheric lenses for myopia

The principle of flattening a curved lens form to make it thinner and then making one surface aspherical to restore the off-axis performance of the flatter form lens can be applied equally to

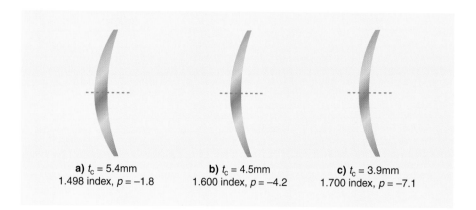

Figure 4.14 Comparison of centre thickness, t_c, of +4.00D lenses made in different media

a) t_c = 5.4mm
1.498 index, p = −1.8

b) t_c = 4.5mm
1.600 index, p = −4.2

c) t_c = 3.9mm
1.700 index, p = −7.1

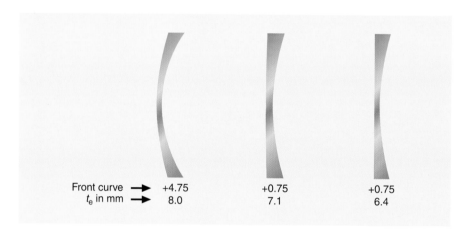

Figure 4.15 Comparison of edge thickness, t_e, for −4.00D lenses made in CR39, 70mm in diameter, with centre thickness 2.0mm, in various forms

Front curve → +4.75 +0.75 +0.75
t_e in mm → 8.0 7.1 6.4

minus lenses. For example, the reduction in thickness obtained for −4.00D lenses made in CR39 material with uncut diameters of 70mm and centre thickness of 2.0mm is shown in Figure 4.15.

It can be seen that the traditional best-form design made using spherical surfaces might employ a +4.75D base curve, when the resultant edge thickness would be 8.0mm. Then, flattening the base curve to +0.75D produces an edge thickness of 7.1mm, which is a saving of 0.9mm at the edge.

Finally, making aspheric the flatter form lens to provide the same off-axis performance as the best-form spherical design results in an edge thickness of 6.4mm, this is a further saving of 0.7mm – the final aspheric design being 1.6mm thinner than the traditional spherical form.

The author's original proposal for the correction of myopia was to employ a concave hyperboloidal surface, but lens manufacturers prefer to make the convex surface of the lens aspherical, since it is easier to incorporate the cylinder on the concave surface as a minus-base toric.

Several aspheric minus lens series, therefore, incorporate a convex aspherical surface, the purpose of which is to increase the convexity of the front surface towards the edge of the lens (Figure 4.16). Typically, a convex oblate ellipsoid might be used as its tangential curvature increases at a faster rate than that of a spherical surface of the same vertex radius, as illustrated in Figure 4.16. Usually, however, a two- or three-term polynomial convex curve is chosen, since this does not place a restriction on the maximum diameter of the lens.

For higher power minus lenses, the principle of blending has been applied to the workshop-flattened lenticular lens to produce a blended concave lenticular lens with a truly invisible dividing line. These blended lenticulars for myopia, such as the *Wrobel Super-lenti* and the Rodenstock *Lentilux* designs, enjoy excellent cosmetic properties and allow very high minus prescriptions, in excess of −20.00D, to be dispensed in relatively thin and lightweight form.

Distortion in aspheric lenses

The aberration distortion causes a change in shape of the image of an object produced by an optical system. Typically, a plus spectacle lens with spherical surfaces causes an image of a square object viewed through the lens to take on a characteristic pincushion shape.

In the case of high-power plus lenses, such as those considered earlier for the correction of aphakia, as pointed out earlier, the use of an aspherical surface reduces the amount of pincushion distortion that the wearer experiences. The reduction in distortion occurs because there is a significant reduction in the tangential power of the deep convex surface when the eye rotates away from the vertex of the curve. In the case of a convex spherical surface, the tangential surface power increases as the eye uses zones of the lens further and further from the optical centre of the lens. This is because the angles of incidence and refraction, and thus the deviation produced by the surface, increase as the ocular rotation increases.

In the case of lenses for the normal power range, however, there is no significant improvement in the distortion exhibited by the lens. Indeed, the distortion is very slightly worse than it is for the more steeply curved traditional lenses that employ spherical surfaces.

The tangential surface power of the front surface of a lens is given by the relationship:

$$F_{IT} = n \, \sin(i - i')/r_{IT} \, \cos^2 i'$$

where i and i' are the angles of incidence and refraction at the front surface and r_{1T} is the tangential radius of curvature of the surface at the point in question. Table 4.1 lists the tangential front surface powers and the distortion for the +12.00D post-cataract lenses considered in detail earlier in this chapter.

Inspection of Table 4.1 shows quite clearly that, in the case of the spherical lens, the tangential surface power increases quite significantly as the eye uses zones further from the optical axis and that this increase is accompanied by a large increase in distortion. In the case of the aspheric lens, the tangential power of the convex prolate ellipsoidal surface decreases as the surface flattens away from the vertex of the curve. The surface is still undercorrected for spherical aberration, which indicates that it remains afflicted with pincushion distortion, but the distortion is considerably reduced when compared with the spherical surface.

Table 4.2 lists the tangential front surface powers and the distortion for the +4.00D lenses made with –1.50D back curves in the spherical and aspheric forms considered above.

Inspection of Table 4.2 shows that the distortion of the flatter spherical lens form (Form 1) is considerably worse than the best-form spherical lens (Form 3), which indicates that the deviation of the light is greater for the flat-form lens. When the front curve is made aspherical to neutralize the oblique astigmatism of the flat-form lens, the reduction in the tangential power of the front surface indicated for Form 2 brings about a reduction in distortion almost to the same level as that exhibited by the traditional spherical lens.

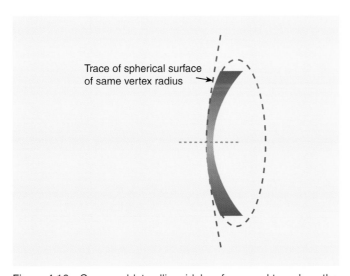

Trace of spherical surface of same vertex radius

Figure 4.16 Convex oblate ellipsoidal surface used to reduce the edge thickness of a minus lens. Such a surface introduces positive surface astigmatism to neutralize the negative astigmatism of oblique incidence that arises from the flat-form lens

When a suitable target, such as graph paper, is viewed through an aspheric lens of moderate power, the lens having been turned back-to-front and held at arm's length, the lens exhibits less distortion when used as a spectacle magnifier than as a traditional spherical lens. However, under these circumstances, the entrance pupil of the system is not in the same position as when the lens is mounted close to the eye and used as a spectacle lens. One cannot deduce from this demonstration that an aspheric lens exhibits less distortion than a spherical lens. Table 4.2 indicates quite clearly for the forms under consideration that it does not, and it is important to bear this in mind, and to be careful in what claims are made to patients when using aspheric lens demonstrators of this kind! It would be very easy for the client to infer that there is less distortion if an aspheric design is chosen.

Choice of aspheric base curve

The possibility of using an aspherical surface offers another degree of freedom in the search for the optimum form of lens for a given prescription. When the designer is restricted to the use of spherical surfaces, the sole freedom is the bending of the lens, but the use of an aspherical surface frees the designer from traditional forms, and enables a combination of bending and asphericity to be employed to improve off-axis performance. As a general rule, the designer could choose any form for a given power and then determine the asphericity required for that particular choice of bending to eliminate, for example, oblique astigmatism.

An important aspect of aspheric lens design is to select the correct asphericity for the given degree of bending for each lens power. When the original lens manufacturer is able to provide finished uncuts to the glazing laboratory, the correct combination of asphericity and curve is obtained automatically, since the manufacturer will faithfully comply with the design requirements. However, when a speedy supply is required, it is not always convenient to wait for the original manufacturer to produce lenses to individual prescription requirements. It is commonplace for prescription houses to stock a series of semi-finished lenses from which they can select a blank with a suitable base curve and complete the concave surface to obtain an individual prescription. In the case of aspheric lenses it is essential that the base curve interval is small; certainly the interval should not be more than about 1.00D.

A typical series of base curves and the group of powers that each curve is designed to cover is shown in Table 4.3. Note in particular the close interval of the curves for the plus power range. It can be seen that each base curve is designed to be used for a small power range. This is an essential feature of aspheric lens design since, in cases where there is a difference in power between the two eyes, such that different base curves are necessary, it is essential that the design characteristics of each power do not differ too widely.

Table 4.1 Comparison of tangential front surface powers and distortion for +12.00D lenses made in spherical and aspherical forms. Each lens has a –3.00 base curve and a front surface power at the vertex of +13.63D. The p-value of the aspherical surface for the aspheric lens is +0.65

Lens zone (°)	Spherical lens		Aspheric lens	
	F_{1T}	Distortion (%)	F_{1T}	Distortion (%)
40	+14.21	20.84	+11.63	14.45
30	+13.88	10.22	+12.42	7.18
20	+13.73	4.15	+13.06	2.93
10	+13.65	0.99	+13.49	0.70
0	+13.63	0.00	+13.63	0.00

Table 4.2   Comparison of tangential front surface powers and distortion for +4.00D lenses made in spherical and aspheric forms. Forms 1 and 2 have −1.50 base curves and the front surface powers at the vertex of these two forms are given for the 0° lens zone. The *p*-value for the aspherical surface of the aspheric lens is −1.8. Form 3 is the traditional steeply curved point-focal form with spherical surfaces with the performance that the aspheric design is to match

Lens zone (°)	Form 1 Spherical −1.50 base		Form 2 Aspheric −1.50 base		Form 3 Spherical −5.25 base	
	F_{1T}	Distortion (%)	F_{1T}	Distortion (%)	F_{1T}	Distortion (%)
40	+5.82	11.88	+4.62	8.79	+9.07	8.18
30	+5.67	5.66	+5.00	4.31	+9.01	4.11
20	+5.52	2.24	+5.23	1.75	+8.95	1.69
10	+5.42	0.53	+5.35	0.41	+8.95	1.69
0	+5.38	0.00	+5.39	0.00	+8.88	0.00

Table 4.3   Base curve range for a typical series of aspheric lenses

Nominal base curve	Typical power range
+0.50	−10.00 to −5.50
+1.50	−5.25 to −2.50
+2.50	−2.25 to −0.25
+3.50	Plano to +1.00
+4.00	+1.25 to +2.00
+5.00	+2.25 to +4.00
+6.00	+4.25 to +5.25
+7.00	+5.50 to +6.00
+8.00	+6.25 to +7.00

Although, for obvious proprietary reasons, an exact mathematical description of these curves cannot be given, the +1.50D base curve does not differ markedly from the asphere described by the series:

$$x = Ay^2 + By^4 + Cy^6$$

where $A = +1.14 \times 10^{-3}$, $B = +1.69 \times 10^{-7}$ and $C = +5.01 \times 10^{-11}$.

Figure 4.17 illustrates a field diagram for a −4.00D lens made using this curve, from which it can be seen that the off-axis performance is remarkable for such a shallow-form lens.

CD-ROM

Aspheric surfaces for myopia are considered in more detail on the CD-ROM

Atoric lenses

Aspherical surfaces of the type described so far provide excellent imaging properties for any lens power, provided the prescription is spherical. Clearly, in the case of astigmatic prescriptions, the asphericity of, say, a conicoidal surface can only be correct for one principal meridian of the lens. The other principal meridian requires a different eccentricity, or different *p*-value, for the power along this meridian.

For example, in the case of the prescription +2.00/+2.00 × 180, which has been made as an aspheric lens with a −1.50 base curve, the principal meridians of the lens have powers of +4.00 and +2.00. As already pointed out, the +4.00 meridian that requires the −1.50 base curve would be point-focal if the front curve has a hyperbolic section with a *p*-value of −1.8. Accurate trigonometric

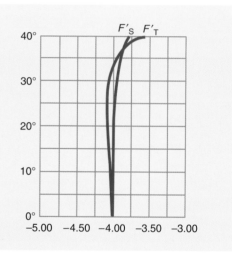

Figure 4.17   Field diagram for a −4.00D lens made in CR39 material with a convex polynomial surface of the form, $x = Ay^2 + By^4 + Cy^6$

ray tracing shows that the +2.00 meridian with a cross-curve of −3.50 would need a *p*-value of +0.45 if this meridian is also to remain point focal for the 35° zone of the lens. Such a surface is depicted in Figure 4.18, which illustrates a convex *atoroidal* surface in which the 'toricity' is caused by a change in asphericity from one meridian to a second meridian at 90° to the first. It should be understood that the surface illustrated in Figure 4.18 has no cylindrical power in the usual sense of the term, since the curvatures of the surface at the vertex along the two principal meridians are identical. The cylindrical component of the lens is provided in the usual way by grinding a toroidal surface on the back of the lens. One might argue that the term *atoroidal* is not really a good description for this type of surface and a better definition for the surface might be a *non-rotationally symmetric aspherical surface*. However, this term also describes many other forms of surface, including progressive power surfaces, and the term *atoroidal* seems to have entered the literature.

Such a surface is employed for the Zeiss *Hypal* series of lenses when dispensed for astigmatic prescriptions. For spherical prescriptions the convex surface of the *Hypal* design is simply an aspherical surface that is virtually indistinguishable from a conicoid.

A general equation to any meridian of such a surface inclined at θ to the principal meridian, which is parallel to the concave base curve meridian (on the other surface of the lens), the convex

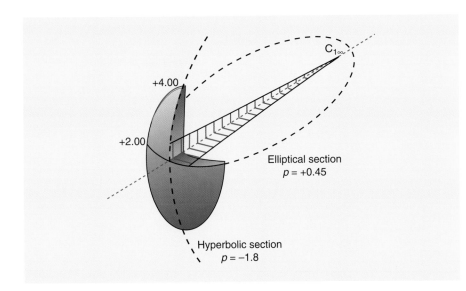

Figure 4.18 Non-rotationally symmetric aspherical surface such as that used for the Zeiss *Hypal* designs. This convex aspherical surface was introduced by Carl Zeiss in 1986 for the *Hypal* lens, which was the first low-power aspheric design on the UK market (1987). In the case of spherical prescriptions, the convex surface is simply aspherical, that is rotationally symmetrical, and virtually indistinguishable from a hyperboloid. For astigmatic prescriptions, however, the principal meridians of the convex surface have different asphericities, each one apposite for the principal power in question. In the case of the lens illustrated here, the asphericity is greater in the vertical meridian (power +4.00D) than in the horizontal meridian (power +2.00D)

surface having a power F_0 at its vertex and asphericity p_B along the base curve meridian, can be written in the form:

$$x = Ay^2 + By^4 + Cy^6 + Dy^8 + \ldots$$

where:

$$A = F_0/N + \left(N^2 - PF_0^2y^2\right)$$
$$N = 10^3 \times (n-1)$$
$$P = p_B - (p_B - p_C)\theta/90$$

The values of B, C, D, etc., and the value of p_C, which is the value of the asphericity for the section of the convex surface parallel with the cross curve that is worked on the concave surface of the lens, are determined by accurate trigonometric ray tracing.

A true atoroidal surface with principal vertex curvatures that differ by the required cylindrical component, in addition to a variation in asphericity for the two principal meridians, is also employed on modern spectacle lens forms.

One proposal for how such a surface might be generated mathematically is disclosed in US Patent 5083859, granted to the author in 1991. The equation to any meridian of the atoroidal surface, inclined at θ to the base curve meridian, which is expressed by its absolute power, F_B, and asphericity, p_B, is given by:

$$x = Ay^2 + By^4 + Cy^6 + Dy^8 + \ldots$$

where:

$$A = Q/N + \surd\left(N^2 - PQ^2y^2\right)$$
$$Q = F_B \cos^2\theta + F_C \sin^2\theta$$

N and P have the same meanings as before. Once more, the values of B, C, D, etc., and the value of p_C, which is the value of the asphericity for the absolute value of the cross curve, F_C, are determined by accurate trigonometric ray tracing.

Atoroidal surfaces of this type have recently become available from Zeiss and Rodenstock to complement the front surfaces of their aspheric progressive power lenses (see below), but, interestingly, they are not the first in the ophthalmic field.

Using their CNC machinery, originally developed for the production of *Varilux* progressive power lenses, Essel Optical Company (now Essilor International) introduced a design in 1970 that

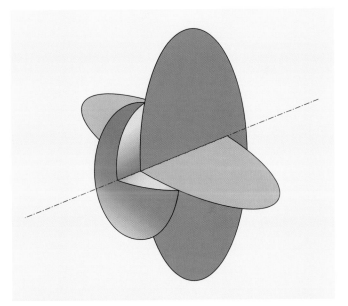

Figure 4.19 Atoral lens. This toric lens with an atoroidal surface was introduced in 1970 by Essel Optical Company (now Essilor International) to improve the optical performance of deep plus astigmatic lenses, required for the correction of aphakia. Each principal meridian of the concave surface is of oblate elliptical cross-section; the *p*-values differ from a minimum along the base curve to a maximum along the cross curve. A progressive version was also made available, the *Atoral Variplas*. This principle was reintroduced by Zeiss in the *Gradal HS* OSD and Rodenstock in the new *Multigressiv* design (1996)

minimized aberrational astigmatism along each principal meridian of a toric lens for the correction of aphakia. This *Atoral* lens design employed a non-rotationally symmetrical surface in which the principal sections were oblate ellipses of different eccentricities along each principal meridian. Between the two principal meridians the eccentricities varied from a minimum along one power meridian to a maximum along the other power meridian (Figure 4.19). The surface was also employed in the *Atoral Variplas* design, a progressive power lens for the correction of aphakia. This concept was revived recently by both Zeiss and Rodenstock, whose progressive designs employ an atoroidal concave surface to optimize the optical performance of astigmatic progressive lenses.

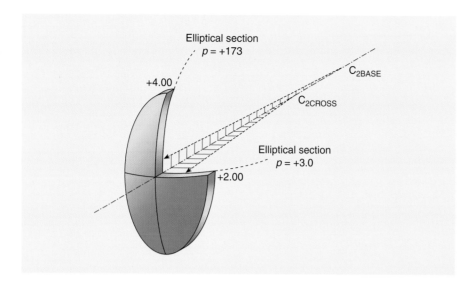

Figure 4.20 Concave atoroidal surface of the type used for the Zeiss *Gradal* and the Rodenstock *Multigressiv* lenses. These state-of-the-art designs have convex progressive surfaces and, in the case of astigmatic prescriptions, concave atoroidal surfaces. Not only do the base and cross curve powers vary along the principal meridians of the lens, but also the asphericities of these meridians are optimized for the principal powers

As mentioned above, the *Hypal* designs from Carl Zeiss employed a non-rotationally symmetrical surface on the convex side of the lenses, in which each principal meridian is indistinguishable from a hyperbolic section, the *p*-values being apposite for each principal power (see Figure 4.18). Recently, Zeiss introduced a concave atoroidal surface that is used in conjunction with a convex progressive surface to provide a progressive power lens with even better imaging properties for astigmatic prescriptions (Figure 4.20). Their *Gradal HS* progressive designs are now all available with Optimum Surface Design (OSD), that is, an atoroidal surface applied automatically to all astigmatic prescriptions in their aspheric series. The *Hypal* single vision design now also employs this type of atoroidal surface.

Rodenstock has also introduced an atoric progressive power lens, their *Multigressiv* design, of which the concave atoroidal surface is optimized for each individual prescription also (Figure 4.20).

In 2001, Hoya introduced a new series of aspheric lenses in their high-index, 1.71 plastics material, Teslalid. The *Nulux LX* lens series was specifically designed to take into account that the lens is likely to be decentred before the eye, for example, to obtain the correct centration for the wearer. In the optimization of the aspherical surfaces in the series, they have taken a decentration of some 2 mm into account.

The Nulux aspheric lens designs employ convex polynomial surfaces[4] of the form:

$$z = y^2 / [r_0 + \sqrt{(r_0^2 - py^2)}] + a_2 y^2 + a_3 y^3$$
$$+ a_4 y^4 + a_5 y^5 + a_6 y^6 + a_7 y^7 + a_8 y^8$$

In the case of the +6.00D lens, the front surface has a radius (r_0) of 79.474 mm, $p = 1.0$, and values for the coefficients are given[4] as:

$a_2 = 0.0$

$a_3 = 0.0$

$a_4 = +3.39527 \times 10^{-7}$

$a_5 = -1.08334 \times 10^{-7}$

$a_6 = +4.00919 \times 10^{-9}$

$a_7 = -6.7018 \times 10^{-11}$

$a_8 = +4.40787 \times 10^{-13}$

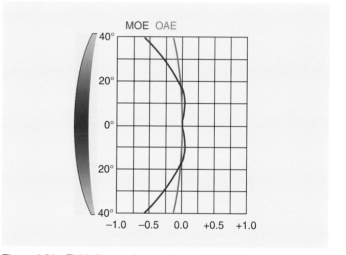

Figure 4.21 Field diagram for a centred +6.00D *Nulux LX* lens made with the convex aspherical surface described in the text, showing plots of the oblique astigmatic error (OAE) and mean oblique error (MOE)

In the case of the −6.00D lens, the front surface has a radius (r_0) of 1002.333 mm, $p = 1.0$ and values for the coefficients are given[4] as:

$a_2 = 0.0$

$a_3 = 0.0$

$a_4 = -4.72996 \times 10^{-7}$

$a_5 = +1.33922 \times 10^{-7}$

$a_6 = -6.36412 \times 10^{-9}$

$a_7 = +1.22833 \times 10^{-10}$

$a_8 = -8.8095 \times 10^{-13}$

Figure 4.21 shows a field diagram for the aspheric *Nulux LX* design of power +6.00D lens made in Teslalid 1.71 index material with the aspherical surface data given above, assuming that the philosophy of the design revealed in the patent is maintained. The axial thickness of the lens is 6.0 mm, and since the lens is flatter in form, its back vertex is assumed to be mounted 26 mm in front of the eye's centre of rotation. The field diagram shows the oblique

Table 4.4   Aberrational data for aspheric *Nulux LX*+6.00D lens ($n=1.71$, $F_1=+8.93$, $c_t=6.0$mm, CRD=26mm)

Ocular rotation (°)	OAE	MOE	TCA (Δ)	Distortion (%)
40	−0.18	−0.66	0.41	+12.6
35	−0.10	−0.42	0.35	+9.0
30	−0.03	−0.26	0.29	+6.3
25	+0.02	−0.12	0.23	+4.3
20	+0.06	−0.03	0.18	+2.7
15	+0.07	+0.03	0.13	+1.5
10	+0.05	+0.04	0.09	+0.7
5	+0.02	+0.02	0.04	+0.2
0	0.00	0.00	0.00	0.0

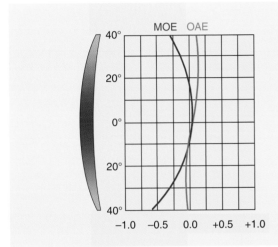

Figure 4.22 Field diagram (showing OAE and MOE) for a decentred +6.00D *Nulux LX* lens made with the convex aspherical surface described in the text. The lens has been decentred 2mm in the vertical meridian. Note the asymmetry in the field plots

astigmatic error (OAE) and the mean oblique error (MOE). The data from which the graphs were plotted are given in Table 4.4.

It is seen in Figure 4.21 that the MOE is positive in sign at the centre of the lens, becoming negative beyond about 17° on either side of the optical axis (see Table 4.4). The aberrational astigmatism is very small, and the design is point focal at about 27° on either side of the optical axis.

The designers of the *Nulux* lens set out to improve the zonal performance of the design when it is decentred before the eye. To achieve this they adjusted the values of the coefficients to the surface to allow the MOE to become positive in the central zone of the lens. This hardly makes any difference to the performance of the *Nulux* lens when it is centred before the eye, but reduces the OAE when the lens is decentred. The field diagram illustrated in Figure 4.22 shows the effect upon the MOE and OAE along the meridian of decentration when the lens is decentred 2mm upwards before the eye.

Bi-aspheric lenses

It was pointed out in the previous section on atoric lenses that when the prescription incorporates a cylindrical correction, an atoroidal surface is necessary to optimize the optical performance along both principal meridians of the lens. Some manufacturers now offer bi-aspheric lenses where the aspherical convex surface is matched with a concave atoroidal surface to ensure that intermediate meridians of the lens also have optimum performance.

The advent of freeform technology has made it possible for surfacing laboratories who have installed CNC generating and polishing machinery to complete the prescription by working the second side of a semi-finished aspheric blank, thus producing a bi-aspheric lens.

Fitting aspheric lenses

For a lens to provide the off-axis performance that its designer intends, the optical axis of the lens should pass through the eye's centre of rotation. In the case of aspheric lenses, in addition to the centre of rotation condition, the optical axis should also pass normally through the pole of the aspherical surface. Whether this condition is achieved or not depends upon any prism that is incorporated in the lens.

As pointed out in Chapter 3, when a spectacle lens is tilted about a horizontal axis in front of the eye by the value of the pantoscopic angle, the optical centre of the lens needs to be decentred downwards, to compensate for the tilt and allow the optical axis of the lens to pass through the eye's centre of rotation. Obviously, if we decentre a lens horizontally, for example to ensure that there is no horizontal prismatic effect at the near centration points, then the lens should be tilted about a vertical axis to compensate for the decentration. Since the decentration is of the order of 2.5mm for each lens, the dihedral angle of the lenses should be about 5°, which corresponds to a reverse bowing of the front of some 10° (Figure 4.23).

Such a drastic step is almost never taken in spectacle frame fitting; indeed, the front is more likely to be given a bow that corresponds with the curve of the face. If this is the case, it has been suggested that the centration of the near vision lenses be made the same as that of the distance pair, that is, no horizontal decentration be given to compensate for the convergence of the visual axes.[5] The purpose of this suggestion is simply to ensure that the optical axis of the lens passes through the eye's centre of rotation and, in the case of a monocular subject, would prove to be a sensible alternative to providing a reverse bow to the front of the frame (Figure 4.24). However, bearing in mind that aspheric lenses are often dispensed to improve the mechanics of medium-to-high power prescriptions, centring near vision lenses of positive power for distance vision will give rise to base-out prism for near. This may prove intolerable in cases of convergence insufficiency and the best expedient is to decentre the lenses inwards as usual, and to reserve the ability to apply a reverse bow to the front to fulfil the centre of rotation condition if it appears that the subject would benefit from such a procedure to improve comfort in near vision.

In the case of minus lenses, no horizontal decentration for near results in a small amount of base-in prism at the near visual points, which is normally quite harmless.

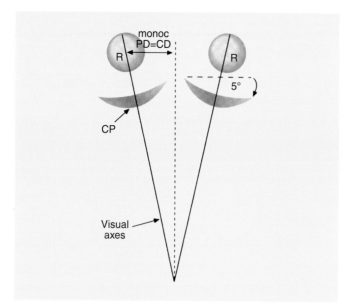

Figure 4.23 Dihedral angle of lenses to satisfy the centre of rotation condition for near vision. The dihedral angle should be 1° for each 0.5mm of inward decentration. Note that the angle is greatly exaggerated in the diagram for clarity

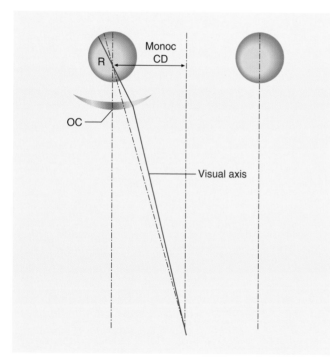

Figure 4.24 Suggested expedient[5] of providing no horizontal decentration for near-in cases in which the horizontal differential prismatic effect is not likely to be troublesome

Prismatic lenses

When an aspheric lens incorporates a prescribed prismatic effect, the optical axis no longer passes through the pole of the aspherical surface since, to view a distant object, the eye will rotate towards the prism apex. It has been suggested[5] that an improvement in the optical performance of prismatic aspheric lenses will be obtained if the lens is decentred in the direction of the prism apex, that is, in the opposite direction to the prism base, the amount of

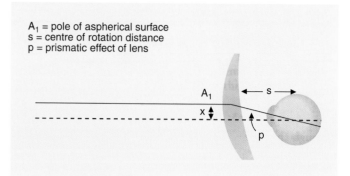

Figure 4.25 Decentration of a prismatic lens to ensure that the pole of the aspherical surface coincides with the visual axis. The decentration, $x = sP/100$, is in the opposite direction to the prism base

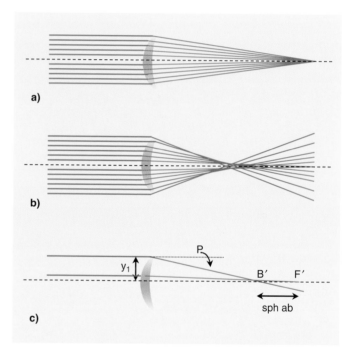

Figure 4.26 Prismatic effect and spherical aberration of a lens: (a) In paraxial theory a lens has no spherical aberration – all rays reunite at the focus; (b) The usual under-corrected form of spherical aberration exhibited by spherical lenses; (c) The relationship between the prismatic effect exerted by the lens and the spherical aberration (sph ab)

decentration depending upon the prism power and the centre of rotation distance. The principle is shown in Figure 4.25, in which it can be seen that the amount of decentration, x, is given by $sP/100$, where s is the distance from the lens to the eye's centre of rotation and P is the prism power.

For an average centre of rotation distance, the value of x is about 0.25 to 0.3mm per prism dioptre and real benefit from this rule is only obtained for lenses that incorporate high prism powers.

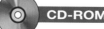

CD-ROM

Centration of aspheric lenses is also considered in detail on the CD-ROM

Table 4.5 Comparison of the prismatic effects and spherical aberration of spherical and aspheric lenses. Columns 2 to 8 give the true prismatic effect obtained when the eye rotates to view through off-axis points of a lens mounted with its back vertex 27mm in front of the eye's centre of rotation and the spherical aberration exhibited by the lens. The final column gives the paraxial value calculated from the simple decentration relationship, $P = cF$

| Decentration (mm) | −4.00D lenses | | | | +4.00D lenses | | | | ±4.00D |
| | Spherical $F_1 = +9.00$ | | Aspheric $F_1 = +5.37$ | | Spherical $F_1 = +4.75$ | | Aspheric $F_1 = +0.75$ | | $P = cF$ |
	P (Δ)	sph ab (mm)	P (Δ)	sph ab (mm)	P (Δ)	sph ab (mm)	P (Δ)	sph ab (mm)	P (Δ)
2.0	0.77	−0.17	0.78	+0.19	0.80	+0.33	0.80	+0.02	0.8
4.0	1.54	−0.70	1.56	+0.76	1.60	+1.31	1.60	+0.09	1.6
6.0	2.32	−1.57	2.34	+1.70	2.41	+2.95	2.40	+0.19	2.4
8.0	3.12	−2.79	3.10	+3.03	3.24	+5.24	3.20	+0.32	3.2
10.0	3.93	−4.36	3.86	+4.73	4.09	+8.19	3.99	+0.45	4.0
12.0	4.76	−6.27	4.60	+6.81	4.97	+11.80	4.79	+0.56	4.8
14.0	5.61	−8.52	5.32	+9.27	5.89	+16.08	5.58	+0.62	5.6
16.0	6.50	−11.12	6.02	+12.11	6.85	+21.02	6.37	+0.57	6.4
18.0	7.43	−14.05	6.70	+15.32	7.87	+26.63	7.15	+0.33	7.2
20.0	8.40	−17.32	7.35	+18.91	8.96	+32.91	7.91	−0.23	8.0

The prismatic effect of aspheric lenses

In paraxial theory, when the eye views through off-axis points on a spectacle lens, the amount of prism that is introduced, P, is simply the product of the decentration, c, expressed in centimetres and the power of the lens, F. The simple decentration relationship, $P = cF$, ignores the spherical aberration of the lens and is, therefore, approximately valid for both spherical and aspheric lenses (Figure 4.26a). When the prismatic effect is calculated by means of accurate trigonometric ray tracing, it is found that it also depends upon the form and thickness of the lens and the type of surface employed. Since the tangential surface power of an aspherical surface differs from that of a spherical surface, a different prismatic effect would be expected to be exerted by an aspheric lens. That this is, indeed, the case is illustrated in Table 4.5, which compares the prismatic effect of the best form +4.00D and −4.00D lenses discussed above. The prismatic effect for each lens, calculated by accurate trigonometric ray tracing at 2mm intervals from the optical axis and the value obtained from the paraxial decentration relationship, $P = cF$, is also given for comparison. The spherical aberration exhibited by the lens for each zone is also tabulated. Spherical aberration opposite in sign to the lens power indicates that it is of the usual, under-corrected form, as normally exhibited by spherical lenses (Figures 4.26b, 4.26c).

The results presented in Table 4.5 offer a good insight into the optical performance of aspheric lenses. Consider first the +4.00D lenses, for which it is seen that the spherical form with a +9.00D front curve exhibits under-corrected spherical aberration, as expected, and that as a result the prismatic effect increases at a faster rate than the paraxial rule predicts. We can imagine, in this case, that the lens becomes more powerful as the light meets it further and further from the optical axis. This is depicted in Figures 4.26b and 4.26c by the foreshortening in the focal lengths of the zonal and marginal rays. Remember that spherical aberration is of very little significance in spectacle lens design, because the pupil of the eye limits the area of the lens that is in use at any one time. That one lens has more spherical aberration than another makes no difference to its optical performance when it is used as a spectacle lens.

The +4.00 aspheric design is seen to behave quite differently as far as spherical aberration is concerned. Table 4.5 shows that the aspheric design with a convex hyperboloidal surface ($F_1 = +5.37$, $p_1 = −1.80$), chosen to provide the same off-axis performance as the spherical design, is *over-corrected* for spherical aberration. The prismatic effect exerted by the lens increases less rapidly than predicted by the decentration relationship and the spherical aberration is now seen to be of slightly greater value than for the spherical design, and of opposite sign. This might have been predicted because there is a significant reduction in tangential power of the aspherical surface as we move away from the pole. What is quite clear is that the aspheric lens is not free from spherical aberration, which some manufacturers' literature quite wrongly implies!

Similar trends are seen for the −4.00D lenses, the performance of which is considered in Table 4.5. Once again, the prismatic effect of the spherical lens increases at a faster rate than is predicted by the paraxial decentration relationship and this design exhibits under-corrected spherical aberration. In the case of the aspheric design, the prismatic effect is much the same as that predicted by the paraxial rule and this aspheric design is corrected well for spherical aberration, there being a change from an under-correction to an over-correction at about 19mm from the optical centre. Clearly, this situation is not achieved for all minus aspheric lenses, it just happens for the power selected that the form and asphericity all but eliminate the spherical aberration.

References

1. Jalie M 1984 Principles of ophthalmic lenses. ABDO, London
2. UK Patent 2030722 1980/US Patent 4289387 1981. Ophthalmic spectacle lenses having hyperbolic surfaces.
3. US Patent 5083859 1992. Ophthalmic spectacle lenses having hyperbolic surfaces.
4. Hoya Corporation. Aspherical Eyeglass Lens International patent application 1997; PCT/JP97/00054
5. Wehmeyer K 1987 Zentrierung von Brillengläsern unter besonderer Berücksichtigung: asphärischer Einstärkengläser. Deutsche Optikerzeitung (Heidelberg), Nr. 9

Reflections from spectacle lens surfaces

The polished surfaces of a spectacle lens reflect light in exactly the same way as plane and curved mirrors. Under certain circumstances they give rise to reflections and ghost images that annoy either the wearer of the lenses, or observers who view the spectacles.[1–3] The intensity of these reflections can be reduced to almost zero by the application of a modern broadband anti-reflection coating to the lens surfaces (these coatings are considered in detail later). We discuss here the reflections themselves, how they arise and how to identify their sources, and what remedies, other than coating the lenses, might be employed to eliminate them.

The formation of the various ghost images is illustrated in Figures 5.1, 5.2 and 5.3.

Figure 5.1 shows the formation of ghost images that arise from sources in front of the lenses. The ghost image illustrated in Figure 5.1a is usually the most troublesome in practice and is formed by total internal reflection at the lens surfaces. This image is referred to herein as ghost image 1. Figures 5.1b and 5.1c illustrate the formation of ghost images that arise from the image of a bright object in front of the lenses. The images are formed by the cornea and the back surface of the lens (ghost image 2), or the cornea and the front surface of the lens (ghost image 3), respectively.

Figure 5.2 shows the formation of ghost images that arise from sources behind the lens and may include images of the wearer's own eyes and their surroundings when the face is strongly illuminated. The ghost image formed by reflection from a source behind the lens at the back surface is referred to as ghost image 4 and that formed by reflection at the front surface as ghost image 5.

Figure 5.3 illustrates the formation of veiling reflections that hide the wearer's eyes or give rise to unsightly reflections from the lenses in photographs, or that arise from the strong lighting used in TV and film studios.

We deal first with the reflections that form ghost images visible to the spectacle wearer. Spectacle lens surfaces must always reflect any available light and, in the presence of any illumination, always form ghost images of the sources before them. Fortunately, these ghost images are not normally visible unless three specific conditions are met.

The first condition concerns the intensity of the ghost with respect to the surrounding illumination and is best understood from the following situation. Imagine you are standing in a room in broad daylight and looking out of a clean window onto a sunny scene. Everything in view should be seen clearly and you may not even be aware of the presence of the window.

Now imagine you are in the same situation at night, with the lights in the room switched on and no illumination within the field of view beyond the window. The window now acts as mirror surface and all you see is a reflection of yourself and everything else in the room beside you. Under these conditions you might think that the window acts as quite an efficient mirror. In fact, the intensity of the reflected images is only some 4% of the illumination of the objects themselves. Nevertheless, at night, the clear glass window pane behaves like quite a good mirror. Typically, a spectacle wearer complains of ghost images of street lamps or car headlights at night because the reflected images are viewed against dark surroundings.

The second condition concerns the vergence of the reflected image. If the wearer's prescription is –4.00D and the vergence of the ghost image is also –4.00D, it will be in sharp focus for the unaccommodated eye. If the vergence of the ghost image happens to be +20.00D, it will be 24.00D out-of-focus for the –4.00D myope and is likely to be too blurred to trouble the wearer. If, however, the vergence of the ghost image is, say, –8.00D, then it will be only 3.00D out-of-focus for the corrected –5.00D myope, who needs to accommodate by only 3.00D to bring the image into sharp focus.

The third condition concerns the position of the ghost image within the field of view. Consider the ghost image of a distant, solitary street lamp at night. If the ghost image of the lamp is superimposed upon the light source itself, it will not be noticed. Neither may it be noticed if it lies at the edge of the field of view, some distance from the refracted image of the source, but if it lies close to the refracted image, say just to one side of it, then it is certain to be noticed at the same time as the source.

Once more, it should be understood that these three conditions must be satisfied simultaneously for the reflected images to

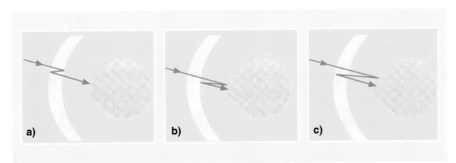

Figure 5.1 Formation of ghost images from sources in front of the lens: (a) ghost image 1; (b) ghost image 2; (c) ghost image 3

a) b) c)

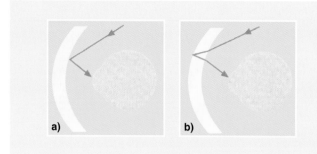

Figure 5.2 Formation of ghost images from sources behind the lens: (a) ghost image 4; (b) ghost image 5

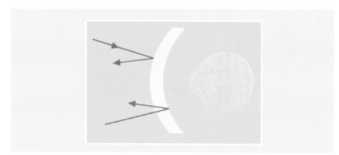

Figure 5.3 Reflections that distract observers

give rise to complaint. It is instructive to examine each condition in a little more detail before describing the various ghost images themselves.

Intensity of the reflected image

When ordinary, unpolarized light is reflected at the polished surface between air and a spectacle lens medium, the reflected light is linearly polarized (Figure 5.4). If the intensity of the incident light is denoted by I_I and the intensity of the reflected light by I_R then the *reflection factor* or *reflectance* of the surface, $I_I/I_R = \rho$, is given by the following expressions shown by Fresnel.

In the plane of incidence (A):

$$I_I/I_R = \rho_{(A)} = \tan^2(i - i')/\tan^2(i + i')$$

and in the plane at right angles to the plane of incidence (B):

$$I_I/I_R = \rho_{(B)} = \sin^2(i - i')/\sin^2(i + i')$$

where i is the angle of incidence at the surface and i' is the corresponding angle of refraction.

Figure 5.5 shows how the reflectances vary with angle of incidence for light incident at the interface between air and a medium of refractive index 1.5. Three items of immediate interest can be seen from this graph. Firstly, when the angle of incidence, i, and consequently the angle of refraction, i', is small, the reflectances in the plane of incidence, $\rho_{(A)}$, and in the plane at right angles thereto, $\rho_{(B)}$, are the same. This is the case for angles of i out, almost, to 20°. For these small angles of incidence, the reflection factors reduce to the single expression given in Chapter 2 for the case of reflectance of a surface for normally incident light, namely:

$$\rho = (n - 1)^2 / (n + 1)^2$$

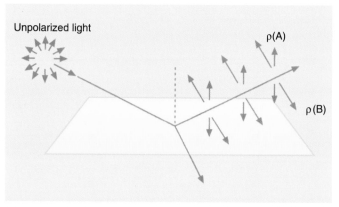

Unpolarized light

$\rho(A)$

$\rho(B)$

Figure 5.4 Plane polarized light formed by reflection: $\rho_{(A)}$ in the plane of incidence; $\rho_{(B)}$ in the plane at right angles to the plane of incidence

The reflectances for various optical media in air are given in Table 5.1.

Secondly, Figure 5.5 shows that for large angles of incidence, the intensity of the reflections increases dramatically. It is well known that, even in broad daylight, it is possible to use a sheet of ordinary glass, such as a window pane, as an efficient mirror simply by tilting the pane of glass so that it is obliquely inclined to the fixation line.

Thirdly, there is a certain angle of incidence for which the reflectance in the plane of incidence becomes equal to zero. This particular angle of incidence, when $\rho_{(A)} = 0$, is known as the Brewster Angle. The reflectance in the plane of incidence vanishes and the reflected light is completely plane polarized. This condition is utilized by a polarizing filter which, when held with its polarizing axis vertically, absorbs the reflectance $\rho_{(A)}$ and causes the reflected light to vanish.

The brightness or intensity of the reflected images depends upon the angle of incidence of the light upon the lens surfaces and the refractive index of the medium from which the spectacle lens is made; the brightness increases as the refractive index of the lens material increases. For normal incidence, the intensities of the various images for different refractive index materials is given in Table 5.2.

Vergence of the reflected image

The second condition that must be satisfied for a ghost image to be troublesome is that the vergence of the light that forms the ghost image must be the same as, or close to, the vergence of the light refracted by the lens. For a distant source of light, this means that the vergence of the reflected ghost image must be the same as the power of the lens.

The reflecting power of a surface, usually referred to as its *catoptric power*, is given by $-2nR$, where n is the refractive index of the medium into which the light is reflected and R is the curvature of the surface, related to the surface powers by the usual expressions:

$$R_1 = F_1/(n - 1)$$

and

$$R_2 = F_2/(1 - n)$$

Figure 5.6 represents a lens for which the refractive index in air is denoted by n, and incident upon which are two rays of light, one

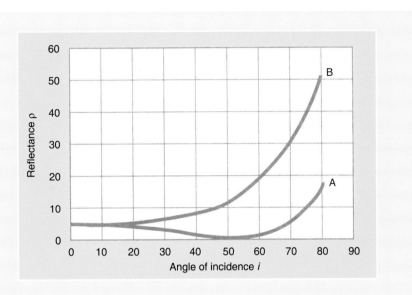

Figure 5.5   Surface reflectance for air–glass, $n = 1.50$

travelling from left to right and the second travelling from right to left, as indicated. Substituting the surface power relationships given above, the catoptric powers of the surfaces are,[2] for light travelling from left to right:

$$F_{1cat} = -2F_1/(n-1)$$
$$F_{2cat} = 2nF_2/(n-1)$$

and for light travelling from right to left:

$$F_{1cat} = 2nF_1/(n-1)$$
$$F_{2cat} = -2F_2/(n-1)$$

These expressions are used to determine the vergences of the various ghost images. If the vergence of the reflected image is similar to that of the refracted light that leaves the lens, which for a distant source is the power of the lens, then the ghost image in question is

Table 5.1   Reflection factors for various media for normally incident light

Medium	Refractive index	Reflectance (%)
Water	1.333	2.04
Corneal tears	1.338	2.09
CR39	1.498	4.00
Spectacle crown	1.523	4.30
Extra dense flint	1.701	6.72
Double EDF	1.800	8.16
Diamond	2.420	17.24

in focus and could be a problem to the wearer. The likely formation of the various ghost images is discussed for each image in turn.

Ghost image 1

It can be seen in Figure 5.1a that ghost image 1 is formed by internal reflection at each of the lens surfaces. It was stated earlier that this image is generally the most troublesome in practice. In view of its low intensity, given in Table 5.2 (of the five possible ghosts, it is only the third brightest), this may seem surprising, but remember that the eye is an excellent detector of any light source within the visual field.

The vergence of this image is found by adding together the dioptric and catoptric powers contributed by each surface. Strictly, an effectivity correction should be made for the optical path through the lens material, but (as shown below) this is unnecessary in view of the likely lens powers for which this ghost might be troublesome.

Referring to Figure 5.1a, there is one dioptric and one catoptric contribution from each surface, so the vergence of this ghost is given by:

$$L_1 + F_1 + F_{2cat} + F_{1cat} + F_2$$

Substituting the values indicated by Figure 5.6 for the catoptric surface powers, taking particular note of the direction of travel of the light, we find the vergence of ghost image 1 to be:

$$L_1 + F(3n-1)/(n-1)$$

where F is the total (thin lens) power of the lens.

Table 5.2   Intensity of the ghost images for various refractive indices

Refractive index	Ghost image intensities (%)				
	1	2	3	4	5
1.500	0.15	0.08	0.08	4.00	3.69
1.523	0.17	0.09	0.08	4.30	3.94
1.600	0.25	0.11	0.10	5.33	4.77
1.700	0.39	0.14	0.12	6.72	5.85
1.800	0.56	0.17	0.14	8.16	6.88

Common sense dictates that L_1 is unlikely to be other than zero, that is, the source would be a distant one, and when $L_1 = 0$, the vergence of ghost image 1 is simply:

$$F(3n-1)/(n-1)$$

For CR39 material with a refractive index of virtually 1.5, the vergence of this ghost turns out to be $7F$, that is, seven times the power of the lens. Since the ghost image is in sharp focus when the catoptric vergence is the same as the power of the lens, this condition can only be fully met when the lens is afocal. This reflection is often commented upon by wearers of plano-sunspectacles, especially dark ones, for sunlenses with low transmittances provide the necessary field of reduced illumination, and a ghost image of a bright source such as the sun may be seen in the field of view.

Ghost image 1 is not entirely restricted to plano-lenses. If a low myope has ample accommodation, it is a simple matter for the eye to accommodate to bring the ghost image into sharp focus. For example, if the subject's prescription is –0.25 and made in glass of refractive index 1.50, then the vergence of the ghost image is –0.25 × 7 or –1.75D. The subject's attention is drawn to the out-of-focus light patch within the visual field and, by exerting just 1.50D of accommodation, ghost image 1 appears in sharp focus.

Table 5.3 gives values for the vergence of ghost image 1 for materials of various refractive indices. It is clear that this image is potentially more troublesome as the refractive index of the lens material increases.

The third condition for a ghost image to be troublesome concerns its position in the visual field. As pointed out above, for the ghost image to attract the wearer's attention it should lie close to, but not superimposed upon, the dioptric image being viewed. A very interesting and instructive observation of both this third condition and of ghost image 1 can be obtained in the consulting room. When the illuminated muscle spotlight is viewed through a plano-prism of power 0.5Δ or 1Δ (no other area of the chart should be illuminated in the darkened room), a ghost image of the spotlight, in sharp focus, is quite visible, always displaced towards the prism apex. The lower the power of the prism, the closer the ghost lies to the spotlight image. Although the precaution of switching off the light in the room must be taken to begin with, once the presence of the ghost image has been detected it will remain visible, although more difficult to see, when the consulting room lights are switched on again. If the experiment is repeated with a 2Δ plano-prism the image is found to be near the ceiling, so far removed from the muscle spotlight itself that some effort has to be made to see it at all.

The formation of this ghost image as a result of the prismatic element of a lens is illustrated in Figure 5.7. It can be shown[2] that the deviation of the ghost image formed by a plano-prism is given by:

$$d_{cat} = (3n-1)a$$

whereas the deviation of the refracted image is $(n-1)a$, so the catoptric image is deviated some seven times more than the dioptric image viewed through the prism. This catoptric property of prisms has important consequences for poorly centred spectacle lenses. Large prismatic errors position the ghost image well away from the fixation line, whereas small prismatic errors may well position the ghost in an unfavourable position close to the object of regard. This form of ghost image 1 is often commented upon by wearers of low-power spectacles that incorporate small prismatic corrections, and is a strong case for dispensing such lenses only in anti-reflection coated form.

So the vergence of ghost image 1 is a function of the lens power and the refractive index of the lens material. It is unaffected by the form and position of the lens. The only practical remedy for eliminating this ghost, if it proves to be an annoyance to the wearer, is to apply an anti-reflection coating to the lens.

CD-ROM

Further consideration of ghost image 1, including how to see it, is given on the CD-ROM

Ghost image 2

The second ghost image, the formation of which is illustrated in Figure 5.1b, is formed by light reflected at the cornea and the back surface of the lens. In view of its low intensity, less than 0.1% for materials with refractive indices below 1.56, it is surprising that it can be observed at all, but it is in focus for high myopes, who may well complain of this particular ghost image.

If it is assumed that the cornea has a radius of curvature of 8mm, then the catoptric power of the cornea is –250.00D and would form an image of a distant source of light, by reflection,

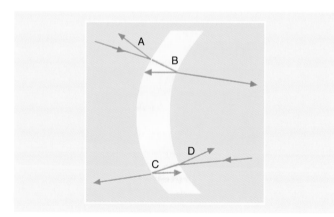

Figure 5.6   Catoptric surface powers:
A = F_{1cat} for light travelling from left to right;
B = F_{2cat} for light travelling from left to right;
C = F_{1cat} for light travelling from right to left;
D = F_{2cat} for light travelling from right to left.

Table 5.3   Vergences of ghost image 1 for various refractive index materials

	Refractive index				
	1.500	1.523	1.600	1.700	1.800
Vergence of ghost image 1 (F is the power of the lens)	7.00F	6.82F	6.33F	5.86F	5.50F

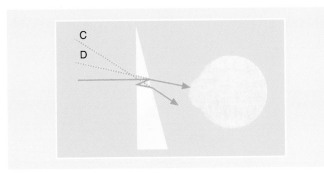

Figure 5.7 Total internal reflection by a prism: C = catoptric (ghost) image, D = dioptric image

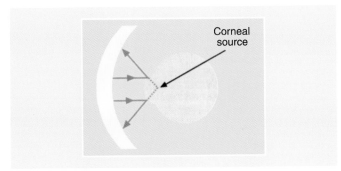

Corneal source

Figure 5.8 Source of ghost images 2 and 3, Purkinje Image No. 1

some 4mm behind the corneal apex (Purkinje Image No. 1). It is the reflection of this image by the back surface of the lens that may be noticed by the wearer (Figure 5.8). The catoptric power of the cornea is so powerful that we can safely ignore any vergence imparted by the lens to the incident light from the original source itself. If the distance from the corneal image to the back vertex of the lens is denoted by z and its reciprocal, in dioptres, by Z, we find the vergence of ghost image 2 to be:

$$-Z + F_{2cat} = -Z - 2F_2/(n-1)$$

If the vertex distance is assumed to be the average value of 12mm, then z is 16mm and Z has the value, 62.50D.

For a material of refractive index 1.5, the vergence of the ghost image is:

$$-62.5 - 4F_2$$

Ghost image 2 is in sharp focus when this vergence is the same as the power of the lens, that is, when $F = -62.5 - 4F_2$.

A moment's thought confirms that this situation can only occur for spectacle lenses of medium-to-high minus power, for example, a −10.50D lens made with a −13.00 back surface or a −12.50D lens made in plano-concave form each fully satisfy the condition.

The coefficient for the back surface power changes, of course, with the refractive index. Table 5.4 shows the coefficients for lenses made in materials of different refractive indices. The value of Z varies with the vertex distance and is found by adding 4mm to the vertex distance of the lens.

Ghost image 2 is very susceptible to either a change in vertex distance of the lens or to a change in lens form. For example, if the vertex distance for the −12.50D lens mentioned above, made in plano-concave form, is changed from 12mm to 14mm, the value of Z becomes 55.56D, and the ghost is thrown out-of-focus by almost +7.00D, which is probably sufficient to make it unnoticeable.

Changing the lens form by 1.00D changes the vergence of this ghost by 4.00D for a material of refractive index 1.5, but this radical solution is almost certainly unnecessary today, for, if the vertex distance cannot be altered significantly, the modern solution is, simply, to apply an anti-reflection coating to the lens.

Ghost image 3

The third ghost image, the formation of which is illustrated in Figure 5.1c, is formed by light reflected at the cornea and the front surface of the lens. From Table 5.2 it is the least bright of all the images. Applying the same reasoning as for ghost image 2, but this time also taking into account the two refractions at the back surface of the lens, the vergence of ghost image 3 is:

$$-Z + 2F_2 + F_{1cat} = -Z + 2F_2 + 2nF_1/(n-1)$$

For a material of refractive index 1.5, the vergence of the ghost image is:

$$-Z + 2F_2 + 6F_1$$

or, since $F = F_1 + F_2$, the vergence of ghost image 3 is simply:

$$-Z + 2F + 4F_1$$

Examination of this statement, and substituting suitable values for Z, leads to the conclusion that this ghost image is in sharp focus only for high-power plus lenses. It can be dealt with in the same way as ghost image 2, either by changing the vertex distance or the lens form or, today, by applying an anti-reflection coating to the surfaces of the lens.

Ghost image 4

The formation of the fourth ghost image is illustrated in Figure 5.2a and is seen from Table 5.2 to be the brightest of all the images. Despite this, reflections that arise from sources behind the lens are probably the least troublesome since, under normal circumstances, the head obstructs most of the possible sources of illumination. Ghost images 4 and 5 are usually only a problem when the lenses are large enough to collect light from behind the head.

The vergence of ghost image 4 is:

$$L_1 + F_{2cat} = L_1 - 2F_2/(n-1)$$

When $n = 1.5$, the vergence of ghost image 4 is:

$$L_1 - 4F_2$$

and may be troublesome when $F = L_1 - 4F_2$.

There are two quite different circumstances when this condition might be satisfied by modern spectacle lenses. The first occurs when the lens is large enough to collect light from a distant source behind the head and the value of L_1 equals zero. Then the condition for the ghost image to be seen in sharp focus is that $F = -4F_2$. This could occur either for high-power plus lenses, for example, a +12.00D made with a −3.00D base curve satisfies this condition, or for modern low-power aspheric lenses, such as a +6.00D lens made with a −1.50 base curve or a +4.00D lens made with a −1.00D base curve, and so on.

The second circumstance under which ghost image 4 might be noticed by a spectacle wearer is when the face is brightly illuminated, either out-of-doors in strong sunlight or, more usually, indoors where, for example, a subject might sit at a desk with

Table 5.4 Coefficients for back surface power, F_2, for ghost images 2 and 4 for various materials

	Refractive index				
	1.500	1.523	1.600	1.700	1.800
Coefficient for F_2	4.00	3.82	3.33	2.86	2.50

a table lamp to one side that illuminates the face and surroundings of the eye. Under these circumstances, L_1 has some finite value in the expression for the vergence of ghost image 4.

For example, the outer canthus might lie 20mm behind the lens, so that if strongly illuminated it acts as a source with an L_1 value of –50.00D. Then a reflection of the outer canthus and its surround is seen in sharp focus when $F = -50 - 4F_2$. This could occur for a –10.00D lens made in plano-concave form or a –8.00D lens made with a –10.50 back surface, and so on. Needless to say, spectacle wearers are unlikely to complain about this novel method of viewing their own eyes. The coefficients for the back surface power for lenses made in materials of other refractive indices are listed in Table 5.4.

For cases in which ghost image 4 proves to be a problem it can be eliminated either by changing the form of the lens or by an anti-reflection coating on the lens.

Ghost image 5

The formation of this ghost image is illustrated in Figure 5.2b and inspection of Table 5.2 shows that this is the second brightest of the five ghost images. Like ghost image 4, it is only likely to be troublesome when the lens is large enough to collect light from behind the head.

The vergence of ghost image 5 is:

$$L_1 + 2F_2 + F_{1cat} = L_1 + 2F_2 + 2nF_1/(n-1)$$

When $n = 1.5$, the vergence of ghost image 5 is:

$$L_1 + 2F + 4F_1$$

and may be troublesome when $F = -L_1 - 4F_1$.

Again, there are two different circumstances when this ghost image may be seen in sharp focus. The first occurs when the lens is large enough to collect light from a distant source behind the head and the value of L_1 equals zero. Then $F = -4F_1$, which might occur for medium- to high-power minus lenses, for example, a –8.00D lens made with a +2.00 front curve or a low-power aspheric –5.00D lens made with a +1.25 front curve, and so on.

As with ghost image 4, there is also the possibility that the face may be illuminated strongly and L_1 may have a finite value. For example, the outer canthus 25mm behind the front surface of the lens gives L_1 the value of –40.00D, and the condition for a reflection of the outer canthus to be seen in sharp focus is $F = 40 - 4F_1$. This condition could be satisfied by plus lenses, for example a +4.00D lens made with a +9.00 front curve or a +6.00D lens made with a +8.50 front curve, and so on.

The remedies for ghost image 5 are the same as those for ghost image 4.

Identification of ghost images

When a subject complains of disturbing reflections it is important to identify the formation of the ghost image. It is simple to elicit information about the position of the source, whether the images

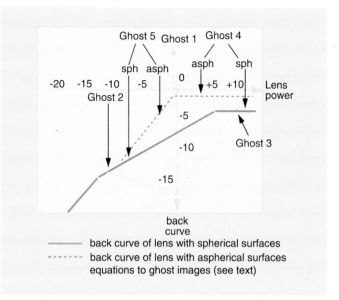

Figure 5.9 Graph to identify ghost images from the power of the lens ($n = 1.5$), with a distant source of light, vertex distance 12mm

appear when the source is in front of the subject or behind, but it can be appreciated from the foregoing discussion that the main clue to the formation of troublesome ghost images is often, simply, the power of the lens.

The graph illustrated in Figure 5.9 should help to identify the probable source of a ghost image. Lens powers are plotted horizontally and the back curves of the lenses vertically. The likely ghost images for each power group are found by plotting the straight-line graphs of the equations for the situations when the reflections are in sharp focus together with the equations for modern spectacle lens forms. The equations for the conditions when the ghost images are in sharp focus are given below. It is assumed that the lenses are thin, made in a material of refractive index 1.5 and fitted at a vertex distance of 12mm. As already pointed out, ghost image 1 is in focus for very low-power lenses, typically +0.50D to –1.00D, and is independent of the form of the lens.

Ghost image 2 equation to line: $F_2 = -0.25F - 15.625$

Ghost image 3 equation to line: $F_2 = 1.25F - 15.625$

Ghost image 4 equation to line: $F_2 = -0.25F$

Ghost image 5 equation to line: $F_2 = 1.25F$

It is immediately seen from the graph, for example, that the wearer of a –12.00D lens who complains of disturbing ghost images is likely to be troubled by ghost image 2.

Reflections from the dividing line of bifocal lenses

The dividing line in flat-top bifocals and trifocals or E-style designs may give rise to the streak reflections illustrated in Figure 5.10.

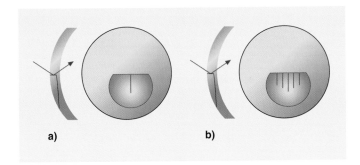

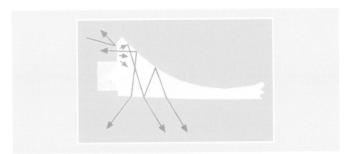

Figure 5.11 Power rings formed by reflections of scattered light from the exposed ground-glass edge of a lens

Each point source gives rise to a separate streak, the length of which depends upon the width of the dividing line. The effect seen by the wearer is a sharply focused vertical bar, or bars, of light, which can be quite disconcerting, say, when driving a car at night along an illuminated street. Figure 5.10 shows that when the dividing line is a plane surface, the vergence of the ghost images is the same as the power of the lens, so that they are always in sharp focus if the wearer does not accommodate. The intensity of the reflections varies with the degree of polish imparted to the bifocal ridge, from a maximum intensity of about 0.16% in the case of fused segments to some 3.9% in the case of the E-style bifocal. Bifocal manufacturers attempt to eliminate this type of reflection by both angling the segment dividing line and applying an anti-reflection coating to the contact edges of the crown and flint components of the composite button before fusion.

Reflections that distract observers

Some reflections do not necessarily annoy the spectacle wearer, but rather observers who view the lenses mounted before the wearer's eyes. The formation of these is illustrated in Figure 5.3. It is well known that lenses with a shallow concave front surface can obscure, very effectively, the wearer's eyes with veiling glare, and thus prevent an observer from viewing, for example, the effect of a conversation with the wearer of the lenses. This puts the observer at some psychological disadvantage if the reaction to what is being said cannot be judged.

Elimination of veiling glare is also very important in photography, theatre and television studios, and there is no doubt that broadband anti-reflection coatings have proved to be a great boon in these situations.

Anti-reflection coatings also offer a dramatic improvement in the appearance of high-power spectacle lenses, simply by making the lenses less visible. In cases of anisometropia, the coatings reduce the difference in appearance of the two lenses and, perhaps

Figure 5.10 Reflections from the dividing lines of straight-top bifocal lenses: (a) reflection from a single source; (b) reflections from multiple sources

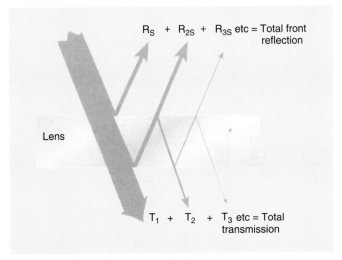

Figure 5.12 Multiple surface reflections

most importantly of all, virtually eliminate reflections of the lens edges in medium- and high-power lenses.

The formation of these power rings is illustrated in Figure 5.11. The ground-glass edge of the lens can pick up light and scatter it in every direction. The edge is, therefore, relatively bright and a reflection of the edge can be seen through the front surface of the lens, the reflection taking place at the back surface of the lens. It is often possible to see a second reflection of the edge that arises from internal reflection at the front surface and again at the back surface. Traditional remedies to eliminate power rings include polishing the bevel or coating it with dark varnish to prevent the edge from picking up light. Dispensing the lenses in a dark, wide-rimmed front is also beneficial, since this prevents the edge from collecting light. Once more, the modern solution is to prevent the lens surfaces from reflecting light by the application of an anti-reflection coating.

Anti-reflection coatings

When multiple internal reflections are taken into account, the total reflection from an uncoated spectacle lens can be calculated by summing the series of multiple reflections, as shown in Figure 5.12. (For tinted lenses, a similar, but more complicated, calculation is used to allow for absorption each time the light ray traverses the tinted lens.)

If there is no internal absorption, then the total front reflection can be calculated from the single surface reflection ratio, ρ_s, by the formula:

Total front reflection ratio, $R_s = 2\rho_s/(1 + \rho_s)$

Table 5.5   Variation in reflectance and transmittance of uncoated spectacle lenses

Material	Refractive index	Reflectance (%)	Transmittance (%)
CR39	1.498	7.6	92.4
Crown glass	1.523	8.2	91.8
Mid-index	1.600	10.1	89.9
High-index	1.700	12.6	87.4
High-index	1.800	15.1	84.9
Diamond	2.417	29.3	70.7

When the intensity of the reflection is low, ρ_S is approximately double the single surface reflection.

The value of the total front reflectance for a selection of clear lens materials is given in Table 5.5. As the index increases, so does the reflectance, and consequently the transmission decreases (the very high reflectance of diamond is one reason for its attraction in the jewellery industry).

Clearly, high-index materials must be anti-reflection coated to achieve an acceptable transmittance and to prevent distracting reflections. In fact, there are other reasons why high-index materials should be coated. High-index glass can be susceptible to staining if not coated and high-index plastics are usually very soft and should be hard coated to prevent scratching.

How to create anti-reflection

There are two known ways by which surface reflections can be reduced. One simple technique (which is rarely used) is to apply a surface layer of a lower refractive index than the basic material. As can be seen from Table 5.5, a lower index material has a lower reflectance. Some hard coats produce this effect; however, there are many practical problems with this method. Not least because if the surface layer is not of precisely equal thickness, and the refractive index of the coating does not match that of the lens, then 'interference colours' can be seen, as on a thin film of oil. This can sometimes be seen on materials such as polycarbonate when a 1.5 index hard coat is applied to the 1.586 substrate material. This effect may become more obvious if an anti-reflection coating is applied on top of a non-matching index hard coat.

The more usual way to create a lower surface reflectance is to make use of the principle of interference technique. This utilizes the fact that light travels as a wave. Although the physics is very complex, and the mathematical formulae for electromagnetic theory are extremely complicated, the theory may be explained simply by reference to Figure 5.13. This shows that if the wave reflections from the front and the back of a coating layer can be made to be out of phase with each other they cancel each other out and no reflection is visible. This is achieved if the reflection from the back of the coating travels half a wavelength further than that from the front, which occurs if the coating is one-quarter of a wavelength thick.

As there is no net reflected energy (and energy must go somewhere), the light that would have been lost by reflection is actually added to the energy transmitted by the lens. A 'perfect' coating therefore has zero reflection and 100% transmission at the design wavelength.

To achieve perfect wave cancellation two things are necessary. Firstly, the two waves must be exactly out of phase and secondly the strength (or amplitude) of the two waves must be identical.

Path condition

To ensure that the two leaves are exactly out-of-phase the thickness of the coating layer must be exactly one-quarter of a wavelength. Strictly speaking, its thickness must be one-quarter of the

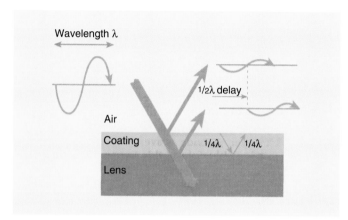

Figure 5.13   Quarter-wave cancellation theory

optical wave thickness, since the length of the wave is affected by the refractive index of the coating. The path condition is satisfied when the thickness of the film is $\lambda/4n_F$, where λ is the wavelength of light chosen in the middle of the visible spectrum, usually around 550nm, and n_F is the refractive index of the coating film.

Amplitude condition

To ensure that the two waves are of equal strength requires that the two reflections be of equal amplitude. It can be shown, by equating the amplitudes of the waves at each surface reflection, that this happens if the refractive index of the coating layer is equal to the square root of the refractive index of the lens, that is, the ideal coating for a 1.5 index lens has an index of 1.22; for a 1.7 index lens the ideal coating index is 1.30 and for a 1.9 index lens it is 1.38. Magnesium fluoride (MgF_2) has an index of 1.38 and is therefore often used to coat glass lenses. Its effectiveness is obviously greater on high-index materials.

Effect of a single-layer coating

In the simple explanation of single-layer anti-reflection coatings given above, it is stated that, ideally, the optical thickness of the coating layer should be one-quarter of a wavelength. However, natural light is made up of a range of different wavelengths, as shown in Figure 5.14, so that a coating of the correct thickness for one colour of light is not correct for other colours of light.

If a single-layer coating is designed to be most effective in the middle of the visible range (i.e. at 550nm), it will be less effective for shorter and for longer wavelengths. In fact, for radiation at double this wavelength (1100nm), wave combination occurs instead of wave cancellation, and the reflection is therefore doubled in strength.

Figure 5.15 shows the effectiveness of a single-layer coating over a range of wavelengths. While no yellow–green light is reflected, there is considerable reflection of blue and red light.

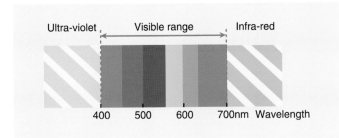

Figure 5.14   The spectrum of light

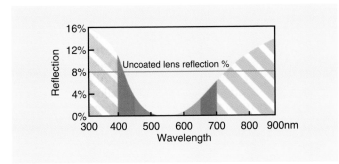

Figure 5.15   Single-layer coating reflection. Note: This and subsequent graphs show the reflectance from both sides of a 1.5 index lens with an uncoated reflectance of 8%. (For accuracy of measurement, reflectance is usually measured in comparison to an uncoated lens)

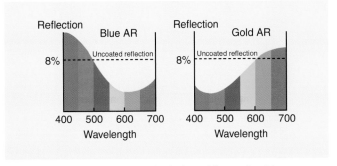

Figure 5.16   Reflection from single-layer blue and gold anti-reflection coatings

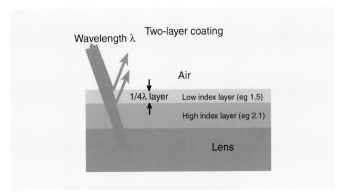

Figure 5.17   Two-layer coating

This produces the classic purple–violet reflection that, typically, is associated with single-layer coatings.

Single-layer blue and gold reflection colours may also be produced using the same technique. By increasing or decreasing the thickness of the coating layer so that its thickness is one-quarter of some other wavelength, the point of minimum reflection can be moved to a different wavelength, as shown in Figure 5.16. (In the two examples shown, the minimum reflectance does not reach zero because the index of the coating layer is not exactly equal to the square root of the index of the lens material.)

Why single layers on glass, but double layers on plastics materials?

As explained above, an effective single-layer coating can be produced easily on glass lenses using a quarter-wave layer of magnesium fluoride.

When coating plastics lenses we are much more restricted in the materials that are available. There are many reasons for this, including difficulties of adhesion, stress differences and because many optical coatings are brittle and they may crack when applied to a flexible plastics material.

Coating materials need to have a lower refractive index than the base-lens material to create an anti-reflective effect. With no known low-index materials physically suitable for coating plastics materials, another solution had to be found. The method is first to apply a layer of material of a higher refractive index to the lens, and then to put the normal refractive index layer on top of that (Figure 5.17). Hence, single-layer coatings on glass have similar optical properties to two-layer coatings on plastics.

A very convenient material of normal index is silicon oxide (SiO_2), commonly known as quartz, which has a refractive index of 1.46. Quartz also has the advantage that it is highly scratch

resistant and forms an ideal top layer to the coating. Another material is required with a refractive index of about 2.13 (the square of 1.46). The oxides of zirconium and titanium are used frequently for this purpose, as they have indices of 2.0 and 2.3, respectively. Both materials are used in coating treatments and each has different advantages. While titanium oxide has a higher refractive index, there is a greater change in its optical properties in the blue spectral region than there is with zirconium oxide.

Multilayer and broadband anti-reflection coatings

Single-layer coatings (on glass) and double-layer coatings (on plastics) can only be effective over a narrow range of wavelengths. Although the reflectance for the design wavelength may be reduced from 8% to zero, hence increasing the transmission from 92% to 100%, the average over the whole of the visible spectrum is little better than half these values. Inspection of these figures, which illustrate the reflection characteristics of violet, blue and gold single-layer coatings, indicates that, typically, the reflectance over the visible range averages 4% and the transmittance, therefore, averages 96%.

To reduce the reflectance over the whole of the visible spectrum requires a sequence of layers so that different wavelengths may be cancelled. This is achieved with multilayer anti-reflection (MAR) coatings. Their effectiveness over a wide waveband, the entire breadth of the visible spectrum, has led to the name *broadband* coatings. A stack of pairs of alternate high and low refractive-index layers is used. Typically, one thicker pair cancels the central spectral range and the other thinner pair cancels the blue and red regions (sometimes three pairs are used). Figure 5.18 illustrates how this produces the typical green broadband reflection.

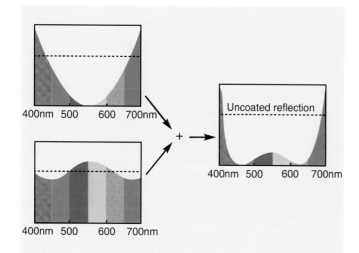

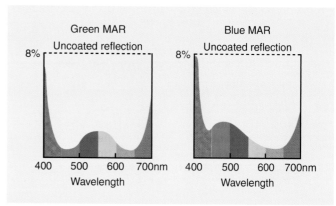

Figure 5.20   Broadband green and blue MAR

Figure 5.18   Multilayer broadband coating

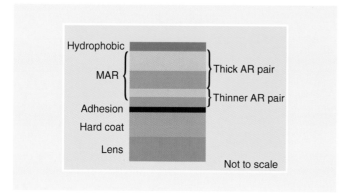

Figure 5.19   Multilayer coating stack

Table 5.6 Percentage of molecules with a mean free path of 1 metre at various pressures	
Pressure (millibars)	Molecules (%) that travel 1 metre
1000	0
1.0	0
0.0001	10
0.00001	78
0.000001	98

design of a very low reflection anti-reflection coating effective over a broad band of the spectrum, while minimizing angular effects, is quite a skilled job. Further complications, such as the variation of refractive index with wavelength for all the coating layers, make the design of multilayer coatings an extremely complex calculation that requires powerful computing facilities.

Vacuum coating

Historically, most anti-reflection coatings were produced using a technique in which the coating material is evaporated in a crucible within a vacuum chamber. The coating material then adheres to the lens. The better the vacuum, the further the coating material travels before it collides with another molecule, and therefore a very good vacuum is required. Table 5.6 indicates what percentage of molecules travel 1 metre in different levels of vacuum (the atmospheric pressure is 1000 millibar).

Vacuum coating machines normally operate at a pressure of around 0.000001 millibar, which is one-thousandth of one-millionth of atmospheric pressure. In industry, this is often referred to as a vacuum of *ten to the six* or 10^{-6}.

Single-layer anti-reflection coating machinery

A small change in coating thickness on single-layer anti-reflection coating does not produce a very obvious effect, so it is possible to manufacture such coatings in relatively simple machines. These machines may also be used to tint glass lenses, as discussed in Chapter 6. The lenses can, therefore, be positioned quite close to the evaporation source. Also, the angular effect of coating the outer part of the lens surface does not make the coating appear significantly different between the centre and the edge of the lens. Since the distance from the evaporation source to the lens is small, the vacuum does not need to be extremely good. A typical belljar coating machine used for single-layer anti-reflection and for glass tinting is shown in Figure 5.21.

As the optical layers are always in pairs, it might be expected that an even number of layers must be used. However, in addition to the optical interference layers, some coating suppliers include in the count extra layers that are added for physical reasons. This is illustrated in Figure 5.19, which shows a four-layer optical coating added to a hard coating layer, an adhesion layer and a hydrophobic top coating. The drawing is not to scale. Typically, the hard-coat layer is 10 times thicker than the anti-reflection layer and the adhesion and hydrophobic layers are extremely thin.

By manipulating the thickness and refractive indices of the multilayer stack it is possible to produce many effects. Typical reflection curves for blue and green reflection multilayer broadband coatings are shown in Figure 5.20.

Angular reflectance

So far, the discussion has assumed that the light is incident and reflected normally. Both the physics and the mathematics become more complicated when reflections at angles of incidence other than normal are considered. Not only does the reflection colour change with the angle of incidence, but the light becomes partially polarized. Water, for example, with a refractive index of 1.33, has a relatively low reflection of 2% when viewed normally, but becomes a very efficient reflector at shallow viewing angles.

With spectacle lenses the lens curvature is also significant, and so it is very difficult to achieve a uniform anti-reflective effect across the lens surface. It is not surprising, therefore, that the

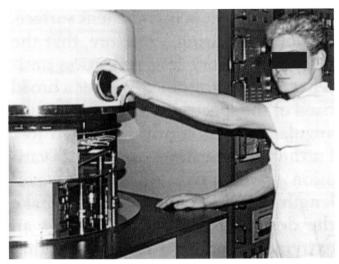

Figure 5.21   Single-layer anti-reflection belljar machine

Multilayer box-coating machinery

To achieve the uniformity of coating necessary to make a satisfactory multilayer broadband anti-reflection coating, extreme accuracy and consistency of coating layer thickness is required. To prevent angular effects with a single evaporation source, it is necessary for the lens to be positioned a large distance (typically 500mm) from the coating material source. This means that MAR machines (which use an evaporation technique) are physically large and can therefore accommodate a large number of lenses. The large box requires a massive vacuum pumping system and outgassing of a large number of plastics lenses in the large chamber means that they need to be dehydrated for many hours before being loaded into the machine. The rate of evaporation of the coating material from the crucible is very variable, which means that an expensive quartz-crystal coating rate-measuring system is required. As they require ultrasonic lens cleaning systems, ultra-clean humidity controlled environments and highly qualified and experienced staff, and with price tags of the order of one million pounds, it is hardly surprising that such machines are only used by the major optical companies. These machines are used by the larger laboratories and require capacities of about 200 pairs or more per day. Figure 5.22 illustrates a large box-coating system.

High-energy IAD PVD coating

By the addition of 'ion assist' or 'plasma assist' technologies, the energy applied during the coating process is increased. This produces a more compact (and harder) coating, often with improved optical properties. High-energy coating is much more compatible with lacquer hard-coated lenses. In fact, as a general rule, ion- and plasma-assisted coatings should only be applied on top of lacquer hard-coated lenses, and the older technology coatings should only be applied on top of non-lacquered lenses.

The increased energy also permits the application of a hydrophobic coating using the same machinery. This is usually done as part of the whole coating process, immediately following the application of the anti-reflection layers. There are a few practical difficulties with ion- and plasma-assisted coatings (see below), but if done correctly these technologies produce an excellent, long-lasting coating.

One difficulty with high-energy coatings is that the increased energy produces a plasma that can move around to the back surface of the lenses while the front is being coated. Coating

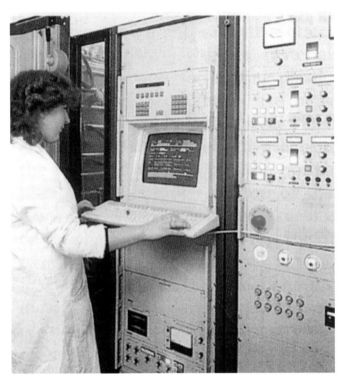

Figure 5.22   Large box-coating machine

companies avoid this problem in special ways, such as by covering the back part while coating the front. This sometimes restricts the process to circular uncut lenses. Lenses that have a hard coat on the front only, and none on the back, should not normally be coated in a high-energy system.

One advantage of the increased energy is that coatings may be applied faster. This is not normally significant, since the major part of the time taken for coating is related to achieving the correct vacuum (with powerful vacuum pumps). However, some companies have used the high energy to apply a 'thick' silicon oxide layer, which can act as a hard coat. As always, there are some problems, such as avoiding reflections when this is carried out on lenses with a different refractive index to that of silicon oxide, but it avoids the need for a separate lacquering process.

Sputter technology laboratory machinery

Conventional box-coaters use heat (generated electrically) to evaporate the coating material from a crucible. Recently, a different method of applying the silicon, zirconium and titanium oxides onto the surfaces of lenses was developed for ophthalmic coatings. This technique has been used for other applications (such as for window glass) for many years. An electromagnetic field is employed to create a plasma that 'sputters' the coating material onto the lenses. Although the production techniques used are different, the alternate low- and high-index optical layers on the lens are the same and hence the resultant anti-reflective effects are identical to those achieved with the evaporation technique.

The main significance to the ophthalmic industry is that it is possible to construct sputter machines that are much smaller and less complex than the conventional box-coater. That a glowing plasma surrounds the lens means it is possible to achieve a uniform coating when the lenses are very close to the source of the coating material. Also, the inherent constant coating rate of such machines means that much of the complex quartz-crystal rate-monitoring electronics is not required, so that sputter machines can be cheaper and simpler.

Prescription laboratories that require a coating capacity of between 20 and 100 pairs can now justify the purchase of their own multilayer coating equipment. Without the need to send lenses to a specialist coating centre, a much more rapid turn round can also be achieved. This coating service is also quicker because the new sputter technique does not need the lenses to be dehydrated for a long time. The small size and relative simplicity of a sputter coating system is shown in Figure 5.23.

Retail anti-reflective coating equipment

Many years ago even the glazing of lenses into frames was carried out remotely from opticians' premises. Gradually, this has changed, and we have seen the installation of in-store surfacing laboratories. With the growth of the number of spectacle wearers who use anti-reflection coatings there is now a desire by the in-store lens makers to provide a fast anti-reflection coating service to complement the fast surfacing that they provide. This has now become possible with coating systems specifically designed for a retail environment. Using the sputter coating technique it is possible to reduce the scale, the complexity and particularly the time required for anti-reflection coatings to the point at which single-pair coating in a few minutes has become possible and also financially viable. An in-store coating system is illustrated in Figure 5.24.

99% plus coatings

If the eye was equally sensitive to all colours and anti-reflection coatings simply reduced the amount of reflection equally for all wavelengths, then a paler white reflection would be produced. The simple concept that transmission (%) plus reflection (%) plus absorption (%) totals 100% would be unambiguous and clearly understood. Unfortunately, this is not the case.

Consider a simple single-layer violet anti-reflection coating with the reflection properties illustrated earlier. Although the minimum point shows no reflection, the average over the visible range is about 5%. This means that the average transmission for an untinted lens would be 95%, which is a typical value for a single-layer anti-reflection coating.

Similarly, for a broadband green or blue MAR coating, such as shown in Figure 5.20, the average reflection is about 1%. This

means that the average transmission for a clear lens would be 99%. Measurement of the transmission at all points over the visible spectral range is usually made on a spectrophotometer, illustrated in Figure 5.25.

From the spectrophotometer measurement, it is possible to calculate the average over the visible range (usually considered as 400–700nm). There is some debate about whether the reflection percentage should be the arithmetical average or the spectrally weighted average. For a broadband multilayer coating the difference in these values is not large; however, they

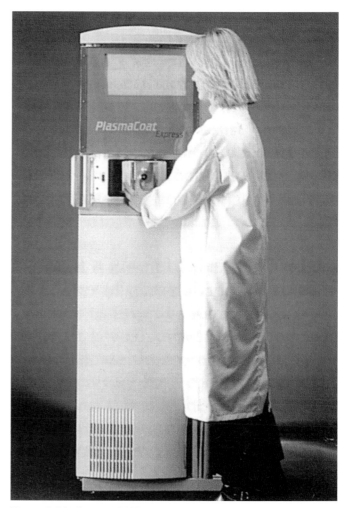

Figure 5.24   In-store MAR coating machine

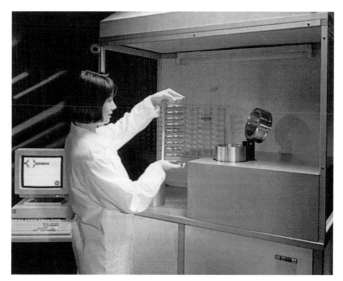

Figure 5.23   Prescription laboratory MAR machine

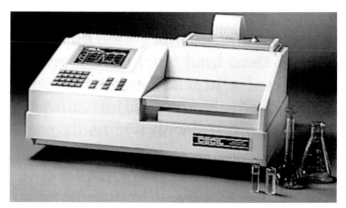

Figure 5.25   Spectrophotometer (to measure reflection)

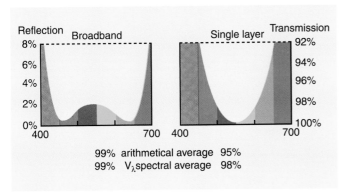

Figure 5.26   Anti-reflection transmission values

could be very different for (non-broadband) single-layer coatings (Figure 5.26).

Drawbacks of the most efficient coatings

The lowest reflection (highest transmission) anti-reflection coating is not necessarily the best. It is necessary to consider other properties, such as ease of cleaning. The lower the reflection value, the more difficult it is to keep a lens looking clean. It is not that the lens is actually any dirtier, just that it appears to be. It is worth pointing out that in Japan, where a high proportion of people wear anti-reflection coatings, the industry normally provides a slightly higher reflection value than in Europe, where anti-reflection coating is not yet so common. When dispensing anti-reflection coatings it may be wise to consider the compromise between a lower reflection and ease of cleaning.

Quality standards for anti-reflection

Standards on the qualities of anti-reflection coatings must consider two important aspects, the optical properties and the physical properties of the coatings.

It is important when considering optical properties that producers make their claims of reflection values on a consistent basis. This is now a requirement of the International Standards on Anti-reflection Optical Quality[4], which states that manufacturers should provide, on request, both the arithmetical and the spectrally weighted values of reflection.

For physical properties, test methods that measure the adhesion and durability qualities of coatings need to be employed. Many test methods are currently available. The quickest and simplest method is to immerse the lenses for a short time alternately in boiling salt water and then in cold water. Failure in this test certainly indicates poor adhesion, but does not guarantee a durable coat. In fact, there is no guarantee, other than subjecting the lenses to many years of real-life situations. Another test, which generally gives results that relate quite closely with real-life, is a cyclic humidity test. Lenses are subjected to a few hours of high humidity at a moderate temperature, followed by a few hours at room temperature, and this is repeated for a few days. At present (2007), the International Standards Organisation (ISO) is developing a standard on Coating Durability. Trials carried out by members of a special ISO committee indicate that the closest correlation with real-life can be achieved by applying heat, humidity and ultra-violet light on a cyclic basis of a few hours, over a number of days.

References

1. Rayton W B 1917 The reflected images in spectacle lenses. J Opt Soc Am 1:137–148
2. Jalie M 1984 Principles of ophthalmic lenses. ABDO, London
3. Bennett A G 1968 Emsley and Swaine's ophthalmic lenses, vol. 1. Hatton Press, London
4. BS EN ISO 8980-4:2000 Ophthalmic optics – Uncut finished spectacle lenses – Part 4: Specifications and test methods for anti-reflective coatings

Surface treatments

Peter Wilkinson, PhD BSc(Eng) CEng MIMechE

The treatment of lens surfaces to reduce reflections by means of single-layer or multilayer anti-reflection coatings is considered in Chapter 5, but surfaces may also be treated to enhance other optical and/or physical properties of lenses. Optical enhancements include tinting, ultraviolet (UV) and mirror treatments, and physical enhancements include hard coats and hydrophobic coatings. Glass lenses may also be specially treated to improve their strength by toughening their surfaces, a process considered later in this chapter.

Hard coating – general

Although some types of glass are softer than others, generally they offer sufficient abrasion resistance not to require a hard surface coating. Some special glasses do require a coating because of their tendency to stain, but these are normally high-index glasses, which would, in any case, usually have an anti-reflection coating.

Turning to plastics and/or resin materials we need to consider, separately, the two families of plastics, thermosetting materials and thermoplastic materials.

A thermosetting material is created in a mould by a chemical reaction, and if subsequently heated will not re-soften. Thermosetting materials include CR39 and most other high-index plastics materials used for spectacle lenses. In chemical terms, a thermosetting material is created by the cross-linking of molecules to form a rigid structure. The main thermosetting optical material, CR39, is reasonably scratch resistant and hard coating it may almost be considered optional. Higher index materials are generally softer and should therefore be hard coated. To distinguish between thermosetting materials and what are usually thought of as plastics, the term resin is normally used. In fact, CR39 stands for Columbia Resin, version number 39.

Thermoplastic materials are those that may be reheated and reformed. They consist of long chains of molecules that do not cross-link with each other. No irreversible chemical reaction is involved. The most common ophthalmic thermoplastic material in use today is polycarbonate, although polymethylmethacrylate (PMMA; Perspex) is still used for special lenses such as aspheric lenticulars, magnifiers and low visual acuity lenses.

All known thermoplastic materials are extremely soft and must therefore be hard coated to resist scratching. Finished single vision polycarbonate lenses are hard coated by the major manufacturers and specially worked lenses must be hard coated after surfacing.

What is meant by the term hard coat is a layer of material applied to a lens surface to improve its abrasion resistance. It is well known that the harder materials are the more brittle they must be. To prevent hard coats from cracking they must therefore be very thin relative to the thickness of the lens. Hard coats are usually between 0.5 micron and 10 microns thick (one micron = 10^{-3} mm). Typically, this is 10 to 20 times thicker than an anti-reflection coating.

Hard coats are made from different materials, but there are two main types. The most common are lacquer hard coats applied by dipping or spinning. Less common are the vacuum-deposited hard coats, which are thinner but of a harder material. The key difference is that dip-spin hard coats can be produced much more cheaply and are normally tintable.

The ability of a hard coat to resist scratching is a difficult property to quantify and is the subject of much debate at scientific meetings. The main problem is that so many different types of scratching can happen. Hard coats are usually very good at preventing the numerous small scratches that occur through general wear and tear, and through lens cleaning, but obviously cannot prevent the deep scratches caused by major abuse. In reality, of course, nothing, not even diamond, is scratch proof.

Another requirement of a hard coat is that it should be permeable to the photographic dyes employed to tint plastics lenses.

Vacuum-deposited hard coats (usually silica) are not tintable. Some makes of lacquer dip-spin hard coats are also non-tintable, depending on the chemicals used. Generally speaking, the non-tintable hard coats offer slightly more scratch resistance than those that tint easily. However, improvements in the chemical structure of dip-spin hard coats over recent years have made them almost as good as the non-tintable versions, with the major advantage of allowing tinting and re-tinting of lenses. Some non-tintable hard coats are only on the front surface of a lens, which permits tinting through the back surface, albeit at a slower tinting speed.

Dip hard coats

The dipping technique of hard coating (Figure 6.1) is usually used for large-volume production. It requires ultrasonic lens cleaning and stain-free drying equipment to prepare the lenses. Also, it is important to control the room temperature and humidity to prevent deterioration of the lacquer in the dipping tank, and ultra-clean conditions are required. A controlled rate of withdrawal is required to achieve constant hard-coat thickness and there are difficulties with the segment tops of bifocals. However, when well controlled by skilled staff, excellent results are achievable. Operating costs are low, but the capital investment is high.

Spin hard coats

The chemicals used for spin hard coating are generally similar to those used for dipping, although, usually, the solids-to-solvent ratio and the viscosity are changed to suit each different production technique. If a spin cleaner is also used, then spin hard coating requires much simpler equipment than does dipping, although the operating costs tend to be higher. A number of companies sell

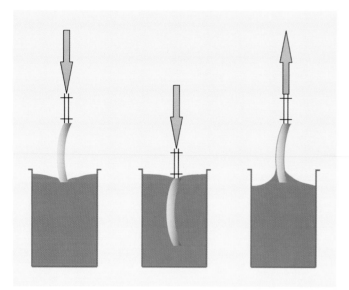

Figure 6.1   Dip coating

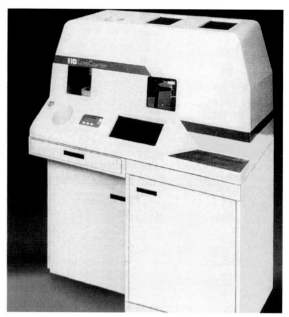

Figure 6.2   Spin hard-coating machine

small-scale hard-coating equipment suitable for coating upwards from 10 lenses per day. A photograph of a laboratory-scale hard-coater is shown in Figure 6.2.

In-mould hard coats

In-mould hard coats are made by forming the hard coat in the mould, at the same time as the lens is formed by a thermosetting process. In principle, this is a good way to make a hard coating since it will inherently bond well to the base lens. However, since in-mould hard coats are usually non-tintable, they are normally used only to make semi-finished lenses, which preferably have a concave hard coat applied after surfacing.

Vacuum hard coats

Vacuum hard coats are not very common, mainly because of the high cost of vacuum equipment. However, when the hard coat is created at the same time as an anti-reflection coating the difference in cost is not quite so significant. As indicated previously, hard coats are typically 10 to 20 times thicker than an anti-reflection coating so that they may require a long time in the vacuum chamber, which obviously must increase the cost.

Merit of hard coating both surfaces of the lens

While everyone agrees that it is important to hard coat the front surfaces of lenses, opinions differ as to the importance of treating the concave surface. Some years ago, when United Kingdom Optical Company (UKO) was developing the *PlasPlus* hard-coating process, they investigated the merits of coating both surfaces of a lens. On examination of a number of lenses that had been worn for some time, it was discovered that the front surface tended to show a few large (abuse!) marks plus a few finer scratches. By contrast the back surface rarely showed large scratches, but tended to have many more finer scratches than the front. Obviously, the power of the lens was also very significant. It was discovered that the fine scratches on the back were caused mainly by lens cleaning, particularly if done dry without previously washing the lens. In some cases, the scratches simply arose through constant contact with the tips of the closed sides when the spectacles were pushed back into the case. Since hard coats are particularly

good at preventing fine scratches, UKO took the view that hard coating the back was just as, if not more, important than hard coating the front surface. Obviously, cost is a factor, but, in general, hard coating both sides is obviously to be preferred.

Optical effect of a hard coat

If the refractive index of the hard coat is identical to that of the lens, and provided it has been applied properly, no optical effect should occur. In particular, it is not normally possible to see a hard coating on a lens, with the possible exception of the edges of bifocal segments. However, if the refractive index is different two effects are possible.

The main effect of a different refractive index in the hard coat to that in the substrate is that the surface reflection is affected (see Chapter 5). This is not usually very significant, as the refractive index of hard coats is very similar to the base lens. When applying anti-reflection coating to plastics lenses, this does offer a practical advantage in that a batch of lenses with different indices, but with identical hard-coat indices, produce anti-reflection coatings with similar reflection colours. This is because the hard coat is relatively thick compared to the anti-reflection coating and so the lens index becomes irrelevant.

The other effect results from the combination of thickness and refractive index. Any thin optical layer produces an optical wavelength interference effect that depends on the coating thickness. Suppose that a lens has a hard coat underneath an anti-reflection coat and the hard coat is exactly 10 times thicker than the anti-reflection coat. Wave-cancellation theory indicates that the hard coat produces 10 times as many wave interferences as the anti-reflection coat. This results in a change of the anti-reflection properties, as seen in Figure 6.3, which shows a spectrophotometer trace for two lenses, one with a hard coat and the other without.

Provided the hard coat is of exactly equal thickness across the lens surface, this does not create a problem with the visual appearance. However, if the hard coat varies in thickness, an interference pattern is seen, similar to the coloured effects produced by a thin film of oil on top of water. Companies involved in hard and anti-reflection coating are aware of this problem and therefore need to know the source of lenses that they are asked to

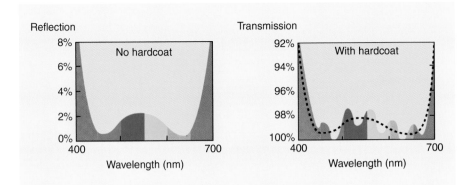

Figure 6.3   Anti-reflection versus wavelength trace with and without a hard coat

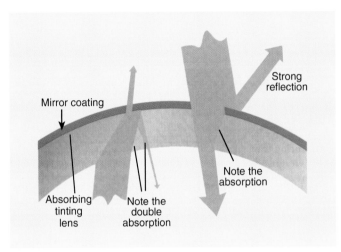

Figure 6.4   Reflection at a mirror coating

coat. This also explains why many prescription laboratories quite reasonably refuse to apply anti-reflection coating to lenses that they have not supplied themselves.

Mirror coatings

Mirror coatings usually combine a highly reflecting front lens surface with a strong absorption tint. In fact, it is not practical to create a mirror on the front of a lens without absorption in the lens, as otherwise the mirror can also be seen by the wearer, who might see a reflection of their own eye. The optics of this situation is illustrated in Figure 6.4.

It is not always appreciated that mirror coatings are not simply a layer of reflective material. In the same way as anti-reflection coatings use quarter-wave cancellation theory to reduce reflections, mirror coatings use half-wave addition theory to double reflections. This allows mirror coatings to be created with distinctive colours. Typical mirror coatings with blue, gold and silver reflections produced in a prescription laboratory anti-reflection coating machine are shown in Figure 6.5.

Hydrophobic coatings

While anti-reflection coatings offer many optical advantages, it is important to keep them clean. The main reason for this is that a very small amount of grease or oil on top of the anti-reflection coating destroys its effect. The result is an increase in reflection, at

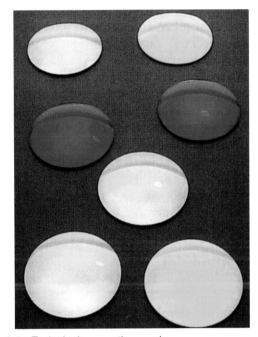

Figure 6.5   Typical mirror coatings on lenses

least back to the uncoated value. The reflection may even be greater because of the high reflectivity of oil or grease. As this does not occur evenly across the lens surface, it can be very annoying and wearers of anti-reflection coatings are often heard to complain that their lenses are difficult to keep clean. In fact, they are actually no dirtier than an uncoated lens, the wearer is just more aware of it.

This problem can be eased if a hydrophobic coating is applied to the lens surface. The basic principle is the same as applying a wax polish to a car, to create a high surface-wetting angle, which allows the water or oil to run off rather than wetting – and then drying on – the surface (Figure 6.6). During their development, hydrophobic coatings are usually quantified by measuring the wetting angle.

Hydrophobic coatings can be applied to lenses by a simple dipping process. However, a hydrophobic coating is so thin that it can easily lose its effectiveness after a short time. Baking after dipping enhances the life, but a better alternative is to apply the hydrophobic in a vacuum chamber as the final stage of a multilayer anti-reflection (MAR) coating process. The thickness of a hydrophobic layer can be measured in numbers of molecules, and so is generally an order of magnitude thinner than an anti-reflection coating, which is itself an order of magnitude thinner than a hard coating.

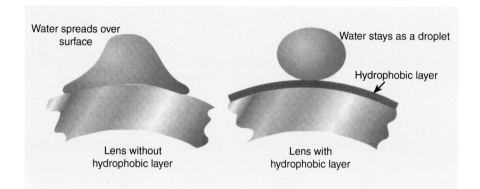

Figure 6.6   The hydrophobic effect

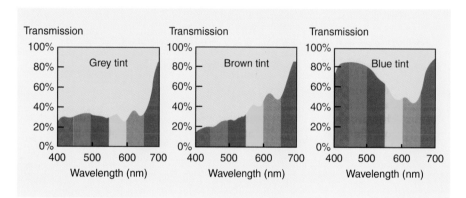

Figure 6.7   Spectral transmission curves for grey, brown and blue tints

Surface tinting of lenses

Tints are simply methods of absorbing light so that transmission is reduced. If all the wavelengths of light are equally absorbed, then a grey (neutral density) tint is produced. If the absorption is different for different wavelengths, then the tint has a particular colour. Figure 6.7 shows typical transmission curves for a grey tint, a brown tint and a blue tint. It is the complementary colours that are absorbed (i.e. a brown tint is produced when light is absorbed mainly from the blue and green regions of the spectrum).

It must be remembered that strongly coloured tints may affect colour vision, which is important in situations such as driving, for which there are legal requirements regarding traffic-signal recognition.

Measuring tint transmission

It is easy to understand the light transmission factor (LTF) for a grey (neutral density) tint, since the transmission is relatively constant across the whole of the visible spectrum. The meaning of LTF for a strongly coloured tint (with varying transmission across the spectrum) is more difficult to appreciate. It depends whether you are measuring the linear average, the spectrally weighted average or just a single value at a single wavelength. To obtain a truly accurate value the spectral curve must be measured with a spectrophotometer to produce the graphs shown in Figure 6.7. In practice, this is too complicated and a simpler instrument, such as the one shown in Figure 6.8, is used. Lenses that have power can also affect some instruments and it may be necessary to measure an equivalent tint in a plano-lens and compare this visually. For the sample tints depicted in Figure 6.7, the values that would be obtained by a simple instrument are given in Table 6.1.

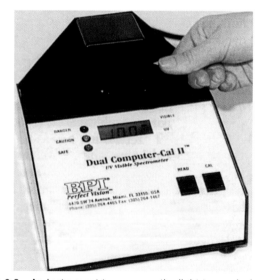

Figure 6.8   An instrument to measure the light transmission factor

Practical tinting of plastics lenses

Tinting plastics lenses is a relatively simple process. The lenses are placed in a suitable bath of hot lens-colouring dye for an appropriate length of time. If the lenses go too dark they may be placed in a bleach to reduce the depth of colour. It is, in fact, good tinting practice to overtint lenses slightly and then to place them in bleach for a few seconds to remove tint from close to the surface. This reduces the tendency for lenses to become paler with time, and is particularly important if lenses are to be placed in an ultrasonic cleaner (i.e. before anti-reflection coating).

Table 6.1　Light transmission factors for the sample tints described in Figure 6.7

	Grey tint (%)	Brown tint (%)	Blue tint (%)
'Visible' LTF	44	38	62
'Blue' LTF	24	33	86
'Green' LTF	36	29	68
'Red' LTF	51	41	63

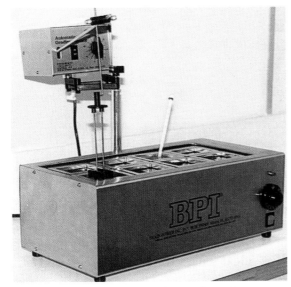

Figure 6.9　Typical plastics-lens tinting equipment

Graduated tints are made by moving the lenses (upside down) into and out of the tint tank so that the upper part of the lens absorbs more colour. Apart from having tint tanks with the common colours, such as grey and brown, it is normal to have some extra tanks with colour-correction dyes, including blue, red, yellow and green.

A typical tinting system is illustrated in Figure 6.9.

Specifying tints and coatings

The most important quality of anti-reflection coatings is the reduction of distracting reflections, so that ideally we should quantify an anti-reflection coating in terms of the strength of the surface reflection. However, most marketing claims are made in terms of the transmission (e.g. 99+ instead of 1% reflection).

There is a similar analogy with tints. What really matters for a tint is the amount of absorption, whereas tint strengths are usually quoted in terms of their transmittance, for example, a pale brown is called Brown 80%, whereas a dark sunglass tint may be a Brown 15%.

This unfortunate practice of specifying absorptive tints in terms of their luminous transmittance and anti-reflection coatings in terms of their transmission creates a particular problem when they are combined. Transmission, reflection and absorption are linked inextricably by the fact that the total energy of a system is constant. The incoming light energy is reflected, or transmitted, or absorbed (Figure 6.10). The light absorbed by a material is actually converted into heat, so that an absorbing lens is very slightly hotter than a non-absorbing one.

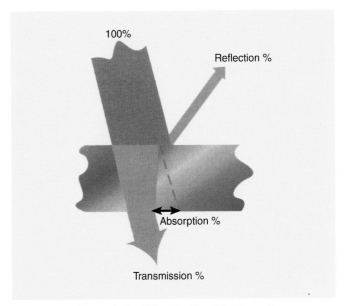

Figure 6.10　Transmission (%)+reflection (%)+absorption (%)=100%, from multiple sources

What this means is that if two lenses both have the same amount of absorbing tint, but only one is anti-reflection coated, then they have different transmission values. The ophthalmic industry convention is that the transmission value of an anti-reflection coating is specified as if the lens had no tint. It is also the convention that the transmission value of a tint is specified as if the lens is made from 1.5 index material and has no anti-reflection coating. This is an important problem when tints and anti-reflection coatings are combined and is best illustrated by the following example.

Suppose that a prescription order specifies a 99% MAR and a pale grey 75% tint, but these are to be supplied on a 1.6 index lens. The laboratory actually understands this to mean an anti-reflection coating that would give a 1% reflection on a clear lens, combined with a tint to produce a 75% transmission on a 1.5 index uncoated lens.

First, consider the tint. Since a clear 1.5 index lens reflects about 8% of the light, its untinted transmission is 92%. To achieve the 75% transmission, it is necessary to incorporate 17% absorption (92–75%; Figure 6.11a). In this case the laboratory first tints the lens to obtain this amount of absorption. The 1.6 index lens at this stage would be as shown in Figure 6.11b.

After the tinting has been completed, the anti-reflection coating is applied next, and reduces the normal reflectance to 1% (Figure 6.11c). The lens still has an absorption of 17%, but with a reflection of 1% it is easy to calculate that the transmission has increased to 82%. The finished lens therefore has the 1% reflection and 17% absorption implied by the order for a 99% MAR and 75% LTF tint; however, its actual light transmission value is 82%.

In fact, the actual situation is even more complicated because the specified coating reflection is divided between the two sides of the lens and the tint affects the surface reflections. This becomes more significant for darker tints. To prevent confusion, it is best both to discuss the precise requirement with the prescription laboratory so that they understand the requirement, and to use tinted samples to illustrate the actual absorption required.

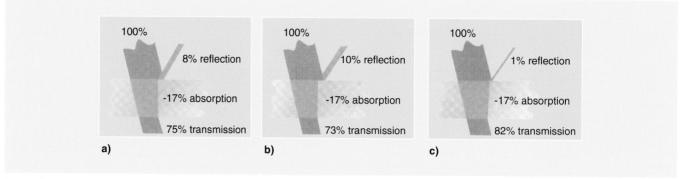

Figure 6.11   Transmission for a coated and an uncoated lens with the same absorption: (a) tinted 1.5 index lens; (b) tinted 1.6 index lens; (c) tinted and anti-reflection coated lens

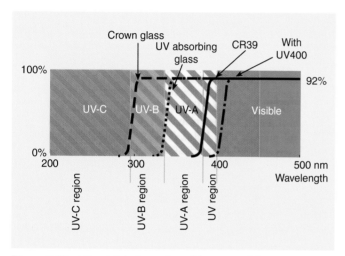

Figure 6.12   Ultraviolet absorption of lens materials

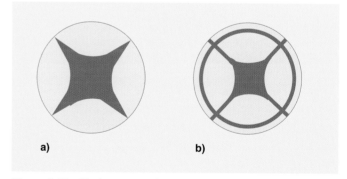

Figure 6.14   Resistance to force: (a) non-toughened glass; (b) toughened glass

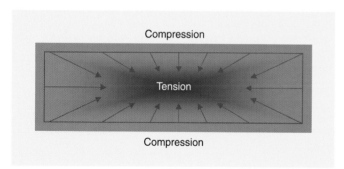

Figure 6.13   Toughened glass

Figure 6.15   Strain patterns in toughened lenses: (a) plus lens; (b) minus lens

Ultraviolet absorption

CR39 lenses already absorb some UV radiation, up to about 370nm, but the cut-off point may be moved to a higher wavelength by placing the lenses into a suitable dye. It is important that this is done correctly and that some check is made of the absorption properties after tinting. If the UV cut-off point is brought close to 400nm, then the lens still retains a white colour, but as soon as the absorption moves above 400nm lenses begin to show some yellowing. It is a requirement that any lens with a strong tint should also incorporate an UV absorber. The pupil of the eye increases in size in response to a dark tint and could therefore receive excessive amounts of UV radiation (see Chapter 7).

Transmission curves for materials typically used for clear lenses are shown in Figure 6.12.

Surface tinting of glass lenses

Glass lenses are less common now, particularly those with fixed tints. While mass-manufactured glass sunglare lenses are still available, non-photochromic tinted glass suitable for making prescription lenses is obsolete. An alternative technique is to use a vacuum-coating method to apply a tint to glass. Care should be taken to ensure that adequate UV blocking is provided by this method of tinting. Surface tinting has the advantage of allowing a

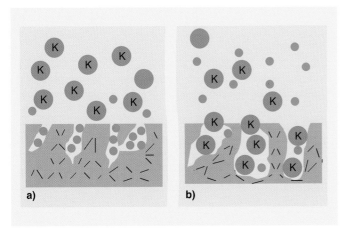

Figure 6.16 Schematic representation of ion exchange during chemical toughening: (a) before ion exchange; (b) after ion exchange

variety of colours to be produced, including gradient tints. Relatively small-scale glass-tinting machines are still used for this purpose by a few companies.

Toughening glass lenses

When glass has to be supplied as the lens medium, it can be strengthened by a toughening process. *Thermally toughened* lenses are produced by heating the finished lens to its softening point, followed by rapid cooling, either by a stream of cold compressed air directed at the surfaces or by submerging the lens in oil. The result of this treatment is to build up great compressive strength in the glass, since the outer region of the lens material cools more rapidly than the interior, which remains hotter and more fluid for some time. When the interior finally cools it contracts and exerts tension on the rigid outer surface to produce an exterior compressive envelope that encloses an interior under great tensile stress (Figure 6.13). When toughened glass receives a blow that would fracture ordinary glass, the compressive stress opposite the point of impact takes up the tension that the force exerts on the lens. Provided the tension exerted by the blow is less than the degree of compression, the lens does not break (Figure 6.14).

Toughened glass lenses are far more durable than ordinary glass lenses, for not only are they more difficult to break, but also they are more resistant to scratches because of their increased surface hardness. Furthermore, when a toughened lens does break it shatters into relatively harmless cubes of glass, which greatly decreases the danger from sharp splinters. The strain pattern in air- or oil-quenched thermally toughened lenses can be detected with a polariscope or strain tester. The patterns are frequently used to confirm the degree of toughening that the lens has received. The patterns from spherical lenses are quite characteristic (typical strain patterns are illustrated in Figure 6.15), but, in general, the strain pattern depends upon the power and shape of the lens.

Glass can also be toughened by a chemical process, in which a compressive envelope is produced by ion exchange as a result of a hot dip of the finished lens into a salt bath. For example, potassium ions in the bath can be exchanged for sodium or lithium ions in the glass. The smaller sodium or lithium ions near the glass surface are replaced by larger potassium ions, which squeeze their way into the glass surface and induce compressive stress (Figure 6.16). The usual bath composition is 99.5% potassium nitrate and 0.5% silicic acid heated to some 470°C. Temperature must be controlled carefully and the length of stay in the bath is critical, as the ion-exchange process is quite lengthy; the lenses need to remain in the bath for 16 hours. *Chemically toughened lenses* are stronger than air-quenched toughened lenses, but their strain pattern is not detectable in a strain tester.

Tinted lenses

Chapter 7

Trevor White, BA FBDO(Hons)

Light is a non-ionizing electromagnetic radiation produced naturally by thermonuclear reactions in the sun (or by other natural sources, such as lightning flashes) and artificially by incandescence, for example by a candle flame, the filament of a bulb, or by arcing between anode and cathode. Radiation is characterized by its wavelength; the radiation from the sun that reaches the earth's atmosphere extends from about 290nm to 20000nm in the infrared.

The optical range of radiation extends from about 100nm in the ultraviolet (UV) region of the spectrum up to 10^6nm in the infrared (Figure 7.1). The visible waveband, the part of the electromagnetic spectrum that stimulates the eye and gives rise to the sensation of vision, lies between 380nm and 780nm.

Although the eye is sensitive only to electromagnetic radiation within the waveband 380nm to 780nm, it is not uniformly sensitive to this waveband. When the visual response to a daylight source is plotted against wavelength, we obtain the spectral luminous efficiency for the daylight source shown in Figure 7.2. It can be seen that the wavelength that evokes the maximum response from the eye is at about 555nm, in the yellow–green portion of the spectrum.

Solar radiation

Light from the sun reaches the earth's surface according to the absorption and scattering characteristics of the earth's atmosphere. At any given time and particular position on the earth's surface, atmospheric effects depend on the elevation of the sun in the sky and daylight spectral power distribution varies with the time of day and the season of the year. Variations in the amount of light reflected by the terrain, such as woods, mountains, snow fields, sand or concrete expanses, lakes, etc., also contribute to the eventual daylight spectrum.

For all practical purposes, the shortest wavelength of solar radiation that reaches the earth's surface is 280nm. There is no conveniently definable upper limit, and only the narrow waveband from 380nm to 780nm gives rise to the sensation of vision.

Notice that the scale for the optical range of radiation, illustrated schematically in Figure 7.1, is not linear. The UV region is divided into three zones, but only two have biological significance, the short waveband UVC being absorbed by the earth's atmosphere.

Radiation within the UVB band (280–315nm) is absorbed substantially at the surface of the cornea, but energy at wavelengths from 295nm to 315nm can penetrate the interior of the eye and reach the retina. This waveband has a high photochemical activity and sunglass filters must be used to attenuate this region of the spectrum. Recommended maximum transmittance values for this waveband are specified in Table 7.1.

Radiation within the UVA band (315–380nm) penetrates more deeply into the eye as wavelength increases, so that crystalline lens and retinal damage can be caused by excessive exposure. Photochemical activity is lower than for UVB and permanent effects, such as cataract development or a reduction in transmittance of the ocular media, are seen to be accelerations of natural ageing processes over the years. Protection for this region is also essential and recommended maximum transmittance values for UVA are again specified in Table 7.1.

As said, it is the narrow waveband, 380–780nm, that gives rise to the sensation of light. Any discomfort within this visual spectrum is defined as glare. This occurs in strong sunlight, particularly when light is reflected at either specular or diffuse surfaces and notably when the dark-adapted eye is suddenly exposed to bright sources.

In recent years, concern has been expressed over the potential effects upon the eye of short-wave visible radiation. The blue-light hazard remains a controversial topic and, at present, it is suggested in the appropriate literature that under normal

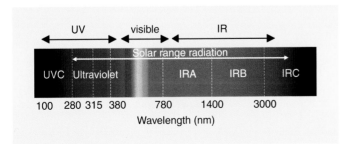

Figure 7.1   Optical range of radiation

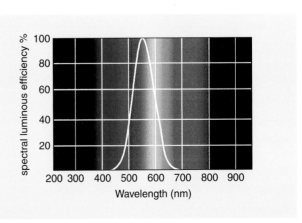

Figure 7.2   Graph of the spectral luminous efficiency function

97

Table 7.1   Categories for luminous transmittances and the related permissible transmittances in the ultraviolet solar spectral range

Categories	Visible spectral range (range of luminous transmittance) τ_V (%)	Ultraviolet spectral range (maximum value of solar transmittance) UVA from 315nm to 380nm	Ultraviolet spectral range (maximum value of solar transmittance) UVB from 280nm to 315nm
0	80–100		τ_V
1	43–80		
2	18–43	τ_V	$0.125\tau_V$
3	8–18	$0.5\tau_V$	
4	3–8		1.0% absolute

circumstances no risk is expected. However, modern standards on sunglass lenses do include a definition of blue-light transmittance and suggest how it should be expressed.

Radiation at wavelengths longer than over 780nm can also be categorized into zones according to the biological effects, but it is rare, if ever, for natural solar radiation to exceed the maximum permissible exposure level for this region. When a sunglare filter is claimed to have an infrared radiation protection quality, the infrared transmittance should not exceed the luminance transmittance.

The main purpose of sunglare filters is to protect the human eye against excessive solar radiation so as to reduce eyestrain and increase visual perception. To ensure fatigue-free vision, especially for prolonged usage, the choice of filter depends on the ambient light level and the individual's sensitivity to glare. Filters are now attributed to five luminance transmittance categories, as specified in Table 7.1.

It is worth noting that the new categories given in the Standards will replace the former categories:

A   (100 to 80%)
AB   (80 to 58%)
B1   (58 to 43.2%)
B2   (43.2 to 29.1%)
C   (29.1 to 17.8%)
D   (17.8 to 8%)

A tinted lens is defined in BS 3521 Part 1:1991 as a lens (generally an absorptive lens) that has a noticeable colour in transmission. Tinted lenses may either be of fixed colour or they may be photochromic. Such lenses may be supplied for cosmetic purposes, for the attenuation of unwanted radiations or for the modification of the incident radiation profile for various practical reasons.

Even in the case of lenses supplied for cosmetic purposes, the dispenser must be aware of the performance of the tint and be able to advise the patient, if necessary, on any problems with the lens, such as the distortion of signal colours. In the case of tints supplied for a specific 'clinical' purpose, since most of the relevant standards are registered under the Consumer Protection Act, a precise knowledge of the performance of the tint is essential.

Information for the specification of tinted lenses is contained in several Standards; Table 7.2 lists British, European and International Standards that contain information relevant to the specification and use of tinted lens materials.

Several artificial sources may give rise to radiation hazards. For example, UV radiation may be met in UV clinics, physiotherapy, from arc lights in film and TV studios and from the intense arc lights used in welding.

In ordinary circumstances solar infrared is unlikely to give rise to ocular problems, unless a subject stares hard at the sun, in which case macular lesions are likely to occur, but since exposure to infrared is invariably accompanied by the sensation of warmth, there is immediate awareness of the hazard.

Infrared radiation also occurs in industries in which furnaces are employed. Furnace workers, such as glass blowers, have long

Table 7.2   Standards relating to filter lenses

Standard	Date	Title
BS EN 169	2002	Personal eye-protection. Filters for welding and related techniques. Transmission requirements and recommended use.
BS EN 170	2002	Personal eye-protection. Ultraviolet filters. Transmission requirements and recommended use.
BS EN 171	2002	Personal eye-protection. Infrared filters. Transmission requirements and recommended use.
BS EN 174	2001	Personal eye-protection. Ski goggles for downhill skiing.
BS EN 207	1999	Personal eye-protection. Filters and eye protection against laser radiation (laser eye protectors).
BS EN 379	2003	Personal eye-protection. Automatic welding filters.
BS EN 1836	2005	Personal eye-equipment – Sunglasses and sunglare filters for general use and filters for direct observation of the sun.
BS 7394: Part 2	1994	Complete spectacles: specification for prescription spectacles
BS EN ISO 8980-3	2004	Ophthalmic optics – Uncut finished spectacle lenses-Part 3 Transmittance specifications and test methods.
BS EN ISO 13666	1999	Ophthalmic optics – Spectacle lenses – Vocabulary
BS EN ISO 14889	2003	Ophthalmic optics – Spectacle lenses – Fundamental requirements for uncut finished lenses.

been recognized as typical subjects for radiation cataract, so protection against infrared is usually provided in the workplace for these industrial activities.

Table 7.3 lists the terms used to discuss tinted lenses and deal with attenuation by filters.

Basic definitions

Attenuation of radiation is obtained either by absorption within the lens material or by reflection from the lens surfaces. The transmittance of a filter for a specified wavelength, $\tau_F(\lambda)$, is known as

Table 7.3 Tinted lens terminology

Radiant flux	Power emitted, transferred or received in the form of radiation
Luminous flux	Quantity characteristic of radiant flux that expresses its capacity to produce visual sensation, evaluated according to the figures of relative luminous efficiency for the light-adapted eye adopted by the Commission Internationale de l'Eclairage
Absorption	Reduction of radiant flux during its passage through a medium, not including loss by reflection
Transmission	Passage through a medium of radiant flux without change of frequency of its monochromatic components
Transmittance	For a specified wavelength, the ratio of the radiant flux transmitted by a lens to the incident radiant flux
Transmission curve	Graph in which the transmittance is plotted against wavelength
Luminous transmittance (τ_V)	Ratio of luminous flux transmitted by a lens to that which it receives
Optical density	Logarithm to the base 10 of the reciprocal of the appropriate transmittance
Filter	Device that changes the intensity and may also change the spectral distribution of the light passing through it
Sunglasses	Spectacles or attachments to spectacles that incorporate a filter to attenuate natural solar radiation
Anti-actinic	Absorbing ultraviolet radiation to a markedly greater extent than does white spectacle glass
Equitint	Of even coloration, notwithstanding thickness variations in different parts of the lens
Graduated tint	Having a controlled variation of tint over the whole or part of the lens
Coated lens	Lens to which one or more surface layers have been applied to alter one or more of the properties of the lens
Evaporated coating	Thin layer of a metal, or of a compound, deposited on the surface of a lens or screen by volatilization in a vacuum
Metallized lens	Lens upon which a metallic film has been formed by methods that include chemical deposition, evaporation in a vacuum and cathodic sputtering
Sputtered lens	Form of metallized lens
Surface-tinted lens	Lens that incorporates a surface layer to obtain an equitint effect
Flashed glass	Glass of one kind to which a thin layer of glass of another kind has been fused
Polarizing lens	Lens that shows different absorption according to the plane of polarization of the incident light
Photochromic lens	Lens made, completely or partially, from material that reversibly changes its transmission characteristics dependent upon the intensity of the radiation
Solid tinted lens	Lens in which the tint is incorporated throughout
Dyed lens	Plastics lens with the surface tint obtained by dipping into a dye
Shade number (N)	Indication of the transmittance of a filter defined by the equation: $N = 1 + (7/3)\log_{10}(1/\tau_V)$

the *spectral transmission factor* and is simply the ratio of the radiant flux transmitted by the lens to the incident radiant flux. A transmission curve (such as those shown in Figures 7.3 and 7.4) is a plot of the spectral transmission factors usually drawn for the waveband 300–800nm. Transmission curves are obtained by means of a spectrophotometer, which records the amount of radiant flux that falls on a photocell and produces a plot of the transmission for the filter under test.

That quantity characteristic of radiant flux that evokes the sensation of vision, evaluated according to the figures of spectral luminous efficiency for the light-adapted eye by the Commission Internationale de l'Eclairage (CIE), is called *luminous flux*. Spectral luminous efficiency is assumed to be that of a standard observer viewing a standard source, which is taken to be the day-light source CIE Standard Illuminant D65.

As pointed out above, the eye's visual system is not uniformly sensitive to the visible spectrum (illustrated by the graph of the spectral luminous efficiency function in Figure 7.2). The graph, which refers to photopic vision, shows that the eye is most sensitive to radiation with wavelength of about 555nm. The response

to the extreme red and blue ends of the visible spectrum is very low.

The ratio of the luminous flux transmitted by a lens to that which it receives is known as the *luminous transmittance*. Luminous transmittance is the ratio of the total amount of luminous energy received by a standard eye viewing a standard source through a filter to the amount of energy received directly.

The luminous transmittance is determined from the equation:

$$\tau_V = \frac{\int_{380nm}^{780nm} S_{D65}(\lambda)\,\tau_F(\lambda)\,V(\lambda)\,d(\lambda)}{\int_{380nm}^{780nm} S_{D65}(\lambda)\,V(\lambda)\,d(\lambda)}$$

where $s_{D65}(\lambda)$ is the spectral distribution of radiation of CIE standard illuminant D65, $V(\lambda)$ is the spectral luminous efficiency for photopic vision and $(\tau)_F(\lambda)$ is the spectral transmittance of the sun glare filter.

In practice, factors are supplied for the waveband 380–780nm in 10nm steps, which when multiplied by the spectral

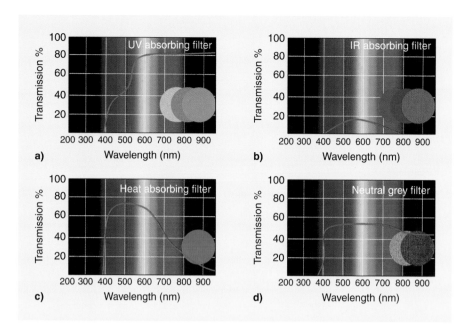

Figure 7.3   Transmission curves for various types of filter: (a) UV-absorbing filters; (b) infrared-absorbing filters; (c) heat-absorbing filters; (d) neutral grey filters

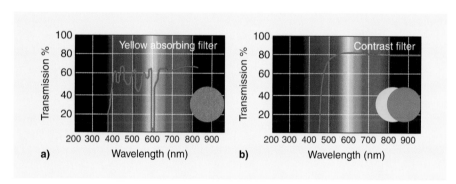

Figure 7.4   Transmission curves for special types of filters: (a) yellow-absorbing filter; (b) contrast filter

transmittances for these wavelengths can be summed to provide the luminous transmittance of the filter.

The *mean ultraviolet transmittance*, τ_{UVA}, of a filter is deduced from seven values taken from a spectral transmittance curve between 315nm and 375nm, at 10nm intervals. The mean UVA transmittance is obtained from the equation:

$$\tau_{UVA} = \frac{10\left[0.5\tau_{315} + \sum\limits_{325}^{375}\tau_F(\lambda)\right]}{65}$$

Mean blue range transmittance, τ_B, is the mean of the spectral transmittances taken at 13 wavelengths from 380nm to 500nm in 10nm intervals:

$$\tau_B = \frac{\sum\limits_{380}^{500}\tau_F(\lambda)}{13}$$

To ensure that a filter does not distort colour values, the *relative visual attenuation coefficient* (Q) for four signal colours, red, yellow, green and blue, is determined:

$$Q = \frac{\tau_{sign}}{\tau_V}$$

where τ_{sign} is the luminous transmittance of the sunglare filter for the spectral power distribution of the signal light and

τ_V is the luminous transmittance of the sunglare filter for CIE Illuminant D65. The recommendation is that the coefficient should not be less than a given amount for each of the signal colours. In short, the luminous transmittance of the filter for the specified signal lights must not be less than a given percentage of the luminous transmittance.

If a filter is claimed to attenuate infrared radiation associated with daylight, the *mean infrared transmittance* should not exceed τ_V when determined from:

$$\tau_{SIR} = \frac{\sum\limits_{780}^{2000}E_\lambda\tau_\lambda}{\sum\limits_{780}^{2000}E_\lambda}$$

where τ_λ is the spectral transmittance of the material and E_λ is the spectral irradiance, expressed in MWm^{-3}, for the infrared spectral range 780–2000nm.

Types of filters

An ideal filter for sunglass use should attenuate UV radiation, reduce transmittance to a comfortable level without distorting colour values and maintain good visual acuity across the spectrum. Since no risk is expected from the infrared portion of the spectrum, even under extreme illuminance conditions, infrared attenuation is not essential in ordinary sunglass lenses.

Filters can be classified conveniently as being either absorptive or reflective.

Absorptive tints absorb the light that passes through them and converts it into another form of energy. All solid tints and dyed plastics tints are absorptive.

Absorptive glasses

Most absorptive glass tinted lenses are of solid materials, and have the tint distributed uniformly through the material during the manufacturing process. In the case of photochromic materials, absorption is accompanied by a change in the colour of the filter. Coloration of the tinted material is caused by the addition to the glass melt of compounds designed to produce attenuation of different wavebands. Typical examples are given in Figures 7.3 and 7.4.

Figure 7.3 illustrates the transmission curves of common glass filters used to attenuate sunlight. The pink filters simply absorb UV radiation. Notice that the darker shades of pink are a warm brown colour. The green filters absorb both UV and infrared, and the darker shades of green take on a smoky brown appearance. The neutral grey filter absorbs UV and, since its transmission curve is fairly even throughout the visible spectrum, should not distort colour values.

Figure 7.4 illustrates the transmission curves of two specialist filters. The yellow-absorbing filter contains didymium, which causes the filter to absorb strongly in the yellow region of the spectrum. It has been suggested that use of such a filter may enhance colour discrimination between the red and blue ends of the spectrum.

The contrast filter absorbs strongly at the blue end of the spectrum, and thus enhances contrast, for example, in hazy weather. Such filters, however, do disturb colour discrimination.

The transmittance of an absorptive material depends upon the lens thickness. This is a problem with prescription lenses, since they exhibit uneven transmittance as the thickness varies. Even for lower power lenses, since the variation of thickness with transmission is not linear, this can cause difficulties for the practitioner who requires a specific transmittance, but only knows the transmittance of a given lens at a different thickness to that of the finished prescription. A number of methods[1,2] to determine the transmittance of a given lens at a new thickness have been described, but perhaps one of the simplest ways is to use the surface transmittance (T_S), which is simply (1 – the reflectance). Then, if the transmittance (T) of a lens at thickness t is known, its transmittance (T') at a new thickness (t_n) is given by:

$$T' = T_S^2 \left(T/T_S^2\right)^{(t_n/t)}$$

When the transmittance of a solid tint at a new thickness needs to be known, this expression can be programmed readily into a spreadsheet and the calculations carried out quickly and with the minimum of tedium. The example below shows the transmittance calculated for thicknesses between 1mm and 5mm of a spectacle crown glass lens known to have a transmittance of 0.57 at 2mm. Approaching the calculation this way has the advantage that, when the spreadsheet is written, the lens parameters simply have to be changed to produce the data for another lens just as quickly.

An example is given to demonstrate how the transmittance at the different wavelengths is calculated for a new thickness of, say, 4mm.

We are given that:

$$n = 1.523 \quad t = 2$$
$$T = 0.57 \quad t_n = 4$$

$$T_S = 1 - \left(\frac{1 - 1.523}{1 + 1.523}\right)^2$$
$$= 0.9570$$

$$T_S^2 = 0.916$$

$$T' = 0.916 \times \left(\frac{0.57}{0.916}\right)^{(4/2)}$$
$$= 0.355$$

Absorptive plastics

Plastics filters are produced by dyeing either the parent material or the finished lenses by a hot dip in photographic dyes; the dye penetrates the surface up to a depth of about 1mm. In some cases the dye is designed to penetrate only a coating applied to the lens.

Unlike a glass filter, the colour of plastics filters is not a reliable indication of its transmission properties and a transmission curve for the filter should be consulted to determine the transmission properties. UV attenuation can be increased by adding a UV inhibitor to the white lens monomer.

Reflecting filters

Reflecting filters protect the eyes by reflecting away unwanted radiation. The reflectivity of one surface is increased deliberately by coating the surface under high vacuum with a very thin film of a metallic substance. The mechanical properties required for the film are the same as those required for an anti-reflective film (hard, strongly adherent, etc.). The first reflecting filters were all brown in colour and available in any percentage transmission (e.g. 75%, 50%, 25%, etc.). Now, almost any colour is available and in recent years strongly reflecting mirror coatings have been applied to the convex surface of plastics lenses (see Chapter 6).

Reflecting filters use coatings of high refractive index to reflect away the unwanted radiations. Most coated tints are reflective, although it is possible to produce absorptive coatings.

Absorptive coatings

Absorptive coatings are usually made from chromium or NiCr with MgF_2 or SiO (or SiO_2). They must be evaporated with substrate temperatures of 250 to 300°C, and are therefore unsuitable for use with plastics lenses.

Reflective coatings

Usually, reflective coatings are basically chromium or NiCr, which have good adherence even if the substrate is almost unheated. They can therefore be used satisfactorily with plastics lenses, but their low hardness normally results in the deposition of a quartz layer over them.

When a single layer of high refractive index material, n_f, is deposited on glass of refractive index n_g, the reflectance, ρ, is given by:

$$\rho = \left(\frac{n_g^2 - n_f}{n_g^2 + n_f}\right)^2$$

For example, zinc sulphide (ZnS), $n_f = 2.3$, on glass of $n_g = 1.5$ produces the result, $\rho = 31\%$.

Since the rear surface of the film is highly reflective (in contact with air), it is usual to deposit a second coat of magnesium fluoride – the usual anti-reflective coating substance – on top of the reflective coat to decrease reflections from the back surface into the eye. Some reflective tints can, however, be produced

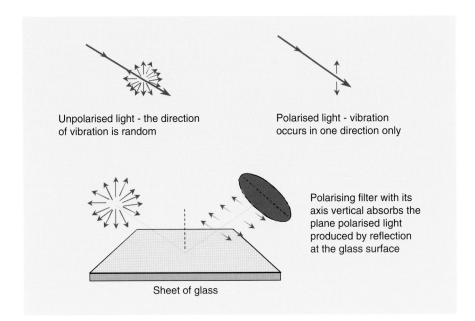

Figure 7.5 Polarized light produced by reflection

Unpolarised light - the direction of vibration is random

Polarised light - vibration occurs in one direction only

Polarising filter with its axis vertical absorbs the plane polarised light produced by reflection at the glass surface

Sheet of glass

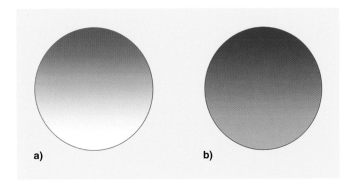

Figure 7.6 Gradient filters: (a) dark to clear; (b) two-colour (rainbow) filter, blue to pink

without the characteristic appearance of an anti-reflection coating, so called 'bloom-free' coatings, by the incorporation of multiple layers in the stack.

Polarizing filters

It can also be helpful to supply sunglasses that eliminate horizontally reflected radiation from water, snow or metalled roads. Polarizing sunglasses fulfil this function. These absorb, in addition to unwanted radiation, the plane polarized light usually produced by reflection from the surfaces mentioned. Polarized light is different from ordinary or unpolarized light. Ordinary light may be represented by a wave motion that vibrates in all directions (Figure 7.5). Plane polarized light can be imagined as a vibration in one direction only.

When light is reflected, the degree of polarization depends upon the angle of incidence. It reaches a maximum when the angle between the refracted and reflected rays is 90° (see Chapter 5). The light reflected is then totally plane polarized, the plane of the vibration being parallel to the reflecting surface (i.e. horizontal). When the polarizing axis of the filter is set vertically, the reflected light is absorbed. The filter therefore eliminates reflected glare and enables the eye to view objects illuminated by unpolarized light. Anglers, in particular, find these filters useful, since with them they can see below the surface of the water.

Gradient filters

Gradient filters have a progressive variation in luminous transmission, usually from darkest at the top to lightest at the bottom of the filter (Figure 7.6). They may be single colour, as depicted in Figure 7.6a, or they may produce a so-called rainbow effect, as in Figure 7.6b. Glass gradient filters can be produced by a bonding process or by vacuum coating. Plastics lenses are produced in gradient form easily by withdrawing the filter from the dye bath at a controlled steady rate.

Assessment of performance

The old Standard relating to Spectacle Lens Materials, BS 3062:1985, (now obsolete) required the supplier of spectacle lens material to provide:

- Nominal spectral transmittance graphs over the wavelength 380nm to 800nm for a 2mm (or another specified) thickness.
- Nominal luminous transmittance for CIE illuminant C for a 2mm (or another specified) thickness.
- If ultraviolet absorbing properties are claimed, then the graph must be extended from 380nm to 280nm.
- If infrared absorbing properties are claimed, then the graph must be extended out to 2000nm.

In assessing the performance of a spectacle lens, the prescriber has available the spectral and luminous transmittances. It is also a requirement that a tinted prescription lens that is intended for use when driving should not have a luminous transmittance of 8% or less at the design reference point, that the spectral transmittance, $\tau(\lambda)$, at any wavelength in the range 500nm to 650nm shall not be less than $0.2\,\tau_V$. In addition, if the lenses are to be used for driving at night the luminous transmittance should not be less than 75% at the design reference point. Lenses that are intended to be used for driving must also conform to the signal and colour recognition requirements of BS EN ISO 14889. The *relative visual attenuation coefficient*, Q, for the four signal colours is defined above. The Standard requires Q to be not less than 0.8 for the red and yellow signal colours, not less than 0.6 for green and not less than 0.4 for the blue signal light.

As has already been stated, tinted lenses are supplied largely to attenuate unwanted radiations or to alter the profile of radiations that reach the eye. There are a number of common situations in which this is required.

Attenuation of radiation

Ultraviolet

UV radiation relevant to tinted lenses is divided into UVB (280–315nm) and UVA (315–380nm). The danger of UV radiation is now well understood by both patients and prescribers. The question of whether UVB is the only source of danger, or whether UVA may also be considered dangerous, remains contentious. However, a research report by the National Radiological Protection Board casts some doubt on the view that the only radiation likely to cause problems is UVB.[3] A UV filter, therefore, should obstruct all radiations below 360nm at least. Figure 7.3 illustrates a transmission curve for a typical filter that attenuates UV. It is often feasible, of course, to provide this degree of UV protection without the use of a filter, but if protection is desired from the start of the visible spectrum, then some residual colour in the lens is inevitable.

BS 7394 specifies the terminology, described below, for UV-absorbing lenses (Table 7.4).

Infrared

Infrared radiation has wavelengths between 760nm and approximately 500000nm, and usually arises from industrial processes such as furnace working. It is generally reckoned that wavelengths of about 1400nm are the most hazardous, and for any filter claimed to have specific infrared-absorbing properties, the manufacturer is required to extend the spectral transmission chart from 780nm to 2000nm. Such filters are most often supplied as plano-goggles or face shields, but if required in spectacles, most usually the lenses need to be glass, since CR39 does not make a good basis for an infrared-absorbing filter as the heat tends to degrade the material. However, polycarbonate can be used to some degree to provide infrared absorption and at least one such lens is commercially available. Glass infrared-absorbing filters are generally green in colour as they contain ferrous oxide (Figure 7.3).

Heat

Filters specified as heat absorbing are also infrared absorbing, but they are designed to allow as much light through as possible. They are usually pale blue or green in colour and have a peak transmission at 500–550nm, after which transmission falls rapidly to virtually zero at about 800nm, and remains so into the far infrared. A typical transmission curve for a heat-absorbing filter is illustrated in Figure 7.3.

Table 7.4	Ultraviolet absorption	
	Minimum absorption (%) at any wavelength within the range	
	UVB	UVA
UVB absorber	99	50
UVA absorber	99	95

Yellow light

Yellow has the highest luminosity of all the colours and effectively is most likely to cause dazzle. Filters that absorb yellow reduce glare and also increase discrimination between the red and the blue ends of the spectrum. They can also be of some use in certain cases of colour defectiveness. Solid-glass filters that contain didymium can be obtained and provide a high degree of yellow absorption (Figure 7.4).

Blue light (contrast filters)

Although the extent of the 'blue-light hazard' is a matter of dispute, it has been known for many years that reducing the transmittance at the blue end of the spectrum increases contrast and eases the eye's ability to distinguish between light and dark areas. Such filters, which are available in both glass and plastics, vary in colour from yellow to red, depending on the amount of absorption required. As a minimum, a contrast filter should be expected to absorb all radiation below about 450nm and rise to a peak transmission at about 525nm, and thereafter remain virtually constant (Figure 7.4).

The use of contrast filters has been advocated recently to reduce the troublesome effects of flickering fluorescent lighting in offices. Fluorescent lighting has peaks of power both in the UV and the blue region of the spectrum, and it is claimed that when these peaks of flickering are removed, the total effect of the flicker is less noticeable. This appears to work for a number of people, but (like all contrast filters) they distort the spectral distribution and may therefore be unacceptable to the patient.

Photochromic lenses

The purpose of any sunglass filter is to provide protection from harmful radiation and comfort to the eyes under all conditions of illumination. In theory, this ideal is more nearly attainable with photochromic filters, which darken automatically in bright sunlight and lighten automatically when the exciting radiation is removed (Figure 7.7). In bright sunlight and in conditions under which the illumination level is constant, fixed-tint filters offer immediate relief from the sun's glare. In conditions under which illumination levels vary, however, fixed-transmission filters may be too dark or too light for a particular scene. The self-adjusting nature of the photochromic phenomenon lends itself well to variations in ambient illumination.

The phenomenon of photochromic behaviour (literally, coloured by light) may be described as the modification of the light-absorbing characteristics of a material under the influence of radiation from the sun. In the best-known photochromic process, used in photographic film, the light-sensitive film is a mixture of silver halide crystals, usually bromide with a little iodide, embedded in gelatine on a cellulose acetate base. When light strikes the silver halide crystals they undergo a chemical change, so that during the developing process the liberated metallic silver forms the image on the film.

The photochromic behaviour of glass lenses is produced by the addition of silver halide crystals to the glass melt. When photochromic glass is exposed to short-wave visible light and, notably, UVA radiation, the crystals disperse minute silver particles (about 100nm in size) into the glass mass. This metallic silver absorbs light and causes a tint to appear in the lens. The crystals remain decomposed in the presence of the exciting radiation, but when the source is removed the silver held within the glass matrix is available to recombine with the halogens and the glass recovers to its clear state. Control of the size and number of these particles

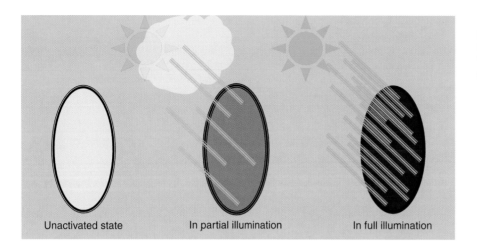

Figure 7.7 The photochromic phenomenon. As the intensity of the radiation increases, the lens darkens further. The tint fades when the exciting radiation is removed

Unactivated state   In partial illumination   In full illumination

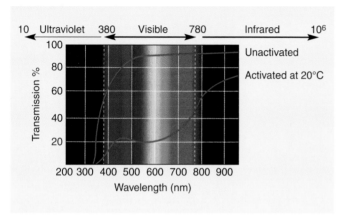

Figure 7.8 Transmission curves for Photogray Extra glass at 2mm thickness in unactivated and activated states

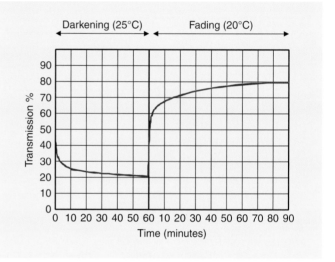

Figure 7.9 Speed of photochromic reaction in the darkening–fading cycle for Photogray Extra glass

ensures the reproducibility of the colour and darkened transmittance of photochromic glass.

The ideal size for the silver halide crystals suspended in the glass is between 800nm and 1500nm.[4] Below 800nm the photochromic effect is insignificant and above 1500nm the glass tends to become opalescent. The ideal separation of the silver halide crystals is given as approximately 10000nm.

The photochromic reaction in silver glasses is, in general, quite slow and it is normal to add small amounts of copper to the glass mix as a catalyst. Many other factors affect the darkening and fading rates, such as levels of lead, boric acid and alkali in the mix, the temperature of the material and the precise nature of the heat treatment during the annealing process.

Absorption of UVA and light from the blue region of the spectrum is the trigger for the photochromic process, and that these wavebands are absorbed is confirmed by the typical transmission curve for a photochromic glass material, Corning's Photogray Extra, illustrated in Figure 7.8.

In the activated state it can be seen that the glass absorbs strongly both the UVA radiation and the blue region of the visible spectrum. Removal of these wavebands is exactly what is required to protect the eyes from harmful radiation, so the photochromic reaction is visible proof that the lenses actually protect the eyes.

The photochromic performance of glass depends upon several factors:

- **The amount of light** – darkening occurs far more quickly with a clear blue sky than in overcast conditions or inside a motor car.

- **The type of radiation** – the activating waveband is within the UVA and blue region of the visible spectrum. Conditions in which there is a large amount of this waveband (e.g. at high altitudes) enhance the speed of darkening.
- **The temperature of the lens** – photochromic performance increases as the temperature of the lens decreases. The performance is enhanced by the cold.
- **The thickness of the lens material** – the thicker the lens the greater the density of the halide crystals and the darker the lens becomes.
- **The history of previous cycles** – the photochromic behaviour of the lens is enhanced by continuous darkening and fading cycles. The glass requires a conditioning period to work at full performance. Glass lenses can be artificially restored to their original clear state by immersion in boiling water in a glass beaker for 30 minutes.

Photochromic glasses first appeared in 1964, but it took a further 10 years of development to produce the sophisticated fast-acting glasses from which today's lenses are made. The speed at which the photochromic reaction occurs in Corning's Photogray Extra material is shown in Figure 7.9. After just 20 seconds' exposure the material has darkened to 30% transmission and reaches 25% transmission after 10 minutes.

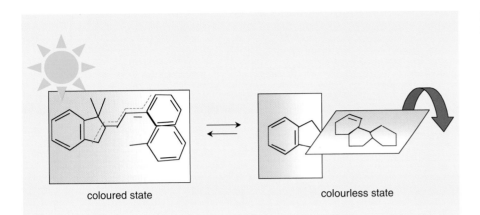

coloured state   colourless state

Figure 7.10   Mechanism of photochromic response in spiropyrans

On removal from light, fading is slightly slower, with the glass recovering to about 65% after 5 minutes and approaching 80% transmission after 90 minutes in the dark. These transmission details vary with the temperature of the lens. As a general rule, photochromic lenses darken more in low temperatures and fade more rapidly as the temperature increases.

Photochromic glasses are available for prescription use in normal 1.523 index and mid-index 1.600 material, in grey and brown versions. Pre-tinted pink and brown glasses are also available for sunglass use.

The hardness of glass lenses provides the advantage that they are resistant to surface scratching, but the drawback that they break if subjected to shock. They can be treated for impact resistance by toughening. With heat toughening, the treated lenses darken rather more in response to sunlight and clear a little more slowly. Anti-reflection treatment also affects the speed of reaction.

The photochromic molecules are distributed evenly throughout the volume of the glass. In the case of prescriptions for moderate-to-high power, with thickness that varies from centre to edge and required in photochromic form, it is necessary to bond a thin photochromic shell to a base white lens. A specially designed glass is available when this bonding process is necessary, which still develops a good depth of tint at thicknesses below 2mm. This can be bonded to either normal index crown glass or to 1.70 high-index glass to obtain even thinner equitint prescription lenses.

Photochromic plastics materials

The vast majority of spectacle lenses dispensed today are made from plastics materials, since these are much lighter and inherently safer than glass. It took many years of research to obtain a photochromic process for plastics lenses that would perform in the same way as that in glass. The first photochromic plastics lenses appeared during the 1970s, but real success was not achieved until 1990 when the first Transitions lenses were introduced.[5]

The photochromic process in plastics materials is quite different from that in glass. Photochromic materials, such as oxazines, pyrans and fulgides, are added to the lens material. The exciting wavelengths that activate the photochromic behaviour are usually more specific than is required for glass. The mechanism of the photochromic response of spiroxazines is similar to that of the spiropyrans. When the molecules are exposed to UV radiation a portion of the molecule rotates, which causes the material to darken and absorb strongly in the UV and blue wavebands. Removal of the exciting wavelengths allows the molecules to flip back to their original orientations and the material fades back to its original transmittance (Figure 7.10).

The photochromic compounds are applied to a plastics lens by a coating process. If dip-coating or spin-coating methods are

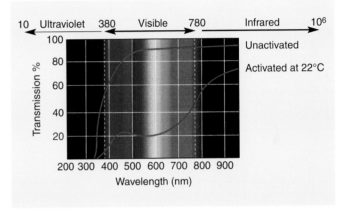

Figure 7.11   Transmission curves for *Transitions III* lenses at all thicknesses in unactivated and activated states

employed, the photochromic layer is too thin, so it is usual to allow the photochromic compounds to penetrate the plastics substrate by a dyeing process. To optimize performance, it is essential to ensure uniformity in depth and density of penetration. This involves careful preparation of the original monomer and closely controlled time and temperature cycles during the imbibition process. The photochromic dye penetrates just 100μm to 150μm beneath the surface of the lens and so the dyed lens is always of equitint form, even if the thickness of the material varies. This is of enormous advantage to the wearers of moderate and high-power prescriptions, since the colour of their photochromic lenses does not vary with the depth of tint.

Absorption of UVA is the trigger for the photochromic process, and the transmission curve for *Transitions III*, depicted in Figure 7.11, illustrates that the activated lens also absorbs strongly in the blue waveband.

The factors that affect the photochromic reaction in plastics lenses are much the same as those for glass. High levels of UV radiation and cold temperatures enable the lenses to darken optimally. The speed at which the photochromic reaction occurs in *Transitions III* material is shown in Figure 7.12. The reaction time for the darkening cycle is almost as fast as for glass lenses. The values for the transmission indicated in Figure 7.12 assume an ambient temperature of 22°C. At colder temperatures the lens darkens even further; for example, at 10°C the material darkens to about 25%. Fading is somewhat slower, but (as with glass lenses) speeds up as the temperature increases.

A darker version of Transitions is also available in the form of *Transitions XTRActive*, with a transmission swing from about 75% in the faded state to 20% in the darkened state.

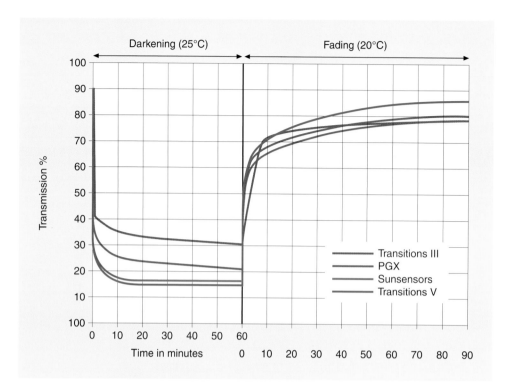

Figure 7.12   Speed of photochromic reaction in the darkening–fading cycles for *Transitions III* and *Transitions V Next Generation* lenses

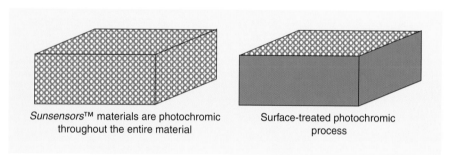

Figure 7.13   *SunSensors*™ material is photochromic throughout the entire material

Photochromic plastics lenses are available for prescription use in CR39 material, 1.54 and 1.56 index materials and now mid-index 1.59 polycarbonate, all in either grey or brown versions.

The latest version of Transitions lenses, known as *Transitions V*, has a luminous transmittance of 92% in the unactivated state, darkening to 30% after 15 seconds exposure, with the transmission dropping to 15% after just 5 minutes exposure to the exciting radiation (Figure 7.12). This new product performs like a white lens indoors and darkens to either deep brown or deep grey to provide true sunglass protection out-of-doors. It will eventually replace earlier versions of Transitions, since it darkens more quickly, lightens more quickly and is less temperature dependent than earlier generations of plastics photochromic materials. The Trans-Bonding™ process, suitable for high-index plastics and polycarbonate, as well as CR39 material, enables the lens to receive proprietary surface treatments that provide scratch resistance and anti-reflection coatings over the imbibed photochromic layer.

New photochromic plastics materials have been developed by Corning (the originators of photochromic glass spectacle lenses), Hoya, Optical Dynamics and Rodenstock, and are photochromic throughout the entire mass. Corning scientists spent 5 years developing their new material and, along the way, registered no fewer than 25 patents in relation to it. Being photochromic through and through, it is likely to retain its photochromic properties for a long time without a noticeable loss of light response (Figure 7.13).

Table 7.5   Technical details of SunSensors™

n_d	n_e	v_d	Density
1.555	1.559	38	1.17

The Corning material, SunSensors™, has been designed primarily for the prescription lens market, and is available in both grey and brown. Technical details of the material are given in Table 7.5. It is a mid-index plastics with an extremely low density and is compatible with anti-reflection coating procedures. The resultant prescription lenses are thinner and lighter than when made in normal CR39.

For example, a +2.00D lens at an uncut diameter of 65mm with an edge thickness of 1.2mm has a centre thickness of 3.2mm and a weight of 8.7g. The same lens in CR39 has a centre thickness of 3.5mm and a weight of 10.4g, almost 20% heavier!

Its fashionable colours, an attractive 'blue–green' grey and a warm brown, and its sunglass-style darkening are designed to enable ametropes to enjoy the full benefits of photochromic lenses, clear indoors and comfortable absorption in strong sunlight. The transmission characteristics of the two versions at 22°C are shown in Figure 7.14 and Table 7.6.

There can be no doubt that photochromic lenses are by far the most popular form of prescription sun lens in use. Although

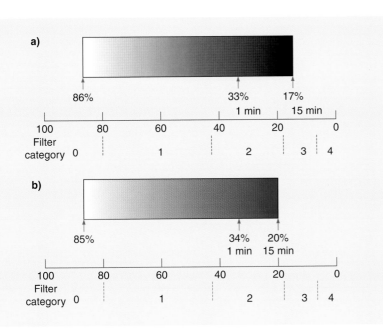

Figure 7.14 Transmission characteristics of SunSensors™ material: (a) grey; (b) brown

Table 7.6 Transmission characteristics of SunSensors™

	SunSensors™ grey (%)	SunSensors™ brown (%)
Transmission in clear state	85	85
Transmission after 60 seconds	33	34
Transmission after 5 minutes	20	22
Transmission after 16 minutes	17	20

Table 7.7 Classification of photochromic filters

Classification	Luminous transmittance
Light	≥80
Medium	≥40 but <80
Dark	≥15 but <40
Extra dark	<15

state-of-the-art technology, their performance can be seen and understood by the ordinary spectacle wearer. They absorb the harmful radiation encountered in the usual environment and have no adverse effects upon the eye.

The specification of photochromic materials

EN ISO 13666:1999[6] describes a photochromic material as a material which reversibly changes its luminous transmittance characteristics depending upon the intensity and wavelength of the radiation falling upon it, adding the note that the material is designed to react principally to the wavelengths within the solar spectral range, 300–450nm, and the transmission properties are usually temperature dependent.

A material can claim to be photochromic if the ratio of the luminous transmittance in its faded state, $\tau_V(0)$ and after 15 minutes irradiation, $\tau_V(15)$, in its darkened state is at least 1.25.

Photochromic fatigue is also defined in the Standard as an irreversible change in luminous transmission characteristics of a photochromic material with time, usually after prolonged cumulative and/or repeated exposure to radiation.

EN ISO 8980-3:2004[8] defines a method of measuring the transmittance of photochromic lenses. This recommended method, when used universally, will prevent lenses from different manufacturers appearing to possess slightly different properties.

BS 7394 Part 2:1994 extends the definition of a photochromic lens to include the wavelength of the incident radiation as being a factor that affects the transmission characteristics. Also, the standard endeavours to overcome the problem of classification of photochromic lenses by type. Traditionally, such lenses have been known as wide-swing or narrow-swing depending on the photochromic range. This might lead to confusion because 'comfort' lenses and sunglass lenses might both be narrow-swing. The standard endeavours to overcome this problem by providing a series of classification terms as shown in Table 7.7. Luminous transmittance is required to be determined at 25°C ± 2°C.

Thus a lens with a faded transmittance of 90% and a darkened transmittance of 50% is classified as light/medium, whereas a lens with a faded transmittance of 50% and a darkened transmittance of 10% is classified as medium/extra dark.

Ordering tinted lenses

BS 7394 Part 2 is limited in its recommendations for the specification of tinted lenses, suggesting that when a tint is required for cosmetic purposes, it should be ordered by reference to the manufacturer's code and that the effect of any additional treatment should be noted. It goes on '…If particular transmission or absorption characteristics are required … specific values should be quoted in the prescription or prescription order. To avoid ambiguity it is recommended that such requirements should be quoted by reference to the LTF.' The reasons for limiting the recommendations are hinted at in the introduction to the standard, but are spelt out in greater detail here.

If a lens is ordered with reference to the manufacturer's code or name, there should be little difficulty in providing a match. Problems are likely to arise when either a plastics lens sample

Table 7.8 Filter categories and descriptions

Filter category	Description	Range of luminous transmittance, τ_V	
		from over (%)	to (%)
0	Clear or very light tint	80	100
1	Light tint	43	80
2	Medium tint	18	43
3	Dark tint	8	18
4	Very dark tint not suitable for driving and road use	3	8

Note: for photochromic filters the filter category for labelling and marking is defined by the luminous transmittance values in the faded state and in the darkened state.

is old and may have faded, or when an anti-reflection or other coating is added to a tinted lens. In the latter case the coating also affects the appearance of the lens, from the point of view of either colour or transmittance. Both problems are anticipated easily by the prescriber.

If a particular transmittance is required and a coating is to be added to the lens, the problem may not be solved quite so easily. If the lens is ordered with reference to its uncoated luminous transmittance, clearly the anti-reflection coating will change this unacceptably. It may also alter the perceived colour of the tint. If, however, the transmittance of the completed lens is to be specified, it is possible that the relationship between the two luminous transmittances may not be as obvious as that between the spectral transmittances at a selected wavelength. The concept of luminous reflectance may help to make this matter easier for the practitioner, but where the final luminous transmittance or the transmittance profile is critical, good liaison between the prescriber and the manufacturer is the best solution.

Sunglass lenses

The term 'sunglass lenses' refers to non-prescription (plano), tinted lenses, which are sold universally, generally over the counter, by retail stores, chemists and other non-optical outlets. Of course, they may also be sold at optical outlets.

Recommendations for the use of sunglare eye protection are contained in Appendix E of the relevant British Standard on sunglasses[9]. This Standard is intended to be read and applied by all vendors (and users!) of sunglasses and it is important that the ophthalmic profession be aware of the information which might accompany retail sales from non-optical outlets.

Table 7.8 gives details of the filter categories and descriptions.

Recommended information that should be supplied by the manufacturer or the supplier of sunglass spectacles is given below. The written information which must be supplied applies equally to plano sunglasses which are supplied by an optician.

Complete spectacles

Information to be supplied with each sunglass and eye protector for direct observation of the sun, in the form of a marking on the sunglass frame, an affixed label or packaging, or any combination thereof, in the language where the product is destined to be sold.

(a) identification of manufacturer or supplier
(b) filter category number (according to Table 7.8)
(c) number and year of the Standard
(d) in the case of filter category 4 or a filter which does not meet the requirements for driving detailed above under the heading

'Assessment of performance', the warning 'Not suitable for driving and road use' in the form of an approved symbol or in writing
(e) in the case of eye protectors for direct observation of the sun; the warning that direct viewing of the sun is dangerous. Projection techniques are safe. Alternatively adequate eye protection specifically designed for viewing the sun is essential and must be worn so that no direct radiation from the sun can reach the eye
(f) unless specifically designed for this purpose (generally, τ_V less than 0.0012%) the warning: 'Not for direct viewing of the sun.'

The following information should also be supplied by the manufacturer or supplier:

(a) name and address of the manufacturer or supplier
(b) type and performance of the filter, e.g.:
  (1) photochromic
    – luminous transmittance in the faded state, t_0
    – luminous transmittance in the darkened state, t_1; and
    – photochromic range, R_P, as a measure of the photochromic performance
  (2) polarizing: the degree of polarization in percent
  (3) gradient
(c) instructions for care and cleaning
(d) explanation of the markings
(e) optical class
(f) in cases where the reference point is different from the defined one, the position of the reference point as specified in the technical file
(g) nominal value of luminous transmittance.

Standards for sunglass lenses

The basic Standard for sunglass lenses is BS EN 1836:2005. Personal eye-equipment – Sunglasses and sunglare filters for general use and filters for direct observation of the sun.

This defines various standards for lens properties and quality; the transmission requirements are summarized here and in Table 7.9.

Spectral transmittance

Filters suitable for road use and driving shall be of Categories, 0,1, 2 or 3 (see Table 7.9) and shall additionally meet the requirement that for wavelengths between 500nm and 650nm the spectral transmittance of filters suitable for road use and driving shall not be less than $0.2 \times$ the luminous transmittance, τ_V.

Table 7.9 Transmittance for sunglare filters for general use

	Requirements						
	Ultraviolet range Maximum value of				Visible range of luminous transmittance τ_V		Enhanced infrared absorption Max. value of solar IR transmittance* τ_{SIR}
Filter category	spectral transmittance $\tau_F(\lambda)$		solar UVA transmittance τ_{SUVA}				
	280 to 315nm	315 to 350nm	315 to 380nm		from over (%)	to (%)	
0					80	100	
1		τ_V	τ_V		43	80	
2	$0.1\tau_V$				18	43	τ_V
3					8	18	
4		$0.5\tau_V$	$0.5\tau_V$		3	8	

*Only applicable to sunglare filters recommended by the manufacturer as a protection against infrared radiation.

Table 7.10 Measurement conditions for the different luminous transmittance values for photochromatic materials

Luminous transmittance	Surface temperature of the test specimen °C	Illumination at the surface of the sample lux
τ_0	23 ± 1	0 in the faded state
τ_1	23 ± 1	$50\,000 \pm 5000$
τ_W	5 ± 1	$50\,000 \pm 5000$
τ_S	35 ± 1	$50\,000 \pm 5000$
τ_a	23 ± 1	$15\,000 \pm 1500$

Luminous transmittance

The standard CIE observer is employed together with standard illuminant D65. Note that some manufacturers specify the *absorptance* (or absorption) of the filter where the absorptance is the difference, 1 minus the transmittance minus the reflectance, i.e.

$$\text{absorptance} = 1 - \tau_V - p$$

where p is the reflectance of the surface.

For photochromic lenses, it is recommended that the luminous transmittance is evaluated over a range of temperature and light intensities to provide a fairer picture of the performance of the filter in different conditions. Luminous transmittance is specified in the faded state and at four other states as described in Table 7.10. The five values selected are:

- τ_0 – luminous transmittance in the faded state at 23°C after specified conditioning;
- τ_1 – luminous transmittance in the darkened state at 23°C after specified irradiation simulating mean outdoor conditions;
- τ_W – luminous transmittance in the darkened state at 5°C after specified irradiation simulating outdoor conditions at low temperatures (e.g. in winter);
- τ_S – luminous transmittance in the darkened state at 35°C after specified irradiation simulating outdoor conditions at high temperatures (e.g. in high summer or the tropics)
- τ_a – luminous transmittance in the darkened state at 23°C after specified irradiation simulating reduced light conditions (e.g. when driving in a closed car).

The conditioning which is suggested to obtain the faded state for a photochromic sunglare filter requires the sample to be stored in the dark at 65°C for 2 hours followed by a further 12 hour period in the dark at 23°C.

The photochromic range, R_P for a photochromic sunglare filter is given by:

$$R_P = (\tau_0 - \tau_1)/\tau_0$$

the value giving an indication of the change in transmission between the faded and darkened states. For example, a filter whose transmittance in the faded state, τ_0, is 90% and in the darkened state (as defined above for τ_1) is 20%, the photochromic range would be expressed as 0.78 whereas if the variation was from 90% to 50%, the photochromic range would be expressed as 0.44.

Recognition of signal lights and colours

To determine the ability of the filter to discriminate between the four signal colours, red, yellow, green and blue, the relative visual attenuation coefficient, Q, must be determined. The coefficients are the same as those specified earlier for prescription sunglass lenses.

Shade numbers

The shade number of a tinted lens as an alternative method to classify its transmittance properties has had limited acceptance by the suppliers of tinted materials. The shade number, N, is given by:

$$N = 1 + (7/3)\log\left[100/\tau_V\,(\%)\right]$$

Although the value can describe the transmittance precisely in terms of optical density, it is not as meaningful as the transmission value expressed as a percentage.

Polarizing filters

A polarizing sunglare filter is defined as a filter of which the transmittance is dependent upon the polarization of the radiation. The degree of polarization, P, is determined from:

$$P = \left(\tau_{Pmax} - \tau_{Pmin}\right) / \left(\tau_{Pmax} + \tau_{Pmin}\right)$$

where τ_{Pmax} is the maximum value of luminous transmittance and τ_{Pmin} the minimum value of luminous transmittance as determined with linearly polarized radiation.

Polarizing sunglare filters must be mounted in the frame such that the plane of polarization does not deviate from the horizontal direction by more than ±5°. Any misalignment between the plane of polarization of the right and left filters shall not be greater than 6°.

The Standard also stipulates that the plane of polarization of an uncut polarizing filter should be marked to enable the lens to be mounted correctly and that the ratio of the luminous transmittance values parallel and perpendicular to the plane of polarization shall be greater than 8:1 for filter categories 2, 3 and 4 and greater than 4:1 for category 1.

References

1. Jalie M 1984 The principles of ophthalmic lenses. ABDO, London
2. Fanin T E, Grosvenor T 1987 Clinical optics. Butterworths, London
3. Driscoll B et al. 1994 A critique of recommended limits of exposure to ultraviolet radiation with particular reference to skin cancer. HSE, London
4. Araujo R J 1977 Photochromic glass. In: Prichard M J (ed) Treatise on materials science and technology: interaction with electromagnetic radiation: glass I. Academic Press, London, p 91–122
5. Crano J C, Welch C N 1991 Plastics photochromic lenses. Properties, measurement and preparation. Optical World, July/August:12–14
6. BS EN ISO 13666:1999 Ophthalmic optics – Spectacle lenses – Vocabulary
7. BS EN ISO 14889:2003 Ophthalmic optics – Spectacle lenses – Fundamental requirements for uncut finished lenses. BSI, London
8. BS EN ISO 8930-3:2004 Ophthalmic optics – Uncut finished spectacle lenses – Part 3: Transmittance specifications and test methods. BSI, London
9. BS EN 1836:2005 Personal eye-equipment – Sunglasses and sunglare filters for general use and filters for direct observation of the sun. BSI, London

Dispensing in myopia

Full-aperture lenses of high power made in normal-index materials are thick, heavy and unsightly. Even quite moderate prescriptions, when dispensed in frames of large aperture, may result in thick and heavy lenses. Various courses of action may be taken through the judicious selection of frames and lenses to ensure that the outcome results in a comfortable pair of spectacles.

As a general rule, the smaller the size and the more symmetrical the choice of lens shape, the thinner, lighter and better looking are the lenses. Interestingly, since the mid-1990s, following the very large eye sizes of the 1970s and 1980s, the trend in frame design has been towards smaller frames.

The mechanical problems encountered in dispensing for myopia and hypermetropia differ somewhat, simply because the cross-sectional shape of minus and plus lenses is different. The cross-sectional shape of minus lenses (Figure 8.1a) lends itself well to a method of supply whereby a finished range of uncut lenses may be employed to produce a series of glazed lenses of different shapes. The edge thickness of a minus lens reduces as it is edged down to fit the frame. Thus, provided the centre thickness of the lens is a minimum and the size is kept as small as possible, a reasonable lens may be obtained from a stock uncut.

Plus lenses, on the other hand, do not lend themselves so readily to this convenient method of supply. Figure 8.1b indicates what happens when a plus lens is edged down to produce the final lens for mounting. For a given centre thickness, the edge thickness increases as the diameter of the lens is reduced, so the only way in which the optimum lens can be obtained is to surface the lens to provide the required edge thickness for the finished diameter once full details of the prescription, decentration and frame size are known (Figure 8.1c).

Before deciding the optimum lens for any given prescription the following should be taken into account:

- form of the lens
- material of the lens
- field of view
- optimum centre thickness
- resultant edge thickness
- weight of the lenses
- disturbing reflections
- surface treatments.

As is shown later, some of these considerations may well influence the choice of spectacle frame, and some designs are less suitable than others for any given specification.

The choices of lens form and material are dealt with in Chapter 2, so only a summary of the pertinent points is given here.

Lens form

Lens manufacturers supply lenses in one of two ways. They may supply the prescription house with semi-finished blanks, with a front surface that is completely finished, and the final prescription is obtained by the surfacing workshop, which completes the second side. Or, the lens manufacturers may supply the glazing department with finished stock uncut lenses, which sets them as required and edges them to the final size and shape for mounting into the spectacle frame. The reasons for the likely surface curves that may be used for any given power are discussed in Chapter 2.

Spectacle lenses are numbered in terms of their back vertex power; in the case of a minus lens, this is virtually the same as the sum of the two surface powers. The surface powers chosen for any given back vertex power are usually those that make the power during oblique gaze as close as possible to the power obtained when the eye views along the optical axis of the lens.

The lens may be designed to be free from oblique astigmatism, in which case it is described as a point-focal lens form, or it may be designed to be free from mean oblique error, in which case it is described as a Percival lens form. Today, a lens is likely to be designed to be free from tangential error at a given vertex distance. This so-called minimum T-error form has the advantage that, if it is fitted at a longer vertex distance than the designer intended, it tends to behave like a point-focal lens form, whereas if it is fitted at a shorter vertex distance it tends to behave like a Percival lens form.

When finished lenses are dispensed from a stock range of finished uncuts, the surface curves conform to the design criteria chosen by the manufacturer. The lenses are certain to provide good off-axis performance. When lenses need to be specially surfaced, the form is selected from the range of semi-finished blanks held in stock by the surfacing workshop. A typical range of semi-finished sphere blanks suitable for minus lenses made in spectacle crown glass or CR39 material with spherical surfaces is given in Table 8.1.

These curves assume the use of normal index materials ($n_d < 1.54$) and, as a general rule, as the refractive index increases, so should the true front base curve, to maintain the same off-axis performance as the crown glass lens. The higher the myopia, the closer the lens becomes to the theoretical ideal. For example, a lens of power −20.00D, made in crown glass in plano-concave form, is virtually point-focal (i.e. it has no oblique astigmatic error, and virtually no mean oblique error for a distant object).

Normally, it is wise to dispense lenses in best-form curvatures, for then not only are off-axis errors minimized, but also different series do not differ much in form from one another and, in particular, the distortion is about the same for a given power.

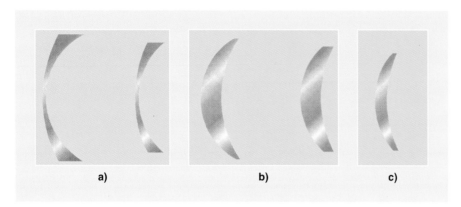

Figure 8.1 Cross-sectional views of minus and plus lenses: (a) the edge thickness of a minus lens reduces as the lens is edged smaller; (b) the edge thickness of a plus lens increases as the lens is edged smaller; (c) the optimum plus lens is produced by surfacing when all its parameters are known

a)   b)   c)

Table 8.1   Base curves for minus spherical lenses

Nominal base curves	To work powers in the range
+6.00	−0.25 to −1.00
+5.00	−1.25 to −2.00
+4.00	−2.25 to −6.00
+3.00	−6.25 to −9.00
+2.00	−9.25 to −12.00
+1.00	−12.25 to −14.00
Plano	Over −14.00

Myopes who become accustomed to a particular lens form are often dissatisfied when their lens form is changed; usually, the only solution to their problem is to provide a new pair of lenses in a similar form to their previous pair. Typically, a myope may have become accustomed to wearing flat-form lenses so, although theory shows that curved-form lenses provide better off-axis performance, many myopes will not tolerate a change from their flat-form design.

Astigmatic lenses for myopia provide the best optical performance when the cylinder is incorporated on the back surface, the lenses being supplied as minus-base toric designs.[1] Ideally, the toroidal surface should be of barrel form, which is possible with singly worked lenses if toroidal tools are maintained by the surfacing house in barrel form. Minus-base toric construction also improves the appearance of the lens, since the variation in edge thickness that occurs along different power meridians can be hidden on the back of the lens.

For very deep minus lenses, it is easier for the manufacturer to incorporate the cylinder on the front surface of the lens, in the form of a plano-convex cylindrical surface.

When the refractive index of the lens material changes, the lens form also needs to change to provide the same off-axis powers. Table 8.2 indicates the form required for various lens powers that have approximately the same off-axis performance as plano-concave forms made in spectacle crown glass or CR39 material. Needless to say, the transverse chromatism exhibited by the lens is dependent upon the Abbe number of the material and will only match if the Abbe number of the new material matches that of crown glass or CR39.

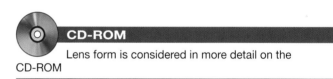

CD-ROM

Lens form is considered in more detail on the CD-ROM

Aspheric lens forms for myopia

For any given lens power, the flatter the lens form is made, the smaller the edge thickness of the lens will be. However, flat-form lenses do not provide good off-axis performance if spherical surfaces are used. Lens forms flatter than the Percival design for the power under consideration are afflicted with negative aberrational astigmatism. By employing an aspherical surface that itself possesses positive surface astigmatism, it is possible to restore the off-axis performance, since the asphericity of the surface can be chosen so that the positive surface astigmatism neutralizes the negative astigmatism of oblique incidence.

A typical surface is illustrated in Figure 8.2. This is a convex oblate ellipsoidal surface and Figure 8.2 shows that the increasing convexity of the surface reduces the edge thickness of the lens even more, and thereby offers a further saving from that obtained by flattening the lens from its traditional spherical form.

Table 8.2   Form of higher-index lenses

Lens power (D)	Original front curve (1.498/1.523)	Required front curve when new refractive index is:			
		1.600	1.700	1.800	1.900
−4.00	Plano	+0.25	+0.50	+0.75	+1.00
−6.00	Plano	+0.25	+0.75	+1.25	+1.62
−8.00	Plano	+0.37	+0.87	+1.50	+2.00
−10.00	Plano	+0.37	+1.00	+1.75	+2.25
−12.00	Plano	+0.37	+1.00	+1.75	+2.50

Lens material

Table 8.3 gives a typical selection of lens materials and lists certain physical properties of the materials pertinent to the choice of material. The significance of the physical data is discussed in full in Chapter 2. The curve variation factor (CVF) for the material enables a direct comparison of the thickness of lenses when made in materials of different refractive index.

For example, a 1.701 index material has a CVF (Table 8.3) of 0.75, which informs us that the reduction in thickness is some 25% if this material is substituted for crown glass. A 1.600 index material has a CVF of 0.87, so that use of this material provides a thickness reduction of 13%, and so on.

Density determines how heavy a material is, and a comparison of densities indicates the likely change in weight to be expected from using a given material. The value given is the mass per unit volume of the material and is almost exactly the same as the weight in grams of one cubic centimetre of the material. Densities of materials of high refractive index may be compared directly with that of crown glass to determine whether lenses made in high-index materials will be much heavier than their crown glass counterparts.

The Abbe number or V-value of the material is a measure of the optical properties of the material rather than its mechanical characteristics. As pointed out in Chapter 2, the transverse chromatic aberration exhibited by a spectacle lens is inversely proportional to the Abbe number of the lens material (the higher the Abbe number the less the chromatism).

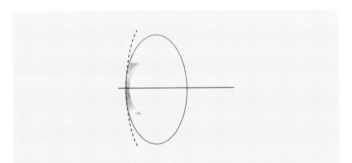

Figure 8.2   Minus lens with convex aspherical surface similar in form to a convex oblate ellipsoid

The reflectance, ρ, indicates the percentage of normally incident light reflected at each lens surface; one purpose of an anti-reflection coating is to reduce the intensity of this reflectance almost to zero.

Field of view

Figure 8.3 shows that myopes enjoy a wider real field of view in the object space than implied by the aperture diameter of their frame or lens. For example, in Figure 8.3 an apparent angular field of view of 73° corresponds to a real angular field of 86°. The real macular field of view of a spectacle lens of power, F, and diameter, $2y$, mounted 27mm in front of the eye's centre of rotation can be found from:

$$\tan\theta = y\,(37-F)/1000$$

where θ is half the field of view. Hence, a −10.00D lens edged 40mm round has a real angular field of 86°.

A −15.00D lens made in lenticular form with a 30mm round aperture has a real field of view of some 76°. This same field of view is provided by a plano-lens of 42mm diameter or a +5.00D lens of about 49mm diameter, assuming each lens to be placed 27mm in front of the eye's centre of rotation.

To obtain the maximum field, whatever the size of the aperture might be, the lens should be fitted as close to the eyes as the lashes permit. In cases of very high myopia, a close fit has the added advantage of increasing the retinal image size, a point of some importance where there is poor retinal sensitivity.

Lens thickness

A very important role of the dispensing optician is to assist a subject in choosing a frame design that is suitable, not only from a cosmetic point of view on the face, but also for the prescription with which the frame is to be glazed. For this second condition, the finished spectacles must be visualized. Several sources now supply computer software that allows the lens prescription and frame data to be input, from which the program calculates the thickness and weight of the finished lenses. This information is

Table 8.3 Physical data for typical lens materials						
Medium	n_d	n_e	CVF	Density	Abbe number	ρ
Glasses						
White crown	1.523	1.525	1.00	2.5	59	4.3
Light flint	1.600	1.602	0.87	2.6	42	5.3
1.7 glasses	1.701	1.706	0.75	3.2	42	6.7
1.8 glasses	1.802	1.808	0.65	3.7	35	8.2
1.9 glasses	1.885	1.892	0.59	4.0	31	9.4
Plastics						
PMMA	1.490	1.492	1.07	1.2	58	3.9
CR39	1.498	1.500	1.05	1.3	58	4.0
Trivex™	1.532	1.534	0.98	1.1	46	4.4
Sola Spectralite	1.537	1.540	0.97	1.2	47	4.5
PPG HIP	1.560	1.563	0.93	1.2	38	4.8
Polycarbonate	1.586	1.589	0.89	1.2	30	5.2
Polyurethane	1.600	1.603	0.87	1.3	36	5.3
	1.660	1.664	0.79	1.4	32	6.2
Hoya Teslalid	1.710	1.715	0.74	1.4	36	6.9
Nikon	1.740	1.745	0.71	1.4	32	7.3

output to the VDU screen and the patient and practitioner can review the likely outcome before the lenses are actually made. A typical output is illustrated in Figure 8.4.

In the absence of this computer software, it is possible to estimate lens thickness to within two- or three-tenths of a millimetre by a simple mental calculation. This estimation is very useful at the dispensing table where, obviously, it is unnecessary to calculate lens thickness with absolute accuracy when all that is required is to provide the subject with some idea of how their new spectacles might look.

To estimate the thickness of a minus lens, two items need to be known – the centre thickness of the lens and the sag of the lens power at the diameter in question.

Centre thickness of minus lenses

When lenses were edged by hand, high-power minus lenses were made with a minimum centre thickness of 0.6mm.

With a modicum of care, lenses with such a thin centre could be hand edged without fear of breakage. With the advent of automatic edging equipment, in which lenses are clamped by their centres, such a small centre thickness might cause the lens to shatter from the stress imposed during the edging cycle. As a result, today's stock glass minus lenses have a minimum centre thickness of 1.0mm. As a general guide, the centre thickness varies from 2.0mm down to 1.0mm – the value decreasing as the power increases.

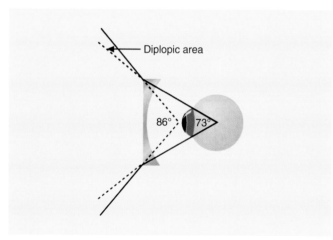

Figure 8.3 Increased field of view of a minus lens.

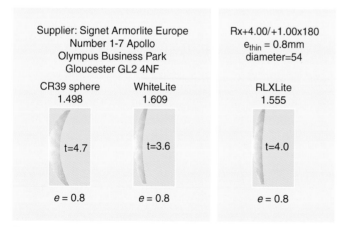

Figure 8.4 Computer-generated thickness comparisons as an aid to dispensing

A typical series of centre thicknesses, t, for glass lenses is given by the rule:

$$t = 2.0 + 0.2 \times \text{power of lens}$$

Thus, we might expect a glass lens series to have centre thicknesses given in Table 8.4.

An exception to these values occurs for tinted lenses. If the power is less than −2.00D there is usually no problem in dispensing a fixed tint or a photochromic tint with a centre thickness following those suggested above. For stronger powers, the minimum centre thickness should not be less than 1.6mm to ensure an adequate thickness of glass at the centre of the lens.

For higher powers, in general, it is better to provide tinted lenses in equitint form so that the transmittance is the same across the whole lens. Glass equitints can be provided by bonding a 1.6–2.0mm thick layer of tinted material to a white glass carrier lens, although this technique does result in somewhat thicker lenses.

Plastics lenses made in CR39 material are not normally supplied with centre thicknesses less than 2.0mm since, being less rigid than glass, they would flex under pressure from the mount when fitted to a plastics or metal full-rimmed frame. For this reason CR39 lenses made with spherical surfaces are invariably thicker than their crown glass counterparts. Polyurethane plastics materials are more rigid than CR39, so lenses made from these materials may be obtained with thicknesses similar to those of glass lenses.

Tinted plastics lenses are normally produced by dyeing a finished white lens, the dye being allowed to penetrate the white lens for a length of time that depends upon the transmittance required. This process automatically results in an equitint lens.

Sag factors for crown glass lenses

The thickness of a lens resulting from its power can be estimated as a simple function of the lens power. The method employs the use of a sag factor, which is related to the lens diameter.[1] Sag factors for various useful diameters are shown in Table 8.5. It is only necessary to multiply the sag factor by the lens power to obtain the thickness of the lens for the diameter under consideration.

From Table 8.5, at a diameter of 45mm the sag factor is 0.5. This value indicates that, for this diameter, lens thickness increases at the rate of 0.5mm per dioptre of lens power. Hence:

sag 1.00 at 45 = 0.5mm
sag 2.00 at 45 = 1.0mm
sag 3.00 at 45 = 1.5mm
sag 8.00 at 45 = 4.0mm

and so on.

This simple method of finding the thickness of a lens works well, provided the product of the power and the lens diameter does not exceed the value 500. Thus, for the 45mm diameter

Table 8.4 Centre thicknesses of glass lens series	
Power (D)	**Centre thickness (mm)**
−0.50	1.9
−1.00	1.8
−1.50	1.7
−2.00	1.6
−3.00	1.4
−4.00	1.2
−5.00 and over	1.0

Table 8.5 Sag factors for crown glass lenses

Lens diameter (mm)	Sag factor
20	0.1
30	0.2
35	0.3
40	0.4
45	0.5
50	0.6
54	0.7
57	0.8
60	0.9
63	1.0
66	1.1
70	1.2

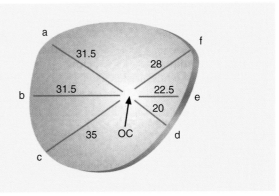

Figure 8.6 Typical spectacle lens shape in which the lens has been decentred. The distances shown represent the distances from the optical centre to the lens edge

The edge thicknesses at points 'b' to 'f' are:

'b', $1.2 + 4 \times 1.0 = 5.2$mm

'c', $1.2 + 4 \times 1.2 = 6.0$mm

'd', $1.2 + 4 \times 0.4 = 2.8$mm

'e', $1.2 + 4 \times 0.5 = 3.2$mm

'f', $1.2 + 4 \times 0.8 = 4.4$mm

In the case of minus lenses, at the dispensing table it is probably necessary only to consider the maximum edge thickness, which for a spherical lens lies at the furthest point on the lens periphery from the optical centre.

By measuring the frame rim thickness the overhang of the lens can be indicated immediately if the subject chooses the frame in question. As pointed out above, myopes are particularly interested in the edge thickness of their finished spectacles, but can hardly refuse to accept them if they were warned beforehand that the lenses would be thick and overhang the frame rim.

Sag factors for other lens materials

The sag factors given in Table 8.5 relate only to spectacle crown glass of refractive index 1.523. However, they can be used for lenses made in other materials provided that the power is first converted into its crown glass equivalent. This is done simply by multiplying the power of the lens by the CVF quoted for the material.

Suppose the use of a 1.701 index material is considered for the –4.00D specification described above. The crown glass equivalent is 4.00×0.75 or –3.00D. In other words, use of this material of high refractive index enables the thickness of the –4.00D lens to vary in the same way as a –3.00D lens made in crown glass. The centre thickness, however, still remains at 1.2mm.

The variation in edge thickness around the lens periphery of this 1.701 index –4.00D lens would be:

'a', $1.2 + 3 \times 1.0 = 4.2$mm

'b', $1.2 + 3 \times 1.0 = 4.2$mm

'c', $1.2 + 3 \times 1.2 = 4.8$mm

'd', $1.2 + 3 \times 0.4 = 2.4$mm

'e', $1.2 + 3 \times 0.5 = 2.7$mm

'f', $1.2 + 3 \times 0.8 = 3.6$mm

The advantage of using a glass of high refractive index for this specification is immediately apparent. The maximum edge thickness decreases from 6.0mm to 4.8mm, a reduction of some 20%.

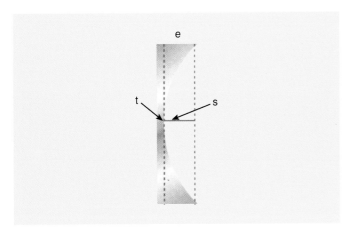

Figure 8.5 Edge thickness of a minus lens, $e = t + s$

chosen as an example, the sag factor 0.5 can be used up to an 11.00D curve, since $11.00 \times 45 = 495$.

Edge thickness of minus lenses

To determine the edge thickness of a minus lens it is necessary to add the thickness resulting from the power to the centre thickness of the lens (Figure 8.5). Thus, a –5.00D lens made in crown glass and edged 45mm in diameter would have an edge thickness of 3.5mm. This value is obtained by adding sag 5.00 at 45 (5×0.5) to the likely centre thickness of a –5.00D lens, 1.0mm, obtained from Table 8.4.

Similarly, the thickness at a point on the edge of a –3.00D lens 30mm away from its optical centre is 4.1mm (sag 3.00 at $60 = 3 \times 0.9 = 2.7$mm, and the centre thickness is 1.4mm).

Consider the lens shape depicted in Figure 8.6. It is a typical modern quadra shape, of box dimensions 60×50, and the specification includes 4.5mm of inward decentration. The dimension of the lens along the horizontal centre line is 54mm.

The distances shown on Figure 8.6 represent the distances from the optical centre to the lens periphery. Naturally, these distances should be doubled to determine the diameter and its associated sag factor. Suppose the power of this lens is a –4.00D sphere. The centre thickness for this power is 1.2mm.

The edge thickness at point 'a' on the lens periphery is the sum of the centre thickness and sag 4.00 at 63. The sag factor for this diameter is 1.0, and hence at 'a' the edge thickness is $1.2 + 4.0 = 5.2$mm.

If the same −4.00D specification was dispensed in CR39 material, its crown glass equivalent would be −4.20, the CVF for this material being 1.05. Clearly, this CR39 plastics lens is thicker than its crown glass counterpart for two reasons. The crown glass equivalent power is somewhat greater than −4.00D and the centre thickness of a CR39 lens needs to be increased to prevent the lens from flexing under pressure from the frame mount.

Typically, a −4.00D lens made in CR39 material has a centre thickness of 2.0mm and the variation in edge thickness for the lens is:

'a', $2.0 + 4.2 \times 1.0 = 6.2$mm
'b', $2.0 + 4.2 \times 1.0 = 6.2$mm
'c', $2.0 + 4.2 \times 1.2 = 7.0$mm
'd', $2.0 + 4.2 \times 0.4 = 3.7$mm
'e', $2.0 + 4.2 \times 0.5 = 4.1$mm
'f', $2.0 + 4.2 \times 0.8 = 5.4$mm

The maximum edge thickness of this plastics lens has increased at point 'c' from 6.0 to 7.0mm.

Table 8.6 shows how the maximum edge thickness at point 'c' for this specification for a −4.00D lens varies for different materials. The CVFs and centre thicknesses used are given for convenience.

Astigmatic lenses

The edge thickness of astigmatic lenses can be predicted using exactly the same sag factors as those for spherical lenses, but, of course, these must be associated with the correct principal powers of the lens. The power along the axis meridian of an astigmatic lens results from the sphere alone, whereas the power at right angles to the axis is the sum of the sphere and the cylinder.

Thus, for the prescription −4.00/−2.00 × 90 made in spectacle crown glass with a centre thickness of 1.2mm and edged to a 45 × 40 oval shape, the thin-edge substance at the extremities of the vertical meridian would be:

$$1.2 + 4.00 \times 0.4 = 2.8 \text{mm}$$

and the thick-edge substance at the extremities of the horizontal meridian would be:

$$1.2 + 6.00 \times 0.5 = 4.2 \text{mm}$$

Along intermediate meridians we must first determine the notional power of the lens along the meridian in question. To calculate the lens thickness, we can assume that the power varies by the square of the sine of the angle between the cylinder axis and the meridian. Thus, at 30° from the cylinder axis we would add one-quarter of the cylinder power to the sphere to determine the notional power of the lens along this meridian.

To determine the notional power at 45° to the cylinder axis, add one-half of the cylinder power to the sphere, and at 60° to the direction of the cylinder axis, add three-quarters of the cylinder power to the sphere.

Consider the prescription −3.00/−2.00 × 30 to be dispensed in the lens shape depicted in Figure 8.6. Assume that the meridian 'c–f' lies along 30°. The power along this meridian is −3.00D.

The notional power of the lens along the 180 meridian, 'b–e', which lies at 30° to the cylinder axis, is one-quarter of the power of the cylinder plus the power of the sphere, which is −3.50D.

Suppose that the meridian 'a–d' lies along 150°; the notional power along 150, which lies at 60° to the cylinder axis, is three-quarters of the cylinder power plus the power of the sphere, which is −4.50D.

If the lens is made in spectacle crown glass with a centre thickness of 1.4mm (obtained from the rule, $t = 2 + 0.2F$, applied to the sphere of the minus cylinder transposition of the prescription), the edge thicknesses at the six points on the lens periphery are:

'a', $1.4 + 4.5 \times 1.0 = 5.9$mm
'b', $1.4 + 3.5 \times 1.0 = 4.9$mm
'c', $1.4 + 3.0 \times 1.2 = 5.0$mm
'd', $1.4 + 4.5 \times 0.4 = 3.2$mm
'e', $1.4 + 3.5 \times 0.5 = 3.2$mm
'f', $1.4 + 3.0 \times 0.8 = 3.8$mm

The maximum edge thickness lies at point 'a', where it is 5.9mm.

Clearly, the position of the maximum edge thickness varies with the cylinder axis direction. In general, the maximum power of the lens lies at right angles to the direction of the minus cylinder axis. If the maximum power meridian lies close to the maximum diameter of the lens, then the edge thickness will be at its greatest for the shape in question. Whenever possible the lens shape chosen for an astigmatic prescription should have its maximum diameter coincident with the minimum power meridian of the lens.

If the prescription of the lens considered above is changed to −3.00/−2.00 × 150, which is a change only in cylinder axis direction from the previous specification, then the power of the lens along meridian 'a–d' becomes −3.00D and the notional power along 'c–f' is −4.50D.

The edge thicknesses at the lens periphery become:

'a', $1.4 + 3.0 \times 1.0 = 4.4$mm
'b', $1.4 + 3.5 \times 1.0 = 4.9$mm
'c', $1.4 + 4.5 \times 1.2 = 6.8$mm
'd', $1.4 + 3.0 \times 0.4 = 2.6$mm
'e', $1.4 + 3.5 \times 0.5 = 3.2$mm
'f', $1.4 + 4.5 \times 0.8 = 5.0$mm

Table 8.6	Variation in edge thickness with refractive index		
Refractive index	CVF	Centre thickness (mm)	Edge thickness at 70mm diameter (mm)
1.498	1.05	2.0	7.0
1.523	1.00	1.2	6.0
1.600	0.87	1.2	5.4
1.701	0.75	1.2	4.8
1.802	0.65	1.2	4.3
1.900	0.58	1.2	4.0

The maximum thickness on the edge now lies at point 'c' and is seen to be nearly 2.0mm greater than when the axis lay at 30°.

The appearance of minus lenses depends, to a large extent, upon the edge form chosen, and whether any steps are taken to diminish power rings, which are reflections of the edge at the lens surfaces. The formation of power rings is illustrated in Figure 8.7. The edging process leaves a fine ground-glass edge, which acts in the same way as any diffusely reflecting surface. It picks up any available illumination and scatters it in every direction. The edge is, therefore, relatively bright and a reflection of the edge at the back surface can be seen through the front surface of the lens. In some cases it is possible to see a second and third reflection of the edge, which arise from total internal reflection at the front and back surfaces of the lens.

These unsightly reflections are greatly reduced by preventing the edge from scattering light and/or by reducing their intensity. Traditional remedies include polishing the bevel, which is much simpler with a plastics lens than with one made of glass, or painting the edge with dark varnish to prevent the light from reaching the edge. A simple technique that 'ages' a freshly ground lens edge is to rub graphite (pencil lead) all over the edge before mounting the lens in the frame.

A spectacle frame with a wide dark rim also reduces the area of exposed edge. Avoidance of a conventional V-bevel design also helps; the minibevel technique reduces the amount of grey edge that can be seen through the lens and is often the only method that can be used to mount a lens successfully in a metal front.

In the case of rimless lenses, a thick edge can be disguised by providing a decorative faceting to the front edge of the lens. The faceting hides a pronounced chamfer on the back surface, which can be polished using the same technique described below for hand-edged lenticular lenses.

An anti-reflection coating produces a dramatic improvement in the appearance of a minus lens by reducing the intensity of the reflections to the point that they are almost invisible. Needless to say, the more efficient the coating, the better the result.

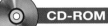

CD-ROM

The thickness of minus lenses is also considered in detail on the CD-ROM

Weight of lenses

Ideally, spectacles should be as light in weight as possible to prevent discomfort to the wearer. The weight of the front of the spectacles is generally borne entirely by the bearing surface of the frame on the bridge of the nose.

As a general rule, the larger the bearing surface, the more evenly the weight of the front is spread around the bearing surface of the nose. Glass lenses in large eye sizes fitted to frames with small pads on arms are the worst possible scenario.

The weight of a pair of spectacles is made up from the weight of the spectacle frame and the weight of the lenses. The weight of the frame depends upon the materials used in its construction and varies from the featherweight three-piece rimless mount or very thin, fully rimmed titanium frame to the heavyweight plastics library frames with thick rims made from cellulose acetate. In theory, the higher the prescription the sturdier the mount should be to ensure that the lenses are held at the correct vertex distance and at the correct pantoscopic angle before the eyes. As already noted, a dark, thick-rimmed front prevents the lens edge from picking up light, and thus prevents the formation of power rings.

The weight of a spectacle lens is calculated by multiplying the volume of the lens by the density of the lens material. The volume of a circular lens is found from the sum of the volumes of the two spherical caps that comprise the lens surfaces.

The rules used to ensure that spectacle lenses are as light as possible are the same as those used to obtain thin lenses. The eye size should be kept as small as possible; symmetrical shapes should be chosen and, wherever possible, the horizontal centre distance of the frame should match the subject's centration distance to avoid decentration of the lenses.

Table 8.7 compares the weight in grams of lenses made in various materials at 40 and 50mm diameter. The lenses are assumed to be round in shape and made with typical curved forms and centre thicknesses. Table 8.7 shows how important it is, in cases where weight is a significant factor, to try to dispense the smallest possible eye size. When the lens diameter is increased from 40mm to 50mm, the weight of the lens doubles.

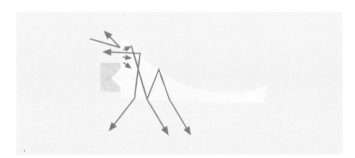

Figure 8.7   Power rings formed by reflections of scattered light from an exposed ground-glass edge of the lens

Table 8.7	Weight (g) of minus lenses at 40 and 50mm diameters											
Material	CR39		1.523		1.600		1.600		1.700		1.800	
Density	1.32		2.54		1.30		2.60		3.0		3.7	
Diameter (mm)	40	50	40	50	40	50	40	50	40	50	40	50
Power (D)												
−4.00	4.7	8.6	6.4	12.3	3.4	6.4	6.2	11.7	6.7	12.5	7.9	14.5
−6.00	5.4	10.4	7.0	14.5	3.6	7.3	6.6	13.5	7.1	14.1	8.2	16.0
−8.00	6.1	12.1	8.3	17.7	4.2	8.7	7.8	16.3	8.2	16.8	9.4	18.9
−10.00	6.8	13.8	9.6	21.0	4.8	10.1	8.9	19.1	9.3	19.6	10.6	21.8
−12.00	7.5	15.7	10.8	24.0	5.4	11.5	10.0	22.0	10.4	22.3	11.7	24.8

Lenticular lenses

As pointed out above, to obtain thin lightweight lenses, the eye size should be kept as small as possible, symmetrical shapes should be chosen and decentration should be avoided. It is also shown above that for a lens of power −10.00D, an increase in lens size from 40mm to 50mm causes the edge thickness of a normal index lens to increase by some 40% and the lens weight to double. The advent of glasses of very high refractive index (e.g. 1.8 and 1.9 indices) has made it possible to reduce the edge thickness of full-aperture, moderate power minus lenses to such an extent that the use of a full-aperture design is still practicable. The modern trend in frame design to use smaller eye sizes, coupled with the use of multilayer anti-reflection coatings to improve the appearance of lenses, has done much to assist the myope to obtain spectacle lenses that do not look as though they were made from beer-bottle bottoms!

A −10.00D lens dispensed in a fashionable 45-eye oval frame in a 1.90 index material and with no decentration has a maximum edge thickness of just 3.9mm. This is an enormous improvement upon the same power dispensed in CR39 material at 50mm diameter with 3mm of inward decentration, in which case the maximum edge thickness would be 10.4mm. In cases of high myopia, it is always sensible to consider the saving in thickness obtained by employing a high index ($n \geq 1.64$ but ≤ 1.74), or very high index ($n \geq 1.74$) material, especially when combined with one of the techniques for improving the appearance of the edge of a minus lens, discussed earlier in this chapter.

Some instances will still remain, usually because of the wearer's insistence that a particular size or type of frame should be used, in which the edge thickness and weight of full-aperture lenses become unacceptable. In such cases, the only way to obtain thin, lightweight lenses is to dispense them in a reduced aperture or lenticular form. These designs are particularly useful for high-power minus prescriptions, since not only can most designs be produced in the surfacing workshop using ordinary machinery (and are, therefore, easy to obtain), but also the real field of view provided by a high-power minus lens is much wider than the apparent field.

It can be seen in Figure 8.8 that the use of small aperture lenticular lenses is justified in cases of high myopia. Using the relationship given earlier to calculate the real angular field of view of a spectacle lens, a −15.00D lens dispensed with just a 28mm aperture offers the same real field of view as a +5.00D lens at 45mm aperture.

From a cosmetic point of view, the best lenticular designs are those that are blended to make the dividing line between the aperture curve and marginal curve invisible.

Lenticular designs may be obtained with a round aperture. However, in the case of non-blended designs, a profile aperture, in which the shape of the aperture follows the shape of the edged lens, offers the best cosmetic solution (Figure 8.9).

Bearing in mind that the great majority of modern spectacle shapes have a longer horizontal than vertical dimension, an oval aperture design is the next-best choice, with the round aperture design being used in the last resort unless, of course, a round-eye frame is selected.

Several lenticular designs can be produced by flattening a finished full-aperture lens with a third curve, with this third surface forming the margin of the lens (Figure 8.10).

The simplest lenticular design is the workshop-flattened lenticular lens with convex flattening, depicted in Figure 8.10a. The convex margin is ground with a plus tool, the power of

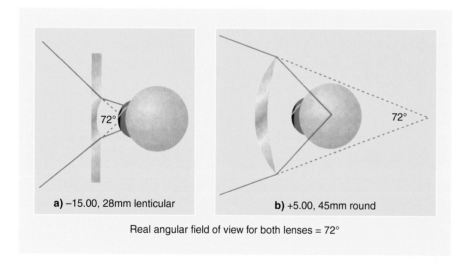

a) −15.00, 28mm lenticular   b) +5.00, 45mm round

Real angular field of view for both lenses = 72°

Figure 8.8 Increased field of view of a minus lenticular lens: (a) a −15.00D lens made as a 28mm aperture lenticular lens offers the same field of view as (b) a +5.00D lens at 45mm diameter

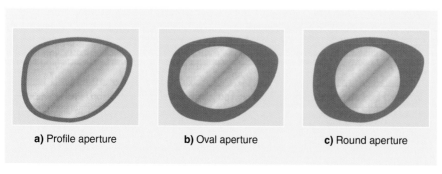

a) Profile aperture   b) Oval aperture   c) Round aperture

Figure 8.9 Profile, oval and round aperture lenticular designs

which is chosen to produce a given aperture diameter together with the required edge thickness at the given uncut diameter. Any aperture diameter can be produced, and this design enables a thin edge to be obtained regardless of the diameter of the aperture.

As inspection of Figure 8.10a shows, only one flattening tool produces the desired aperture diameter at the same time as a given edge thickness. Suppose the flattening tool used for the design in Figure 8.10a is +6.00D. If a steeper tool had been employed and the same aperture diameter produced, then the edge thickness would be less than that shown. On the other hand, if a shallower tool had been employed and the same aperture diameter achieved, then the edge thickness would be greater than that indicated. The required flattening tool can be deduced by applying the sag formula. The relationship between the required marginal tool and the aperture diameter can be deduced as follows. If the lens form is plano-concave, as shown in Figure 8.10a, then the sag of the marginal curve at the lens diameter, d, minus the sag of the marginal curve at the aperture diameter, a, plus the edge thickness, e, is the same dimension as the sag of the back curve at the aperture diameter plus the centre thickness, t.

Using symbols:

$$\text{sag } F_M \text{ at } d - \text{sag } F_M \text{ at } a + e = \text{sag } F_2 \text{ at } a + t$$

Rearranging this statement:

$$\text{sag } F_M \text{ at } d - \text{sag } F_M \text{ at } a = \text{sag } F_2 \text{ at } a - (e - t)$$

With the aid of a table of sags, the right-hand side of this expression can be evaluated immediately and the left-hand side, sag F_M at d – sag F_M at a, extrapolated from the table by finding which curve differs in sag between the full lens diameter and the aperture diameter by the value of the right-hand side of the expression.

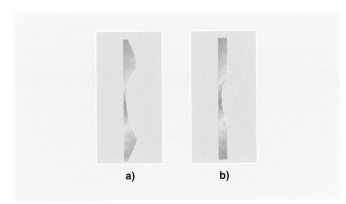

a)   b)

Figure 8.10   Workshop flattened lenticulars: (a) with convex flattening; (b) with plano flattening

For example, suppose that a –15.00D lenticular lens with a 30mm aperture diameter needs to be produced in spectacle crown glass and in plano-concave form. The centre thickness of the lens is to be 1.0mm and the edge thickness at an uncut diameter of 60 is to be 1.2mm.

From the relationship given above:

$$\text{sag } F_M \text{ at } 60 - \text{sag } F_M \text{ at } 30 = \text{sag } 15.00 \text{ at } 30 - (1.2 - 1)$$

From the sag tables for 1.523 index glass:

$$\text{sag } F_M \text{ at } 60 - \text{sag } F_M \text{ at } 30 = 3.39 - 0.2 = 3.19$$

Inspection of the sag tables shows that the sag of a +4.75 curve at 60 is 4.17mm and the sag of the same curve at 30 is 1.03mm. The difference is 3.14mm, which is very close to the required value of 3.19mm, so this tool should be used to work the marginal curve.

A neater design is obtained by flattening the concave surface with a tool of the same curvature as the front surface to produce an afocal margin, as depicted in Figure 8.10b. The cosmesis of these designs is discussed below.

If a spherical tool is used to flatten the concave surface, the resultant aperture is circular. If a cylindrical or toroidal tool is used to flatten the concave surface, an oval aperture results. Naturally, the difference between the horizontal and vertical dimensions of the oval aperture depends upon the cylindrical power of the tool.

In the case of an oval aperture design, an excellent cosmetic result is obtained when the difference between the horizontal and vertical dimensions of the oval is chosen to duplicate the shape difference of the lens. Several different methods can be used to produce an oval aperture, but the simplest is to employ a plano-convex cylindrical margin, with the axis of the cylinder coinciding with the horizontal meridian of the lens.

The result of the cylindrical flattening can be deduced from Figure 8.11, from which the following relationship may be established:

$$\text{sag } F_M \text{ at } a_V = \text{sag } F_2 \text{ at } a_H - \text{sag } F_2 \text{ at } a_V$$

F_M is the power of the cylindrical flattening tool, F_2 is the power of the concave surface and a_H and a_V are the horizontal and vertical aperture dimensions, respectively. With the aid of a table of sags, no calculation other than simple addition is necessary to determine the required cylinder power.

For example, suppose a –15.00D surface is to be flattened to produce a 34×30 aperture. We find from the sag tables:

$$\text{sag } 15.00 \text{ at } 34 = 4.43\text{mm}$$
$$\text{sag } 15.00 \text{ at } 30 = 3.39\text{mm}$$

Hence, sag F_M at $30 = 4.43 - 3.39 = 1.04\text{mm}$.

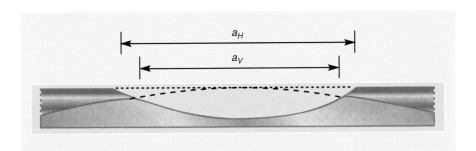

Figure 8.11   Determination of the cylindrical flattening curve

It is now only necessary to determine from the sag table, under the column headed 30mm, which curve has a sag of 1.04mm at 30mm diameter. Extrapolating from the tables, the curve is seen to be +4.75D, so the flattening tool required to produce a 34×30mm aperture for a −15.00D surface is $+4.75DC \times 180$.

Clearly, this specification requires quite a high-powered cylindrical curve. Furthermore, if a greater difference in horizontal and vertical dimensions is specified, then the cylindrical power required would be higher still.

For example, if an oval aperture of 34×26 is specified for the −15.00D surface considered above, the necessary flattening tool is found to be $+11.37DC \times 180$. It is most unlikely that the surfacing house would carry such a high-powered cylinder tool, and would probably reject the job as being impractical.

In general, the steeper the concave surface and the greater the difference between the horizontal and vertical aperture diameters, the greater becomes the power of the cylindrical flattening tool. An approximate, but useful, guide to the power of the necessary cylinder tool is as follows:

To obtain a 4 difference oval $F_M = 0.3F_2$

To obtain a 6 difference oval $F_M = 0.5F_2$

To obtain an 8 difference oval $F_M = 0.75F_2$

These rules indicate the region of the necessary cylindrical tool. Applied to the two examples considered above, we obtain +4.50 for the 34×30 aperture and +11.25 for the 34×26 aperture oval designs for −15.00D concave surfaces.

The workshop-flattened designs described so far have various cosmetic drawbacks in wear. The visibility of the dividing line, of course, depends upon the difference between the aperture and marginal curves, which is marked when a concave surface is flattened with a convex curve. The dividing line is very visible with these designs.

In wear, the eye itself is seen through the aperture and will appear minified viewed through a negative aperture. The surroundings of the eye, on the other hand, will be viewed through the margin of the lens, which has positive power and will magnify those regions viewed through it.

Furthermore, the convex margin presents a forward-facing concave reflecting surface, which gives rise to unsightly reflections. An enormous improvement can be obtained by anti-reflection coating the lens.

A significant cosmetic improvement in lenticular design is obtained by flattening the lens to obtain an afocal margin. These plano-flattened designs have the concave surface flattened with a tool of equal but opposite surface power to the front surface of the lens. The margin, therefore, is virtually afocal.

In the case of an astigmatic prescription, the cylinder is incorporated on the front surface as a plano-convex cylindrical surface or as a shallow plus-base toric. The flattening curve is chosen to match the base curve of the front surface, which results in a plano-cylindrical margin. This design is very neat in appearance. The edge substance is thin, the lens is light in weight and the dividing line is inconspicuous. In wear, observers see the surroundings of the eye and orbit unmagnified through the margin.

To maintain a thin margin, the aperture of the lenticular lens must be kept quite small, usually in the region of 22–26mm diameter. Assuming that the design is made in plano-concave form, it can be seen from Figure 8.10 that the edge substance is simply the sum of the centre thickness and the sag of the concave surface at the aperture diameter.

Table 8.8 Aperture diameters (maximum recommended) for plano-flattened lenticular lenses in various refractive indices

Power (D)	Refractive index				
	1.498	1.523	1.600	1.700	1.800
−10.00	27	28	30	33	35
−12.00	25	26	28	30	32
−14.00	23	24	25	28	30
−16.00	22	22	24	26	28
−18.00	–	–	22	24	26
−20.00	–	–	–	23	25
−22.00	–	–	–	22	23
−24.00	–	–	–	–	22

A reasonable margin (and edge) thickness for this design is 3.0mm. Assuming a centre thickness of 1.0mm, a typical range of aperture diameters for the design in various materials is given in Table 8.8, which shows that by increasing the refractive index, it is possible to provide a larger diameter without an increase in edge thickness. If the aperture diameter is increased above the values given in Table 8.8, the edge thickness and, of course, the weight of the lens increase.

Aperture diameters less than 22mm are not listed in Table 8.8.

Large diameters result in a thicker margin and, if required, it would be preferable to flatten the margin with a convex curve to reduce the edge thickness and weight of the lens. Once again, by employing a material of higher refractive index it is possible to obtain larger apertures without an increase in marginal thickness.

Blended lenticulars

Modern manufacturing methods enable lenticular designs to be produced with afocal margins that have invisible dividing lines made by blending the aperture curve with the marginal curve. The blending process literally rubs out the dividing line to give the design the appearance of a low-power full-aperture single-vision lens. The dividing line is replaced by a convex curve continuous with both the aperture curve and the marginal curve, and hence the dividing line is truly invisible.

The blended annulus is highly astigmatic and, just like the marginal portion of the design, useless for clear vision. However, since myopes obtain a wide field of view even when fitted with small aperture lenticulars, the enormous cosmetic advantage of a truly invisible dividing line enables many high myopes to wear large eye-size frames without the usual drawbacks of thick unsightly lenses.

Solid concave lenticulars

Solid lenticulars are so called because they are made with the same machinery as that required to produce solid bifocals. The form of the lenticular is illustrated in Figure 8.12, which shows that the edge of the aperture stands proud from the back marginal surface in the form of a ridge. The design is very useful for disguising strong prisms, since when the prism is incorporated on the aperture curve, the thickness difference is apparent only on the ridge.

Profile aperture lenticulars

As already pointed out, in cases in which the lenticular dividing line is visible, the best cosmetic designs are those in which the shape of the aperture follows the shape of the edged lens. Various forms of profile aperture designs are illustrated in Figure 8.13.

Figure 8.13a illustrates a hand-edged lenticular produced in the glazing department by skilful hand flattening of the edged lens, in the form of a heavy chamfer. The chamfer, which should be free from facets, is subsequently polished on a polishing mop lubricated with cerium oxide or other lens-polishing compound, care being taken not to allow the mop to mark the concave surface of the lens. The aperture follows, approximately, the shape of the edged lens.

A modern version of the hand-edged lenticular design is often supplied in rimless form, with the lens edge scalloped with a series of semi-circular facets and the lenses mounted in a lightweight three-piece rimless mount (Figure 8.13b).

When hand-edged lenticulars are to be mounted in supra-frame designs, a neater cosmetic result may be obtained by flattening only the lower portion of the lens; the top portion, which is surrounded by the frame rim, retains its full-aperture form. These half-flattened designs are known as hand-edged semi-lenticulars (Figure 8.13c). Often the optical centre of the lens is positioned some 5mm above the horizontal centre line to reduce the edge thickness at the top of the lens.

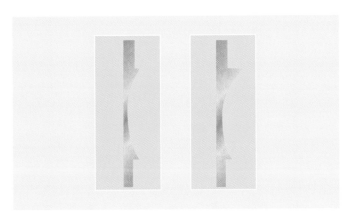

Figure 8.12   Solid concave lenticular lenses, with the lens on the right incorporating base up prism on the aperture

Figure 8.13d illustrates a bonded profile lenticular in which the effective aperture and carrier portions are worked separately, with their contact surfaces having the same curvature. The aperture is reduced to the desired size and shape by hand edging, and bonded to the carrier lens by means of a UV-cured resin. Cylindrical power may be worked on the front surface of the carrier or on the concave surface of the aperture. This design offers a neat method for producing an equitint design, since the carrier alone may be tinted.

Various lens manufacturers offer profile lenticular designs in which the edged lens has a chamfer machined round the edge, which is subsequently brightened (non-optical polishing) to produce a polished margin round an aperture that follows the same shape as the lens.

Reflections that may disturb myopes

Ghost images, which may appear in the field of view and cause annoyance to spectacle wearers, are discussed in detail in Chapter 5, but a review of the reflections that cause a particular problem to the wearers of high-power minus lenses is useful here. We have already considered the formation of reflections of the lens edge, so-called power rings, which occur when the lens edge is exposed to light, as it might be when the edge thickness of the lens exceeds the thickness of the frame rim (Figure 8.7).

Myopes may complain of troublesome reflections[1,2,3] or ghost images that appear in the visual field under certain conditions, usually indoors or in a lighted street at night, where there are bright sources of light in conditions of low illumination. The four likely causes of ghost images in cases of myopia are depicted in Figure 8.14.

Figure 8.14a illustrates the formation of a ghost image of a source in front of the lens by total internal reflection at the lens surfaces. The intensity of this ghost image is only 0.15% of the original intensity of the source for a material of refractive index 1.5, and 0.39% for a material of refractive index 1.7. It can be shown that the vergence of this ghost image, for a distant point

Figure 8.13   Profile lenticulars

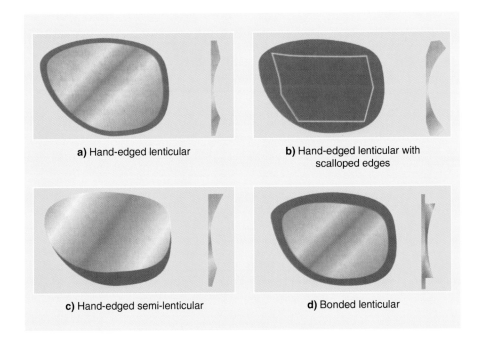

a) Hand-edged lenticular

b) Hand-edged lenticular with scalloped edges

c) Hand-edged semi-lenticular

d) Bonded lenticular

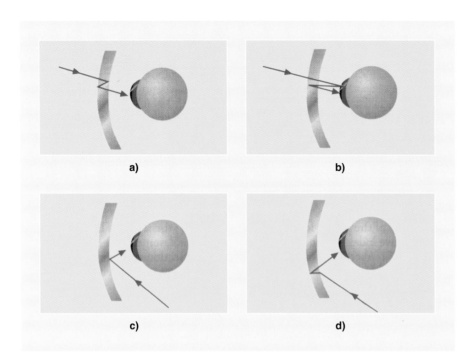

a)   b)

c)   d)

Figure 8.14 Source of ghost images in myopia: (a) image formed by total internal reflection; (b) image formed by reflection at cornea and F_2; (c) image formed by reflection at F_2; (d) image formed by reflection at F_1. Note that ghost images (a) and (b) are images of sources in front of the lens, whereas ghost images (c) and (d) are images of sources behind the lens

source of light, L'_c, depends only on the refractive index of the lens material, n, and the power, F, of the lens,

$$L'_c = [(3n-1)/(n-1)]F$$

For glass of refractive index 1.5, $L'_c = 7F$ and for glass of refractive index 1.7, $L'_c = 5.86F$.

For the ghost to be seen in sharp focus, the vergence L'_c should be the same as the power of the lens, F, or capable of being made the same by accommodation of the eye. We may conclude, therefore, that this ghost is usually well out of focus except for lenses of very low power.

For instance, in the case of a –0.50 myope with ample accommodation who wears CR39 lenses ($n = 1.5$), the vergence of this ghost image would be –3.50D. Despite the very low intensity of the image (0.15%), it may be bright enough to stand out from the background illumination. For example, when facing a solitary distant street light at night, the myope would be aware of a faint out-of-focus bright patch (or ghost image) in the field and would only need to accommodate by 3.00D to bring the ghost image into sharp focus.

This problem is aggravated by the presence of small prismatic corrections, since the ghost image is no longer superimposed upon the refracted image and is always displaced, in the direction of the prism apex, from the refracted image. This often occurs simply from poorly centred lenses in which the ghost image is always displaced in the direction of the apex of the induced prismatic effect. Only by ensuring that all lenses are centred correctly can this problem be reduced.

The remedy for this ghost image is to use an anti-reflection coating, which reduces the intensity of the reflected ghost image to negligible proportions. A broad-band multilayer coating should eliminate the problem entirely.

In the case of lenses of high refractive index, the problem with this ghost image is exacerbated, since it is brighter and, at the same time, less accommodation is required to bring the ghost into sharp focus. As already pointed out, an anti-reflection coating should always be considered for high-index

lenses, not just to reduce the intensity of reflected images, but also to prevent the surfaces staining in abnormal atmospheric conditions.

Figure 8.14b illustrates the formation of a ghost image of a source in front of the lens by reflection at the cornea and subsequent reflection at the back surface of the lens. The intensity of this ghost image is only 0.08% of the original intensity of the source for a material of refractive index 1.5, and 0.14% for a material of refractive index 1.7. It can be shown that the vergence of this ghost image is given by:

$$L'_c = -Z - 2F_2/(n-1)$$

The distance z is the sum of the vertex distance and half the radius of curvature of the anterior surface of the cornea, with the source of the ghost taken to be the reflection at the anterior corneal surface of the original source of light in front of the eyes. Taking an average value for the vertex distance of 14mm and 8mm for the corneal radius, $z = 18$mm and $Z = 55.56$D ($Z = 1/z$), and if $n = 1.5$ we have the condition for the ghost image to be in sharp focus when:

$$F = -55.56 - 4F_2$$

Examination of this statement leads to the conclusion that this ghost image will be troublesome for high myopes only; for example, a –11.50D lens made in plano-concave form would almost completely satisfy the condition. This ghost image can be defocused by altering the vertex distance or eliminated by anti-reflection coating the lens.

Figure 8.14c illustrates the formation of a ghost image of a source behind the lens by reflection at the back surface of the lens. Although the intensity of this ghost image is the greatest of all, being 4% of the original intensity of the source for a material of refractive index 1.5, and 6.7% for a material of refractive index 1.7, the image is likely to be the least troublesome, since myopes simply see a reflection of their own eyes and surroundings when the face is strongly illuminated.

It can be shown that the vergence of this ghost image is given by:

$$L'_c = L_1 - 2F_2/(n-1)$$

or when $n = 1.5$:

$$L'_c = L_1 - 4F_2$$

This is seen in sharp focus when:

$$F = L_1 - 4F_2$$

If a point on the face 20mm behind the lens is strongly illuminated, $L_1 = -50.00$D and the image of this point is in sharp focus when $F = -50 - 4F_2$. This condition would be satisfied by a -10.00D lens made in plano-concave form or a -8.00D lens made with a -10.50 back curve and so on. The intensity of this ghost image can be reduced by means of an anti-reflection coating.

Figure 8.14d illustrates the formation of a ghost image of a source behind the lens by reflection at the front surface of the lens. The intensity of this ghost image is 3.7% of the original intensity of the source for a material of refractive index 1.5, and 5.9% for a material of refractive index 1.7. This ghost image is only likely to be troublesome for myopes if they have been dispensed lenses large enough to collect light from behind the head.

It can be shown that the vergence of this ghost image is given by:

$$L'_c = L_1 + 2F_2 + 2nF_1/(n-1)$$

or when $n = 1.5$:

$$L'_c = 2F + 4F_1$$

The ghost will be troublesome when $L'_c = F$, or when:

$$F = -L_1 - 4F_1$$

For a distant object, this could occur for a -10.00D lens made with a $+2.50$ front curve or a -12.00D lens made with a $+3.00$ front curve and so on. Again, the remedy is to anti-reflection coat the lens.

References

1. Jalie M 1984 Principles of ophthalmic lenses. ABDO, London
2. Rayton W B 1917 The reflected images in spectacle lenses. J Opt Soc Am 1:137–148
3. Bennett A G 1968 Emsley and Swaine's ophthalmic lenses, vol. 1. Hatton Press, London

Dispensing in hypermetropia

Chapter

9

In Chapter 8, which considered in detail the dispensing of lenses for myopia, the point was made that the mechanical problems encountered in dispensing for myopia and hypermetropia differ somewhat, simply because the cross-sectional shape of minus and plus lenses is different. The cross-sectional shape of minus lenses (Figure 9.1a) lends itself well to a method of supply whereby a finished range of uncut lenses may be employed to produce a series of glazed lenses of different shapes. The edge thickness of a minus lens reduces as it is edged down to fit the frame so, provided that the centre thickness of the lens is minimum and the size is kept as small as possible, a reasonable lens may be obtained from a stock uncut.

Plus lenses, on the other hand, do not lend themselves so readily to this convenient method of supply. Figure 9.1b indicates what happens when a plus lens is edged down to produce the final lens for mounting. For a given centre thickness, the edge thickness increases as the diameter of the lens is reduced, and the only way in which the optimum lens may be obtained is to surface the lens to provide the required edge thickness for the finished diameter when full details of the prescription, decentration and frame size are known (Figure 9.1c). This chapter considers the problems encountered with plus lenses and in particular the dispensing of full-aperture lenses for hypermetropia.

Full-aperture lenses of high power, made in normal-index materials, are thick, heavy and unsightly. Even quite moderate plus prescriptions, when dispensed to frames of large aperture, may result in thick and heavy lenses. Additionally, in hypermetropia, the magnification effects of the lenses detract from the overall appearance of the wearer, as the eye and its surroundings appear more prominent since they are enlarged. Various courses of action may be taken by way of judicious selection of frames and lenses to ensure that the outcome results in a neat and comfortable pair of spectacles.

As a general rule, the smaller the size and more symmetrical the choice of lens shape, the thinner, lighter and better looking become the lenses. Following the very large sizes of the 1970s and 1980s, frame design today offers ranges of sizes at least 10mm smaller in diameter.

Before deciding the optimum lens for any given prescription the following should be taken into account:

- form of the lens
- material of the lens
- field of view
- optimum centre thickness
- resultant edge thickness
- weight of the lenses
- disturbing reflections
- surface treatments.

As this chapter shows, some of these considerations may well influence the choice of spectacle frame, with some designs being less suitable than others for a given specification.

The choice of lens form and material have been dealt with in detail in Chapter 2 and only a summary of the pertinent points is given here.

Lens form

The supply of spectacle lenses by lens manufacturers to the profession is in one of two ways. They may supply the prescription house with semi-finished blanks on which the front surface is completely finished and the final prescription is obtained by the surfacing workshop, which completes the second side. Or, they may supply the finished stock uncut lenses to the glazing department, who set them as required and edge them to the final size and shape for mounting into the spectacle frame. The reasons for the likely surface curves that may be used for any given power are discussed in Chapter 2.

Spectacle lenses are numbered in terms of their back vertex powers. Unlike minus lenses, the back vertex power of plus lenses is not the sum of the two surface powers. The effect of the thickness of the lens, t, also has to be taken into account. If the individual surface powers of the lens, F_1 and F_2, are known, together with the refractive index of the lens material, n, then the back vertex power of the lens, F'_V, is given by:

$$F'_V = \left[F_1 + F_2 - (t/n)F_1 F_2 \right] / \left[1 - (t/n)F_1 \right]$$

For example, if the individual surface powers are +8.76 and −5.00, respectively, and the lens is made in a material of refractive index 1.5, with an axial thickness of 4.5mm (which must be substituted as 0.0045 metres in the expression), then the back vertex power of the lens is found from:

$$F'_V = \frac{8.76 - 5 - (0.0045/1.5) \times 8.76 \times -5}{1 - (0.0045/1.5) \times 8.76}$$

$$= 3.891/0.9737$$

$$= +4.00D$$

The influence of the lens thickness in this example is quite apparent; it has contributed +0.24D to the power of the lens. The sum of the individual surface powers as might be read with the aid of a lens measure would result in a lens power of just +3.75D.

The form of the lens chosen for any given back vertex power is usually that which makes the power during oblique gaze as close as possible to the power obtained when the eye views along the optical axis of the lens.

The lens may be designed to be free from oblique astigmatism, in which case it is described as a *point-focal* lens form, or it may be designed to be free from mean oblique error, in which case it is described as a *Percival* lens form. Alternatively, it may be designed

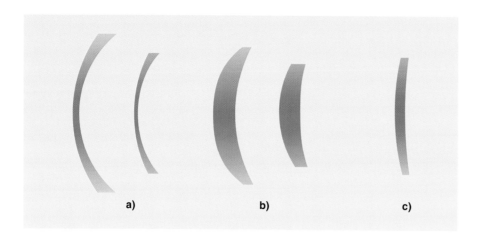

Figure 9.1 Cross-sectional views of minus and plus lenses:
(a) the edge thickness of a minus lens reduces as the lens is edged smaller;
(b) the edge thickness of a plus lens increases as the lens is edged smaller;
(c) optimum plus lens produced by surfacing when all its parameters are known

Table 9.1   Base curves and typical thicknesses for plus spherical CR39 lenses

Nominal base curves	Exact base curves	Range of centre thicknesses (mm)	To produce powers in the range	Error
+6.00	+5.94	0–6.2	+0.25 to +1.00	±0.09
+7.00	+6.90	0.4–5.8	+1.25 to +3.00	±0.09
+8.00	+7.80	2.0–7.5	+3.25 to +4.00	±0.12
+9.00	+8.75	2.5–6.9	+4.25 to +5.00	±0.12
+10.00	+9.62	4.1–7.7	+5.25 to +6.00	±0.12
+11.50	+10.80	7.1–9.8	+6.25 to +7.00	±0.12

to be free from tangential error at a given vertex distance. This so-called *Minimum T-error* form has the advantage that when fitted at a longer vertex distance than the designer intended, it tends to behave like a point-focal lens form, whereas when fitted at a shorter vertex distance it tends to behave like a Percival lens form (see Chapter 2).

When finished lenses are dispensed from a stock range of finished uncuts, the surface curves conform with the design criteria chosen by the manufacturer. The lenses are certain to provide good off-axis performance. When lenses need to be specially surfaced, the form is selected from the range of semi-finished blanks held in stock by the surfacing workshop. A typical range of semi-finished sphere blanks with spherical surfaces suitable for plus lenses made in spectacle crown glass or CR39 material up to a power of about +8.00D is given in Table 9.1. Recall from Chapter 2 that lenses over this power can only be made in a good optical form if one surface of the lens is aspherical.

Table 9.1 also gives the likely true front curves of the lenses, together with the ranges of centre thicknesses over which the power of the lens will not fall outside the current British Standard tolerances, if the back curve of the lens is assumed to be simply the difference between the back vertex power and the nominal front curve of the lens.

For example, to make a lens of power +5.00D, selecting a +9.00 front curve as suggested in Table 9.1, the required back curve would be:

$$+5.00 - +9.00 = -4.00D$$

provided that the centre thickness of the finished lens lies within the range 2.5mm to 6.9mm. Since the permissible tolerance in back vertex power for a +5.00D lens is ±0.12D (see Table 9.1), and assuming the other lens parameters to be correct, the lens

will vary in power from +4.87D, when the thickness is 2.5mm, to +5.12D, when the thickness is 6.9mm.

The information presented in Table 9.1 assumes the use of CR39 material of refractive index 1.498. Similar curves would be used for all normal-index materials (n_d <1.54) and, as a general rule, as the refractive index increases, so should the true front base curve to maintain the same off-axis performance as the normal-index lens.

Normally, it is wise to dispense lenses in best-form curvatures, for not only are off-axis errors minimized, but also different series do not differ much in form from one another and, in particular, the distortion is about the same for a given power.

Astigmatic lenses for hypermetropia provide the best optical performance when the cylinder is incorporated on the convex surface, the lenses being supplied as plus-base toric designs. Ideally, the toroidal surface should be of barrel form, which is possible with singly worked lenses if a set of toroidal tools is maintained by the surfacing house in barrel form. Plus-base toric construction, however, requires the surfacing workshop to hold a large range of toric tools, each individually compensated for an assumed value of centre thickness. Most laboratories, given the choice, incorporate the cylinder on the concave surface of the lens as a minus-base toric. In the case of strong cylinders this procedure, at least, improves the cosmetic appearance of the lens, since the variation in edge thickness that occurs along different power meridians is then hidden on the back of the lens.

When the refractive index of the lens material changes, the lens form needs to change to provide the same off-axis powers. Table 9.2 indicates the form required for various lens powers to have approximately the same off-axis performance as forms made in spectacle crown glass or CR39 material with base curves selected from Table 9.1. As with minus lenses, the transverse chromatism exhibited by the lens is dependent upon the V-value of the material, so when the material is changed this chromatism remains

Table 9.2 Form of higher-index lenses

Lens power (D)	Original front curve (1.498/1.523)	Required front curve when new refractive index is			
		1.600	1.700	1.800	1.900
+2.00	+6.90	+8.00	+9.12	+10.50	+11.50
+3.00	+6.90	+8.00	+9.12	+10.37	+11.37
+4.00	+7.80	+8.87	+9.75	+11.00	+12.25
+5.00	+8.75	+9.87	+11.00	+12.12	+13.25
+6.00	+9.62	+10.75	+11.87	+13.12	+14.25
+7.00	+10.80	+11.87	+13.00	+14.12	+15.37
+8.00	+10.80	+11.75	+12.62	+13.75	+14.75

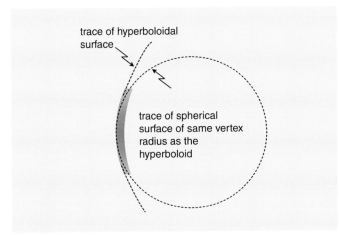

Figure 9.2 Plus lens with convex aspherical surface similar in form to a convex hyperboloid with an asphericity chosen so that the surface astigmatism neutralizes the astigmatism of oblique incidence

the same only if the V-value of the new material matches that of crown glass or CR39.

Aspheric lens forms for hypermetropia

For any given plus lens power, the flatter the lens form is made, the less the centre thickness of the lens may become. However, flat-form lenses do not provide good off-axis performance if spherical surfaces are used. Forms that are flatter than the Percival design for the power under consideration are afflicted with positive aberrational astigmatism. By employing an aspherical surface, which itself possesses negative surface astigmatism, it is possible to restore the off-axis performance, since the asphericity of the surface can be chosen so that the negative surface astigmatism neutralizes the positive astigmatism of oblique incidence.

A typical surface is illustrated in Figure 9.2. This is a convex hyperboloidal surface and Figure 9.2 shows that the decreasing convexity of the surface reduces the centre thickness of the lens even more, which offers a further saving in thickness over that obtained by simply flattening the lens from its traditional spherical form.

Needless to say, any higher order aspherical surface could be used, but, in practice, it does not depart significantly from a hyperboloid, since this curve regulates the astigmatism at the correct rate.

The optical performance of an aspheric design can be made to match any design philosophy. The lens may be made point-focal, or it may be made in Percival form or, more typically,

a compromise bending between these two forms is used to provide a reasonable performance over a wide range of fitting distances.

An even greater saving in thickness is obtained when a higher refractive index material is used. If a base curve of the same power is used the saving is two-fold. Firstly, there is the obvious reduction in the sags of the curves, since longer radii of curvature are employed.

Secondly, the use of the same power base curve on a higher refractive index material requires a longer radius of curvature at the vertex, r_0, so that, effectively, the lens is flatter still and requires greater asphericity on its convex surface to restore the off-axis performance.

This is illustrated in Figure 9.3, which compares the centre thicknesses of +4.00D lenses made in 1.50, 1.60 and 1.70 index materials, each with a diameter of 70mm and an edge thickness of 1.0mm. The asphericity of each of the convex surfaces, indicated in Figure 9.3, is chosen to provide the same off-axis performance for each lens.

Another important advantage of the low-power aspheric designs for hypermetropia can be gleaned from Figure 9.3. A best-form +4.00D design made in CR39 with spherical surfaces requires a centre thickness of 6.6mm to obtain an edge thickness of 1.0mm at 70mm diameter. If this uncut lens is edged down to a finished diameter of 50mm, it will have an edge thickness of 4.1mm, which is not at all acceptable for a lens of this power.

The aspheric design made in 1.60 index material, on the other hand, has a centre thickness of 4.5mm and an edge thickness of 2.6mm when edged down to a finished diameter of 50mm. As the front curve is flatter, aspheric lens designs lend themselves far better to a system of supply of large-diameter plus uncut lenses that need to be edged to smaller diameters depending upon the choice of shape and size of the lens.

An enormous cosmetic advantage with the use of flatter aspheric lens forms for the correction of hypermetropia is that not only is the plate height of the lens smaller, which makes them appear less bulbous, but also they lie closer to the eyes. This means that the appearance of the wearer's eyes and the surrounding portions of the face are seen with less magnification than with more steeply curved lenses with spherical surfaces.

Lens material

Table 9.3 gives a typical selection of lens materials and lists physical properties of the materials that are pertinent to the choice of material. The significance of the physical data is discussed in full in Chapter 2.

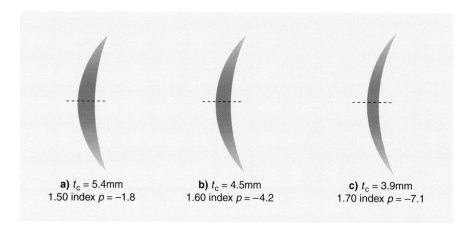

Figure 9.3 Comparison of the centre thicknesses, t_c, of +4.00D lenses made in 1.50, 1.60 and 1.70 materials with convex hyperboloidal surfaces with asphericities, p, chosen to provide the same off-axis performance for each design

a) t_c = 5.4mm
1.50 index $p = -1.8$

b) t_c = 4.5mm
1.60 index $p = -4.2$

c) t_c = 3.9mm
1.70 index $p = -7.1$

Table 9.3   Physical data for typical lens materials

Medium	n_d	n_e	Curve variation factor	Density	Abbe number	p
Glasses						
White crown	1.523	1.525	1.00	2.5	59	4.3
Light Flint	1.600	1.602	0.87	2.6	42	5.3
1.7 glasses	1.701	1.706	0.75	3.2	42	6.7
1.8 glasses	1.802	1.808	0.65	3.7	35	8.2
1.9 glasses	1.885	1.892	0.59	4.0	31	9.4
Plastics						
PMMA	1.490	1.492	1.07	1.2	58	3.9
CR39	1.498	1.500	1.05	1.3	58	4.0
Trivex	1.532	1.534	0.98	1.1	46	4.4
Sola Spectralite	1.537	1.540	0.97	1.2	47	4.5
PPG HIP	1.560	1.563	0.93	1.2	38	4.8
Polycarbonate	1.586	1.589	0.89	1.2	30	5.2
Polyurethanes	1.600	1.603	0.87	1.3	36	5.3
	1.660	1.664	0.79	1.4	32	6.2
Hoya Teslalid	1.710	1.715	0.74	1.4	36	6.9
Nikon	1.740	1.745	0.71	1.4	32	7.3

Field of view

Figure 9.4 shows that hypermetropes suffer a loss in their real field of view in the object space. For example, in Figure 9.4 an apparent angular field of 73° for a +5.00D lens at 40mm diameter corresponds to a real angular field of only 65°. Figure 9.4 shows an area surrounding the edge of the lens from which no light can enter the eye. With the example illustrated, the angular extent of this ring scotoma is 4°, which is half of the difference between the real and apparent fields. Since 4° is very nearly equal to 7Δ, the linear extent of this ring scotoma on a Bjerrum screen mounted 1 metre in front of the subject is 7cm. The loss is 70cm at 10 metres away, more than enough to obscure a motorist's view of a pedestrian waiting at the kerb to cross the street. These figures ignore both the thickness of the rim of the frame and spherical aberration, the effects of each of which increase the size of the scotoma. The ring scotoma is stationary while the head remains stationary. When the head is turned the ring scotoma also turns, roaming around the field of vision; for obvious reasons, this phenomenon is referred to as a *roving ring scotoma*.

A secondary problem for the hypermetrope is the sudden disappearance and reappearance of objects as they pass through the ring scotoma, a phenomenon known as the *jack-in-the-box* effect.

The characteristic head swing, which is evident in many hypermetropes when they wish to view laterally placed objects, is obviously developed to minimize the effects of the roving ring scotoma.

The real macular field of view of a spectacle lens of power, F, and diameter, $2y$, mounted 27mm in front of the eye's centre of rotation is given by:

$$\tan \theta = y(37 - F)/1000$$

where θ is half the field of view. Hence, a +10.00D lens edged 40mm round has a real angular field of view of 57°. A +12.00D lens made in lenticular form with a 32mm round aperture has a real field of view of just 44°.

To obtain the maximum field, whatever size the aperture might be, the lens should be fitted as close to the eyes as the lashes permit. In cases of high hypermetropia and aphakia, a close fit has the added advantage of reducing the retinal image size and the magnification of the eye and surroundings viewed through the lens.

Lens thickness

It has already been pointed out that although minus lenses lend themselves well to a method of supply in which uncuts can be stocked in any diameter, with the edge thickness of a minus lens

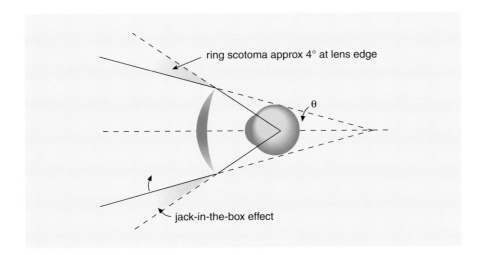

Figure 9.4   Decreased field of view of a plus lens. Note the area that forms the ring scotoma and causes the jack-in-the-box effect at the edge of the lens. θ is the semi-angular real field of view

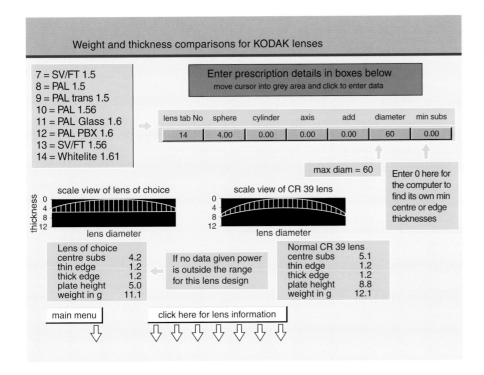

Figure 9.5   Computer-generated thickness comparisons as an aid to dispensing (courtesy of Signet Armorlite Europe Ltd)

reducing as its diameter reduces, this is not the case for plus lenses. In an ideal world, where the goal is to supply the thinnest, lightest possible lenses for every plus prescription, each lens should be custom designed when all the details of the prescription, centration and eye size are known. The use of stock uncuts for powers over about +2.50D cannot lead to the optimum lens thickness for the prescription, which can only be obtained by surfacing each lens individually when all the prescription data are to hand.

Just as with minus lenses, it is very useful for the dispensing optician to be able to visualize the finished spectacles. Computer software, available from several sources, allows the lens prescription and frame data to be input, whereupon the program calculates the thickness and weight of the finished lenses. This information is output to the VDU screen and the patient and practitioner can review the likely outcome before the lenses are actually made. A typical output is illustrated in Figure 9.5.

In the absence of the computer it is possible to estimate lens thickness to within two- or three-tenths of a millimetre by a simple mental calculation using the sag factors detailed in Chapter 8 and again described below for convenience.

To estimate the thickness of a plus lens, two items need to be known – the edge thickness of the lens and the sag of the lens power at the diameter in question.

Edge thickness of plus lenses

The edge thickness of a plus lens depends, in the main, upon the mount to which the lens is to be fitted. In the case of glass lenses, which are rigid and do not flex under pressure from the mount, an edge thickness of 1.0mm is all that is required (provided that the centre thickness is not less than about 2.0mm) when the lens is to be bevelled and fitted to a plastics frame. If a glass lens is to be fitted to a metal-rimmed frame, it is safer to allow an edge thickness of 1.8mm, and for lenses that have to be drilled for a rimless mount or grooved to take a supra cord, it is usual to allow a minimum edge thickness of 2.0mm.

These minimum edge thicknesses can also be used for plastics lenses with the proviso that the compression exerted by the mount should not cause the lens to flex. Mounted plastics lenses should always be inspected for evidence that they might have been over-glazed, optical discontinuities such as waves being quite apparent, especially near the edge of the lens.

As a general guide, for both edged and uncut lenses the edge thickness varies from 2.0mm down to 1.0mm, the value decreasing as the power increases. A typical series of edge thicknesses, e, for either glass or plastics lenses is given by the rule:

$$e = 2.0 - (0.2 \times \text{power of lens})$$

Thus, we might expect a series of uncuts to have the edge thicknesses shown in Table 9.4.

It has already been pointed out that it is not good practice to attempt to stock plus uncut lenses over about +5.00D, since details of the final lens diameter and decentration are unknown.

Sag factors for crown glass lenses

The thickness of a lens resulting from its power can be estimated as a simple function of the lens power. The method employs the use of a sag factor that is related to the lens diameter.

Sag factors for various useful diameters are shown in Table 9.5. It is necessary only to multiply the sag factor by the lens power to obtain the thickness of the lens from the power, for the diameter under consideration.

From Table 9.5, at a diameter of 45mm the sag factor is 0.5. This value indicates that, for this diameter, lens thickness increases at the rate of 0.5mm per dioptre of lens power. Hence,

sag 1.00 at 45 = 0.5mm
sag 2.00 at 45 = 1.0mm
sag 3.00 at 45 = 1.5mm
sag 8.00 at 45 = 4.0mm

and so on.

This simple method of finding the thickness of a lens works well provided that the product of the power and the lens diameter does not exceed the value 500. Thus, for the 45mm diameter chosen above, the sag factor 0.5 can be used up to an 11.00D curve, since $11.00 \times 45 = 495$.

Thickness of plus lenses

To determine the centre thickness of a plus lens it is necessary to add the thickness from the power to the edge thickness of the lens (Figure 9.6).

Thus, a +5.00D lens made in crown glass and edged 45mm in diameter that is to be fitted to a plastics frame needs a centre thickness of 3.5mm. This value is obtained by adding sag 5.00 at 45 (5×0.5) to the likely edge thickness for a +5.00D lens, which is 1.0mm, obtained from Table 9.4.

If, in an attempt to supply this lens quickly, it was obtained from a 60mm diameter uncut, edged down to 45mm diameter, then, assuming the edge thickness of the uncut to be 1.0mm, the centre thickness of the uncut would be 5.5mm ($5 \times 0.9 + 1.0$). The resultant edge thickness of the lens when edged down to a diameter of 45mm would be 3.0mm ($5.5 - 5 \times 0.5$). This is not at all satisfactory for a lens of this power.

Consider the lens shape depicted in Figure 9.7. It is a typical modern *quadra* shape, of box dimensions 60×50, and the specification includes 4.5mm of inward decentration. The dimension of the lens along the horizontal centre line is 54mm.

The distances shown on Figure 9.7 represent the distances from the optical centre to the lens periphery. These distances should be doubled to determine the diameter and its associated sag factor. Suppose the power of this lens is +4.00D sphere and a minimum edge thickness of 1.0mm is required to glaze the lens into a plastics frame. The minimum edge thickness is located at the point on the lens periphery that lies furthest from the optical centre of the lens, which is seen in Figure 9.7 to be point 'c' on the lens periphery.

Hence, the necessary centre thickness for the lens is the sum of the edge thickness and sag 4.00 at 70 = ($1.0 + 4 \times 1.2$), or 5.8mm.

The edge thicknesses at the other points on the lens periphery can be found by subtracting the sags caused by the power from the centre thickness, 5.8mm.

The edge thickness at point 'a' on the lens periphery is 5.8 – sag 4.00 at 63. The sag factor for this diameter is 1.0, and hence at

Table 9.5   Sag factors for crown glass lenses

Lens diameter (mm)	Sag factor
20	0.1
30	0.2
35	0.3
40	0.4
45	0.5
50	0.6
54	0.7
57	0.8
60	0.9
63	1.0
66	1.1
70	1.2

Table 9.4   Power of lens and edge thicknesses

Power (D)	Centre subs (mm)
+0.50	1.9
+1.00	1.8
+1.50	1.7
+2.00	1.6
+3.00	1.4
+4.00	1.2
+5.00	1.0

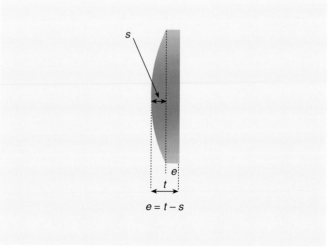

$$e = t - s$$

Figure 9.6   Edge thickness of a plus lens, $e = t - s$

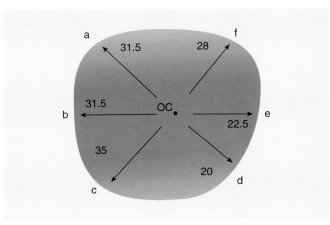

Figure 9.7 Typical spectacle lens shape in which the lens has been decentred. The distances shown represent the distances from the optical centre to the lens edge

'a' the edge thickness is 5.8 – 4.0 = 1.8mm. The edge thicknesses at the other points are:

'b', 5.8 — 4 × 1.0 = 1.8mm

'd', 5.8 — 4 × 0.4 = 4.2mm

'e', 5.8 — 4 × 0.5 = 3.8mm

'f', 5.8 — 4 × 0.8 = 2.6mm

At the dispensing table, in the case of plus lenses, it is usually necessary to consider only the maximum edge thickness, which in the case of a spherical lens lies at the closest point to the optical centre of the lens periphery.

By measuring the frame-rim thickness one can immediately point out the overhang of the lens if the subject were to choose the frame in question. For the example in hand, this lies on the nasal side of the lens between points 'd' and 'e' and an edge of this thickness is certain to cause disappointment to the wearer, especially if the lens is mounted in a thin-rimmed frame.

Sags for other lens materials

The sag factors given in Table 9.5 relate only to spectacle crown glass of refractive index 1.523. However, they can be used for lenses made in other materials provided the power is first converted to its crown glass equivalent. This is done simply by multiplying the power of the lens by the curve variation factor quoted for the material.

Suppose the use of a 1.66 index plastics material is considered for the +4.00D specification described in Figure 9.7. The crown glass equivalent is +4.00 × 0.79 or +3.2D. In other words, the use of material with a high refractive index enables the thickness of the +4.00D lens to vary in the same way as a +3.2D lens made in crown glass. Assuming the minimum edge thickness at point 'c' remains 1.0mm, the centre thickness of the lens is 1.0 + sag 3.2 at 70 = (1.0 + 3.2 × 1.2) = 4.8mm. The variations in edge thickness around the lens periphery of this 1.66 index +4.00 lens are:

'a', 4.8 — 3.2 × 1.0 = 1.6mm

'b', 4.8 — 3.2 × 1.0 = 1.6mm

'c', 4.8 — 3.2 × 1.2 = 1.0mm

'd', 4.8 — 3.2 × 0.4 = 3.5mm

'e', 4.8 — 3.2 × 0.5 = 3.2mm

'f', 4.8 — 3.2 × 0.8 = 2.2mm

The advantage of using material of higher refractive index for this specification is immediately apparent. The maximum edge thickness has decreased from 4.2mm to 3.5mm, a reduction of some 17%.

If this same specification is now produced in a 1.66 index material in aspheric form, the centre thickness of the lens reduces to 4.2mm and the edge thicknesses around the lens, with the thickness at point 'c' remaining 1.0mm, are:

'a', = 1.5mm

'b', = 1.5mm

'c', = 1.0mm

'd', = 3.1mm

'e', = 2.8mm

'f', = 2.1mm

The advantage of using the high-tech aspheric design is immediately apparent, as the maximum edge thickness of this plus lens is nearly 30% thinner than its crown glass counterpart.

Thickness of astigmatic lenses

The edge thickness of astigmatic lenses can be predicted using exactly the same sag factors as for spherical lenses, but, of course, these must be associated with the correct principal powers of the lens. The power along the axis meridian of an astigmatic lens results from the sphere alone, whereas the power at right angles to the axis is the sum of the sphere and the cylinder.

Consider the astigmatic lens +4.00/+2.00 × 90. The principal powers of this lens are +4.00D along 90 and +6.00D along 180. When the lens is circular in shape and without decentration, it is the meridian of greatest power that controls the thickness of the lens, which in this case is the horizontal meridian. Thus, for the prescription +4.00/+2.00 × 90 made in spectacle crown glass with a thin-edge thickness of 1.0mm and edged to a 45 × 40 oval shape, the centre thickness, controlled by the horizontal meridian, is given by the sum of the thin-edge substance and sag 6.00 at 45, that is, 1.0 + (6.00 × 0.5) = 4.0mm. The thick-edge substance at the extremities of the vertical meridian is given by the difference between the centre thickness and sag +4.00 at 40, that is 4.0 – (4.00 × 0.4) = 2.4mm.

Suppose that the cylinder axis lay at 180 instead of 90 for the above specification. The principal powers of this lens are +4.00D along 180 and +6.00D along 90. The meridian that now controls the thickness of the lens is the meridian that has the greatest sag, so it is necessary to begin by determining which is the greater, sag 4.00 at 45 or sag 6.00 at 40. Using sag factors, sag 4.00 at 45 is 2.0mm, whereas sag 6.00 at 40 is 2.4mm, so the +6.00D meridian again controls the thickness of the lens and the thinnest point on the edge of this lens now lies at the extremities of the vertical meridian. The centre thickness of the lens is the sum of the thin-edge substance and sag 6.00 at 40 = 1.0 + (6.00 × 0.4) = 3.4mm. The thick-edge substance now lies at the extremities of the horizontal meridian, and is given by the difference between the centre thickness and sag 4.00 at 45, which is 3.4 – (4.00 × 0.5) = 1.4mm.

These examples assume that the meridian that controls the thickness of the lens can be determined by inspection, or by the comparison of sags along the principal that the meridians of the lens. As has just been pointed out, this is easy with circular lenses or with oval lenses when the cylinder axis lies at 90 or 180.

When the cylinder axis is oblique, or decentration is required, a little more thought is necessary to dispense the optimum spectacles. When a plus astigmatic lens is surfaced such that it has zero edge thickness all round its periphery (i.e. it is knife-edged), it becomes oval in shape with the short axis of the oval coinciding with the minus cylinder axis direction of the prescription (Figure 9.8). Ideally, the frame shape chosen for these lenses should correspond with the longest and shortest dimensions of the knife-edge uncut.

It can be shown[1] that the major axis, a, of a knife-edge oval astigmatic uncut is given by:

$$a = b\sqrt{\left[(S+C)/S\right]}$$

where b is the minor or short axis of the oval and S and C are the spherical and cylindrical powers of the lens, respectively.

If the ratio between the long and short dimensions of the knife-edged astigmatic oval uncut is known, it is possible to visualize or to sketch the oval superimposed upon the shape in question. The thinnest edge of the lens must lie where the knife-edged astigmatic oval uncut just touches the edge of the shaped lens. It is quite easy to estimate the minimum diameter of the short axis that just encompasses the shape.

For demonstration purposes, we consider here the prescription +5.00/+2.00 × 150 to be surfaced to produce a thin-edge substance of 1.0mm on the edge of the 42 × 35 quadra shape illustrated in Figure 9.9, the specification also incorporating 3mm inwards decentration.

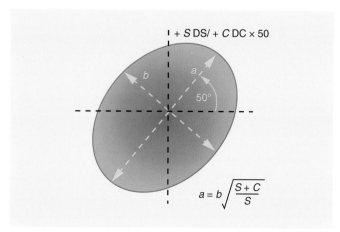

Figure 9.8 Plus astigmatic uncut lens, +S DS/ +C DC × 50 with zero edge thickness. A plus astigmatic lens with an edge thickness of zero all round its periphery is elliptical in shape. The major axis of the ellipse is $\sqrt{[(S+C)/C]}$ times the minor axis, where S and C are the spherical and cylindrical powers of the lens

At present, the position of the thinnest point on the edge of the finished shape is unknown.

The ratio:

$$a = b\sqrt{\left[(S+C)/S\right]}$$

indicates that the oval, astigmatic, knife-edged uncut will have a long axis, along the 150° meridian, of:

$$a = b\sqrt{\left[(5+2)/5\right]} = 1.18b$$

The long axis is 1.18 times the short axis. The short axis, obviously, lies along the 60° meridian.

In Figure 9.9b, an oval of the correct dimensions has been superimposed in the correct position with its long axis lying along the 150° meridian and with its geometrical centre decentred 3mm inwards to coincide with the required optical centre position. Figure 9.9b shows that the thin edge for the specification lies where the oval uncut just touches the shape and that this point lies down and out along 35° from the optical centre of the lens.

To establish the optimum uncut specification, the short-axis diameter must be determined and measurement of the superimposed oval indicates that the short-axis diameter must be 48mm.

Assuming nominal curves and that the lens is to be made as a −3.00 base toric, in CR39 material, and with a thin-edge substance of 1.0mm, the necessary centre thickness, t, is given by:

$$t = \text{sag } 10.00 \text{ at } 48 - \text{sag } 3.00 \text{ at } 48 = e_{\text{thin}}$$
$$= 6.2 - 1.7 + 1.0$$
$$= 5.5\text{mm}$$

The edge thickness all round the periphery of the oval uncut is 1.0mm.

Owing to the thickness of the lens, the true front-surface power is +9.67D and the actual centre thickness, by accurate transposition, is 5.2mm.

Problems of this nature occur frequently in the surfacing workshop and are not confined to strong plus lenses.

The correct proportions of the oval are obtained by measuring the distance OB (20mm) along the 60° meridian (Figure 9.9b) and constructing OA (20 × 1.18 = 24mm) to obtain the long- and short-axis dimensions of the dashed oval outline shown in Figure 9.9b. The oval was then expanded in the same proportion to determine the position of e_{thin}.

Figure 9.9 Determination of the position of the thin edge for the specification +5.00/+2.00 × 60, which is to be edged to a 42 × 35 quadra shape

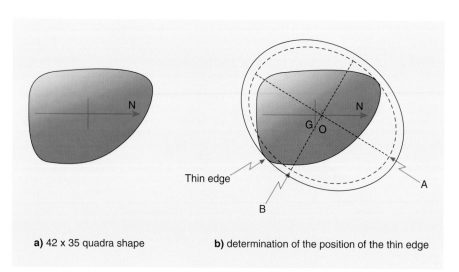

a) 42 × 35 quadra shape   **b)** determination of the position of the thin edge

In 1977 Bennett and Crockford[2] offered a practical solution to this astigmatic lens design problem with their ALTO (Alpha lens thickness optimization) system, which consisted of a series of transparent plastic templates with ovals of the correct proportions inscribed upon them. The templates could be held over the frame or glazing former and the correct short-axis dimension determined by inspection.

Today, thickness optimization of astigmatic lenses involves tracing the lens shape from the frame or the former by means of a frame tracer and the thickness optimized from the digitized shape information. Essentially, the computer calculates and compares the lens thickness along different meridians of the lens and decides which meridian controls the lens thickness. It can then assign a minimum edge thickness along the thin-edge meridian and compute the centre thickness and vertex power allowance for this centre thickness. Most of the major lens manufacturing companies offer thickness optimization packages, such as NIDES (Norville integrated design and edging system), METS (minimum edge thickness system) from Hoya, PRECAL (precalibrated lens system) from Essilor, OPTIMA from Zeiss, SHAPE TO SHAPE from Rodenstock and so on.

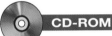

CD-ROM

The thickness of plus lenses is also considered in detail on the CD-ROM

Weight of plus lenses

It is pointed out in Chapter 8 that spectacles should be as light in weight as possible to prevent discomfort to the wearer. The weight of the front of the spectacles is generally borne entirely by the bearing surface of the frame on the bridge of the nose.

As a rule, the larger the bearing surface the more evenly the weight of the frame is spread around the bearing surface of the nose. Glass lenses fitted to large eye-size frames that have small pads on the arms is the worst possible scenario.

The weight of a pair of spectacles is made up from the weight of the spectacle frame and the weight of the lenses. The weight of the frame depends upon the materials used in its construction and varies from the featherweight three-piece rimless mount, or very thin metal fully-rimmed frame, to the heavyweight plastics library frame with thick rims made from cellulose acetate. In theory, the higher the prescription, the sturdier the mount should be to ensure that the lenses are held at the correct vertex distance and at the correct pantoscopic angle before the eyes. If the shape of the lens is such that there is an appreciable edge substance at any

zone around its periphery then, just as with minus lenses, a dark thick-rimmed front prevents the lens edge from picking up light, and thus avoids the formation of power rings.

The weight of a spectacle lens is calculated by multiplying the volume of the lens by the density of the lens material. The volume of a circular lens is found from the sum of the volumes of the two spherical caps that comprise the lens surfaces.

The rules that ensure spectacle lenses are as light as possible are the same as those used to obtain thin lenses. The eye size should be kept as small as possible, symmetrical shapes should be chosen and, wherever possible, the box centre distance of the frame should match the subject's centration distance to avoid decentration of the lenses.

Table 9.6 compares the weight in grams of lenses made in various materials at 40mm and 50mm diameter; the lenses are assumed to be round in shape and made in typical curved forms with edge thicknesses as indicated. This table shows how important it is, in cases where weight is a significant factor, to use not just the lightest lens material, but also to dispense the smallest possible eye size. When the lens diameter is increased from 40mm to 50mm, the weight of the lens virtually doubles.

Reflections that may disturb hypermetropes

Ghost images that may appear in the field of view and cause annoyance to spectacle wearers are considered in detail in Chapter 5, but a review of the reflections that cause a particular problem to the wearers of plus lenses may be useful here.

Hypermetropes may complain of troublesome reflections or ghost images that appear in the visual field under certain conditions, usually indoors or in a lighted street at night where there are bright sources of light in conditions of low illumination. The four likely causes of ghost images in cases of hypermetropia are shown in Figure 9.10.

Figure 9.10a illustrates the formation of a ghost image of a source in front of the lens by total internal reflection at the lens surfaces. The intensity of this ghost image is only 0.15% of the original intensity of the source for a material of refractive index 1.5, and 0.39% for a material of refractive index 1.7.

It can be shown[3] that the vergence of this ghost image for a distant point source of light, L'_c, depends only on the refractive index of the lens material, n, and the power, F, of the lens:

$$L'_c = \left[(3n-1)/(n-1)\right]F$$

For glass of refractive index 1.5, $L'_c = 7F$, and for glass of refractive index 1.7, $L'_c = 5.86F$.

Table 9.6	Weight (g) of plus lenses at 40 and 50mm diameters											
Material	CR 39		1.523		1.600		1.600		1.700		1.800		
Density	1.32		2.54		1.30		2.60		3.00		3.70		
Diameter	40	50	40	50	40	50	40	50	40	50	40	50	Edge
Power (D)													
+2.00	3.4	6.0	6.4	11.3	3.2	5.5	6.4	11.0	7.1	12.2	8.6	14.6	1.6
+4.00	3.4	6.6	6.4	12.3	3.1	5.8	6.2	11.7	6.7	12.5	7.9	14.5	1.2
+6.00	3.4	7.4	6.4	13.7	3.0	6.3	6.0	12.5	6.3	12.9	7.3	14.5	0.8
+8.00	3.7	8.5	6.7	15.5	3.1	6.9	6.1	13.8	6.3	13.9	7.0	15.3	0.5
+10.00	4.4	10.3	8.0	18.8	3.6	8.3	7.3	16.7	7.4	16.6	8.2	18.2	0.5

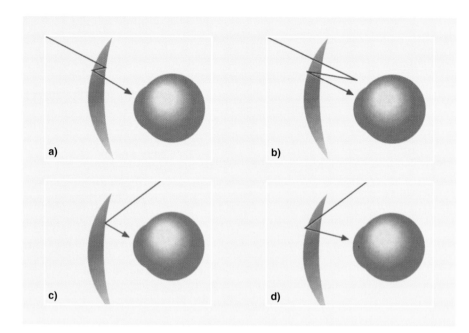

a)

b)

c)

d)

Figure 9.10   Source of ghost images in hypermetropia:
(a) image formed by total internal reflection
(b) image formed by reflection at the cornea and front surface of the lens
(c) image formed by reflection at the back surface of the lens
(d) image formed by reflection at the front surface of the lens.
Note. Ghost images (a) and (b) are images of sources that lie in front of the lens, whereas ghost images (c) and (d) are images of sources that lie behind the lens

For the ghost to be seen in sharp focus, the vergence L'_c should be the same as the power of the lens, F, or capable of being made the same by accommodation of the eye. We may conclude, therefore, that this image is usually well out of focus except with lenses of very low power.

For instance, in the case of a +0.25 hypermetrope who wears CR39 lenses ($n = 1.5$), the vergence of this ghost image would be +1.75D. Despite the very low intensity of the image (0.15%), it may be bright enough to stand out from the background illumination as a slightly out-of-focus bright patch. For example, when facing a solitary distant street light at night the wearer might be aware of a faint out-of-focus bright patch (or ghost image) in the field.

This problem is aggravated by the presence of small prismatic corrections, since the ghost image is no longer superimposed upon the refracted image and is always displaced, in the direction of the prism apex, from the refracted image.

This often occurs simply from poorly centred lenses, in which the ghost image is always displaced in the direction of the apex of the induced prismatic effect. Only by ensuring that all lenses are centred correctly can this problem be reduced.

The remedy for this ghost image is to use an anti-reflection coating that reduces the intensity of the reflected ghost image to negligible proportions. A broad-band multilayer coating should entirely eliminate the problem.

For lenses of high refractive index, the problem with this ghost image is exacerbated since it is brighter and, at the same time, less accommodation is required to bring the image into sharp focus. In general, an anti-reflection coating should always be considered for high-index lenses, not just to reduce the intensity of reflected images, but also to prevent the surfaces from staining in abnormal atmospheric conditions.

Figure 9.10b illustrates the formation of a ghost image of a source in front of the lens by reflection at the cornea and subsequent reflection at the front surface of the lens. The intensity of this ghost image is only 0.08% of the original intensity of the source for a material of refractive index 1.5, and 0.12% for a material of refractive index 1.7.

It can be shown that the vergence of this ghost image is given by:

$$L'_c = -Z + 2F_2 - 2nF_1/(n-1)$$

The distance Z is made up from the sum of the vertex distance and half the radius of curvature of the anterior surface of the cornea. The source of the ghost image is taken to be the reflection at the anterior corneal surface of the original source of light in front of the eyes.

Examination of this statement and substituting suitable values for Z leads to the conclusion that this ghost will only be in focus for high-power plus lenses. It can be dealt with by changing the vertex distance of the lens or by anti-reflection coating on the lens surfaces.

Figure 9.10c illustrates the formation of a ghost image of a source behind the wearer produced by reflection at the back surface of the lens. The intensity of this ghost image is the greatest of all, being 4% of the original intensity of the source for a material of refractive index 1.5, and 6.7% for a material of refractive index 1.7. However, the image is only likely to be troublesome if the lens is large enough to collect light from a distant object behind the head.

It can be shown that the vergence of this ghost image is given by:

$$L'_c = L_1 - 2F_2/(n-1)$$

or, when $n = 1.5$:

$$L'_c = L_1 - 4F_2$$

It will be seen in sharp focus when:

$$F = L_1 - 4F_2$$

For a distant object, $L_1 = 0$, and the condition for this ghost image to be troublesome is that $F = -4F_2$.

This could occur either for high-power plus lenses (e.g. a +12.00D lens made with a −3.00D base curve exactly satisfies the condition) or for low-power aspheric lenses (such as a +6.00D lens made with a −1.50 base curve, or a +4.00D lens made with a −1.00D base curve, and so on). The intensity of this ghost image can be reduced by means of an anti-reflection coating.

Figure 9.10d illustrates the formation of a ghost image of a source behind the lens by reflection at the front surface of the lens.

The intensity of this ghost image is 3.7% of the original intensity of the source for a material of refractive index 1.5, and 5.9% for a material of refractive index 1.7.

It can be shown that the vergence of this ghost image is given by:

$$L'_c = L_1 + 2F_2 + 2nF_1/(n-1)$$

or, when $n = 1.5$:

$$L'_c = L_1 + 2F + 4F_1$$

The ghost will be troublesome when $L'_c = F$, or when:

$$F = -L_1 - 4F_1$$

This ghost is likely to be troublesome for a hypermetrope only if the face is strongly illuminated, for then L_1 will have a finite value.

For example, the outer canthus 25mm behind the front surface of the lens would give L_1 the value −40.00D and the condition for a reflection of the outer canthus to be seen in sharp focus would be:

$$F = 40 - 4F_1$$

This condition could be satisfied by a +4.00D lens made with a +9.00D front curve or a +6.00D lens made with a +8.50D front curve, and so on. The remedy is to apply an anti-reflection coat to the lens.

Near vision effectivity errors with plus lenses

The back vertex power of a lens represents the vergence on leaving the lens when the light originates from a distant object. In near vision, the light originates from a point that lies at a finite distance in front of the lens and the vergence leaving the back surface now depends not just on the back vertex power, but also on the form and thickness of the lens. For lenses with an axial thickness that cannot be ignored when considering the lens power, such as plus lenses over about +3.00D, the vertex power notation gives only an approximate indication of the performance of the lens in near vision.

The vergence leaving the back surface of the lens, L'_2, that has arrived from a near object lying at L_1 dioptres in front of the lens, is given by:

$$L'_2 = (L_1 + F_1)/\left[(1 - t/n)(L_1 + F_1)\right] + F_2$$

When L_1 is zero, this expression reduces to the expression given earlier for the back vertex power of the lens, as expected.

The difference between the vergence leaving a lens when the light originates from a near object, L'_2, and the anticipated vergence obtained from the sum of the incident vergence and the back vertex power, $L_1 + F'_V$, is called the near vision effectivity error (NVEE) of the lens.

It can be shown that the NVEE is given by the approximate relationship:

$$NVEE = (t/n)L_1(L_1 + 2F_1)$$

NVEE is usually only a problem when the thickness of the lens becomes appreciable, which occurs with plus lenses of moderate-to-high power. Its significance is that lenses of the same back vertex power but of different forms are not interchangeable in near vision. Typically, trial case lenses are either plano-convex in form, with the curved surface designed to face the eye, or they may be symmetrical, equi-convex in the case of plus lenses. However, the final lens that is eventually dispensed is certain to be curved in form with its concave surface facing the eye. For a trial lens of power +10.00D employed for near vision, the power of the final curved-form lens dispensed needs to be increased by about +0.50D from that of the flat-form trial lens. The use of the above expression is illustrated in Chapter 13, which deals specifically with strong plus lenses for the correction of aphakia. Some manufacturers include tables in their technical literature that detail the errors likely to be found in trial lenses and in their own lens series. As a rule, they propose a correction factor that can be added to the back vertex correction to ensure that the final lens duplicates the effect of the trial lens. It goes without saying that the person who has prescribed the near-vision prescription should inform the dispensing optician whether a correction for NVEE has been included, or whether the modification needs to be made at the time when the lenses are ordered.

CD-ROM

Near vision effectivity errors are also considered in detail on the CD-ROM

References

1. Jalie M 1981 Prescription lens design. Manufacturing Optics International 34:7
2. Bennett A G, Crockford E 1977 Second International Symposium on Manufacturing Optics, London
3. Jalie M 1984 Principles of ophthalmic lenses. ABDO, London

Bifocal lenses

When a subject requires a separate correction for distance and near vision, the two prescriptions may be provided as one pair of spectacles in the form of bifocal lenses, various types of which are illustrated in Figures 10.1 and 10.2.

The area of the lens used for distance vision is called the *distance portion*, or DP, and the area used for near vision is called the *near* or *reading portion*, NP. The larger of these two portions is referred to as the *major portion*. It is very useful, when considering the theory and performance of bifocal lenses, to assume that the lens is made up of two distinct components, a *main lens*, which is usually the distance portion (the exception being the upcurve bifocal illustrated in Figure 10.1d), attached to which is a supplementary segment lens, the power of which is the addition for intermediate or near.

British Standards terminology relating to bifocal lenses is given in Table 10.1 and the definitions included there are taken from BS 3521 Part 1:1991. Abbreviations suggested in the Standard are included and terms that appear in italic are defined elsewhere in the Standard.

Some of the terminology is relatively new and it should be found worthwhile to read the definitions given in Table 10.1 carefully and to compare them with any older definitions that the reader might be familiar with. When the new terminology has gained universal acceptance and becomes commonly employed, it is certain to aid communication between the practitioner and the workshop. Most of the dimensions that are peculiar to bifocal lenses are illustrated in Figures 10.3 to 10.5.

Bifocal types

Bifocal lenses can be classified in several ways, one of the most useful being by method of construction. The earliest bifocals were *split bifocals* (Figure 10.2), in which two separate lenses for distance and near vision were fitted edge-to-edge in a single rim. This design is often referred to as a *Franklin bifocal*, since Benjamin Franklin, in a famous letter (dated August 21, 1784) to his 'Dear Old Friend', the philanthropist, George Whately, wrote:

> '...I cannot distinguish a Letter even of Large Print; but am happy in the invention of Double Spectacles, which serving for distant objects as well as near ones, make my Eyes as useful to me as ever they were: If all the other Defects and Infirmities were as easily and cheaply remedied, it would be worthwhile for Friends to live a good deal longer...'[1]

It is notable that Franklin does not claim to have invented bifocals, but rather to be 'happy in the invention'. History records that several other contemporaries of Franklin wore 'double spectacles'. It would appear that the term bifocal was first applied by John Isaac Hawkins (1772–1855), the inventor of trifocal lenses.[2]

Since the distance and near portions of the split bifocal are formed from two separate lenses, this design allows the distance and near portions to be centred separately, with the distance optical centre located in the distance visual zone and the near optical centre in the near visual zone. This fundamental optical requirement of all bifocal lenses is not usually achieved in other bifocal designs.

In its simplest form, the split bifocal is dispensed most easily in a metal frame when the two components, carefully flat-edged along their contact edges, can be screwed up against one another in the metal rim. If they must be dispensed in a plastics frame they can be bonded together along their contact edges before assembling them into the frame. A particularly neat form of split-bifocal design can be obtained by bonding the two components together in a semi-finished blank form, before working the second side (normally the concave surface). This enables the thickness to be reduced to a minimum, but does not normally allow independent centration of the DP and NP.

An improved form of split bifocal, the *perfection bifocal*, has one component bevel-edged to fit into a groove on the contact edge of the other component. The dividing line need not have a straight top; it could be a downcurve segment with a circular dividing line.

Figure 10.1 Bifocal designs: DP, distance portion; NP, near portion

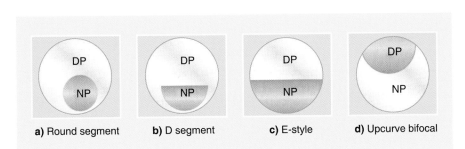

a) Round segment   **b)** D segment   **c)** E-style   **d)** Upcurve bifocal

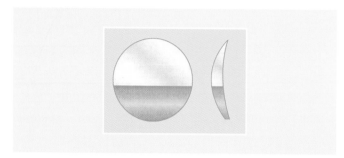

Figure 10.2   Split bifocal (Franklin design)

The second class of bifocals is the *cemented bifocal* in which a segment is cemented to the main lens. Until about 1960, the adhesive in common use was Canada balsam, a resin exuded by the balsam fir tree. Canada balsam was easy to apply, and to reapply when its adhesion deteriorated after being subjected to mechanical, thermal or chemical shock. More recently, ultraviolet-cured epoxy resins have replaced Canada balsam and provide excellent long-term adhesion of glass components. This has enabled several forms of tinted equitint and prism-controlled bifocal designs to be made. A very neat form of cemented design is the *wafer bifocal*, in which the segment is worked on a temporary support until it is extremely thin and then slid onto the main lens. The edge of the wafer segment is often so thin that it is difficult to distinguish from a solid bifocal.

In theory, cemented bifocal segments can be produced in any shape and size, but for the dividing line to remain invisible (i.e. as inconspicuous as is possible), the segment should be round in shape with its optical centre coinciding with its geometrical centre.

The reading portion of a *fused bifocal* is constructed from a button of high refractive index that is fused at high temperature to a depression curve worked on the main lens, made from glass of a lower refractive index (Figure 10.6). After completion of the segment side, the segment surface is continuous over the DP and NP so the dividing line cannot be felt. The reading addition, A, obtained depends upon the power of the DP surface, F_1, the power of the original depression curve, F_C, and the fused bifocal *blank ratio*, which is a function of the refractive indices of the two glasses used (i.e. n for the crown glass main lens and n_S for the higher refractive index segment glass).

The blank ratio is the quantity:

$$(n-1)/(n_S-n)$$

which is usually denoted by k, and the near addition is given by:

$$A=(F_1-F_C)/k$$

In theory, different reading additions can be obtained by using just one glass type of high refractive index for the segment and varying the powers of the DP curve and the depression curve, but in practice it is now usual to use a number of different glasses for the segment. A typical range of segment glasses used in Europe to produce various reading additions is given in Table 10.2.

The method of construction of the fused bifocal lends itself well to the production of shaped segments, such as straight-top, D-segments, curved-top, C-segments and B (ribbon) segments. A composite button that employs two glasses of different refractive indices is fused to the depression curve, the crown component of the button 'disappears' after fusion since it has exactly the same

refractive index as the crown glass employed for the main lens (Figure 10.7). By combining a third glass, *trifocal* designs are possible in fused form. Fused bifocals are currently available in the following segment diameters:

22 B segments	28 D and C segments
22,24,25,26 round segments	30 B segments
25 D and C segments	34,35 D segments
26 B segments	40 C segments

To cope with the demand for large eye sizes, the blank manufacturer supplies the prescription industry with semi-finished blanks in which the segment is decentred down and in from the geometrical centre of the blank (Figure 10.8). Typically, the segment top might lie 6mm down and 6mm inwards from the blank centre. When completing the second side, the surfacing laboratory must work prism to shift the distance optical centre to its required final position, say 4mm above the segment top and 2mm outwards from the segment centre, to provide a *segment drop* of 4mm and a *geometrical inset* of 2mm. *Solid bifocals* are made of a single piece of material in which the reading addition results from different curvatures on one surface of the lens. The reading addition of this design is given by the difference between the near portion curve (NPC) and the distance portion curve and can be read off by means of a lens measure (Figure 10.9). Plastics bifocals are all solid in form and are produced by casting the monomer in a concave mould, which itself is produced using normal surfacing machinery. Glass solid bifocal production, however, is one of the most skilful of all surfacing operations, and requires specialized machinery and working procedures.

Plastics bifocals can be obtained with either round or shaped segments; the following diameters and sizes are currently available:

22,24,25,26 round segments	28 D and C segments
38,40,45 round segments	30 B segments
25 D and C segments	35 D segments
26 B segments	40 C segments

Glass solid bifocals are only made with round segments and, although in the past a wide selection of diameters were produced, currently the following are available:

30 round segments	40 round segments
38 round segments	45 round segments

Since most surfacing houses now work only the concave surface of semi-finished blanks, some series of glass solid bifocals are produced with the segment on the convex surface, similar to most plastics solid bifocals.

E-style, or *Executive* bifocals (Figure 10.10a), which have wide near portions, are solid visible no-jump bifocals in construction and are available in both glass and plastics form. Mechanically, the E-style design can be looked upon as a near vision lens to which is added a minus segment for distance vision (Figure 10.10b), which results in the upper edge of the blank becoming thicker than the lower portion. The edge thicknesses of the blank at the top and bottom can be made the same by *prism thinning*, in which a vertical prism is worked across the blank to reduce the thickness, usually of the distance portion. The amount of prism used depends upon the reading addition and is usually in the region of $yA/40$, where y is the distance from the dividing line to the top of the finished lens and A is the reading addition. Since the reading addition is almost always the same for each eye, the same amount of prism thinning is applied to each lens. Lenses

Table 10.1 Terms relating to bifocal lenses

Term	Definition
Group A. Descriptive	
Bifocal lens	A lens having two discrete portions of different *focal power*, usually for distance and near vision
Multifocal lens	A lens designed to provide correction for two or more discrete viewing ranges (for example, *bifocal* and *trifocal*)
Progressive power lens	A special type of *multifocal lens* designed to provide correction for more than one viewing range and in which the power changes continuously rather than discretely
Distance portion, DP	That portion of a lens having the *correction* for distance vision
Near portion, NP (reading portion)	That portion of a lens having the *correction* for near vision
Major portion	That portion of a lens with the larger or largest *field of view*
Main lens	The lens to which one or more *segments* are added to make a *bifocal* or *multifocal* lens
Dividing line	The boundary line between two adjacent portions of a *bifocal* or *multifocal* lens
Invisible	Describing a *multifocal* lens in which every *dividing line* is inconspicuous
Segment	A supplementary lens added to the *main lens* by cementing or fusing, or a supplementary surface on the *main lens*, for the purpose of providing the desired difference in *power*
Segment side	That side, front or back, of a *bifocal* or *multifocal* lens on which the *segment* is situated
DP surface	The surface of the *distance portion* on the *segment side*
Segment surface	The exposed surface of the *segment*
Contact surface	The surface of contact between an added *segment* and the *main lens*
Segment circle	The circle concentric with the *optical centre* of the *segment* considered in isolation and just large enough to include the finished *segment* (see Figure 10.3)
Segment diameter	The diameter of the circle of which the boundary of the finished *segment* forms a part (see Figure 10.4). Note 1. Except in the case of *invisible bifocals*, the *segment diameter* is not necessarily the same as the *segment circle* diameter. Note 2. The *segment diameter* should, where possible, be specified for a *bifocal* or *multifocal* lens. The use of the terms 'round segment' and 'crescent segment' as defining particular *segment diameters* is deprecated
Segment top (segment extreme point)	The point of contact of the curve that forms the upper boundary (imaginary if broken by a re-entrant arc) of the *segment* with its horizontal tangent or, in the case of a *straight-topped segment*, the mid-point of the straight top (point T in Figure 10.4). Note. Applicable only to a *segment* in the lower portion of the lens
Segment top position (segment extreme point position)	The vertical distance of the *segment top* above or below the *horizontal centre line*. Note 1. This dimension is frequently given as in the example 'Segment 2 below horizontal centre'. Note 2. In the absence of instructions to the contrary, this dimension is assumed to apply to the highest *segment* of a *multifocal* lens
Segment height	The vertical distance of the *segment top* above the horizontal tangent to the lens periphery at its lowest point (see Figure 10.4). Note. If the lens is bevelled the periphery is taken to be the peak of the bevel
Segment depth	The vertical extent, measured through the *segment top* or the *segment bottom*, whichever applies, of a *segment* that nowhere extends to the periphery of the lens
Segment bottom	The point of contact of the curve that forms the lower boundary of the *segment* with its horizontal tangent or, in the case of a straight-bottomed *segment*, the mid-point of the straight bottom. Note. Applicable only to a segment in the upper portion of the lens
Segment bottom position	The vertical distance of the *segment bottom* above or below the *horizontal centre line*
Segment size	Specification consisting of the *segment diameter* and the *segment depth* (applicable only to a *shaped segment*)
Segment drop	Vertical height of the distance *optical centre* above the *segment top*. Note. It is essential to specify the *segment drop* when ordering one lens of a pair to avoid introducing vertical differential prism
Round segment	A *segment* with a *dividing line* that is a single circular arc
Straight-top segment	A *segment* with a straight *dividing line* (see Figure 10.4)
D-segment	
flat-top-segment	
Curved top segment	A variation of a *straight-top segment* in which the *dividing line* is a shallow circular arc.

(Continued)

Table 10.1   Terms relating to bifocal lenses—cont'd

Term	Definition
E-style bifocal Executive	A type of monocentric visible *solid bifocal* lens in which the *distance* and *near portions* are separated by a straight *dividing line* going right across the lens
Group B. Relating to optical properties and focal properties	
Addition (Add)	The magnitude of the *power* that when added to the *power* of the *distance portion* gives the *power* of the *near portion* or of an *intermediate portion*. Note. When the *segment* is incorporated on the *front* surface of a lens, the *focal power* of the addition is measured as the difference between the *front vertex powers* of the distance and corresponding *segment portions*. When the *segment* is incorporated on the *back* surface of the lens the addition is measured as the difference between the *back* vertex powers of the *distance* and corresponding *segment* portions
Intermediate addition	The *addition* for an *intermediate portion*
Near addition (reading addition)	The *addition* for a *near portion*
Distance optical centre	The *optical centre* of the *distance portion*
Intermediate optical centre	The *optical centre* of an *intermediate portion*
Near optical centre (reading optical centre)	The *optical centre* of the *near portion*
Segment optical centre	The *optical centre* of the supplementary lens (real or imaginary) that forms the *segment*, the *segment* being considered as an entity and in isolation from the *main lens*
Distance visual point, DVP	An assumed position of the *visual point* on a lens that is used for distance vision under given conditions, normally when the eyes are in the *primary* position
Near visual point, NVP	An assumed position of the *visual point* on a lens that is used for near vision under given conditions
Insetting	Displacing a *bifocal segment* towards the nose, usually without reference to the effect on the *near optical centres*, with the purpose generally of bringing the right and left reading fields into coincidence. Note. This term should not be used for an inward *decentration* of the *distance optical centres*
Geometrical inset, G in	The distance between vertical lines through the *distance centration point* and the midpoint of the *segment diameter* (see Figure 10.5). Note. For lenses with round *segments*, the conventional method of insetting in workshop practice is by rotation about the distance *centration point* and is frequently based upon the measurement JK of Figure 10.5, where the distance CJ is arbitrary and usually about 15mm
Optical inset, O in	The horizontal displacement relative to the distance *centration point* of the *near* or *intermediate optical centre* with any prescribed prism being neutralized (see Figure 10.5)
Jump	The abrupt displacement of the image when vision passes from one portion to another because of a sudden change of prismatic effect at the *dividing line*
Fitting cross	A reference point (indicated by two intersecting lines) on a *progressive power lens* that is specified by the manufacturer. Note. The *fitting cross* is usually coincident with the start of the progression
Prism reference point	The point stipulated by the lens manufacturer for checking the prescribed relative prism between a pair of *progressive power lenses*. Note. It is essential to stipulate the prism required at the prism reference point when ordering one lens of a pair to avoid introducing vertical differential prism

that are prism thinned should always be anti-reflection coated to eliminate any problem that might occur with the ghost image[3] formed by total internal reflection at the two lens surfaces (see Chapter 5).

Prismatic effect at the near visual point of a bifocal lens

One of the most important optical considerations in the performance of bifocal lenses is the amount of prismatic effect that occurs in the near visual zone of the lenses. When determining the prismatic effect in the near portion, it is very convenient to consider that a bifocal lens is made up from two separate components: a main lens, with a power that is usually the distance prescription, added to which is a supplementary segment lens with a power equal to the reading addition (Figure 10.11).

The optical centre of the main lens, the distance optical centre, is referred to as O_D, and the optical centre of the segment lens as O_S. The total power of the near portion is the sum of the distance portion power and the reading addition of the lens, and the prismatic effect at some point in the near portion is given by the sum of the prismatic effect of the distance portion and the prismatic effect of the segment.

Consider the bifocal lens depicted in Figure 10.11. The prismatic effect at the NVP, 8mm below the distance optical centre and 5mm below the segment top, can be determined as follows.[4] Consider, first, the main lens of power +3.00D. The prismatic effect at a point 8mm below the optical centre of a +3.00D lens can be found from the decentration relationship, $P = cF$, where

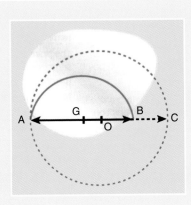

Figure 10.3 Segment circle (a specification used mainly for prism-controlled bifocals). AC is the segment circle diameter and O the optical centre of the segment. G is the geometrical centre of the finished segment of diameter AB. Illustrated is the difference between the segment circle and the segment diameter dimensions for the specification: 38mm segment Add +2.00 and 2Δ base in for near vision.

The 2Δ base in for near vision could be achieved by a horizontal inward decentration of the segment OC of 10mm. The segment circle diameter is 58mm. The finished 38mm could be cut from a circle diameter of 58mm

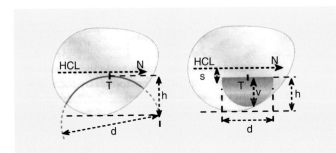

Figure 10.4 Segment dimensions. The horizontal centre line and nasal side of the lens are indicated: T, segment top; d, segment diameter; h, segment height; s, segment top position; v, segment depth

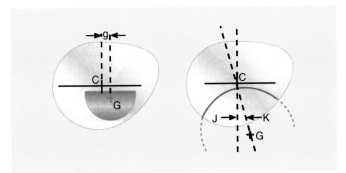

Figure 10.5 Geometrical inset, g. C is the distance centration point, G is the geometrical centre of the finished segment. JK is the conventional inset for crescent segments

c is the decentration in centimetres and F is the power of the lens. Hence, $P = 0.8 \times 3.00 = 2.4\Delta$ base up.

If the hypermetropia had been corrected in the past, before the subject became presbyopic, he or she would almost certainly have become accustomed to some base-up prism when using spectacles

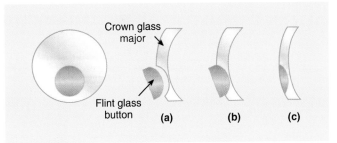

Figure 10.6 Fused bifocal: (a) flint glass button fused to crown glass major of lower refractive index; (b) rough fused bifocal blank; (c) semi-finished fused bifocal

Table 10.2 Compatible flint series for fused bifocal lenses

Adds	Segment glass	Blank ratio
+0.50 to +1.25	1.588	8.0
+1.50 to +2.75	1.654	4.0
+3.00 to +4.00	1.700	3.0

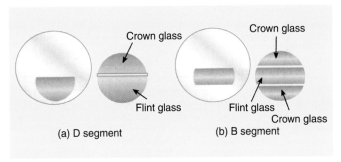

Figure 10.7 Composite buttons for production of shaped fused bifocals: (a) D-segment composite button; (b) B-segment composite button

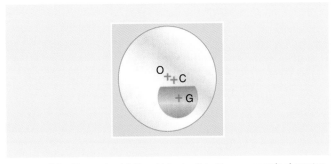

Figure 10.8 Decentred bifocal blank: O is the geometrical centre of the blank; G is the geometrical centre of the segment (the segment lies 6mm down and 6mm in from O); C is the distance centration point at which O_D is to be located, typically 2mm down and 4mm inwards from O

for near vision. The effect of prescribing a bifocal correction might be to alter the amount of prism at the NVPs. For example, if the subject was prescribed a crescent segment for near purposes, as depicted in Figure 10.11, the segment would exert base-down prism at the NVP, which would tend to neutralize the base-up effect of the main lens.

The prism from the segment can be deduced as follows. Suppose the segment diameter is 38mm. The distance from the

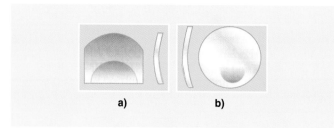

Figure 10.9   Solid bifocals: (a) glass solid 38 bifocal with segment on back surface; (b) plastics 25 D-segment with segment on front surface

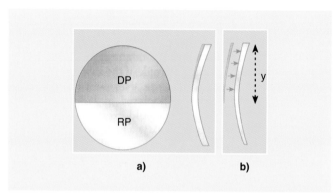

Figure 10.10   (a) E-style (executive) bifocal. (b) For thickness purposes an E-style bifocal can be looked upon as a near vision lens to which is added a minus segment lens for distance vision. The thickness at the top and bottom edges of the lens can be equalized by working a thinning prism of power $yA/40$, where y is the distance from the dividing line to the top edge of the finished lens and A is the reading add

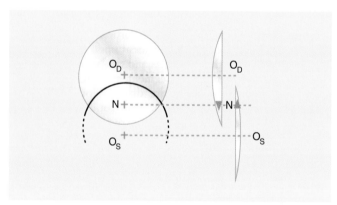

Figure 10.11   Prismatic effect at the near visual point, N, of a bifocal lens: O_D is the optical centre of the distance portion; O_S is the optical centre of the segment element

dividing line to the geometrical (and optical) centre of the segment is 38/2 or 19mm. Since the NVP lies 5mm below the segment top, it must lie 14mm, or 1.4cm, above the segment centre. Hence, the prism from the segment is $1.4 \times 2.00 = 2.8\Delta$ base down. (The base direction is indicated by the cross-sectional shape of the lens in the Figure 10.11.)

The total prismatic effect at the NVP is the sum of 2.4Δ base up and 2.8Δ base down, which is 0.4Δ base down. From an optical point of view, the centration of the near portion is better with the bifocal segment *in situ*, since an ancillary effect of the segment is to create a new optical centre for the near portion, O_N, which lies, in this instance, just 0.8mm below the NVP. Normally, the

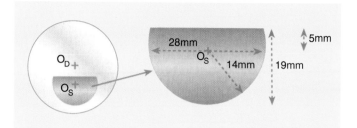

Figure 10.12   Geometry of shaped segment, 28×19: O_S, the optical centre of the segment element, lies 5mm below the segment top and coincides with the NVP

centration of the near portion of an invisible bifocal is dependent upon the power of the main lens and the power and diameter of the segment, and often, particularly when the distance prescription is negative, O_N does not lie in the near portion at all. To control the position of the optical centre of the near portion it is usually necessary to use a *prism-controlled* bifocal.

Consider now the D-segment bifocal lens depicted in Figure 10.12. In this case, a shaped segment has been prescribed of segment size 28×19. If we suppose that the NVP is located in exactly the same position, 8mm below O_D and 5mm below the segment top, clearly the optical centre of the segment, O_S, now coincides exactly with the NVP and the segment adds no prism at this point. Hence, if this shaped segment is dispensed for the prescription, +3.00 Add +2.00, the prismatic effect at the centre of the near visual zone would be the same as it would have been if the segment did not exist. This is an important advantage of shaped bifocal segments and is one of the reasons why this design is so popular around the world.

It can be seen from Figure 10.11 that, when the distance prescription is positive, the base-up effect of the main lens in the near portion is counteracted by the base-down effect of a downcurve circular segment, resulting in a reduced amount of prism in the near visual zone.

If the prescription for the bifocal type depicted in Figure 10.11 is −3.00D Add +2.00, then the prismatic effect at the NVP from the main lens would be 2.4Δ base down. If a 38mm downcurve segment is prescribed for this case, then adding the prismatic effect from the segment, 2.8Δ base down, would increase the total prism at the NVP to 5.2Δ base down. The large increase in the prismatic effect encountered by a subject wearing minus *downcurve* bifocals should be avoided; it is largely for this reason that flat-top and curved-top shaped segments are preferred by myopes who need bifocal spectacles. As has just been pointed out, a 28×19 shaped segment adds no prismatic effect to that of the distance portion.

Some bifocal designs, such as no-jump bifocals, incorporate segments that exert base-up prism in the near visual zone. Such a design is the E-style bifocal depicted in Figure 10.13. The optical centre of the segment of this design is positioned on the dividing line, which is the condition that must be satisfied to obtain no jump. The optical centre of the segment lies above the NVP and, since the power of the segment lens is positive, the segment can be seen to exert base-up prism.

For the example, −3.00 Add +2.00, assuming the same position for the NVP as before, the segment would exert 1.0Δ base up at the NVP, which reduces the overall prism at this point to 1.4Δ base down.

The control of prismatic effect at the NVP is one of the important factors to be taken into account when selecting the best

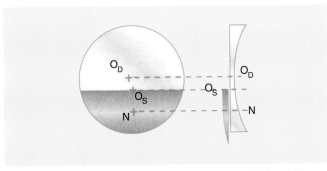

Figure 10.13 Centration of the E-style (executive) bifocal. The segment element exerts base-up prism at the NVP

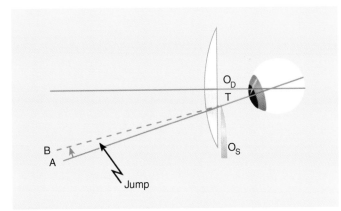

Figure 10.14 Jump at the bifocal dividing line. Jump = TO$_S$ (cm) × Add

type of bifocal design for a given prescription. The suggestions made later in this chapter for the suitability of bifocal designs for various prescriptions are based, mainly, upon the prismatic effects exerted by different types of segment.

It is also important to be able to control any vertical differential prism that might occur in the near visual zones, a topic considered in the section on prism-controlled bifocals.

Jump in bifocal lenses

When the eyes transfer from the distance portion to the near portion of a bifocal lens, they encounter a change in prismatic effect through the sudden introduction of base-down prism by the segment as the eye crosses the dividing line. Figure 10.14 shows how this prismatic effect occurs.

The segment exerts prism at all points just inside its circumference; the base of this prismatic effect lies at the optical centre of the segment, O$_S$. Consider an eye viewing through the distance portion. As the gaze is lowered, the eye encounters an ever-increasing prismatic effect as it rotates away from the optical centre of the distance portion. When the eye enters the near portion it suddenly encounters the base-down prism exerted by the segment at the segment top.

The effect upon the wearer is two-fold. Firstly, objects that actually lie in the direction AT, appear to lie in the direction BT. Apparently, they have jumped to a new position! Secondly, light from the angular zone BTA, around the edge of the segment, cannot enter the eye. The segment dividing line causes an annular scotoma within which objects are completely hidden until the

wearer moves his or her head to shift the zone in which jump occurs.

The amount of jump is simply the magnitude of the prismatic effect exerted by the segment at its dividing line, that is the product of the distance from the segment top to the segment optical centre, in centimetres, and the power of the reading addition.

For a round invisible segment the distance from the segment top to the optical centre of the segment is simply the segment radius and so, for circular, invisible segments:

$$\text{jump} = \text{segment radius in cm} \times \text{Add}$$

Clearly, the jump is completely independent of the power of the main lens and the position of the distance optical centre.

Jump increases as the distance from the segment top to the segment optical centre increases, that is, in the case of round segments, as the segment diameter increases.

If the reading addition is +2.00, the jump exerted by a 24mm segment is 2.4Δ base down. If the segment diameter is increased to 38mm, the jump increases to 3.8Δ base down.

In the case of shaped segments, the optical centre of the segment lies much closer to the dividing line. For example, with a D-shape segment of size 28 × 19, illustrated in Figure 10.12, the segment centre lies just 5mm below the segment top. For a reading addition of +2.00 the jump would be only 1.0Δ base down, less than half of that which occurs for a 24mm round segment. Reduced jump is yet another reason why shaped segments have proved to be so popular.

To eliminate jump in a bifocal lens it is necessary to work the segment in such a fashion that its optical centre, O$_S$, coincides with the segment top. As is shown shortly, this can be accomplished in several ways, either by the manufacturer of the bifocal surface, or by the surfacing workshop when completing the second side. Several proprietary no-jump bifocals are also available from various sources, such as the E-style, or Executive bifocals illustrated in Figure 10.13.

Optical performance of the near portion

When the eye views through the near portion of a bifocal lens it uses extra-axial zones of the main lens, which in most cases incorporate the distance prescription. It is pointed out in Chapter 2 that the off-axis performance, that is the real effect of the lens, depends upon the form of its individual surface powers. The real effect an eye obtains when viewing through the near portion of various bifocal designs is considered in detail below, where it is seen that, just as when using a single-vision lens, there is a zonal variation in power across the segment area. Notwithstanding this difficulty, bifocal blank manufacturers have to label their products with a nominal value for the reading addition that the lens will provide when it is completed on its second side. We consider, first, how this nominal addition is defined and how we can ensure that the addition that is provided actually matches the effect of the trial lens prescription.

Reading addition of a bifocal lens

The reading addition of a bifocal lens is defined as the difference between the vertex powers of the near and distance portions, measured from the surface upon which the segment is incorporated. Hence, in the case of the great majority of today's bifocal

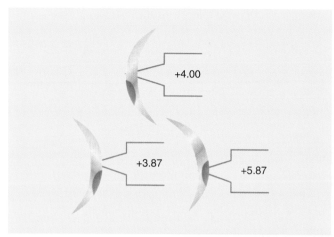

Figure 10.15   Measurement of the reading addition when the segment is situated on the front surface. The reading addition is defined as the difference between the front vertex powers of the distance and near portions. The prescription of the lens depicted is +4.00 Add +2.00. The author refers to this value as the nominal addition of the lens

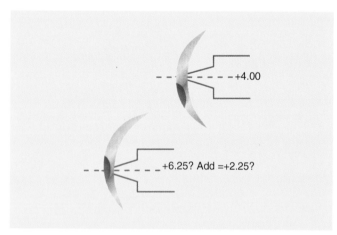

Figure 10.16   Reading the difference between the back vertex powers of the distance and near portion leads to an incorrect measurement of the reading addition when the segment is situated on the front surface of the lens. The measured addition in this case may not indicate the true effect of the segment

designs, in which the segment is situated on the front surface, the addition for near is the difference between the *front vertex powers* of the near and distance portions. This method of measurement can give rise to difficulties in practice, especially in the case of bifocal lenses in which the distance portion is positive and the thickness of the lens plays an appreciable part in its power.

The problem is illustrated in Figure 10.15, which indicates the readings that would be obtained when the prescription +4.00 Add +2.00 is checked by means of the focimeter. If the lens has been correctly made the back vertex power of the distance portion will read +4.00D.

The addition provided by the manufacturer is defined as the difference between the front vertex powers of the near and distance portions, which must be read with the spectacles reversed in the instrument. If the lens has been correctly made then the difference between these two readings should be +2.00D, as indicated in Figure 10.15.

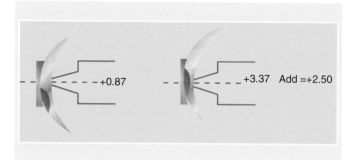

Figure 10.17   Measurement of the mechanical addition of a bifocal lens. An auxiliary lens of power –3.00D held in contact with the front surface of the lens under test provides a close approximation to the actual addition the subject will obtain at the near visual point for plus lenses

If the spectacles were not reversed, the difference between the *back vertex powers* of the near and distance portions would be measured and the readings would indicate that the addition is too strong (Figure 10.16). In the case illustrated in Figure 10.16, we might deduce that the reading addition measured from the back of the lens, and the addition which the patient might actually be given, is +2.25D.

A better indication of the real effect of the segment in near vision is obtained by measuring the *mechanical addition* of the lens. The term mechanical addition relates to the actual ray path of the light through the distance and near portions when the lens is used for near vision. It is defined as the difference between the vergences that leave the near and distance portions when the vergence incident upon the front surface is supposed to arrive from the near point.

It is possible to measure the vergence that leaves a lens under near-vision conditions by employing an auxiliary lens placed in contact with the front surface of the lens under test and designed to simulate the ray path in near vision[5] (Figure 10.17). For near vision at 33.3cm, a –3.00D auxiliary lens would be held in contact with the front surface of the lens when it is placed in the focimeter. For near vision at 40cm, a –2.50D auxiliary lens would be used, and so on. Strictly, the auxiliary lens should be plano-concave in form and placed with its concave surface in contact with the front surface of the lens under test. However, since the auxiliary lens is of low power and likely to be thin, from a practical point of view, its form is immaterial.

The mechanical addition can be measured with the assistance of an auxiliary lens used as described above, and represents the real difference between the vergences that leave the near and distance portions in near vision. In other words, it indicates the effect obtained when the wearer looks through the segment compared with the effect that would be obtained if the segment was not there (i.e. the effect of a single vision lens with a power and form that matches that of the distance portion). It takes errors of near vision effectivity into account. These errors arise from the thickness of the lens and are usually negligible when the distance portion is of minus power. However, as is shown shortly, the actual reading addition obtained in the case of minus bifocal lenses is not easily predictable when the off-axis effects of the lens are taken into account.

The mechanical addition is measured by reading the vergences that leave the back surface of the lens through the distance and near portions with an auxiliary minus lens held in contact with the front surface of the lens under test (Figure 10.17). The bifocal lens should not be reversed in the focimeter.

The significance of the mechanical addition is understood by considering the values tabulated in the examples below, which result from the measurement of various types of bifocal lenses and employ an auxiliary –3.00D lens to obtain the values for the vergence that leave the back surface, L'_2.

Example i

Glass solid bifocal – segment on the concave surface

axial thickness = 4.0mm, back surface = –6.00D

	DP	NP	NP–DP
measured BVP	+4.75	+7.50	+2.75
measured L'_2	+1.62	+4.37	+2.75

In this first example, the segment is situated on the concave surface of the lens and the measured addition is the same, with or without the auxiliary lens. This is as expected, since the near vision effectivity error (NVEE, –0.12D) is the same for both the distance and near portions.

Example ii

Plastics solid bifocal – segment on the convex surface

axial thickness = 4.0mm, front DP suface = +8.75D

	DP	NP	NP–DP
measured BVP	+4.00	+6.62	+2.62
measured FVP	+3.87	+6.37	+2.50
measured L'_2	+0.87	+3.37	+2.50

In this second example, in which the segment is situated on the convex surface of the lens and the axial thickness is not too great, the mechanical addition is the same, to within the accuracy of measurement, as the measured difference between the front vertex powers of the lens. High-power plus lenses are relatively uncommon, so this example goes some way towards justifying the convenience of expressing reading additions in terms of the vertex powers of the lens.

Example iii

Plastics lenticular bifocal – segment on the convex surface

axial thickness = 9.7mm, front DP suface = +16.37D

	DP	NP	NP–DP
measured BVP	+16.00	+19.75	+3.75
measured FVP	+14.00	+17.00	+3.00
measured L'_2	+12.37	+15.87	+3.50

In this example, the part that the axial thickness plays in contributing towards the lens power cannot be ignored. The mechanical addition is +0.50 greater than the measured difference between the front vertex powers of the two portions.

To avoid this *overplus syndrome*, which is a well-known source of difficulty in practice, a correction factor can be applied to the prescribed reading addition in those cases in which the bifocal design chosen has its segment on the front surface. A suitable correction is obtained for lenses of refractive index in the region of 1.50 (e.g. CR39 and crown glass lenses), from the expression:

$$\text{correction} = -tA_BF_1/750$$

where t is the axial thickness of the lens, A_B is the required reading addition and F_1 is the front DP surface of the lens.

Since reading additions are normally manufactured in +0.25D intervals, a suitable expression for the correction factor is:

$$-INT\left[4 \times t \times A_B \times \left(F_1/750\right) + 0.5\right]/4$$

This statement may be easily incorporated into a computerized ordering system for the lens manufacturer.

Correction factors for examples (ii) and (iii) above would be 0 and –0.75, respectively. Values for these correction factors have been published by various lens manufacturers.[6]

Optical performance of bifocal lenses

In general, the surface powers selected for the main lens, and thus determining the form of a bifocal lens, are those that provide the best form for distance vision. As a rule, this is very sensible since it is in distance vision that the eyes demand optimum visual acuity.

Reading tasks are generally quite coarse and, if very fine detail needs to be observed, a magnifying device can be employed in near vision. The optical performance of the near portion of a bifocal lens depends, therefore, not just upon the bifocal type and segment details, but also upon the form of the distance portion and upon which surface the segment is incorporated.

As pointed out in Chapter 2 (which considers the best form of single-vision lenses), the off-axis performance of an ideal spectacle lens should not differ from its paraxial performance.

When considering the near vision performance of spectacle lenses, it is the tangential and sagittal *oblique vertex sphere image vergences* that should remain the same for all directions of gaze. Figure 10.18 illustrates the ray path from a near object point through the near portion of a bifocal lens. The vergence that arrives at the front surface is L_1 (= $1/l_1$) and the vergence in the fan of rays that leaves the back surface of the lens, as it crosses the vertex sphere, in the plane of the paper is the *tangential oblique vertex sphere image vergence*, L'_T. The refracted ray is likely to be afflicted with aberrational astigmatism, so the vergence of the refracted rays in the sagittal plane, at right angles to the plane of the paper, differs from that in the tangential plane. The vergence in the plane at right angles to the tangential plane is the *sagittal oblique vertex sphere image vergence*, L'_S. The difference between the two values, L'_T and L'_S, is the oblique astigmatic error (OAE), and the average vergence in the refracted pencil at the vertex sphere, $(L'_T + L'_S)/2$, is called the mean oblique image vergence (MOIV). The author has suggested[7] that a better idea of the reading addition a lens provides, taking into account the off-axis effects, would be given by the difference between the MOIV and the vergence that would leave the back surface from the same near object point if the segment were not there. If this is measured in the paraxial region of the distance portion, it is the value, L'_2, for the DP. The MOIV varies with the zone of the segment under

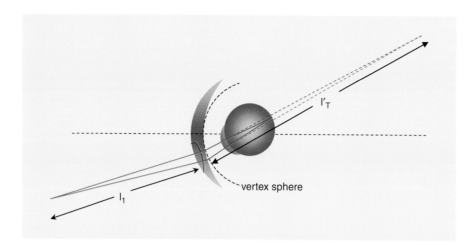

Figure 10.18 The ray path through the near portion of a bifocal lens. The object distance from the near point to the lens, measured along the oblique ray path, is l_1 and the position of the image in the tangential plane is l'_T. The tangential oblique vertex sphere image vergence, L'_T, is $1/l'_T$. The sagittal oblique vertex sphere image vergence, in the plane at right-angles to the plane of the paper, is L'_S. Ideally, these values should differ from the paraxial vergence, L'_2, leaving the distance portion from the near object by the value of the reading addition

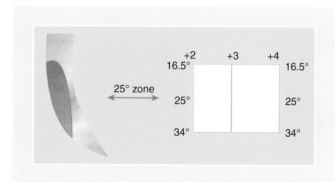

Figure 10.19 Field diagram for the ideal near portion of a flat-top bifocal with a power of +4.00 Add +2.00. The vergence that leaves the near portion is +2.88D, which is the sum of the incident vergence, L_1 (= −3.00), the back vertex power of the NP (= +6.00) and the NVEE (= −0.12). The vergence that leaves the distance portion in the paraxial region for the same object vergence is +0.88 (= $L_1 + F'_V + $ NVEE)

consideration and so the true reading addition provided by any bifocal lens also varies across the segment.[8]

From the foregoing, it can be understood that, when discussing the term *reading addition*, since, by its very purpose, we are dealing with zonal effects of a bifocal lens, it is quite difficult to provide a specific definition of the term. At present, there is no universally accepted definition of the term reading addition that really indicates the actual effect for the wearer of adding a segment to their distance prescription. In the case of a bifocal lens, in addition to the ideal DP performance outlined earlier being obtained when the eye is using the near portion, the requirement for an ideal design is also that the oblique vertex sphere image vergences in the tangential and sagittal meridians should remain equal for all directions of gaze within the segment area.

Figure 10.19 shows a field diagram, drawn specifically for the segment area, to illustrate the ideal off-axis performance of the near portion of a flat-top bifocal lens with a prescription of +4.00 Add +2.00. To be helpful, the segment area is also indicated so that the zone of the segment in use can be visualized at the same time. The field diagrams represent the optical performance obtained along a straight line that joins the distance and segment opthical centres, and ignore skew rays through the near portion. To obtain this ideal performance, it is supposed that the wearer views a near object at 33.3cm from the front surface of the

segment and that the NVEE[4] of the near portion is −0.12D, so the paraxial vergence expected to leave the near portion is +2.88D. This value arises from the sum of the vergence L_1 (−3.00), F'_V (+6.00) and NVEE (−0.12).

Since the near portion of a bifocal lens is usually identified by its reading addition, it is more useful when discussing the optical performance of the near portion[8] to illustrate the departure of the reading addition from its ideal value. Since any departure from the prescribed value actually expresses the variation in MOIV, it is also useful to plot the OAE of the near portion alongside.

This is done in Figure 10.20, which indicates both how the reading addition varies from its prescribed amount, δA, and how the OAE varies within the segment area. The distance portion power is plotted along the top of the field diagrams and the error is shown to the same scale along the usual x-axis of the graphs. Figure 10.20a illustrates the ideal situation in which there are no field errors, and Figure 10.20b gives a typical case for a flat-top bifocal of fused design, with the segment situated on the front surface of the lens.

The values from which these curves are plotted were obtained by accurate trigonometric ray tracing through the near portions of various segment designs, assuming the eyes to have rotated 16.5°, 25° and 34° downwards from the optical axis of the distance portions of the lenses. These ocular rotations correspond approximately with points 8mm below, 13mm below and 18mm below the distance optical centres of bifocal lenses with a segment drop of 2mm in each case.

The optical performance of the near portion of the lens depicted in Figure 10.20b is quite good. The error in the reading addition is quite small, there being no appreciable error in addition when the eye enters the near portion at the top of the segment, and the error reaching a maximum value of −0.12D at the bottom of the segment area. In short, this bifocal design provides an addition of +2.00D in the upper portion of the segment, the add reducing to +1.87D as the eye sweeps down to the bottom of the segment. The second graph indicates the oblique astigmatism that the eye encounters in the near portion, which is also negligible for the design and the powers in question.

Figure 10.21 illustrates the optical performance of the same bifocal design shown in Figure 10.20, of DP power +4.00D, but this time showing how the near portion performance varies with the reading addition. Three different additions are illustrated, +1.00, +2.00 and +3.00D, to represent the range. Inspection of the graphs indicates that in the case of a +3.00D addition, the MOIV increases slightly as the eye sweeps down through the segment,

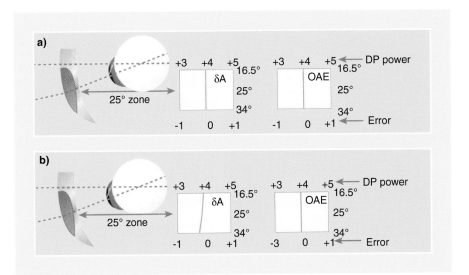

Figure 10.20 Field diagrams that show variation in reading addition, δA, and oblique astigmatic error in the near portion of flat-top bifocal segments: (a) field diagram for an ideal bifocal near portion (δA = 0, OAE = 0); (b) field diagram for a flat-top fused bifocal of power +4.00 Add +2.00, 22 × 16 segment. At the centre of the near visual zone, δA = −0.10, OAE = 0

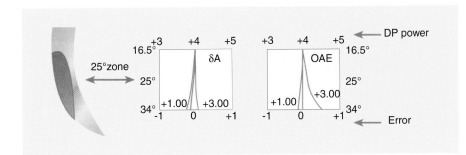

Figure 10.21 Field diagram showing variation in reading addition, δA, and OAE in the near portion of flat-top bifocals with segments on the convex surface of the lenses, with DP power +4.00D and three different reading additions, +1.00, +2.00 and +3.00D

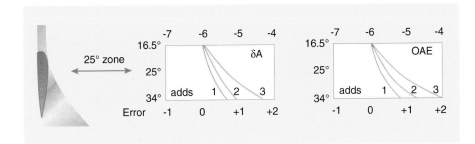

Figure 10.22 Field diagram showing variation in reading addition, δA, and OAE in the near portion of flat-top bifocals with segments on the convex surface of the lenses, with DP power −6.00D and three different reading additions, +1.00, +2.00 and +3.00D

the addition reaching a value of about +3.12D. The oblique astigmatism encountered in the segment area also increases for an addition of +3.00D and is of the order of +0.37D. These values are not dramatically different from those encountered in the middle of the segment, the area most used for near vision purposes.

Figure 10.22 compares the optical performance of the same bifocal design, but this time the power of the distance portion is −6.00D and the performances for the three additions, +1.00, +2.00 and +3.00D, are given. It is seen that the peculiar gain in plus power exhibited by single-vision minus lenses[4,8] as the eye rotates away from the optical centre of the lens is also demonstrated by minus bifocal lenses. In the case of the +2.00D addition design the real addition, which is obtained at the centre of the near visual zone, is +2.50D and the astigmatism in this zone is also of the order of +0.50D. At the bottom of the segment these values increase to an add of +3.00D with accompanying oblique astigmatism, OAE, of +1.12D. To say the least, the optical performance of the near portion of this design is not very good.

Figure 10.23 compares the optical performance of bifocal lenses with a distance prescription, again of −6.00D, and with the additions +1.00, +2.00 and +3.00D for the same segment design, a flat-top fused, but this time with the segment located upon the back surface of the lens.

It is immediately apparent that the optical performance of this design is not the same as the performance obtained when the segment is situated on the convex surface of the lens. With the segment on the concave surface, the reading addition again increases as the eye rotates downwards through the segment area, but more slowly than when the segment is incorporated on the front surface of the lens. In the case of the +2.00D addition, at the centre of the segment the addition is about +2.25D and the astigmatism just under +0.25D. At the bottom of the segment the errors reach about +0.50D each.

A study of the optical performance of the reading portion of various types of bifocal design can be undertaken with the assistance of Figures 10.24 to 10.26, which illustrate the optical performance of the near portion of various designs with front and

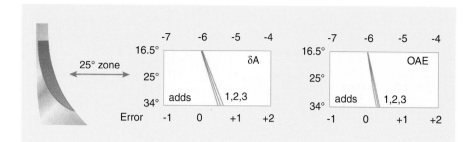

Figure 10.23   Field diagram showing variation in reading addition, δA, and OAE in the near portion of flat-top bifocals with segments on the concave surface of the lenses, with DP powers −6.00D and three different reading additions, +1.00, +2.00 and +3.00D

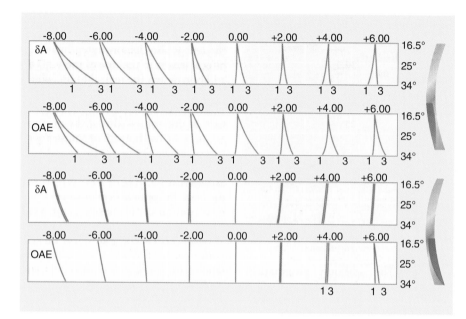

Figure 10.24   Field diagrams showing variation in reading addition, δA, and OAE in the near portion of flat-top bifocals with segments on the convex and concave surfaces of the lenses, for DP powers +6.00 to −8.00D and two different reading additions, +1.00 and +3.00D (+2.00D additions are extrapolated easily from these figures)

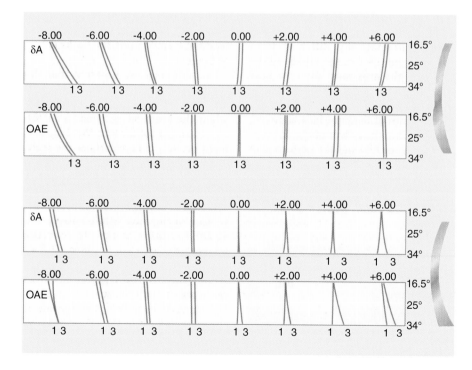

Figure 10.25   Field diagrams showing variation in reading addition, δA, and OAE in the near portion of solid 22 bifocals with segments on the convex and concave surfaces of the lenses, for DP powers +6.00 to −8.00D and two different reading additions, +1.00 and +3.00D

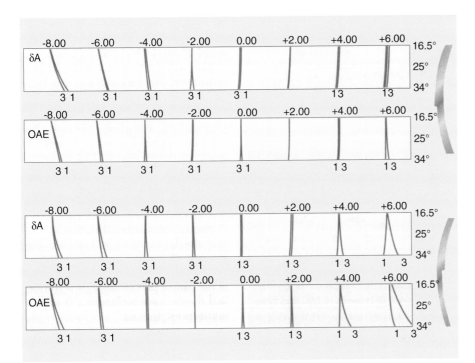

Figure 10.26 Field diagrams showing variation in reading addition, δA, and OAE in the near portion of E-style bifocals with segments on the convex and concave surfaces of the lenses, for DP powers +6.00 to –8.00D and two different reading additions, +1.00 and +3.00D

back surface segments. Figure 10.24 gives the near vision performance of the same designs given in Figures 10.22 and 10.23, fused flat-top bifocals, but for distance portion powers from +6.00 to –8.00D in 2.00D intervals. The performance is given for the two reading additions, +1.00 and +3.00D.

Inspection of the graphs leads to the important conclusion that, as a general rule, it is better to incorporate the segment on the major surface of the lens. The major surface is the convex surface in the case of plus distance prescriptions and the concave surface in the case of minus prescriptions.

As we should expect, this rule becomes increasingly important as the distance portion increases in power. Certainly, it is possible to obtain round bifocal segments on the convex surface, which is the usual case for plastics bifocals, and round segments on the concave surface, which is the usual case for glass bifocals. Since glass solid bifocals are available with 22mm diameter segments, this diameter was chosen for the comparison illustrated in Figure 10.25.

Shaped segments are also available in glass on either the convex (normal) or the concave surface (see the Zeiss catalogue). The E-style design, with the performance illustrated in Figure 10.26, is also available with the segment on the convex surface (usual) or the concave surface.

Figure 10.26 indicates quite clearly that the best optical performance in the near portion is provided by bifocals of the no-jump variety, such as the E-style illustrated. As stated above, the E-style bifocal may be considered to be a near vision lens to which is added a minus segment for distance vision. Hence, when the near portion is negative in power, the higher the reading addition, the weaker the near portion becomes. Unlike the other dependent bifocals illustrated in Figures 10.24 and 10.25, the graphs show that the off-axis errors of the E-style design become smaller as the addition increases.

In view of the differences that occur in the near vision performance of bifocal designs if the segment is incorporated on the convex or the concave surface, we might anticipate problems if a subject changes from one design to another without adjustment being made to the reading addition to compensate for the difference in performance. For example, suppose a subject is wearing the prescription –6.00 Add +2.00 in the form of a glass solid bifocal with a 22mm diameter segment on the concave surface of the lens. At the centre of the segment, the actual reading addition the subject obtains is seen (from Figure 10.25) to be about +2.25D. If the subject is switched to a plastics bifocal design with a segment incorporated on the convex surface of the lens, the actual reading addition at the centre of the segment is seen to be almost +2.50D. Clearly, the *overplus* phenomenon, which is often encountered in practice, is not restricted to thick plus lenses.

Bifocal fitting

Bifocal segments must be positioned so that the distance and near portions of the lens provide adequate fields of view for distance and near vision. It is convenient to consider the positioning of the segment in the vertical and horizontal meridians separately. In the vertical meridian, bifocal lenses prescribed for general purpose use are usually mounted before the eyes so that the segment top is tangential to the lower edge of the iris (Figure 10.27a). In most cases, the position of the lower edge of the iris also corresponds with the line of the lower eyelid when the head is held in the primary position. This position is the norm for the great majority of bifocal wearers and certainly the safest position for the segment top in the case of first-time wearers. If any doubt exists in the fitter's mind as to the best segment height to provide, the lenses may be dispensed in a frame that permits easy vertical adjustment of the height if the wearer finds that the normal position is unsuitable.

If the bifocals are prescribed mainly for near vision, then the segment top might be fitted a little higher, say midway between the lower edge of the pupil and the lower edge of the iris (Figure 10.27b). If the lenses have been prescribed for some vocational purpose and are to be designed for only occasional near vision use, then the segment tops might be fitted 3–5mm lower than the norm (Figure 10.27c).

These suggested positions of the segment top assume that the head is held in the subject's primary position with the eyes viewing a distant object. Dispensing aids have been proposed from time

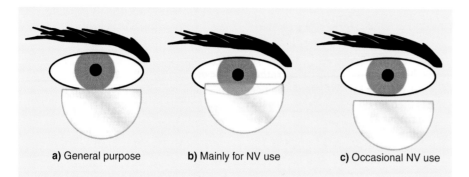

a) General purpose   b) Mainly for NV use   c) Occasional NV use

Figure 10.27   Bifocal segment positioning (NV, near vision)

Table 10.3   Insetting of bifocal segments

| Lens power (D) | Monocular centration distances | | | | | | | | | |
	28	29	30	31	32	33	34	35	36	37
	Geometrical inset in mm for working distance of 33.3cm									
+12.00	3.0	3.1	3.2	3.3	3.4	3.5	3.6	3.8	3.9	4.0
+10.00	2.8	2.9	3.0	3.1	3.2	3.3	3.4	3.5	3.6	3.7
+8.00	2.6	2.7	2.8	2.9	3.0	3.1	3.2	3.3	3.4	3.5
+6.00	2.5	2.6	2.6	2.7	2.8	2.9	3.0	3.1	3.2	3.3
+4.00	2.3	2.4	2.5	2.6	2.7	2.8	2.8	2.9	3.0	3.1
+2.00	2.2	2.3	2.4	2.4	2.5	2.6	2.7	2.8	2.8	2.9
0.00	2.1	2.2	2.3	2.3	2.4	2.5	2.6	2.6	2.7	2.8
−2.00	2.0	2.1	2.1	2.2	2.3	2.4	2.4	2.5	2.6	2.6
−4.00	1.9	2.0	2.0	2.1	2.2	2.3	2.3	2.4	2.5	2.5
−6.00	1.8	1.9	2.0	2.0	2.1	2.2	2.2	2.3	2.3	2.4
−8.00	1.8	1.8	1.9	1.9	2.0	2.1	2.1	2.2	2.3	2.3
−10.00	1.7	1.7	1.8	1.9	1.9	2.0	2.0	2.1	2.2	2.2
−12.00	1.6	1.7	1.7	1.8	1.8	1.9	2.0	2.0	2.1	2.1

to time to assist in the fitting of bifocal lenses (e.g. segment height determinators) and other forms of bifocal fitting instruments, but most practitioners obtain excellent and consistent results by simply measuring the segment height with a millimetre ruler. Ideally, the segment height should be converted into a segment top position in relation to the horizontal centre line (HCL) of the frame.

A typical routine for taking the measurement is:

1. Choose the final frame and adjust it to fit the subject correctly.
2. If the frame is empty, attach vertical strips of transparent adhesive tape to each eye of the frame to enable reference points to be marked.
3. Replace the frame on the subject's face and direct the subject to look straight into your eyes. If necessary, adjust the height of your stool so that your eyes are on exactly the same level as those of the subject.
4. Direct the subject to look straight into your open left eye and, using a fine-tip marking pen and, preferably a light-coloured ink, place a mark at the same height as the lower edge of the subject's right iris. This point often coincides with the line of the lower lid.
5. Direct the subject to look straight into your right eye, without moving his or her head, and place a second mark in front of the subject's left lower iris margin.
6. Remove and replace the frame on the subject and repeat the procedure, this time without making any marks, to ensure that the marks do lie directly in front of the lower edges of the irides.

7. Record the segment heights or top positions with respect to the HCL and use a blank sizing chart to ensure that the lenses can be obtained from the blank diameters available for the design in question.

Whenever bifocal lenses are ordered, it is better to give the prescription laboratory the segment top position (the height of the segment top above or below the horizontal centre line), rather than, simply, the segment height, since there is then no doubt as to whether the measurement has been specified properly from the lower horizontal tangent to the lens periphery.

With experience, the transparent tape may be dispensed with and the segment top position recorded simply with the ruler.

The horizontal positioning of the segment (i.e. the geometrical insetting required to bring the near fields into coincidence) depends upon the power and position of the main lens in front of the eye, and the assumed position of the near point. Segment insetting is discussed in Chapter 3, and Table 10.3 is reproduced here for convenience without further comment. It was customary[9] for the prescription house to advise opticians that they need not state an inset on their bifocal orders unless an unusual specification was required. Otherwise, the insetting suggested in Table 10.3 would be provided automatically.

Table 10.3 has been compiled from the relationship for various lens powers and a working distance of 33.3cm. Since the geometrical inset is a function of the monocular centration distance, it cannot properly be expressed in terms of the binocular CD and so is listed in the Table 10.3 for various monocular centration distances.

Vocational design of the lens

Bearing in mind that the great majority of bifocal prescriptions are dispensed to replace two separate pairs of spectacles, it is useful to begin by supposing that the areas of the lenses devoted to distance and near vision should relate to the amount of use each portion will receive (Figure 10.28). Thus, if the lens is designed to be used mainly for near vision, large segments set somewhat higher than the norm will satisfy this requirement (Figure 10.29). Alternatively, if the lens is designed for some vocational purpose, to be used mainly for distance vision, small segments set lower than usual or in some unusual position on the lens might be suggested (Figure 10.30). It is important to bear in mind that no single pair of spectacles can be expected to provide the best vocational design for every purpose. The two quite ordinary, everyday tasks of changing a light bulb in a ceiling holder and of lying in bed watching the late-night news, which a spectacle wearer might reasonably expect to be able to perform with bifocal lenses, really require, to be able to accomplish either in comfort, two quite different forms from the usual bifocal design.

Figures 10.28, 10.29 and 10.30 illustrate various bifocal designs currently available that might be used for the purposes suggested next.

Figure 10.28 shows various designs commonly prescribed for general-purpose wear. Figures 10.28a,b depict round and flat-top segments, in which most of the lens is devoted to distance vision, but the segment, with diameters in the range 22mm to 28mm, provides ample field of view for near vision. Figures 10.28c,d depict designs with larger segments, but still most of the lens is devoted to providing distance vision.

The E-style design in Figure 10.28d might well be prescribed for a moderate myope, since the segment exerts base-up prism in the near visual zone to counteract the base-down prism of the main lens.

Figure 10.29 illustrates various bifocal designs that might be prescribed mainly for intermediate or near vision. Figure 10.29a depicts a downcurve solid bifocal with an extra-deep segment, which provides better centration in the near portion for moderate plus prescriptions than an E-style design, in which the additional base-up prism from the segment increases the base-up effect from the main lens. Figure 10.29b illustrates a large flat-top segment set high in the lens area, which is ideal for those who work at a computer terminal all day. Typically, the segment incorporates an intermediate addition for comfortable viewing of both the screen and the desktop area, or in cases of advanced presbyopia, the lens is prescribed for specific use at the terminal and could incorporate an intermediate prescription in the main lens and a near prescription in the segment area. Such designs are often provided in tinted form to reduce the effects of glare and/or flicker from the screen.

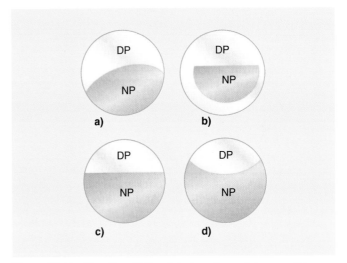

Figure 10.29   Vocational bifocal designs for mainly near vision use: (a) extra-deep downcurve crescent segment; (b) flat-top design set high in the lens area for use at a computer terminal; (c) E-style segment set high in the lens area for use at a desk; (d) upcurve bifocal mainly for near vision use

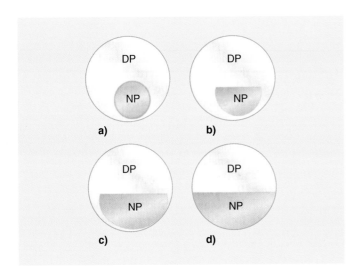

Figure 10.28   Bifocal designs for general purpose use: (a) 24 round segment; (b) 25 flat-top segment; (c) 35 flat-top segment; (d) E-style segment

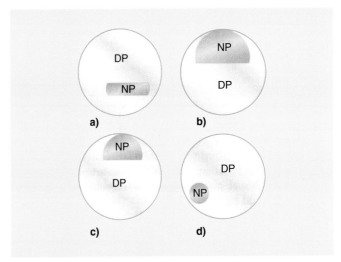

Figure 10.30   Vocational bifocal designs for occasional near vision use: (a) B-shape (ribbon) segment allows distance vision to be obtained beneath segment; (b) reversed downcurve bifocal with intermediate or near portion at the top of the lens; (c) reversed downcurve bifocal for golfer; (d) small fused segment offset for occasional near vision use

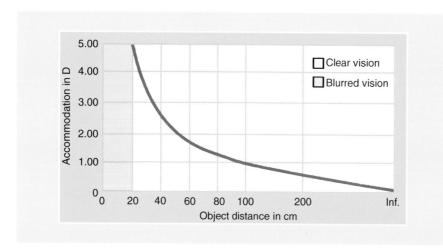

Figure 10.31 Accommodative demand before the onset of presbyopia. It is assumed that the subject has an amplitude of accommodation of +5.00D and that no accommodative effort is required to see a distant object. If the total amplitude is exerted the near point will lie at 20cm. Slightly more accommodative effort is required by a hypermetrope, because of the forward position of the spectacle lens, so the curve plotted for a hypermetropic eye would lie slightly higher than the curve shown here. Conversely, the curve would be lower for corrected myopia

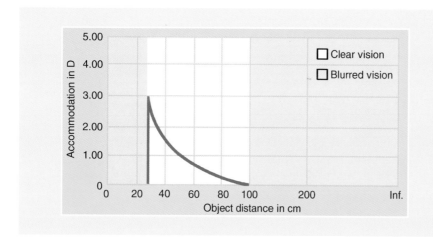

Figure 10.32 Accommodative demand with the aid of a +1.00D single-vision lens for near vision. The +1.00D near vision lens makes the subject artificially myopic for distance vision. The artificial far point lies 100cm in front of the lens. When the subject exerts the total amplitude of +3.00D, the near point lies at 25cm from the lens

Figure 10.29c depicts an E-style design with the major portion of the lens to be used for near vision; an *executive* design in every sense of the term. Such a lens fitted with the segment top midway between the lower edges of the pupil and the iris (Figure 10.27c) is ideal for use in occupations in which a large clear field of view is required for near vision.

Figure 10.29d illustrates an upcurve bifocal in which the reading portion occupies the major portion of the lens and just occasional distance vision is required. Upcurve bifocals are particularly suited to minus prescriptions, since the main lens (the near portion) exerts base-up prism at the distance visual point, which can be counteracted by the base-down effect of the minus distance segment.

Figure 10.30 illustrates various bifocal designs that might be prescribed for occasional intermediate or near vision purposes. Figure 10.30a depicts a B-shape, or ribbon, segment that provides useful distance vision below the segment area and is useful for occupations in which it is inconvenient to have the near portion cover the entire lower regions of the lens. Figures 10.30b,c illustrate *reversed downcurve bifocals*, that is, bifocal designs that have been turned upside down for specific purposes. The design illustrated in Figure 10.30b might be used by a teacher, for whom the segment could incorporate an intermediate prescription for comfortable viewing of the blackboard, with the main area of the lens being used to survey the class. Figures 10.30c,d are both designs that would be found useful for golf. The design in Figure 10.30c enables the golfer to use the entire lower portion of the lens to address the ball and, hopefully, follow the path of its flight down the fairway. The reversed downcurve segment set high in the lens area enables the

scorecard to be marked, simply by holding up the card above eye level when entering the scores. Only one lens, before the dominant eye, really needs the segment. (The thought occurs, ruefully, to the author as he writes this sentence that the cost of such a useful golfing aid is about half that of the cost of the golf shoes or club that the player wears or holds!) Figure 10.30d illustrates a different lens design for a right-handed golf player, a design supposed to be worn monocularly in front of the right eye. The rest of the lens area, together with the whole of the left lens, may be used for distance vision and the scorecard marked by rotating the head to the left.

Ranges of vision and accommodative demand with bifocals

Before the onset of presbyopia, the eye exerts an ever-increasing amount of accommodation to view objects that lie closer and closer to the eye. A graph of the accommodative demand against the object distance shows a smooth hyperbolic curve (Figure 10.31). No accommodation is assumed necessary for an infinitely distant object and accommodation of +5.00D is required when the object lies 20cm in front of the eyes. The curve is similar for corrected ametropes, but shifted slightly upwards for the hypermetropic eye, or downwards for the myopic eye, the shift depending upon the amount of ametropia.

On reaching presbyopia, a near vision correction is required to assist the eye to focus upon near objects. If this is supplied in the form of a single-vision lens then, when wearing the near vision correction,

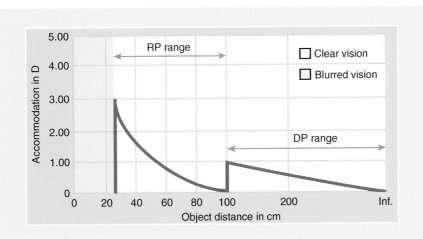

Figure 10.33 Accommodative demand with the aid of a bifocal with Add +1.00. The DP range of vision extends from infinity to 100cm and the near portion (RP) range, obtained through the near portion, extends from 100cm to 25cm

the accommodative demand follows the same form as the curve before presbyopia (Figure 10.32). An ancillary effect of the near vision correction is to render the subject artificially myopic by the magnitude of the reading addition. In Figure 10.32, a near correction of +1.00D is supposed to have been supplied. With accommodation relaxed, the furthest point that the subject can see distinctly, ignoring depth of field considerations, lies 100cm in front of the eyes.

When the near vision correction is provided in the form of a bifocal lens, the subject's accommodative demand varies as shown in Figure 10.33. Assuming that the subject has a total amplitude of accommodation of 3.00D, and that objects beyond 100cm are viewed through the distance portion, when transferring to the near portion, the subject needs exert no accommodation for objects at 100cm and the curve from 100cm to 25cm indicates the effort required for these object distances. This altered demand upon the accommodative faculty is just one more adaptation problem for the new bifocal wearer, and one of the many advantages for the wearer of progressive power lenses is that the accommodative demand with a progressive lens is not very different from the curve before presbyopia.

Prismatic effect at the near visual points

When the eye uses the near portion of a bifocal lens it views through an extra-axial zone of the main lens and encounters a prismatic effect exerted by the distance portion. Determination of prismatic effects at the NVP is considered above, where it is pointed out that the total prismatic effect at the NVP is the sum of the prismatic effect of the main lens and the prismatic effect, if any, of the segment lens.

The prismatic effect at the NVP of a bifocal lens can be determined immediately by means of Tables 10.4 to 10.6, which assume that the NVP lies 8mm below and 2mm inwards from the distance optical centre and that the segment drop is 2mm. Table 10.4 gives the prismatic effect from the spherical component of the prescription. Fractional components of the power can be added to obtain the prismatic effect from the sphere.

Note that the prismatic effect is given for plus lenses, which exert prism base up and out at the NVPs. For minus spherical powers the base directions should be reversed.

Table 10.5 gives the prismatic effect from each +1.00D of cylinder power. For other cylinder powers the value given in Table 10.5 must be multiplied by the cylinder power. Again, Table 10.5 gives the base directions for plus cylinder powers. For minus cylinders, the base directions should be reversed, or the prescription

Table 10.4 Prismatic effect at the NVP from plus spherical power (N.B. for minus powers reverse the base direction)

Sphere power (D)	Prismatic effect (Δ)	
	Vertical	Horizontal
+0.25	0.2 base up	0.05 base out
+0.50	0.4	0.1
+0.75	0.6	0.15
+1.00	0.8	0.2
+1.50	1.2	0.3
+2.00	1.6	0.4
+2.50	2.0	0.5
+3.00	2.4	0.6
+3.50	2.8	0.7
+4.00	3.2	0.8
+4.50	3.6	0.9
+5.00	4.0	1.0
+5.50	4.4	1.1
+6.00	4.8	1.2
+6.50	5.2	1.3
+7.00	5.6	1.4
+7.50	6.0	1.5
+8.00	6.4	1.6
+8.50	6.8	1.7
+9.00	7.2	1.8
+9.50	7.6	1.9
+10.00	8.0	2.0
+10.50	8.4	2.1
+11.00	8.8	2.2

0.25 intervals can be found by simple addition, e.g. +2.75 = +2.50 and +0.25:
– for +2.50: prism from sphere = 2.0Δ base up and 0.50Δ base out;
– for +0.25: prism from sphere = 0.2Δ base up and 0.05Δ base out;
– So for a +2.75D sphere, the prism at the NVP = 2.2Δ base up and 0.55Δ base out.

should first be transposed into its plus cylinder form, in which case Table 10.5 always provides the correct base direction.

Table 10.6 gives the prismatic effect at a point 6mm below the segment top and the jump exerted by the segment for each 1.00D of addition power. For other addition powers the value given in Table 10.6 should be multiplied by the reading addition.

Tables 10.4 to 10.6 can be used to determine the prismatic effect at the NVP on a bifocal lens. Consider the prescription:

R + 3.50/+ 1.50 × 45, L − 1.75/− 1.25 × 165
Add + 2.50, segment 30mm round.

Table 10.5 Prismatic effect at the NVP from each +1.00D of cylinder power (N.B. for minus cylinder powers reverse the base direction)

Axis direction		Prismatic effect in Δ	
R eye	L eye	Vertical	Horizontal
180	180	0.80 base up	0
5	175	0.81 base up	0.07 base out
10	170	0.81	0.14
15	165	0.80	0.21
20	160	0.77	0.28
25	155	0.73	0.34
30	150	0.69	0.40
35	145	0.63	0.44
40	140	0.57	0.48
45	135	0.50	0.50
50	130	0.43	0.51
55	125	0.36	0.51
60	120	0.29	0.50
65	115	0.22	0.47
70	110	0.16	0.43
75	105	0.10	0.39
80	100	0.06	0.33
85	95	0.02	0.27
90	90	0	0.20
95	85	0	0.13
100	80	0	0.06
105	75	0	0.01 base in
110	70	0.03 base up	0.08
115	65	0.07	0.14
120	60	0.11	0.20
125	55	0.17	0.24
130	50	0.23	0.28
135	45	0.30	0.30
140	40	0.37	0.31
145	35	0.44	0.31
150	30	0.51	0.30
155	25	0.58	0.27
160	20	0.64	0.23
165	15	0.70	0.19
170	10	0.74	0.13
175	5	0.78	0.07

For other cylinders, multiply the values given in Table 10.5 by the new cylinder power.

The prismatic effects, read from the tables, may be summed as follows:

R eye :

prism from the sphere = 2.8Δ base up and 0.7Δ base out

prism from the cylinder = 0.75Δ base up and 0.75Δ base out

prism from segment = 2.25Δ base down

total prism at NVP = 1.3Δ base up and 1.45Δ base out

L eye :

prism from the sphere = 1.4Δ base down and 0.35Δ base in

prism from the cylinder = 1.0Δ base down and 0.26Δ base in

prism from segment = 2.25Δ base down

total prism at NVP = 4.65Δ base down and 0.61Δ base in

The jump exerted by each segment is 3.75Δ base down.

For low-power prescriptions, the prismatic effect at the NVP is not great and is usually ignored, provided the magnitude is the same for each eye. The best type of bifocal for a given situation

Table 10.6 Prismatic effect at the NVP, and the jump from each +1.00D of addition power for various segment designs (the NVP is assumed to lie 6mm below the segment top)

Segment diameter or size	Prism at NVP in Δ	Jump in Δ
22	0.5 base down	1.1 base down
24	0.6 base down	1.2
25	0.65 base down	1.25
25 × 17	0.15 base up	0.45
26 × 9	0.15 base up	0.45
28	0.8 base down	1.4
28 × 19	0.1 base up	0.5
30	0.9 base down	1.5
30 × 16	0.5 base up	0.1
30 × 21	0	0.6
30 × 23	0.2 base down	0.8
34 × 22	0.1 base up	0.5
35 × 22	0.15 base up	0.45
38	1.3 base down	1.9
40 × 20	0.6 base up	0
45	1.65 base down	2.25
E-style	0.6 base up	0

Note that the jump is always base down (unless its value is zero).

may then be selected with the vocational requirement for the lens taking prominence. Even with moderate powers, it must be the case that bifocal wearers who have worn a distance correction in the past have become accustomed to the prismatic effect from the distance portion of their lenses. When faced with the selection of a first bifocal design, a sensible guide is to choose a design with a segment that adds little or no prism to that exerted by the main lens.

It can be seen from Table 10.6 that shaped segments, such as the flat (D-shape) and curved-top (C-shape) segments, hardly exert any prismatic effect at the centre of the near visual zone; in general, these have proved to be the most popular design in use. Not only do they not exert much prismatic effect at the NVP, but also the jump encountered at the dividing line when the eyes transfer their gaze from distance to near is only about half that which would be exerted by a round segment of the same diameter.

In the case of high-power prescriptions, much can be said for using the prismatic effect exerted by the segment to counteract the prismatic effect of the main lens. Consider the case of a −8.00D myope who needs an addition of +2.00D. From Table 10.4 the vertical prismatic effect of the main lens is 6.4Δ base down. If the subject requires a large reading zone, we might consider the use of a large diameter segment. Inspection of Table 10.6 shows that if we were to dispense a 45mm downcurve segment, the prism from the segment would be an additional 3.3Δ base down. The total prismatic effect at the NVP would increase to 9.7Δ base down.

Selection of an E-style segment, however, would result in a reduced prismatic effect at the NVP, since this segment design exerts base-up prism at the NVP. For the case in hand, the +2.00D addition would provide 1.2Δ base up at the NVP so that, if an E-style bifocal was selected for this power, the total prismatic effect at the NVP would reduce to 5.2Δ base down. This is almost 50% less than would be obtained with a 45 downcurve segment.

As is shown shortly, a knowledge of the prismatic effect at the NVPs of bifocal lenses assumes great importance in cases of anisometropia. No matter what the magnitude of the prismatic effect, differences between the eyes, particularly in the vertical meridian, may prevent comfortable binocular vision.

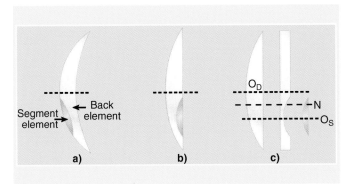

Figure 10.34 Fused bifocal components for the calculation of TCA: (a) the near portion of a fused bifocal comprises two components, a segment element of power $A(k+1)$ and a back element of power $F-Ak$; (b) the power of each of these elements is independent of the form of the lens so, for the calculation of TCA, it is convenient to assume that the lens is made with one plane surface with the segment incorporated on the plane surface; (c) the crown glass element of the bifocal can now, itself, be considered to be made from two separate components of powers F and $-Ak$. The prismatic effect at N is the sum of the prismatic effects of the three components

Chromatic aberration in the near portion

As shown in Chapter 2, when the prismatic effect at a point is known, the transverse chromatic aberration (TCA) at that point can be found by dividing the prismatic effect by the Abbe number, V (i.e. $\text{TCA} = P/V$). This paraxial relationship expresses the chromatism in prism dioptres and the average threshold value is in the order of 0.1Δ; chromatism less than this value is unlikely to give rise to complaints. In the case of solid bifocals, which term here includes both plastics bifocals and glass solid designs, the chromatism can be found simply by dividing the total prismatic effect at the point in question by the Abbe number for the material. Thus, in the case of a plastics solid bifocal of power +5.00 Add +2.00, made with a 24 diameter segment and a segment drop of 2mm, the vertical prismatic effect at a point 6mm below the segment top (from Tables 10.4 and 10.6) is 2.8Δ base up, the horizontal prismatic effect at the point being ignored. The TCA at this point is found by dividing the prismatic effect by the Abbe number, say 58 for CR39 material, which results in 0.05Δ of chromatism; this value at the centre of the near visual zone is hardly likely to be a cause for complaint.

Similarly, if the prescription for the same bifocal design is −5.00 Add +2.00, the prismatic effect at the same point would be 5.2Δ base down and the TCA would be 5.2/58 which is 0.09Δ. Once more, this value is unlikely to be the source of complaints.

In the case of a fused bifocal, in which the near portion combines a crown glass element with a flint glass element of lower Abbe number, the chromatism is the sum of three components, as shown in Figure 10.34. Although the segment might actually be situated on the front surface of the lens, as shown in Figure 10.34a, the powers of the separate segment and back elements of the near portion are not affected if we imagine that the segment has been fused to the back surface of the lens (Figure 10.34b). The crown element of the near portion, which comprises the back element, can itself be split into two separate components, the first of which represents the power of the distance portion, F, and the second represents a centred depression curve of power $-Ak$,

where A is the reading addition and k represents the blank ratio $(n-1)/(n_S-n)$. The power of the segment element can be shown to be given by $A(k+1)$.

At a point, N, in the near portion (Figure 10.34c), three components contribute to the prismatic effect and, hence, to the chromatism at that point. Two components are made from crown glass and the third is the flint glass element of the near portion. If the distance from the distance optical centre to point N is denoted by y, and the distance from N to the segment optical centre by y_S (which must be given a minus sign when O_S lies below N, as shown in Figure 10.34c), then the chromatism at point N is given by:

$$\text{TCA} = yF/V - y_S Ak/V + y_S A\,(k+1)/V_S$$

where V is the Abbe number of the crown glass, and V_S the Abbe number of the segment glass.

Once more, the flat-top fused bifocal design demonstrates its superiority over round segment fused bifocals, since the distance y_S is negligible in the case of most shaped-segment designs, so the low Abbe number of flint glass does not contribute greatly to chromatism in the near visual zone.

In the case of a 24 round segment fused bifocal design made to the prescription +5.00 Add +2.00, using the glasses crown ($V=59$) and flint ($V_S = 36$), and with a blank ratio of 4:1, the chromatism at a point 6mm below the segment top is:

$$\text{TCA} = 0.8 \times 5/59 - (-0.6 \times 2 \times 4)/59 + \big[-0.6 \times 2 \times (4+1)\big]/36$$

which is -0.02Δ, slightly less than found for the solid bifocal design for this power! In the case of a 24 round segment fused bifocal made to the prescription −5.00 Add +2.00, the TCA is found to be -0.15Δ (the minus sign in these values simply indicates that the direction of the resultant prismatic effect is base down). This value is greater than was found for the equivalent solid design; it is well known that chromatism might be a problem in minus fused bifocals, indeed it is usually noticeable on the focimeter target when viewing through the segment zone.

Prism-controlled bifocals

So far we have considered dependent bifocal designs. The term dependent bifocal means a design in which the optical performance of the near portion depends solely upon the powers of the two portions and the diameter of the segment. Bifocal designs that permit control of the prismatic effects in the near portion by the incorporation of prism in the segment are known as prism-controlled bifocals.

We have seen that the prismatic effect at any point in the near portion depends upon the powers of the main lens and the segment lens, and the positions of their individual optical centres in relation to the visual point at which we wish to find the prismatic effect.

It is sometimes necessary to be able to alter the prismatic effect at the NVP, for example, to provide base-in prism for the reading portion only, or to balance the vertical prismatic effects at the NVPs. This can be done by using a bifocal design for which the method of construction allows independent centration of the reading portion. Such a design, called a *prism-controlled bifocal*, is simply a bifocal design constructed such that prism may be incorporated in the segment and be totally independent of any prism included in the main lens.

There are several methods by which prism may be incorporated in the segment only, some of which lead to designs that may be described as being fully prism-controlled and others that are described as being partially prism-controlled.

A fully prism-controlled design is one constructed such that any amount of prism can be incorporated in the segment, with its base set in any direction. One purpose of this prism is to neutralize all prism at the NVP that arises from the distance prescription and the reading addition. When all the prism is neutralized the reading portion has its own optical centre coincident with the NVP. Such designs are often referred to as *centre-controlled bifocals*.

Bifocal designs that permit full centre-control include:

- *Split bifocals* (Figure 10.35) – with distance and reading portions formed from two separate lenses that are cut in half and mounted together in the same eye of the frame. (The prism and prescription possibilities with split bifocals are almost unlimited,

since each eye consists of a pair of single vision lenses for which the powers and centration may be chosen at will.)

- *Cemented or bonded bifocals* (Figure 10.36) – in which a prism segment is attached to the main lens using Canada balsam or a more permanent epoxy resin adhesive. With this design, the prism base represents the thickest point on the dividing line.
- *Solid visible* (or *semi-visible*) bifocals (Figure 10.37) – in which the segment surface is depressed below the level of the distance portion surface, and may be angled to provide any amount of prism and hence any amount of prism control. With this solid prism-controlled segment, the prism base represents the thinnest point on the dividing line. It can be imagined that the segment surface was first depressed into the back surface of the blank and a small prism dropped into the depression.

The method of construction of these centre-controlled designs also permits unusual prescription requirements to be met, such as bifocal designs in which a cylinder is required in the distance or reading portion only, or different cylinder powers or cylinder axis directions in the distance and reading portions.

Some prism-controlled bifocal designs are produced with a given amount of prism incorporated in the segment by the blank manufacturer. For example, the only solid prism-controlled bifocal currently being manufactured in the UK has a 30mm segment diameter and incorporates prism in 0.5Δ steps from 0.5Δ up to 4Δ.

Partially prism-controlled designs include:

- *Solid and fused prism-segment bifocals* with a segment constructed with a fixed range of prisms.
- *Bi-prism bifocals* in which vertical prism has been added to or removed from the reading portion by means of the slab-off technique.

It is shown above that some prism control may be obtained by judicious selection of an appropriate segment diameter. It is shown below that partial horizontal prism control may be obtained by an additional inset of the segment.

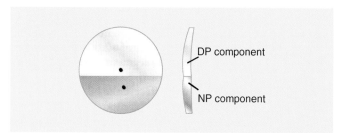

Figure 10.35 Split bifocal: two separate lenses, of powers that correspond with the distance and near prescriptions, are cut in half, flat edged along their contact edges and screwed together in a metal frame. They could also be bonded together along their contact edges and sprung into a plastics frame. If the optical centre of one component is placed at the DVP and the other at the NVP, such a design is automatically centre controlled

Prism control with invisible segments

A downcurve segment with an optical centre that lies below the NVP exerts base-down prism at the NVP, the amount of which depends upon the reading addition (over which there is no control once the prescription has been determined) and the segment diameter, which can be varied (providing that any vocational requirements are met). It is instructive to begin by considering the effect of the segment diameter upon the prismatic effect at the NVP.

Consider the prescription +2.00/+1.00 × 180 Add +2.00 made up with a 24mm segment diameter, with its top 2mm below the

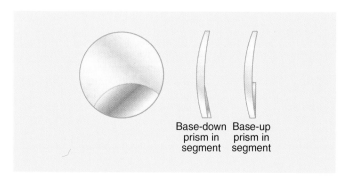

Figure 10.36 Cemented prism segment bifocals: the separate segment lens can incorporate any amount of prism with its base set in any direction. Whenever possible, base-down prism should be incorporated in the segment to position the maximum depth of ridge at the bottom of the segment

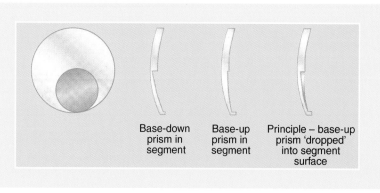

Figure 10.37 Solid prism controlled bifocal: note that, in principle, a depression curve is worked on the DP surface and a small prism dropped into this depression. Whenever possible, base-up prism should be incorporated in the segment to position the maximum depth of ridge at the bottom of the segment

distance optical centre. The prismatic effect at a point in the reading portion 8mm below the distance optical centre can be found from Tables 10.4–10.6 or from first principles as follows:

- The NVP lies 8mm below the optical centre of the main lens, which has a power along 90 of +3.00D. Hence the prism from the main lens is $0.8 \times 3 = 2.4\Delta$ base up.
- The NVP also lies 6mm above the optical centre of the segment element, which has a power of +2.00D, so the prism from the segment is $0.6 \times 2.0 = 1.2\Delta$ base down.
- The total prismatic effect at the NVP is the sum of these two components (2.4Δ base up and 1.2Δ base down), which is a total of 1.2Δ base up.
- The total vertical prismatic effect at the NVP is, therefore, 1.2Δ base up.

It can be seen that the base-down prismatic effect exerted by the segment counteracts the base-up effect of the main lens. This will always be the case when the main lens is positive in power, as the base-down effect of an invisible segment reduces the base-up prism of the main lens.

Clearly, if a larger diameter segment is prescribed then the base-down prism exerted by the segment increases, thereby further reducing the base-up effect of the main lens. If the prism from the segment is increased to 2.4Δ base down it would neutralize completely the base-up effect of the main lens and the optical centre of the reading portion would coincide with the NVP (i.e. the design would be centre controlled). Using the decentration relationship, $c = P/F$, it is an easy matter to determine what segment diameter is needed to centre control the reading portion. The necessary decentration of the optical centre of the segment from the NVP is given by:

Prism from main lens/Reading addition

or, in symbols:

$P/F = 2.4/2.00 = 1.2\text{cm or } 12\text{mm}$

The optical centre of the segment must lie 12mm below the NVP. Since the NVP lies 6mm below the segment top, the radius of the segment must be 18mm and its diameter 36mm. Hence the use of an invisible round segment of diameter 36mm results in a bifocal design in which the near optical centre coincides with the NVP.

This control of prismatic effect at the NVP by a suitable choice of segment diameter is also very useful to control the vertical differential prismatic effect at the NVPs.

In any prescription, if the powers of the lenses differ significantly from one another, the prismatic effects encountered when the eyes look through points away from the optical centres will differ also. Hence, the amounts by which the eyes must rotate to obtain binocular vision will differ also.

In general, the eyes have a much larger tolerance to horizontal differential prismatic effects than to vertical differential prismatic effects. It is generally accepted that the eyes should not be called upon to tolerate more than 1Δ of vertical differential prismatic effect to obtain comfortable binocular vision.

Consider the prescription R -2.00 L -4.00 Add $+2.00$ for near. At NVPs situated 8mm below the distance optical centres the vertical prismatic effect from the distance portion encountered by the right eye is 1.6Δ base down, whereas the vertical prismatic effect from the distance portion encountered by the left eye is 3.2Δ base down. The differential prismatic effect is 1.6Δ base down in the left eye.

If the same diameter segment is given to each eye, the prism from the segment would be the same for each eye and the differential prism would remain 1.6Δ base down.

If a larger segment diameter is given to the right eye, it exerts a larger amount of base-down prism than the left segment and thereby reduces the differential prismatic effect at the NVPs. The difference in segment diameters, $d_1 - d_2$, required to eliminate vertical differential prismatic effect at the NVPs completely can be found from the rule:

$$d_1 - d_2 = (20 \times \text{differential prism})/\text{Add}$$

In this example we find:

$$d_1 - d_2 = (20 \times 1.6)/2.0 = 16\text{mm}$$

For example, a 38mm diameter segment given to the right eye and a 22mm diameter segment given to the left eye would completely eliminate the vertical differential prismatic effect at the NVPs.

This is verified easily by calculating the prism from the segment for each lens. Assuming the NVPs to lie 6mm below the segment tops, the right NVP would lie $(19 - 6) = 13\text{mm}$ above the segment optical centre, whereas the left NVP would lie $(11 - 6) = 5\text{mm}$ above the segment centre.

The prism from each segment would be:

right eye: $1.3 \times 2 = 2.6\Delta$ base down

left eye: $0.5 \times 2 = 1.0\Delta$ base down

and it can be seen that the total prismatic effect at each NVP is now 4.2Δ base down. The use of different-size segments to provide prism control is usually restricted to the use of 38mm and 45mm segments, used in conjunction, since the difference in these diameters is not too obvious. However, the use of this pair in conjunction restricts the amount of prism control to just $0.35 \times \text{Add}$.

Additional insetting to provide base-in prism for near

As shown above, bifocal segments are normally inset to bring the near fields of view into coincidence. Additional insetting of the segment beyond this normal extent creates base-in prism at the NVP. Base-in prism might be useful to relieve convergence insufficiency or simply to counteract the base-out effect, which occurs as a matter of course whenever the main lens is positive. It is curious that, in practice, when dispensing prescriptions for near in single vision form, say BE +5.00DS, the lenses are usually centred for near, by ordering inward decentration of the near optical centres to ensure that the subject is not called upon to overcome base-out prism at the NVPs. Despite this, when dispensing the same prescription in bifocal form the base-out prismatic effect of the distance portion at the NVPs is simply ignored. Additional insetting of the segment, if the segment diameter is large enough, creates base-in prism to counteract the base-out effect of a plus main lens.

The amount of base-in prism can be found from the simple decentration relationship. For example, 2mm of additional insetting, calculated from the geometrical centre of the segment for an addition of +2.50, introduces 0.5Δ base in. It might occur to the reader that this base-in prism could be created by working prism across the entire lens to separate the distance and near centres by an amount that depends upon the powers of the distance and near portions. Suppose we wish to create 1Δ base in for the near portion only, with the prescription, BE +5.00 Add +2.50 for near (Figure 10.38). This could be achieved by working 3Δ base out across the whole lens, the effect of which would be to displace the distance optical centre outwards by 6mm, again using the simple decentration relationship, but the near optical centre would move outwards by only 4mm.

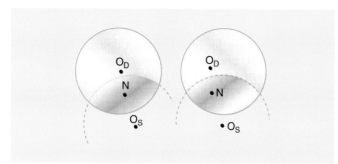

Figure 10.38 Additional insetting to provide base-in prism for near for the Rx +5.00 Add +2.50. Left, the segment has been inset an extra 4mm to create 1Δ base in for the near portion. Right, the same effect can be created by working 3Δ base out across the DP to move the distance optical centre outwards by 6mm and the near optical centre outwards by 4mm. When the lens is decentred inwards by 6mm to restore the position of the distance centre to its correct position, the segment, effectively, is inset by an extra 4mm. This method can be used to provide inset for E-style bifocals

Now, when the bifocal is decentred 6mm inwards to restore the distance optical centre to its rightful position, the near portion will have 1Δ base in at the NVP, 2mm inwards from the distance optical centre. Thus, the segment itself will now be inset by a total of 6mm so the 1Δ base in thus created could equally have been obtained simply by insetting the segment by an additional 4mm in the first place. The amount of prism that needs to be incorporated can be found from the rule:

$$P = \text{inset(cm)} \times \text{DP power} \times \text{NP power/Add}$$

This technique of working prism to split the distance and near centres is useful for providing an inset in the case of E-style bifocals,[10] in which the horizontal inward decentration of the lens to restore the distance optical centre to its correct position does not result in the odd appearance of the segments apparently being in the wrong position in the lens area. Since the dividing line is straight, it is not obvious that the segment has been decentred inwards at all. Obviously, for other segment designs, not only must the blank be large enough to permit the necessary decentration to be obtained, but also the segment needs to be of sufficiently large diameter to provide the subject with an adequate near vision field. For this reason the technique is usually restricted to large crescent segments, 38mm or 45mm diameter, or to 35mm or 40mm flat-top segment designs.

Types of prism-controlled bifocals

The examples above illustrate how it is possible to provide partial prism control by careful selection of the segment diameter and/or by additional inset. Usually, however, it is necessary to control the prismatic effect in the near portion by including a prism in the segment of the lens. Some bifocal designs allow any amount of prism to be incorporated in the segment with the prism base set in any direction. These include solid centre-controlled designs and cemented or bonded segments. Such designs can be used to ensure that the optical centre of the near portion coincides with the NVP.

Consider the prescription –4.00/+1.00 × 180 Add +2.00 to be produced as a centre-controlled bifocal with the optical centre of the near portion coincident with an NVP that lies 8mm below and 2mm inwards from the distance optical centre. The segment specification is 38 × 2 × 2 and the distance optical centre lies 2mm above the segment top.

The prismatic effect at the NVP can be calculated as shown above assuming, to begin with, that an invisible segment is used. From the information given in the specification, the NVP lies 6mm below the segment top and, therefore, 13mm above the optical centre of the segment. From Tables 10.4–10.6, or using the decentration relationship:

prism from main lens	= 2.4Δ base down and 0.8Δ base in
prism from segment	= 2.6Δ base down
so total prism at the NVP	= 5.0Δ base down 0.8Δ base in

To neutralize this prismatic effect, the segment must incorporate 5.0Δ base up and 0.8Δ base out, which, when compounded into a single resultant effect, is equivalent to 5.06Δ up at 99.

This could be incorporated in a bonded segment of power +2.00D, but would result in a thick edge at the top of the segment. A better result is obtained from a solid design, since the minimum depth of ridge lies near the top of the segment.

These centre-controlled bifocal designs are very useful for prescriptions that include prism in the distance portion only or the reading portion only or different prisms in the distance and reading portions. It is possible in these cases to eliminate any other prism at the NVP from the distance portion (i.e. to centre control the design), apart from the prescribed prism at the DVPs or NVPs.

Typical uses for the design include:

● to provide prescribed prism in the DP or NP only, typically to provide prism base in for the near portion only to relieve convergence insufficiency
● to counteract the effects of strong oblique cylinders
● to place the optical centre of the NP at the NVP (i.e., to centre control the NP)
● to eliminate vertical differential prismatic effect in cases of anisometropia
● to produce no-jump bifocals, in which the amount of prism incorporated in the segment is equal and opposite to the jump and places the optical centre of the segment on the dividing line at the segment top.

The following examples illustrate some of these possibilities. The NVP is assumed to be 8mm below and 2mm inwards from the distance optical centre in each case.

Example i

DV	R, +2.50/+1.00 × 180
	L, +1.00/+1.00 × 180
NV	R, +4.50/+1.00 × 180 and 2Δ in
	L, +3.00/+1.00 × 180 and 2Δ in
	Segment 22 × 2 × 2

This prescription might also be written in the form:

DV	R, +2.50/+1.00 × 180
	L, +1.00/+1.00 × 180

Add +2.00 and 2Δ base in NP only

Segment 22 × 2 × 2

Obviously, it is important to state clearly what prism needs to be incorporated in the DP and what prism is required for the NP, which is why it is helpful to write out the distance and reading prescriptions separately and in full.

In this example, prism is required in the reading portion only. The prismatic effects at the NVPs from the main lens are:

R, 2.8Δ base up and 0.5Δ base out

L, 1.6Δ base up and 0.2Δ base out

Assuming that the segment drop is 2mm, the prismatic effect from the invisible 22mm diameter segments is 1.0Δ base down, so the total prismatic effect at the NVPs, before any prism is incorporated in the segments, is:

R, 1.8Δ base up and 0.5Δ base out

L, 0.6Δ base up and 0.2Δ base out

It should be apparent that simply making a pair of prism segments that incorporate 2Δ base in for each eye would not satisfy the prescription requirement at all.

We may proceed in one of two different ways:
1. Make a pair of prism segments that incorporate:

R, 1.8Δ base down and 2.5Δ base in

L, 0.6Δ base down and 2.2Δ base in

This solution offers complete centre control in that the total prismatic effect remaining at the NVPs is just the prescribed 2Δ base in for each eye; all vertical prismatic effect is neutralized.
2. Make a pair of prism segments that incorporate:

R, 1.2Δ base down and 2.5Δ base in

L, 2.2Δ base in

This solution eliminates the vertical differential prismatic effect at the NVPs and provides the prescribed 2Δ base in for each eye at near. It is assumed that bonded prism segments are to be used for this solution. If solid prism segments are employed, a better solution is:

R, 2.5Δ base in

L, 1.2Δ base up and 2.2Δ base in

to ensure that the minimum depth of ridge for the left eye is closer to the top of the segment.

Example ii

DV	R, +1.00/+4.00 × 60 and 1Δ up
	L, +1.00/+4.00 × 120 and 1Δ down
NV	R, +3.00/+4.00 × 60 and 2Δ in
	L, +3.00/+4.00 × 120 and 2Δ in
	Segment 30 × 2 × 2

Strong oblique cylinders give rise to oblique prismatic effects at the NVPs, which might prevent comfortable near vision. This is often the case when the resolved horizontal prism is base out, as in this prescription, since it requires an extra effort of convergence by the eyes. This is the likely reason for the base-in prism requested for near vision only in this specification. However, the prescription also requires vertical prism in the distance portion only, so the segments must also include:

R, 1Δ base down

L, 1Δ base up

to neutralize the DP prism in the reading portion.

The prismatic effects at the NVPs from the main lenses are:
Right eye:

prism from sphere	0.80Δ base up and 0.20Δ base out
prism from cylinder	1.16Δ base up and 2.00Δ base out
Prism in DP Rx	1.00Δ base up
Total prism from	2.96Δ base up and
main lens	2.20Δ base out

Left eye:

prism from sphere	0.80Δ base up and 0.20Δ base out
prism from cylinder	1.16Δ base up and 2.00Δ base out
Prism in DP Rx	1.00Δ base down
Total prism from	0.96Δ base up and
main lens	2.20Δ base out

Assuming that the segment drop is 2mm, the prismatic effect from the invisible 30mm diameter segments is 1.8Δ base down, so the total prismatic effect at the NVPs, before any prism is incorporated in the segments, is:

R, 1.16Δ base up and 2.20Δ base out

L, 0.84Δ base down and 2.20Δ base out

The prism that needs to be added to the segment to provide the prescribed prism of no vertical effect and 2Δ base in is:

R, 1.16Δ base down and 4.20Δ base in

L, 0.84Δ base up and 4.20Δ base in

These are compounded in the usual way to determine the single prismatic effect that must be incorporated in the segment to achieve the effect:

R, 4.36Δ base down at 164.6

L, 4.28Δ base up at 168.7

Example iii
R, +2.00
L, −2.00 Add +2.50
38mm segments
No-jump bifocals

The jump is simply the prismatic effect at the dividing line from the segment and is calculated by multiplying the distance from the optical centre of the segment with the dividing line (in cm) by the reading addition. It is independent of the power of the main lens.

The radius of each segment is 38/2 or 19mm, so the jump is:

1.9 × 2.5 = 4.75Δ base down

To eliminate the jump, the segment must incorporate 4.75Δ base up, the effect of which is to shift the optical centre of the segment to the segment top.

Clearly, a pair of no-jump bifocals cannot be further compensated for vertical differential prismatic effect at the NVPs. In this example, the 3.2Δ difference is certain to prevent comfortable near vision and it would be usual to equalize the vertical prism in cases of anisometropia rather than to eliminate jump.

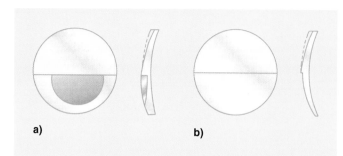

Figure 10.39 Bi-prism bifocals: (a) flat-top D-segment bi-prism design; (b) E-style bi-prism design

Bi-prism bifocals

Prismatic effect in the reading portion of a bifocal lens can be altered by slabbing-off vertical prism from the lower half of the lens. The slab-off process affects only the vertical prismatic effect at the NVP and results in a horizontal dividing line between the two portions, in addition to the segment dividing line (Figure 10.39). For this reason it is customary to restrict the bi-prism technique to bifocal designs, which themselves have a straight dividing line between their distance and reading portions. Flat-top D-segments and E-style segments are ideal for this method of providing partial prism control; in the latter case the bi-prism dividing line can be made to coincide exactly with the horizontal dividing line of the segment.

The amount of prism to be slabbed-off depends, as before, upon the exact prescription requirement. Suppose it is required to produce a pair of D-segment bifocals with no vertical differential prism at the NVPs for the prescription:

R, – 2.50/–2.00 × 180
L, – 1.50/–0.50 × 180
Add + 2.00

The vertical prismatic effect at each NVP from the main lens is:

R, 3.6Δ base down

L, 1.6Δ base down

So the vertical differential prismatic effect is 2Δ base down in the right eye.

To eliminate this differential prism the right eye must incorporate 2Δ base up in the reading portion only or the left eye must incorporate 2Δ base down in the reading portion only.

The slab-off process described above removes base-down prism from the lower half of the lens, so the right eye would be chosen as the bi-prism design.

It is possible, in the case of plastics bifocals, to incorporate a slab-off on the moulded bifocal surface. When the slab-off is worked in-mould, the cast bifocal surface has base-up prism removed from the segment area. If such a design is employed for this example, the left eye of the pair would be the bi-prism design with 2Δ base down added to the reading portion.

Complex prescription requirements

The method of construction of cemented (or bonded) and solid visible bifocals enables complex prescriptions such as cylinders in the distance or near portions only or different cylinders and/or axes in the distance and near portions to be made. The segment elements of these designs may also include separate prismatic effects, for example, to centre control the near portion of the lens.

Consider the bifocal prescription:

DV	R, +2.00
	L, +2.00/+1.00 × 90
NV	R, +4.00/+1.00 × 90
	L, +4.00

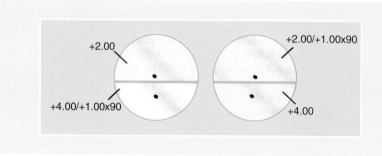

Figure 10.40 Split bifocal made to Rx:

DV   R, +2.00; L, +2.00/+1.00 × 90
NV   R, +4.00/+1.00 × 90; L, +4.00

Four separate lenses are employed and each component may be centred as required

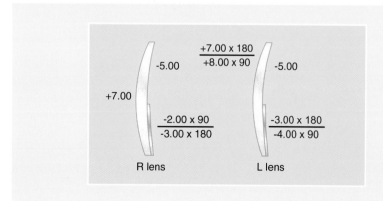

Figure 10.41 Cemented bifocal made to Rx:

DV   R, +2.00; L, +2.00/+1.00 × 90
NV   R, +4.00/+1.00 × 90; L, +4.00

The contact curves are ±5.00D

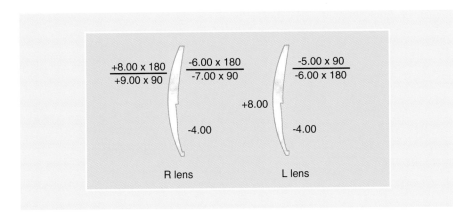

R lens   L lens

+8.00 x 180 / +9.00 x 90   -6.00 x 180 / -7.00 x 90   -5.00 x 90 / -6.00 x 180

+8.00

-4.00   -4.00

Figure 10.42   Solid visible bifocal form of Rx:

DV   R, +2.00; L, +2.00/+1.00×90
NV   R, +4.00/+1.00×90; L, +4.00

The segment curves are −4.00D

Here a cylinder is required in the distance portion only of the left eye and the near portion only of the right eye. This specification could be made easily as a split bifocal design using the components shown in Figure 10.40.

It could also be made in cemented bifocal form as shown in Figure 10.41, in which a ±5.00D contact surface is employed. Or, it could be made as a solid visible design as shown in Figure 10.42, in which a −4.00D spherical NPC is employed.

These methods of construction permit more complex astigmatic requirements to be met, such as providing different cylinder powers and/or different cylinder axes in the distance and near portions.

References

1. Letter to George Whately, London, 15 November 1784. In: Sparks Jared (1856), The Works of Benjamin Franklin … With Notes, 10, 150. Boston
2. Levene J R 1977 Clinical refraction and visual science. Butterworths, London
3. Jalie M 1996 Ophthalmic lenses and dispensing – Part six. Optician 211:24–31
4. Jalie M 1984 Principles of ophthalmic lenses. ABDO, London
5. Jalie M, Wray L W 1996 Practical ophthalmic lenses. ABDO, London
6. Goersch H 1991 Handbook of ophthalmic optics. Carl Zeiss, Oberkochen
7. Jalie M 1989 The spectacle lens in presbyopia. Optician 197:13–18
8. Jalie M 1981 Work reports. 2nd International Symposium on Presbyopia. Essilor, Paris
9. Crundall E 1952 Bifocal lenses. A Stigmat technical publication. Stigmat Ltd, London
10. Sasieni L 1975 Principles and practice of optical dispensing and fitting, 3rd edn. Butterworths, London

Trifocal lenses

As shown in Chapter 10, when a subject requires a separate correction for distance and near vision, the two prescriptions may be provided as one pair of spectacles in the form of bifocal lenses. With increasing presbyopia, the eyes require progressively stronger reading additions to compensate for the lack of accommodation. Eventually, the power of the addition is such that intermediate vision beyond the near point is too blurred to be seen through either the distance portion (DP) or the near portion (NP) of a pair of bifocals. In these cases, a different addition might be suggested to provide clear intermediate vision and the correction may be provided by combining three prescriptions into a single trifocal lens with three distinct portions (Figure 11.1).

The area of the lens used for intermediate vision is called the *intermediate portion* (IP); a trifocal lens has three separate portions of different powers, the DP, the IP and the NP (or reading portion, RP). The addition prescribed for intermediate vision, the IP addition, is often expressed as a percentage of the near addition, known as the IP/NP ratio, where:

IP/NP ratio = IP Add/NP Add × 100%

For example, if a near addition of +2.50D is required, the intermediate addition might be +1.00D, which is an IP/NP ratio of 1.00/2.50 × 100 = 40%. If an IP of power +1.25D is required, this could be described as an IP/NP ratio of 50%, or if +1.50D is required, this could be described as an IP/NP ratio of 60%. The choice of IP/NP ratio depends upon the range of clear intermediate vision the subject is expected to obtain. It is shown later that if the requirement for the IP is to extend the range of clear vision from the distance range closer to, say, arm's length, then a low IP/NP ratio (35–45%) is usually necessary. If, however, the requirement is to extend the near vision range out to arm's length, then

a high IP/NP ratio (60–70%) is needed. Ideally, in any given trifocal design, the IP/NP ratio should be variable.

Ranges of vision and accommodative demand with trifocals

Before the onset of presbyopia, the eye exerts an ever-increasing amount of accommodation to view objects that lie closer and closer to the eye. If accommodative demand is plotted graphically against the object distance, the result is a smooth hyperbolic curve as shown in Figure 11.2. No accommodation is assumed to be exerted for an infinitely distant object and accommodation of +5.00D is required when the object lies 20cm in front of the eyes. The curve is similar for corrected ametropes, but shifted slightly upwards for the hypermetropic eye or downwards for the myopic eye, respectively; the extent of the shift depends upon the amount of ametropia.

On reaching presbyopia, a near vision correction is required to help the eye focus on near objects. If this is supplied in the form of a single-vision lens then, when wearing the near vision correction, the accommodative demand follows the same form as the curve before presbyopia. An ancillary effect of the near vision correction is to render the subject artificially myopic by the magnitude of the reading addition.

The influence of reading spectacles and bifocal lenses upon this curve is considered in Chapter 10, in which it is pointed out that a near vision correction alters the demand upon the accommodative faculty. We now consider the effect upon the accommodative faculty when trifocal lenses are worn.

Take the example of a corrected hypermetrope with a distance prescription of +3.00D and an amplitude of accommodation of +1.00D. Assuming that the subject can exert the full amplitude of accommodation, the range of vision through the distance prescription would extend from infinity down to 100cm. For near vision at one-third of a metre, the subject might be prescribed a near addition of +2.25D. With reading spectacles, or through the NP, if the correction has been dispensed in bifocal form, the range of vision would extend from about 44cm (100/2.25) down to just below 31cm (100/3.25). Ignoring depth-of-field effects, the subject has no optical aid for the range 100cm down to 44cm (Figure 11.3), so to provide vision in this range an intermediate addition is required.

The intermediate addition depends upon the range of clear vision that the subject requires. If an intermediate addition of +1.00D is given, the clear range of vision obtained through the IP extends from 100cm down to 50cm (Figure 11.4), again assuming that the subject can exert the full amplitude of accommodation. This addition enables continuous vision to be obtained from infinity down to 50cm, but still results in a blur range that extends from 50cm to 44cm. Such an IP/NP ratio might be of

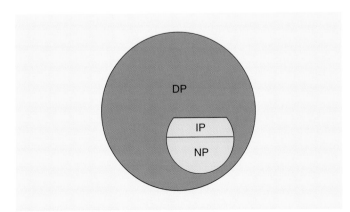

Figure 11.1 Flat-top trifocal design: DP, distance portion; IP, intermediate portion; NP, near portion

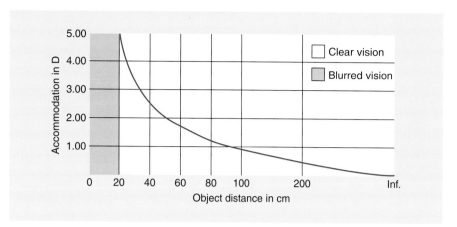

Figure 11.2 Accommodative demand and ranges of vision before the onset of presbyopia

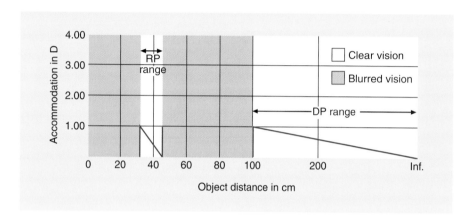

Figure 11.3 Accommodative demand and ranges of vision when corrected by a bifocal lens of power +3.00 Add +2.25. The wearer has a total amplitude of accommodation of +1.00D

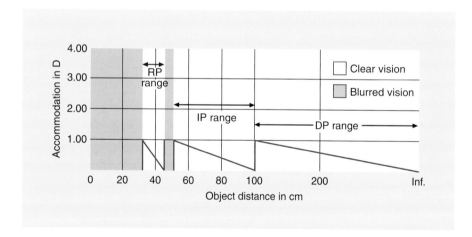

Figure 11.4 Accommodative demand and ranges of vision when corrected by a trifocal lens of power +3.00 Add +2.25 for near with an intermediate addition of +1.00. The wearer has a total amplitude of accommodation of +1.00D

use in some pursuits but, generally, may not prove to be successful since the most common intermediate range requirement is to extend the range of clear vision from the near point out to arm's length.

To achieve this, it is evident that an intermediate addition of +1.25 must be dispensed so that when the subject's own full amplitude of accommodation is exerted, clear vision can be obtained down to 44cm. With this addition, the subject's intermediate range of vision extends from 80cm down to 44cm, but the blur range now remains between 100cm and 80cm (Figure 11.5). It is evident that trifocal lenses may not result in truly continuous vision from the far point to the near point, a condition that can be met either by providing a fourth prescription, in the form of

a second intermediate addition (see 'Quadrifocal designs' below), or (more easily) by dispensing progressive power lenses.

Ideally, it should be possible to vary the IP/NP ratio at will, depending upon the subject's requirements, but with most proprietary trifocal designs the ratio must be predetermined by the blank manufacturer. Thus, the choice of intermediate addition is usually left to the dispensing optician, who selects the particular trifocal design the subject will eventually wear.

The altered demand upon the accommodative faculty is just one more adaptation problem for the new multifocal wearer. One of the several advantages to the wearer of progressive power lenses is that the accommodative demand curve with a progressive lens is not very different from the curve before presbyopia.

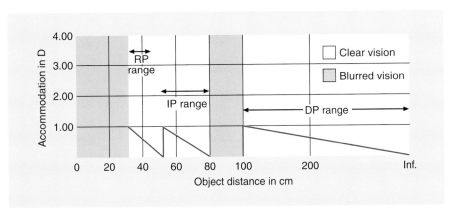

Figure 11.5 Accommodative demand and ranges of vision when corrected by a trifocal lens of power +3.00 Add +2.25 for near with an intermediate addition of +1.25. The wearer has a total amplitude of accommodation of +1.00D

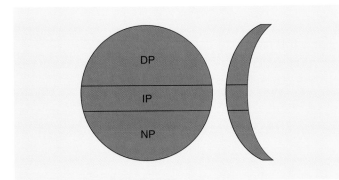

Figure 11.6 Split trifocal (Hawkins' design)

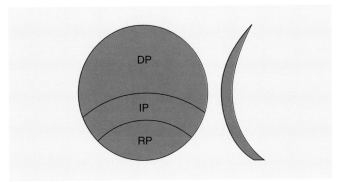

Figure 11.7 Cemented trifocal. This design is constructed from a glass solid bifocal with a crescent segment, which makes up the DP and IP, to which is cemented (or bonded) a circular downcurve segment to make up the NP

Trifocal types

Trifocal lenses can be classified in several ways, one of the most useful being by method of construction. The earliest trifocals were *split trifocals* (Figure 11.6), in which three separate lenses for distance, intermediate and near vision were fitted edge to edge in a single rim. This design was described as early as 1826 by John Isaac Hawkins,[1] who is considered the inventor of trifocal lenses.

Since the distance, intermediate and near portions of the split trifocal are formed from three separate lenses, any IP/NP ratio can be obtained. This design allows each portion to be centred separately, with the distance optical centre located in the distance visual zone, the intermediate optical centre in the intermediate zone and the near optical centre in the near visual zone. This fundamental optical requirement of all multifocal lenses is not usually achieved in other trifocal designs.

In its simplest form, the split trifocal is dispensed most easily using a metal frame into which the three components, carefully flat-edged along their contact edges, can be screwed up against one another in the metal rim. Hawkins, who was an engineer and an inventor of some note, described quite explicitly how the front of the frame that contained his lenses should be angled so that the visual axes were normal to each portion when each was in use. If split trifocals must be dispensed in a plastics frame they could be bonded together along their contact edges before assembling them into the frame.

The second class of trifocal is the *cemented trifocal* in which a segment is cemented to the main lens, which would normally be a downcurve solid bifocal design with a crescent segment (Figure 11.7). The power of the addition for the base bifocal lens is the intermediate addition and the power of the segment that makes up the NP is the difference between the NP and IP additions. Again, this basic trifocal form allows any IP/NP ratio to be obtained. The use of ultraviolet-cured epoxy resins provides excellent long-term adhesion of glass components, and enables several forms of tinted equitint or even prism-controlled trifocal designs to be made.

In theory, the cemented trifocal segment can be produced in any shape and size, but for the dividing line to remain invisible (i.e. as inconspicuous as possible) the segment should be round in shape with its optical centre coinciding with its geometrical centre (Figure 11.7).

The intermediate and reading portions of *fused trifocals* are constructed from a button normally made up from three different glasses, a crown glass of exactly the same material as the main lens and two glasses of high refractive index, chosen to provide the correct IP/NP ratio. The button is fused at a high temperature to a depression curve worked on the main lens, made from crown glass (Figure 11.8). After completion of the segment side, the segment surface is continuous over the DP and NP, so the dividing line cannot be felt. The reading additions, A_I, and A_N, obtained depend upon the power of the DP surface, F_1, the power of the original depression curve, F_C, and the fused bifocal blank ratios for the two glasses used. If the refractive index of the crown glass main lens is denoted by n_1, that of the light flint glass used for the IP by n_2 and that for the glass of highest refractive index, used for the NP, by n_3, then the IP/NP ratio is given by:

$$\text{IP/NP ratio} = (n_2 - n_1)/(n_3 - n_1) \times 100\%$$

Typical segment glasses used in Europe are $n_1 = 1.523$, $n_2 = 1.606$ and $n_3 = 1.654$.

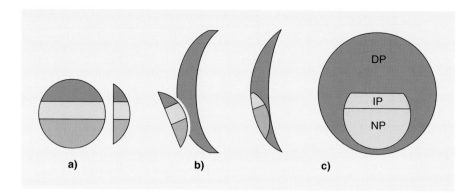

Figure 11.8 Construction of the fused trifocal: (a) a composite flint button comprising three glasses; (b) ready for fusing to a crown glass major; (c) finished fused trifocal

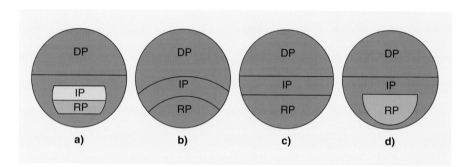

Figure 11.9 Trifocal types: (a) R-segment trifocal; (b) concentric downcurve trifocal; (c) band trifocal; (d) ED trifocal

Since the IP/NP ratios of these designs depend upon the glasses used they are fixed by the manufacturer, usually at 50%, but some designs are available with the IP addition at 40%, 60% or 70% of the near addition.

Fused trifocals are currently available in the following segment diameters and intermediate depths (25 × 7 indicates that the segment diameter is 25mm and the depth of the IP is 7mm):

22,25,28 × 6 D segments
25,28,35 × 7 D segments
25,28 × 8 D segments
25,28,35 × 10 D segments
24 × 7 C segments
25,28,35 × 7 C segments
22 × 6 R segment (Figure 11.9a)

Solid concentric downcurve trifocals are made of a single piece of material in which the reading addition is from different curvatures on one surface of the lens (Figure 11.9b). The intermediate addition of this design is given by the difference between the IP curve and the DP curve and the reading addition is given by the difference between the reading portion curve and the DP curve. These values can, of course, be read off by means of a lens measure. The width of the IP is the difference between the radii of the two segment circles. Thus, if the segment diameters are 38mm for the IP and 22mm for the NP, the width of the IP is (38−22)/2 = 8mm. Glass solid trifocal production requires the same specialized machinery and working procedures as solid bifocals, but, at present, this design is not available in the UK in solid form. If required, this form of trifocal could be made as a cemented design (Figure 11.7).

Plastics trifocals are all solid in form and are produced by casting the monomer in a concave mould, which itself is produced

using normal surfacing machinery. Plastics flat-top trifocals are available in the following diameters and IP depths:

25,28 × 7 D segments
35 × 8 D segment
35 × 14 D segment

Usually, the IP/NP ratio is fixed at 50%, but some designs are available with a 66% IP/NP ratio.

Band trifocals (Figure 11.9c), which have wide portions, are solid, visible no-jump trifocals in construction and are available in both glass and plastics form. The edge thicknesses of the blank at the top and bottom can be made the same by prism thinning, in which a vertical prism is worked across the blank to reduce the thickness, usually of the DP. Since the reading addition is almost always the same for each eye, the same amount of prism-thinning is applied to each lens. Prism-thinned lenses should always be anti-reflection coated to eliminate any problem that might occur with the ghost image formed by total internal reflection at the two lens surfaces, described in Chapter 5. Band trifocals are currently available with either 7mm or 14mm IP depths and with IP/NP ratios of 50%.

ED trifocals combine an E-style dividing line between the DP and IP, and the NP comprises a flat-top, 25 × 17 segment, of which the top lies either 8mm or 13mm below the E-style dividing line (Figure 11.9d). IP/NP ratios of either 50% or 60% are available.

Vocational trifocals

The designs mentioned so far may be described as general purpose designs in that they can be used for most activities. Many trifocal designs have been introduced for specific vocational use.

The *up-and-downcurve trifocal* illustrated in Figure 11.10a is designed for subjects whose main requirement is a large *IP* field in

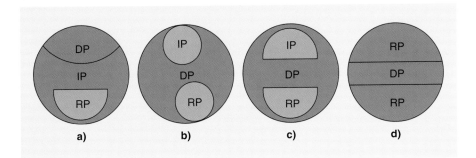

Figure 11.10   Vocational trifocals: (a) up-and-downcurve trifocal; (b) double round segment trifocal; (c) double D-segment trifocal; (d) double E-style bifocal

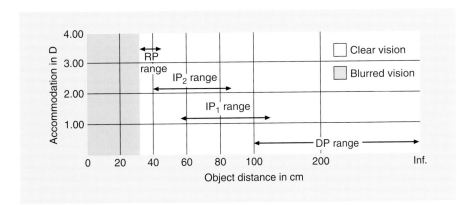

Figure 11.11   Ranges of vision when corrected by a quadrifocal lens of power +3.00 Add +2.25 for near with intermediate additions of +0.75 for middle distance and +1.50 for arm's-length vision. The wearer has a total amplitude of accommodation of +1.00D: DP range of clear vision from infinity to 100cm; IP$_1$ range of clear vision from 133cm to 57cm: IP$_2$ range of clear vision from 67cm to 40cm; NP range of clear vision from 44cm to 31cm

the usual position and occasional distance vision from a portion at the top of the lens. This design should be easy to obtain since it is produced by working an upcurve segment into any downcurve bifocal design. The position and diameter of the DP segment can be varied at will and, since the lenses are individually made to prescription, any IP/NP ratio is available. Normally, the minimum distance between the DP and NP segments is 10mm.

Another group of vocational trifocal designs, sometimes known as combination trifocals, have the IP – or it might be a second reading portion, in which case the design is properly called a double-bifocal – located above the DP of a downcurve bifocal design (Figures 11.10b,c). The upper segment allows intermediate (or near) vision above the distance field. Teachers (for blackboard work), librarians, grocers (for high shelf work) and pilots (for viewing overhead instrument consoles) are just a few examples of those who might benefit from such vocational designs. Double-bifocal lenses are also illustrated in Figure 11.10d, and are designs that provide a second NP at the top of the lens. Clearly, these vocational lenses are designed to be worn for a specific purpose and will not replace the subject's general purpose pair for most other activities.

The frame design for such vocational trifocals should be chosen with care to ensure that it is sufficiently deep to accommodate the three separate portions.

Quadrifocal designs

As indicated above, to provide advanced presbyopes with truly continuous vision from their far points to their near points, a minimum of four different prescriptions are required. This can be deduced from Figures 11.4 and 11.5, which show the ranges of clear vision for the case of a +3.00D hypermetrope who has an amplitude of accommodation of +1.00D and who is prescribed a near addition of +2.25. An intermediate addition of +1.00

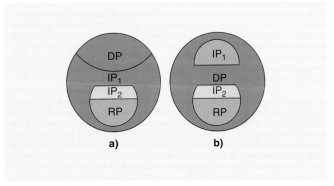

Figure 11.12   Quadrifocal designs: (a) quadrifocal constructed by working an upcurve segment for distance vision at the top of a downcurve trifocal design; (b) quadrifocal design, with main lens designed for distance vision and incorporating a second IP at the top of the lens

provides a range of clear vision from 100cm down to 50cm. A second intermediate addition of +1.25 provides a range of clear vision from 80cm down to 44cm, from which point the near addition can be brought into use. In practice, it is better to provide more overlap of the ranges through each portion, so intermediate additions of +0.75 and +1.50 would probably provide a more suitable solution (Figure 11.11).

Quadrifocal lenses are commonplace in US lens catalogues; the simplest quadrifocal design is a downcurve trifocal, into the top of which is sunk an upcurve segment for distance vision (Figure 11.12a). The downcurve trifocal design could be of any form. A second quadrifocal design is illustrated in Figure 11.12b, in which the upper segment is designed for intermediate vision. This lens is a glass-fused quadrifocal, but available with any combination of additions for the various portions.

Optical performance of trifocal lenses

It is very useful when considering the theory and performance of trifocal lenses to assume that the lens is made up of three distinct components, a *main lens*, which is usually the DP, attached to which are supplementary segment lenses, with powers that represent the additions for intermediate and near. In general, the optical performance of a trifocal design follows that of the parent bifocal form.

One of the most important optical considerations in the performance of all multifocal lenses is the amount of prismatic effect that occurs in the segment zones of the lenses, since these are dependent upon the powers of the main lens and segments and upon the segment diameters.

The centration of spectacle lenses is considered in detail in Chapter 3 and the following summary draws upon the discussion of bifocal performance in Chapter 10. As shown in Chapter 10, in the case of shaped segments, such as those employed for flat- and curved-top trifocal designs, the centration in the IP and NP does not differ much from the centration of a single-vision lens with the power of the DP, since the segment centre is not far removed from either the intermediate visual point or the near visual point. The jump at each dividing line is also small, since the segment centre is not far removed from the segment tops.

In the case of concentric downcurve segments, the centration in the intermediate and near portions is better when the main lens is positive, since the base-up effect of the main lens is then counteracted by the base-down effects of the segments. The wearer will, however, experience jump at each of the two dividing lines between the three portions.

With band trifocals, which are no-jump in construction, the centration in the intermediate and near portions is better when the main lens is negative, since with this design the base-up effect of each segment counteracts the base-down effects of the main lens.

As already pointed out, the method of construction of the split trifocal and cemented trifocal permits full prism control of these designs, if required.

Trifocal fitting

Trifocal fitting must always be a compromise in that when the height and inset of the IP have been determined, this position also fixes the height and inset of the reading portion. In the case of flat- and curved-top trifocals, which are the most popular in

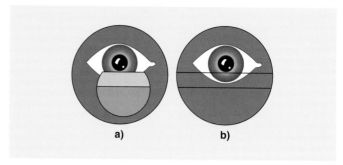

Figure 11.13 Trifocal segment positioning for the two most popular designs: (a) flat-top trifocal; (b) band trifocal

general use, the inset of the intermediate and near portions is exactly the same; it is not possible to inset these two portions separately. The position of one portion of the lens in front of the eye predetermines the position of the other portion.

In the case of trifocals for general purpose use, the IP lies above the reading portion and the eye must pass through the IP before it reaches the NP. The NP is therefore lower than in the case of a bifocal design and the eye needs to rotate downwards somewhat further before it obtains the benefit of the near addition. A good starting position for the IP top is at or just below the lower pupil margin (Figure 11.13), so it is sensible, whenever possible, to dispense a frame that allows some vertical adjustment of the segment height at, or subsequent to, the final fitting. This enables the segment top to be raised or lowered, if found necessary, to hasten adaptation to the new lenses.

Reference

1. Levene J R 1977 Clinical refraction and visual science. Butterworths, London

Progressive power lenses

Chapter

12

As shown in Chapter 11, when a subject requires separate corrections for distance, intermediate and near vision, the three prescriptions may be provided as one pair of spectacles in the form of trifocal lenses. The drawbacks of trifocal lenses are much the same as those of bifocal lenses. The zones of fixed power provide the wearer with a limited focusing range through each zone, jump at the dividing lines (unless visible, no-jump designs are used), and the presence of the segment dividing lines detract from the appearance of the lenses. These drawbacks are all eliminated by dispensing progressive power lenses, the use of which has expanded rapidly in the past few years. Indeed, in their country of origin, France, progressive lenses have become the first choice of multifocal design for the correction of presbyopia.

Progressive power lens design

A progressive power lens is designed to provide continuous vision at all distances, instead of the predetermined working distances of bifocal and trifocal lenses. The lens can be considered to have three distinct zones, just as a trifocal design: a distance zone, a progression zone (or, simply, the progression) and a near zone. Unlike a trifocal lens, the progression provides an increase in reading addition from the distance portion (DP) to the near portion [NP, or reading portion (RP)]. The rate at which the power increases over the progression zone is governed by the power law for the design (Figure 12.1). The power law may be linear, as assumed in Figure 12.1, or it may be more complex to provide a greater or lesser increase in power at the start of the progression (see Figure 12.13).

Compared with bifocal and trifocal designs, the progressive power lens offers:

- vision at all distances – since the addition increases over the progression zone
- more natural use of accommodation – accommodation does not need to fluctuate when vision is transferred from one zone to another
- absence of image jump – there is no abrupt change in power
- the appearance of a single-vision lens, with no dividing lines on the lens.

The second of these benefits is immediately apparent when the accommodative demands and ranges of vision through a trifocal lens and a progressive power lens are compared.

Consider a subject who has an amplitude of accommodation of +1.00D and who is prescribed a correction of +3.00, Add +2.25 for near. The accommodative demands and ranges of vision obtained when this specification is dispensed in trifocal form and progressive power form are illustrated in Figure 12.2.

Figure 12.2a assumes that a trifocal correction with an intermediate addition of +1.25 has been provided. This intermediate

addition provides continuous vision from 80cm down to the near point at 31cm through the intermediate and near portions of the lens.

Figure 12.2b assumes that the correction is dispensed in progressive power form and the accommodative demand is of the same form as that enjoyed by the subject before the onset of presbyopia. Naturally, the actual position of the curve depends upon which zone of the lens the subject happens to be using.

To obtain an idea of the geometry of a progressive surface consider, first, an E-style bifocal with the bifocal surface made from two different spherical surfaces placed together so that their poles share a common tangent at point L (Figure 12.3). Obviously, the two surfaces are continuous only at point L. At all other points there is a step between the two surfaces, which increases as with distance from L. In the broadest terms, if we wish to produce a truly invisible bifocal design (i.e. one in which the dividing line cannot be detected), the two surfaces must be blended together such that the DP surface and NP surface are continuous at all points.

In principle, a progressive lens may be considered to have spherical DP and NP surfaces connected by a surface with tangential and sagittal radii of curvature that decrease according to a specific power law between the distance and near zones of the lens.

In theory, to make a surface with curvature that increases at the correct rate to satisfy whatever power law is necessary, we need to be able to combine small segments of spheres of ever-decreasing radii, all tangential to one another, in a continuous curve. Clearly, these sections will be continuous only along a single, so-called umbilic line, and at all other points on the surface the sections must be blended to form a smooth surface.

The simplest concept of this latter surface is a section taken from an oblate ellipsoid, as illustrated in Figure 12.4, in which

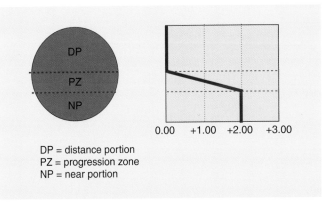

DP = distance portion
PZ = progression zone
NP = near portion

Figure 12.1   Power profile for a progressive lens with a linear power law, 0.00 Add +2.00

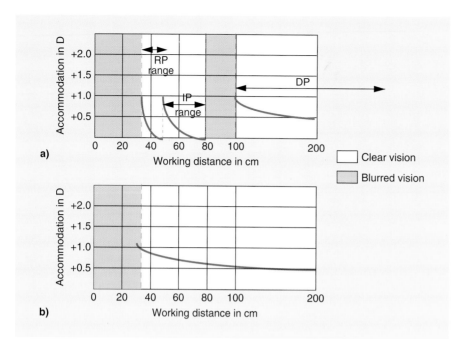

Figure 12.2 Comparison of accommodative demand and ranges of vision through (a) trifocals and (b) progressive power lenses

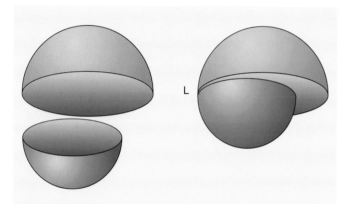

Figure 12.3 E-style bifocal lens made by placing together two spherical surfaces with a common tangent at L

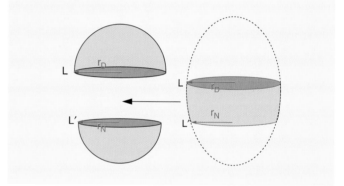

Figure 12.4 Concept of a progressive surface. A section of an oblate ellipsoid is inserted between two hemispheres of radius of curvature, r_D for the distance portion and r_N for the near portion

the radii of curvature of the spherical surfaces that represent the distance and near portions are shown as r_D and r_N, respectively. It can be seen that the solid ovoid obtained by inserting the ellipsoidal section between the two hemispheres shown in Figure 12.4 results in a surface that has no discontinuities.

Along the umbilic line, LL', a cross-section through the surface is circular and the radii of the circles in a plane parallel with either the distance or NP circles do, indeed, decrease from r_D to r_N, continuously.

The ability to cut surfaces of such a complex nature was made possible by the arrival of computer numeric control grinding (CNC) machines. CNC machining methods have made possible the design and production of both progressive and aspheric lens designs in the past 50 years. Basically, the CNC cutter, which could be a single-point diamond tool, cuts a surface under computer control, the cutter sweeping in an arc over the workpiece with the program positioning the cutter in exactly the right place as the cutter traverses the workpiece. This is shown schematically in Figure 12.5, in which it is apparent that the program that provides the machining data must position the single-point diamond tool in the x, y and z planes as the point traverses the workpiece.

The workpiece could be a glass blank or a glass mould from which plastics lenses might eventually be cast, or it could be a ceramic block upon which glass moulds or finished lenses will be slumped with or without vacuum assistance (Figures 12.6 and 12.7).

The drawback to the direct-machining method is that no matter how accurately the surface is generated, it must still be smoothed and polished. These final stages are accomplished using a floating pad system; it is essential to ensure that the pads do not remove any more glass than intended, otherwise an accurate surface geometry will not be maintained.

Slumping uses ceramic slumping moulds, which themselves are produced by CNC cutting, upon which the glass blanks (with carefully polished convex spherical surfaces) are placed (Figure 12.6). The assembly is then heated to the high temperature at which the glass starts to flow. The back surface of the blank then conforms in shape with that of the ceramic mould and the convex surface of the blank, which is the progressive surface, slumps to the required geometry. The initial shape of the mould must be calculated very carefully and highly sophisticated temperature control is necessary to ensure that the glass flows correctly.

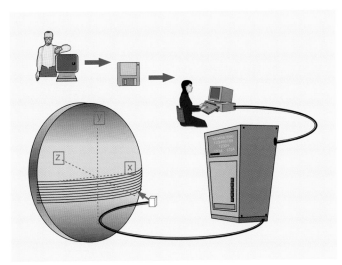

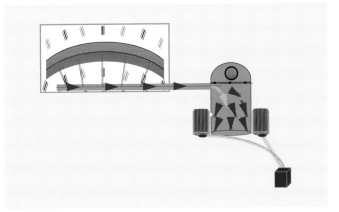

Figure 12.7 Vacuum forming of a glass blank: the glass blank is heated to the softening temperature and a vacuum applied to pull the surface into shape

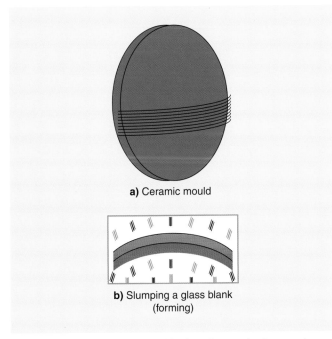

a) Ceramic mould

b) Slumping a glass blank (forming)

Figure 12.6 Slumping a glass blank to the required geometry. (a) A ceramic mould with the convex surface machined to the correct geometry by the CNC machine. (b) The glass blank with a carefully prepared convex spherical surface is mounted on the mould and heated to a high temperature at which the glass begins to flow. The glass slumps and the geometry of the convex surface of the mould is transferred to the convex surface of the blank

Figure 12.5 CNC machining procedure. The design for the progressive surface is fed to the computer that controls the single-point diamond tool. Solid geometry is used to position the tool in the *x, y* and *z* planes

In some cases, the slumping is assisted by vacuum forming, whereby the glass is heated to just beyond its softening point (at which temperature it is unable to flow by gravity alone), whereupon a vacuum is applied to the interface between the forming block and the concave surface of the blank, which effectively sucks the surface into shape (Figure 12.7).

Not least of the difficulties that must be overcome on the production line is to select a test method that can be used to verify the accuracy of the finished surface. Unlike for a rotationally symmetrical aspherical surface, mechanical measurement is useless since, even if a gauge with sufficient accuracy were available, every meridian would have to be checked in turn. Three different optical methods are employed:

- image evaluation by means of the Hartmann Test or by comparing grid patterns
- surface evaluation by interferometric methods
- computer scanning of the power distribution by a specially adapted on-line focimeter.

The actual geometry of a given progressive surface is regarded as proprietary information by lens manufacturers, but some insight into how the design of a surface might proceed can be obtained by developing the concept illustrated in Figure 12.4.

The CNC cutter can be programmed to cut a series of arcs, each one independently controlled but together result in a continuous surface of any geometrical configuration. For example, it is possible to cut a conicoidal surface, such as the oblate ellipsoid, which looks quite promising, at first sight, for a progressive power surface, since both tangential and sagittal surface powers increase quite rapidly with distance from the pole of the surface. The rate of increase in curvature can be controlled by altering the asphericity of this conicoid, and the change can be determined as follows. If an oblique pencil of rays is traced through a spherical lens there is likely to be an error, δT, in the tangential oblique vertex sphere power of the lens. Of course, in the case of a minimum tangential error lens form, the error, δT, may be zero. The ray trace also yields the incidence height, y_1, on the front surface of the lens, the radius of curvature of the front surface, F_1, being denoted by r_1.

It is possible to show[1] that for any given tangential error, there must be a conicoid that will eliminate the error. If the error is positive, a conicoid of p-value < 1 must be employed, whereas, if the error is negative, a conicoid of p-value > 1 would be employed.

If the tangential error is known for a given incidence height on the front surface, the asphericity can be found from the equation:

$$p = 1 + (r_1/y_1)^2 \left\{ 1 - \left[F_1/(F_1 + \delta T) \right]^{2/3} \right\}$$

This relationship provides some of the preliminary information needed to design a progressive power surface. In progressive power surface design we *want* a tangential error to occur, the error being the magnitude of the required reading addition.

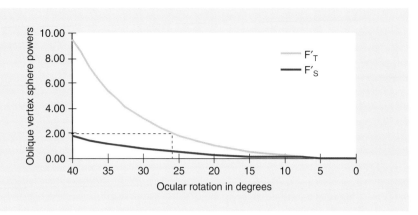

Figure 12.8   Field diagram for a plano-lens made with a convex oblate ellipsoidal surface, $p = +7.2$, to give an add of +2.00D at 14mm below the pole of the surface [$n = 1.5$, $F_1 = +6.00$, $t_C = 3.0$mm, centre of rotation distance (CRD) = 27mm]

Substitution of the add for the tangential error in the above formula gives the required asphericity to reach the value of the addition in the tangential meridian at a given distance below the optical axis of the surface.

For example, in the case of a +6.00D surface worked on a material of refractive index 1.50, an add of +1.00 at 14mm below the pole of the surface requires an asphericity of +4.5. An add of +2.00 needs an asphericity of +7.2 and an add of +3.00 needs an asphericity of +9.4. These p-values describe oblate ellipsoidal surfaces, as depicted in Figure 12.5.

Lenses that employ oblate ellipsoidal surfaces are relatively easy to analyze using ordinary trigonometric ray-tracing techniques. In the case of a plano-lens that employs a convex oblate ellipsoid with a p-value of +7.2 (designed to produce an add of +2.00D, the DP power assumed to be zero), we obtain the field diagram depicted in Figure 12.8. It can be seen that for about a 25° rotation of the eye, which corresponds with a point about 14mm from the pole of the surface, the tangential oblique vertex sphere power is, indeed, +2.00D, the value we set out to achieve.

The ellipsoid alone, however, does not produce a good progressive power surface. Recall from Chapter 4 that the conicoidal surface is astigmatic, the surface astigmatism normally being chosen to eliminate the aberrational astigmatism of oblique incidence.

The field diagram depicted in Figure 12.8 indicates the oblique astigmatism in the refracted pencil; and it can be seen that the astigmatism almost matches the increase in mean oblique power of the surface. Since the field diagram indicates the amount of oblique astigmatic error in the refracted pencil, it actually gives the amount by which the sagittal curvature must be increased to eliminate the astigmatism. For example, at 25°, where the astigmatism is –1.50D, if the sagittal power of the surface is increased by +1.50D this will eliminate much of the astigmatism. The field diagram gives a first indication of the path that the CNC cutter must take as it traverses the progression zone to eliminate the increasing surface astigmatism of the simple ellipsoid.

Progressive lens design, however, does not depend only upon the astigmatism at a single point on the surface, for the power of the progressive surface changes across the refracted pencil. If the power law through the progression zone is linear, then the change in power depends upon the near addition, A, and the length of the progression zone, h. For each 1mm of progression zone the increase in power, δF, through the zone is given by:

$$\delta F = A/h$$

Thus, if the reading addition is +2.00D and the length of the progression zone is 10mm, the surface power through the progression zone must be changing at the rate of 0.20D per millimetre.

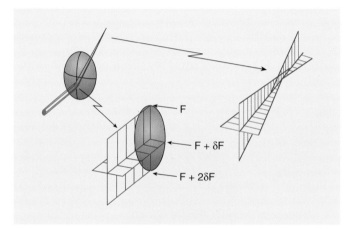

Figure 12.9   Astigmatic nature of the progression zone. The power increase over half the pupil is δF. This represents the astigmatism across the pupil

When the eye uses the progression zone the refracted pencil that fills the pupil must exhibit a skewed form of astigmatism, even along the umbilic line. The astigmatic nature of the pencil is illustrated in Figure 12.9, which depicts the tangential and sagittal fans of a narrow circular pencil of light limited by the eye's pupil, emanating from a region of the progression zone bisected by the umbilic line.

Assuming that the diameter of the beam of light traversing the progression zone is 4mm, with a surface that provides a near addition of +2.00D over a progression length of 10mm, the difference in the tangential and sagittal surface powers across the zone will be 0.40D. If the astigmatism across the pupil is defined as the difference in vergence between the tangential and sagittal fans across the pupil, then the astigmatism is $-2A/hD$. This approximate, but important, rule shows that the astigmatism across the pupil is proportional to the addition, but inversely proportional to the length of the progression zone. In other words, the smaller the addition and the longer the progression zone, the smaller the astigmatism becomes.

As the eye moves away from the umbilic line the total astigmatism increases approximately linearly, but, of course, it is still dependent upon the exact nature of the cross-section of the lens.

The corridor of clear vision through the progression zone is often described as the region in the zone in which the astigmatism does not exceed 1.00D. It is conventional for manufacturers of progressive designs to compare the width of the corridor of clear vision either as a stated number of millimetres or by an

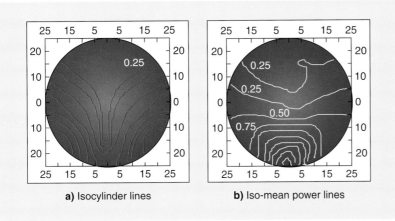

a) Isocylinder lines **b) Iso-mean power lines**

Figure 12.10 (a) Isocylinder and (b) iso-mean power lines for progressive power lens, plano Add +2.00. The intervals between the lines represent a change of 0.25D

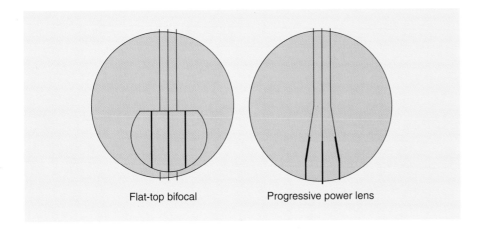

Flat-top bifocal   Progressive power lens

Figure 12.11 Skew distortion in a progressive power lens. The magnification increases through the progression zone

isocylinder diagram in which the contours illustrate the change in surface astigmatism in different zones of the lens. Such a diagram is illustrated in Figure 12.10 together with an iso-mean power diagram, which shows how the power varies across the lens. On the basis of a 1.00D limit on surface astigmatism the lens illustrated in Figure 12.10 is described as having a corridor width of nearly 20mm at 10mm below the geometric centre of the lens.

The iso-mean power diagram illustrates that the surface increases in power slightly as the eye rotates upwards from the geometric centre of the lens, which results from the method chosen to blend the surface between the distance and near portions. Also, the full reading addition of +2.00D is reached at a point 20mm below the geometric centre of the lens.

A second consequence of the progressive surface is depicted in Figure 12.11, which compares the appearance of three vertical lines viewed through a bifocal lens and a progressive power lens. Since an increase in power is inevitably accompanied by an increase in magnification, and it is inevitable that if there is one then there must also be the other, vertical lines viewed through the progression zone exhibit skew distortion.

The directions of the lines can be illustrated with a vector plot that shows how their orientation can be expected to vary in a real image of the lines. The skew effect can be minimized by decreasing the surface curvature as the eye moves away from the umbilic line. The lower down the surface, the greater the reduction in curvature needs to become.

The development of progressive lenses over the past 40 years can be discussed in terms of the way in which the CNC cutter has been employed to blend the DP surface with the NP surface.

In the first commercially successful lens, the *Varilux 1* design from the Essel Optical Company (now part of Essilor International), the DP and NP surfaces were spherical and the CNC followed a path that described circles of ever-decreasing radius as it traversed from the spherical DP to the spherical NP. This necessitated very severe blending of the distance and near portions, with large amounts of surface astigmatism at the peripheries of the progression. However, the DP was almost completely free from surface astigmatism. The second-generation *Varilux 2* design used a series of conic sections of varying asphericity to reduce the astigmatic nature of the earlier design and, at the same time, used aspherical DP and NP surfaces to further reduce the severity of the blend. Without doubt, the *Varilux 2* design pointed the way for later generations of progressive power designs.

Third-generation designs, such as the *Truvision Omni* design, combined aspherical DP and NP surfaces, which spreads the blending further into the DP, softening the definition in the DP, but considerably reducing the astigmatism in the lateral portions of the lens. The power profile of lenses such as the *Omni* can be compared with that of an up-and-downcurve trifocal design with the full distance prescription being obtained near the top of the lens and the near prescription at the bottom. Such a long progression, of course, enables the lens to exhibit remarkably low levels of surface astigmatism in the 'intermediate', peripheral zones. The latest generation of designs combines the features of low-power aspheric lenses with progressive surface design and also adopts different power laws for different near additions.

This feature of progressive lens design, being able to control in which areas of the lens the blending between the DP surface and

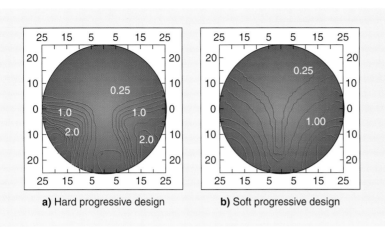

a) Hard progressive design   b) Soft progressive design

Figure 12.12   Comparison of isocylinder lines for (a) hard and (b) soft progressive lens designs of power plano Add +2.00. Isocylinder lines indicate 0.25D contour steps

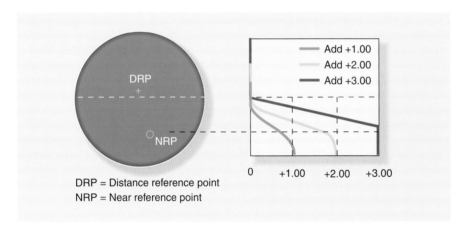

DRP = Distance reference point
NRP = Near reference point

Figure 12.13   Power laws for +1.00, +2.00 and +3.00D additions for a multi-design series of progressive power lenses

the NP surface occurs, enables manufacturers to decide which areas they should prioritize for optimum vision. If the designer requires a large DP with the surface astigmatism confined to the lower portion of the lens, rather like the earliest progressive lens designs, the result is a *hard progressive design*. The arrangement of the surface astigmatism in a hard design is shown in Figure 12.12a. This design enables a large DP area and a relatively large NP area to be obtained, but there are rapid discontinuities in the astigmatism of the lower portion of the lens.

If the designer wishes to reduce the amount of astigmatism that occurs in the lower portion of the lens, to speed the subject's adaptation to progressive lens wear, it can be spread into the DP as indicated in Figure 12.12b. This arrangement results in a *soft progressive design*, and there can be no doubt that when the addition is low, and hence the surface astigmatism is low, the soft progressive design has proved to be the most successful in enabling rapid wearer acceptance of progressive design.

Some manufacturers produce progressive lens series that are deliberately soft in design for the low-addition lenses in the series, the design tending to become harder as the additions increase. These are known as *multi-design* series. Figure 12.13 illustrates how the power law differs with a multi-design series for the additions, +1.00, +2.00 and +3.00D. It can be seen how the length of the progression zone reduces as the addition increases for these series.

Another important feature of progressive power lens design relates to the symmetry of the power distribution across the lens. In Figure 12.14, the eyes are supposed to be viewing an object at B, the visual axes intersecting the lenses at P in the right eye and

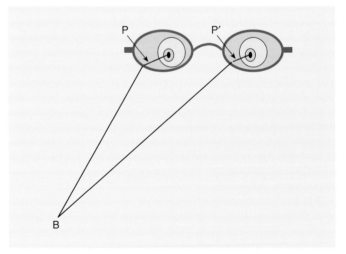

Figure 12.14   Horizontal symmetry at corresponding points on the lens

P' in the left eye. If the surface power at point P differed much in magnitude or orientation from the surface power at P', different prismatic effects will occur at the two points. For ease of fusion in all directions of gaze the vertical prismatic effects at corresponding points must be approximately equal. This is more likely to be the case if each lens is designed individually for the right and left eyes, rather than producing a single design that is rotated inwards, in opposite directions for the two eyes. Progressive lens designs that exhibit approximately equal vertical prismatic effects at corresponding points are said to possess *horizontal symmetry*.

Although isocylinder and vector diagrams are informative, it is foolhardy to suppose that they can be used to predict wearer adaptation and acceptance of the lens.

Despite the consequences of the progressive surface, the brain quickly adapts to the effects of surface astigmatism and skew distortion. The adaptation required of the visual system is probably no greater when a subject wears a first pair of progressive lenses than that required when given a first pair of bifocals. Indeed, if progressive power lenses are introduced at the onset of presbyopia, when the reading addition is low, the adaptation period is probably shorter than it would be for a first pair of bifocal lenses. In an attempt to evaluate the performance of new progressive designs, most manufacturers submit the lenses to clinical trials, the information that the wearers' report being fed back into the design loop.

Subjects who, typically, find it difficult to adapt to progressive lenses are those with high reading additions who have worn bifocal lenses successfully in the past and have become accustomed to a wide reading field of view through a large segment.

Problems with adaptation to progressive lenses almost always result from either an incorrect prescription or poorly fitted lenses.[2,3]

Prism thinning

When a progressive lens is worked to an individual prescription by surfacing the concave surface of the blank, it is usual for the workshop to incorporate a thinning prism in the specification of the back surface. The purpose of the thinning prism is to equalize the edge thickness of the finished lens, and its magnitude depends upon the power of the lens, the cylinder axis direction, if the lens is astigmatic, and the position of the distance reference point with respect to the box centre of the lens (Figure 12.15). Typically, for plus spherical lenses the magnitude of the thinning prism is about two-thirds of the reading addition and its base usually lies at 270°.

It is sensible to apply an anti-reflection coating to any lens that incorporates prism to eliminate the possibility that the ghost image formed by total internal reflection at the lens surfaces will annoy the wearer (see Chapter 5).

Fitting progressive power lenses

A suggested fitting routine for progressive power lenses is as follows:

- Select the final frame that the subject is to wear and adjust it to fit properly. As a general guide, the frame should be closely fitting with the smallest possible vertex distance and the correct pantoscopic angle, and should provide adequate depth beneath the centre of the pupil to accommodate the reading zone of the lens. A minimum depth of 22mm is often suggested.
- If the frame is empty, attach vertical strips of transparent adhesive tape to each eye to enable reference points to be marked. Otherwise the fitting-cross positions can be marked on the existing lenses.
- With the correctly adjusted frame in position, ask the subject to look straight into your eyes. If necessary, adjust the height of your stool to ensure that your eyes are on exactly the same level as that of the subject's eyes.
- Direct the subject to look straight into your open left eye and, using a fine-tip marking pen and (preferably) a light-coloured

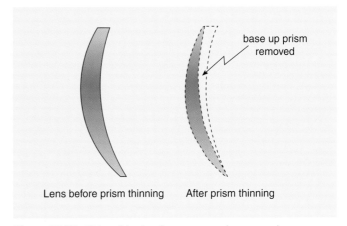

Figure 12.15 Prism thinning for a progressive power lens

ink, place a dot in front of the centre of the subject's right pupil.
- Direct the subject to look straight into your right eye, without any head movement, and place a second dot in front of the centre of the subject's left pupil.
- Remove and replace the frame on the subject's face and repeat the above procedure, this time without making any marks, to ensure the dots that you have marked do lie in front of the centres of the pupils.

Record the fitting-cross positions and check by means of an appropriate blank sizing chart that the lenses can be obtained from the available blank diameters. When ordering the lenses it is necessary to give the progression heights (the heights of the fitting crosses) together with the monocular centration distances (CDs) measured from the centre of the bridge of the frame, which is the reference point for the glazing department. It is very common for the monocular CDs to differ between the right and left eyes. The specification should be written, for example, as 34/32, which indicates that the right eye monocular CD is 34 and the left eye monocular CD is 32. The heights of the pupil centres may also differ for the right and left eyes. Ideally, the progression heights should be specified from the horizontal centre line (HCL) of the frame, such as 4mm above HCL.

It is sensible, whenever possible, to dispense a frame that allows some vertical adjustment of the height of the distance reference point at, or subsequent to, the final fitting. This enables the lenses to be raised or lowered, if this is found to be necessary, to aid adaptation.

Verification of progressive power lenses

Once the lenses have been mounted, they are normally returned with stickers attached to help verify the powers of the lenses and the progression heights. Typically, the lenses appear as shown in Figure 12.16. The upper painted circular line is for the measurement of the distance prescription. The circular sticker at the bottom of the lens is for checking the power of the NP. The prismatic effect of the lens is checked at the painted cross at the geometrical centre of the lens, which is the usual prism reference point. Normally, any prism found at this point is a thinning prism incorporated to equalize the thickness at the top and bottom edges of the lens.

When these lines are removed, the progression height and orientation of the surface can still be determined by locating two small circles that have been engraved on the convex surface 34mm apart on the HCL of the blank. The geometric centre of the original blank lies midway between these two circles. The reading addition of the lens is also permanently engraved under the temporal circle and the manufacturer's identifying mark is engraved under the nasal circle. These markings are easiest to detect by reflected light from a strong source above the lens and with the lens held in front of a black background. In the case of plastics lenses, the engravings are often made easier to detect when a fluorescent dye has been applied to make the engravings fluoresce when illuminated with ultraviolet (UV) radiation from a UV source.

Choice of progressive lens design

The advantages of progressive power lenses over other multifocal designs used for the correction of presbyopia are listed at the beginning of this chapter. These benefits must be weighed against the inevitable optical consequences of the progressive surface, which result in areas on progressive power lenses that may not provide good visual acuity. These areas on a typical progressive lens are illustrated in Figure 12.17. We should expect new wearers of progressive designs to be able to use the zones of the lens that are relatively free of surface astigmatism and skew distortion without too much difficulty. It is the effects manifested in the areas outside the optical zones, where blending of the DP and NP have occurred, that usually require a period of adaptation by the wearer.

A better understanding of the problems of progressive surface design can be obtained by considering how a multifocal design might have its surfaces blended together to form a continuous

surface without any trace of dividing lines. Figure 12.18a illustrates the well-known, E-style trifocal design in which the DP and intermediate portion (IP) surfaces share common tangents at the centre of the lens. Although a trifocal design has been chosen for illustration purposes, the multifocal could have several intermediate bands between the DP and NP, all of which would gradually increase in power from the DP to the NP. At the IP–NP divide the IP and NP surfaces also share a common tangent and, as we move away from these tangent points, the steps that form the dividing lines become deeper and deeper (Figure 12.18b). Imagine that we wish to eliminate these steps simply by reducing their heights until they blend together, with common tangents at every point along their paths. In practice, the CNC cutter effectively blends the curves together as it traverses the workpiece as described above.

If the DP and NP surfaces need to be blended without interfering with the optical properties of the DP of the lens, it is necessary to build up the IP surface to the height of the DP surface and the height of the NP surface to the height of the IP surface. The effect on the optical properties of the lens of blending these regions into a continuous surface is shown schematically in Figure 12.18c. Very severe blending would be necessary near the edges of the lens in which the surfaces have their greatest difference in sag heights, with corresponding optical discontinuities when the eye views through these zones of the lens.

If we are prepared to sacrifice some of the DP of the lens to obtain fewer discontinuities in the intermediate and near zones of the lens, we could reduce the severity of the blending in the lower regions of the lens by reducing the height of the DP surface.

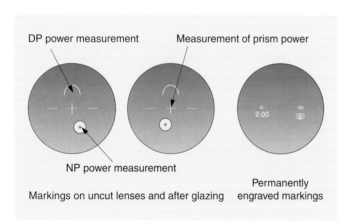

Figure 12.16   Typical markings found on progressive power lenses

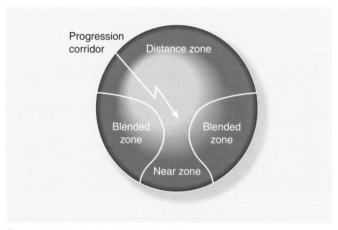

Figure 12.17   Typical positions of the various zones on a progressive power lens. The shapes of the blended zones vary from design to design

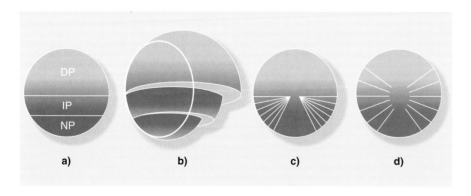

a)   b)   c)   d)

Figure 12.18   Concept of the progressive power lens as a blended multifocal: (a) the design can be imagined to have started out as an E-style multifocal with several portions; (b) to eliminate the dividing lines, the steps between the surfaces must be eliminated: (c) if the IP and NP surfaces are blended by simply raising their heights to the level of the preceding surface, the discontinuities will be severe in the lens periphery; (d) if the blending is allowed to continue into the DP, the DP surface being lowered in height towards its periphery, the discontinuities will be less severe in the lower portion of the lens

The effect of this form of blending is shown schematically in Figure 12.18d, in which it can be seen that the result is to spread the discontinuities into the nasal and temporal areas of the DP surface.

This latter form of blending was used very successfully by the *AO Omni* design, introduced in a patent by John T Winthrop and assigned to American Optical in 1989[4] (Figure 12.19). The patent describes how the designer set out to produce minimum discontinuities throughout the whole lens by blending the surfaces between two poles of power initially arranged as they would be in an up-and-downcurve trifocal design (Figure 12.19a). The necessary blending is shown schematically in Figure 12.19b, and the remarkably low levels of surface astigmatism achieved with this design are illustrated in Figure 12.19c. The reduction in surface astigmatism, however, is not the only requirement for good imaging properties in all zones of the lens. The *Omni* design was one of the first progressive power lenses to combine the progressive surface with the low-base aspheric concept. The tangential flattening of the surface did not allow the periphery of the DP to enjoy the same mean oblique surface power as the central zone of the lens.

Although it is easy to draw some conclusions about the likely performance of one design over another by inspection of isocylinder diagrams, it is more difficult to pontificate over acceptance of the design from these diagrams. Figure 12.12 indicates quite clearly that the soft design has a narrower intermediate channel and a narrower NP than the lens described as a hard design. The widths of these areas could be measured and expressed, for example, in the same way as we would express the diameter of a bifocal segment. However, the significance of this information is not immediately apparent. The author wears several different progressive lens designs, each with different characteristics in their intermediate and near portions, and has no strong preference (at least, none related to the optical performance of the lenses) for any one design over another. If asked to comment on the widths of the intermediate channels of my own progressive lenses I could honestly state that they are as wide as the lenses themselves. Any additional turning of the head that might be necessary to view laterally placed objects within the field is unremarkable from a personal point of view.

Not least, the wearer trials to which prototype progressive designs are subjected must indicate a general preference for the performance of the design that is finally selected. It has been suggested that hard or soft progressive designs might be selected for different purposes. Tunnacliffe,[5] for example, reported findings based upon his personal experience of several designs, and stated that he much preferred soft designs for working at the VDU, but could wear the hard designs for general use where there was no sustained intermediate vision. The wider reading and distance areas of the hard designs were appreciated readily. Based upon his experience that adaptation is easier with soft designs than with hard designs, he

recommends that a hard design be used for someone who is seeking a replacement for bifocal lenses, or for someone who needs a relatively wide NP. He also recommends that wearers be informed of the narrower reading area of progressive power lenses when compared with even the smallest bifocal segment.

Since adaptation takes place in the visual cortex, and there is little understanding, as yet, of the precise mechanism by which this adaptation occurs, it is difficult to lay down any hard and fast rules about patient selection.

Tunnacliffe gives[5] a useful summary of wearer selection and suggests that presbyopic patients who are likely to be successful wearers of progressive power lenses include:

- Current wearers who are satisfied with a previous pair
- Young presbyopes in need of a first near addition
- Subjects who require an intermediate focus in addition to corrections for distance and near
- Subjects who do not want dividing lines on their lenses
- Those whose lifestyle, work or hobbies do not require wide intermediate or near portions on their lenses
- Those who would benefit from the no-jump performance of the lenses
- First-time potential progressive lens wearers who are prepared to gamble on the chance that they will adapt to progressive power lenses.

He suggests that patients who are unlikely to succeed with progressive lenses include:

- Previously failed progressive power lens wearers
- Patients who require a wide near area and cannot or are not prepared to turn the head more for lateral viewing
- Patients who are happy with single-vision, bifocal or trifocal lenses; this includes those who are not disturbed by or conscious of the segment top in multifocals
- Patients who are not prepared to gamble on the chance of adapting to the lenses or who are not prepared to wait an indeterminate time for adaptation to occur.

Perhaps of just as much significance in the successful dispensing and acceptance of progressive power lenses by new wearers is the confidence shown by the practitioner when prescribing this design for the correction of presbyopia and when demonstrating their use at the final fitting. Needless to say, the advantages of progressive designs over other forms of multifocal correction should be spelt out in simple terms at the time of dispensing:

- 'These lenses will enable you to focus at all distances'
- To first-time young presbyopes: 'These lenses will be easier to get used to than bifocal lenses'
- 'In wear, these lenses will restore the vision of youth'
- 'There are no tell-tale dividing lines on the lenses'.

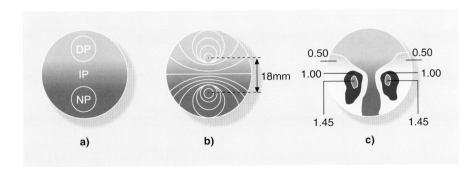

a)   b)   0.50   0.50   1.00   1.00   18mm   1.45   1.45   c)

Figure 12.19 The *AO Omni* design: (a) the power distribution is similar to an up-and-downcurve trifocal lens; (b) blending the surfaces between the poles results in a soft peripheral design; (c) the result is very low levels of surface astigmatism

At final collection it is important to re-emphasize these advantages and demonstrate the use of the lenses.

A suggested routine for the final delivery of progressive lenses to patients when they come to collect their new spectacles is as follows. Firstly, make sure when checking the lenses that not only are the powers at their recommended measuring points and the prism at the prism reference point as ordered, but also that the horizontal painted lines are parallel to the line joining the centres of the engraved circles. Also ensure that the position of the fitting cross on each lens has been restored so that it is clearly visible:

- The frame into which the lenses are mounted should have been set up to fit the subject properly at the time of dispensing. However, the lens-mounting process may have disturbed the initial set-up of the frame, so it is important to ensure that the frame is returned to the adjustment made when the lens measurements were taken. Any small final adjustments that may be needed at the time of final fitting should be undertaken first.
- Verify that the positions of the fitting crosses do coincide with the centres of the subject's pupils. The same procedure as used to dot the desired fitting-cross positions should be adopted.
- Clean off the painted marks completely and ensure that the lenses and frame look like new.
- Direct the subject to look at a distant object directly in front and verify that the anticipated visual acuity is obtained for distance vision.
- Direct the subject to look at a laterally placed object at the same height as the straight-ahead distance target and point out, if required, that it might be necessary to turn the head to obtain optimum acuity for this object.
- Direct the subject to look at a test chart at near, which you should guide into the subject's hands so that it is held directly in front in the usual reading position, and verify that the anticipated acuity for near vision is obtained.
- Direct the subject to move the near chart to one side and again ensure that the subject understands that the head may need to be turned to point the nose in the direction of view to see the near target clearly.
- Move the near test target to a position about 40 to 50 cm directly in front of the subject and just below the original object chosen to verify the distance acuity. Point out that the subject can also see clearly at the intermediate distance, if necessary with a slight adjustment of the visual axes in the vertical meridian. In particular, let the subject confirm that the gaze can be transferred from the distant target to the intermediate target without moving the head, simply by adjusting the direction of gaze of the subject's eyes.
- Point out the visual tasks that are not easy with progressive power lenses, such as reading a notice with small print above head height, reading when lying down or trying to watch television when lying down in bed.

Most important of all is to reassure the subject that the visual tasks are well understood, as is the optical performance of the progressive lenses, and that most people need no more than a short period to become used to this state-of-the-art correction for presbyopia.

In cases of anisometropia, base down prism may be slabbed-off a progressive lens to eliminate vertical differential prismatic effect in exactly the same way as with a bifocal lens. It is possible to blend the bi-prism ridge if it is desired to maintain the appearance of a single vision lens but this leaves a horizontal blended band which, although invisible to observers, the subject must learn to ignore when passing from distance to the progressive intermediate zone.

Occupational progressive power lenses

As presbyopia advances, the drawbacks of a single-vision correction become more obvious. Single-vision lenses do not offer the range of vision required to perform intermediate and near tasks. Progressive power lenses offer a greater working range, but a drawback of these lenses is the narrower intermediate and reading fields they offer when the reading addition increases.

It is stated above that when the reading addition decreases and the length of the progression zone increases, the smaller becomes the blended areas of the lens and the larger the areas of the lens free from surface aberrations. This effect can be achieved by prescribing lenses intended only for intermediate and near use in those circumstances in which a distance vision correction is not needed. Progressive power lenses designed for these purposes are available, either with just intermediate and near portions for use, say, at the computer workstation, or as a half-eye design that also provides some intermediate vision. Some manufacturers even describe these designs as *single-vision lenses for reading*.

The reduction in power provided from near to intermediate has been described as a power *degression*, so that, for example, a progressive power design that has an addition from distance to near of +1.00D might also be described as a design that has a degression of −1.00 from near to distance.

The Essilor *Interview* is designed for use at the workstation, either for desk use or at the VDU. The design has a fixed addition across its progression zone of either +0.80D, or +1.30D obtained at a point 18° below the major reference point, which is designed to be positioned in front of the centre of the pupil (Figure 12.20). The reading prescription is effective at this point.

The power degression of the lens is −0.80D (or −1.30D) from the reading zone to the intermediate zone; it is the relatively small change in surface power, combined with the low level of surface astigmatism, that provides such a wide and stable field of clear vision across the lens.

Adaptation to such a soft design is claimed to be as easy as with single-vision lenses. Also, the wide field of vision means that wearers need only scan from side to side across the lens, rather than having to turn their heads, as would be necessary with the usual progressive designs.

When checking the prescription, the back vertex power measured at the power checking circle should correspond to the ordered near vision prescription. It has been suggested that the advantages of this occupational design can be demonstrated quite quickly to prospective wearers simply by holding up −0.75D lenses in front of the subject's reading correction. The advantages of the increased range of vision should be apparent immediately. The lenses are easy to dispense; the mounting reference line is designed to be fitted so that it is tangential with the lower edge of the iris. It is recommended that the lens be ordered in terms of the subject's reading prescription.

The *Cosmolit P* from Rodenstock is a shallow base, low-power aspheric design described as a variable power lens for near vision, and is recommended for use by VDU users or those who require greater flexibility for near vision than is provided by a simple single-vision lens. The viewing range that the design offers, when prescribed as suggested by Rodenstock, is from some 80 cm to 100 cm in the intermediate field, down to approximately 25 cm in the near field. The lens is especially suited to activities that require

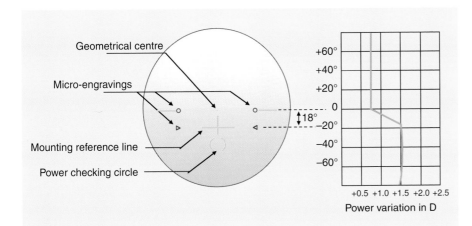

Figure 12.20 Essilor *Interview* 080 occupational progressive design with near vision prescription +1.50D

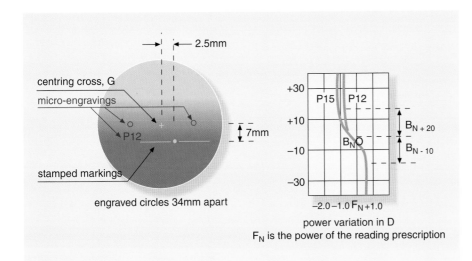

Figure 12.21 *Cosmolit P* occupational progressive power design from Rodenstock

wide viewing fields at intermediate and near, without impairment of visual acuity and with minimum distortion in lateral regions of the lens. Mechanically, the lens is thin and light because of its aspheric form and the incorporation of thinning prism. The power range is from –2.00D to +4.00D in the maximum meridian, with cylinders up to +3.00D and a built-in variation of either 1.25D or 1.50D depending upon the power ordered. The power profile for the *Cosmolit P* design is illustrated in Figure 12.21. The reading prescription is effective at the near reference point, B_N, which lies 7mm below the geometrical centre of the lens, G, and it is the near vision prescription that should be ordered, determined for a working distance of 40cm.

When checking the prescription, the back vertex power measured at B_N should correspond to the near prescription. The power variation provided is indicated on the lens by a micro-engraving. The lens is marked *P12* in the case of the 1.25D power variation or *P15* in the case of the 1.50D power variation.

For near vision powers up to +1.75D, the power variation is 1.25D, and for the near vision power range +2.00 to +4.00D, the power variation is 1.50D. Below the near reference point there is a power increase over 10mm of +0.50D for all powers. Above the near reference point there is a decrease in power of –0.75D in the case of the *P12* designs or –1.00D with the *P15* designs.

When the *Cosmolit P* design is to be mounted in a full-depth frame, Rodenstock recommends that the fitting crosses be centred horizontally, according to the monocular CDs for distance vision. The near reference points are automatically decentred 2.5mm

inwards from these points. In the vertical meridian, the fitting crosses should satisfy the centre of rotation condition, with the same care being taken as with all aspheric lenses.

When the *Cosmolit P* is to be mounted in a half-eye frame, Rodenstock recommends that the fitting cross be positioned 12mm below the top edge of the lens and that there should be a depth of at least 16mm below the fitting cross (i.e. the minimum depth of lens should be 28mm).

The *AO Technica* (available from American Optical) is also designed mainly for intermediate and near use, but (unlike the occupational progressive designs described above) it has a small area on the lens that incorporates the distance prescription. AO is quick to point out that the lens is an occupational lens designed for use when intermediate and near vision is paramount, the small zone for distance vision being available, effectively, only when the subject looks straight ahead (Figure 12.22). The distance reference point and the near reference points are separated by 28mm. Such a design offers a very comfortable solution for a presbyope who spends long periods at the desk or at a computer workstation and is prepared to use a pair of spectacles specifically for work. The narrow distance field, however, prevents the subject from using the lenses, say, for driving.

The areas on the lens at which the blending process produces surface astigmatism are shown in Figure 12.22. Just like its parent design, the *Omni*, the surface astigmatism is quite low, the isocylinder diagram indicating the small areas on the lens where it reaches 1.00D. When used as an occupational design as intended,

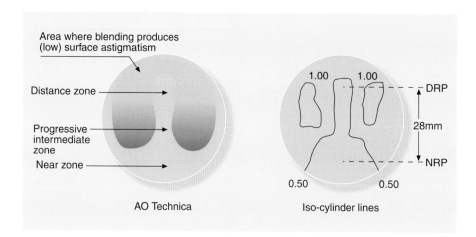

Figure 12.22 The *AO Technica*: an occupational progressive power lens designed mainly for intermediate and near vision use

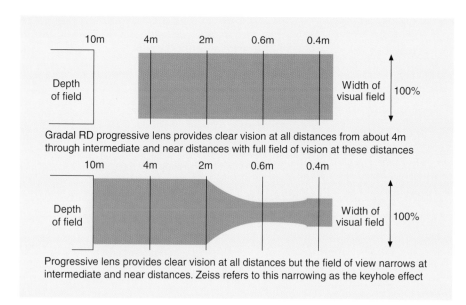

Figure 12.23 Comparison of field of vision and depth of field of progressive design for intermediate and near with the fields provided by a normal progressive lens (after Zeiss)

it provides a more than adequate field of vision for intermediate and near vision.

The Zeiss *Clarlet Gradal RD* is a progressive lens specifically designed for use as an indoor lens. Whatever distance prescription is ordered (currently −7.00 to +6.50D in the strongest meridian, with cylinders to +6.00D), Zeiss add +0.50D of the total reading addition to the DP and the rest of the addition is then provided in progressive addition form. Thus, if the prescription +3.00 Add +2.00 is required, the *Gradal RD* is supplied with a power of +3.50 in the upper portion of the lens and an addition of +1.50 then takes place down to the near reference point, at which the power becomes +5.00D. This expedient ensures wide intermediate and near fields. Zeiss claim that the whole width of the lens offers comfortable vision without the narrowing of field encountered with normal progressive power lenses (Figure 12.23). The design offers good vision at all distances within an indoor environment, with less head movement, faster recognition of detail and freedom of movement when walking around indoors. The elliptical shaped uncut produced using the *Optima* technique ensures that the lens is as thin and light in weight as possible (Figure 12.24). Zeiss suggest that the *Gradal RD* is dispensed as a second, vocational pair of spectacles for subjects who already have a first pair of progressive power lenses for ordinary use.

The Sola *Access* series of reading lenses is designed to provide clear vision from the near point out to about 3 metres. The NP of the design incorporates the full reading correction and the upper portion, designed for mid-range vision, is simply reduced in power by −1.25D. There is a 12mm progression zone between the upper IP and the NP of the design (Figure 12.25).

Sola point out that *Access* is not designed to be a progressive power lens in the same way as lenses intended for distance, intermediate and near use. They describe the design as an improved reading lens, in that the lower portion of the lens can be used for near vision, just like any other conventional correction for presbyopia, but state that the upper portion provides clear intermediate viewing without the need to remove the lenses, as is necessary if single-vision readers are worn.

Fitting the design is claimed to be very easy, with the suggestion that the major reference point (referred to as the fitting point) is fitted 3–5mm below the pupil centre. The fitting point is located at the geometrical centre of the lens (Figure 12.26).

The current prescription range (near vision powers) is from −2.00D to +4.00D with cylinders to +4.00. The lens diameter is 75mm and the lenses can be coated with *Perma Tough* and *UTMC*.

The designers of *Access* deliberately aimed the lens at the late presbyope who does not need, or wear, a conventional multifocal design. Consider a subject who does not need a correction for distance vision and who wears a pair of +2.00D single vision lenses for near. Ignoring depth-of-field effects, when wearing conventional single vision lenses this subject's artificial far point would lie 50cm in front of the lenses. If a pair of *Access* lenses is dispensed, the upper portion of the lens, described as the intermediate viewing area in Figure 12.25, would have a power of only +0.75D (1.25D less than the near correction) and the artificial far point through this design would lie 133cm in front of the lens. Since the 'addition' of this progressive power lens is only +1.25D, the corridor in which the surface astigmatism is low is very wide, just as with the other occupational progressive power lenses considered above.

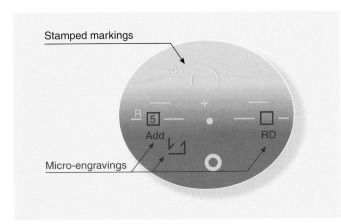

Figure 12.24 Zeiss Clarlet *Gradal RD* occupational progressive power lens

The physiological aspects of the lens should be considered carefully if it is to be dispensed in cases of early presbyopia when the reading addition is low. For example, a low hypermetrope, whose prescription is +0.25 Add +0.75 for near, if dispensed *Access* lenses would effectively be wearing −0.25 Add +1.25 and may not enjoy the benefits to be obtained from a simple +1.00 sphere for near.

The Nikon on*line* design (Figure 12.27) is an occupational progressive lens design available with three different degression powers, 1.00D, 1.50D and 2.00D. If a specific degression is not ordered the following standard values are supplied:

- Adds +1.50 degression = 1.00
- Adds 1.75 to 2.25 degression = 1.50
- Adds 2.50 and above degression = 2.00

However, the degression can be ordered individually as required by the practitioner. For this design, Nikon recommend that the fitting cross be positioned in front of the centre of the pupil and that the ordering data include the distance prescription, the addition power, the required degression power and the individual fitting-point positions.

Availability of progressive power lenses

At the last count, there were some 75 to 80 different 'brands' of progressive power lenses available around the world. However, the casting process for plastics lenses has brought lens production into the era of '*He who has the moulds can make the lenses!*' so

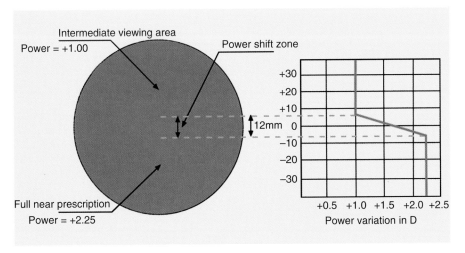

Figure 12.25 Sola *Access* occupational progressive design with near vision prescription +2.25D

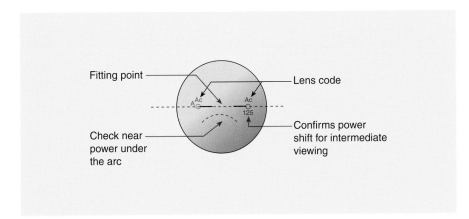

Figure 12.26 Sola *Access* occupational progressive design. The markings in blue are ink markings; those in grey are permanently etched

that, in truth, there are probably no more than 25–30 intrinsically different designs being made. Progressive surface moulds can be bought easily from mould manufacturers such as Shamir/Eyal in Israel, Polycore in Singapore and even in the UK from Crossbows Optical. It should be apparent that the finished progressive lens, brand *X* from company *A*, might also be brand *Y* from company *B*. Partly for this reason, it is very difficult to assess new products in a truly objective way. Neither is it helpful to see the same design being advertised with different isocylinder plots and different claims about its corridor width because different conditions have been applied to the measuring method. More than one new progressive design has been introduced to the marketplace with hype from the distributor, who often does not know the real source of the lens. The supplier (assuming that the distributor did not do the casting) will know from whom the moulds were originally obtained, but the mould supplier will probably not have provided any information from which the design can be assessed. From the prescriber's point of view, the progressive-lens marketplace is a minefield within which the reputation of the manufacturer provides the only real guide to success.

A good demonstration of the difficulties of predicting success with a given type of lens is obtained by considering the isocylinder zones of simpler lens forms, such as single vision designs. Figure 12.28 illustrates the 0.25D isocylinder and iso-mean power plots for a +4.00D spherical lens made with a –1.50D base curve (the optical performance of this design is considered in detail in

Chapter 2). This form is said to provide a flatter, thinner lens than the usual, more steeply curved, best-form design. If the manufacturer decides that the zone of clear vision should be defined as the zone in which the aberrational astigmatism does not exceed 0.50D, it can be seen that the lens might be described as having an effective aperture of some 28mm. Alternatively, if the zone of clear vision is defined as the zone within which the spherical mean power does not vary by more than 0.50D, the lens could be described as having an effective aperture of 35mm.

If, on the other hand, a more enterprising manufacturer decided that the zones of clear vision are those within which the errors do not exceed 1.00D, the lens might be described as having 'an effective aperture of 35mm within which the inevitable cylinder is insignificant...' or, 'an effective aperture of 46mm within which the mean spherical power does not depart significantly from the design value...'.

Recent developments in progressive power lenses

Varilux Panamic

Essilor's policy of striving to perfect the Varilux lens has led to a new design that retains all the benefits of the *Comfort* progressive power lens and achieves an even smoother surface topography

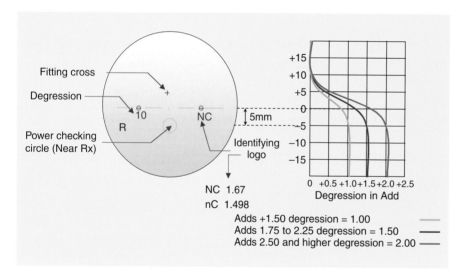

Figure 12.27   Nikon On*line* occupational progressive design

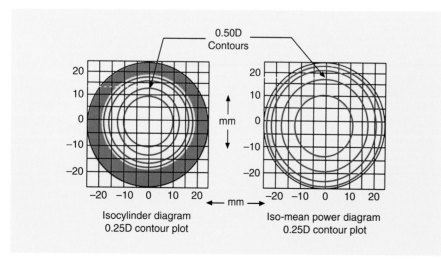

Figure 12.28   Isocylinder and iso-mean power diagrams for +4.00D sphere made with –1.50D base curve

in the periphery of the lens. This enables the designer to address the comfort of the overall field of vision and provide a significant improvement in the overall effect of the lens in wear. *Varilux Panamic* was positioned as the premier Varilux product alongside *Varilux Comfort* and *Varilux Liberty*, which continue to be offered in the Varilux range.

Essilor describe the enhanced performance of the Panamic design as global vision.[6] Just what is meant by this term can be deduced from Figures 12.29 and 12.30.

Ophthalmic lens design is normally concerned only with foveal vision, in which the resolution is highest and the visual acuity is at its maximum. Figure 12.29 shows how the visual acuity varies across the retina out to about 40° from the fixation line, at which the relative visual acuity drops almost to zero. At just 10° from the fixation line the relative visual acuity has dropped to about 0.2.

The criterion for a best-form spectacle lens is that it should produce a good-quality image on the fovea. Provided the distortion produced by the correcting lens is not excessive and, particularly, not significantly different from the distortion to which a subject has become accustomed from a previous pair of spectacle lenses, the brain interprets the scene as rectilinear. It is well known that, in most cases, the brain adapts easily to small changes in distortion.

Figure 12.30 illustrates the concept of global vision. The observer is looking out of a window at a distant scene and fixating the triangular roof of the skyscraper in the middle of the field, which is supposed to be about 1000 metres away (Figure 12.30a). In the horizontal meridian, the fovea subtends about 0.018 radians at the eye's nodal point, which would provide a horizontal field of some 18 metres at 1000 metres, within which the eye could obtain maximum resolution (Figure 12.30b).

The subject may well be aware of an aircraft passing in front of the sun in the peripheral field, especially if the movement of the aircraft is rapid, even though it lies some distance from the line of fixation. If the magnification produced by the lens in the peripheral field is irregular, because of rapid changes in the shape of the surface, peripheral objects will appear to change direction. This is often described as a 'swimming' effect by the new wearer of progressive lenses, as images viewed through peripheral portions of the right and left lenses apparently move at different speeds.

The swimming effect is a combination of distortion produced by the increasing power between the distance and near portions and changes that take place in surface topography as a result of trying to achieve the correct blend between the various zones of the lens. The influence of distortion is summarized in Figure 12.31. In general, minus lenses produce barrel distortion, whereas plus lenses produce pincushion distortion (Figures 12.31a–c). With low-power lenses these effects are rarely noticed. In the case of progressive lenses, the power of the lens increases from distance to near by the value of the addition. There is an accompanying increase in magnification, which causes vertical lines viewed through the progression zone to slant (Figure 12.31d). In designing the *Panamic* lens, Essilor developed a new ray-tracing system that gives the position in space of the various components of the visual scene. A net, rather like the object shown in Figure 12.31a, is superimposed upon the visual scene and the positions of the intersections of the net in the image space calculated by ray

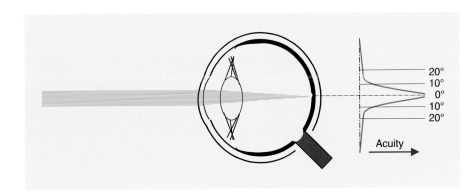

Figure 12.29 Variation in visual acuity across the retina. Maximum acuity occurs in foveal vision, an area that subtends some 0.018 by 0.012 radians at the nodal point. At 10° from the fovea the relative visual acuity falls to 0.2. Note the section chosen does not pass through the optic disc, at which the acuity would fall to zero

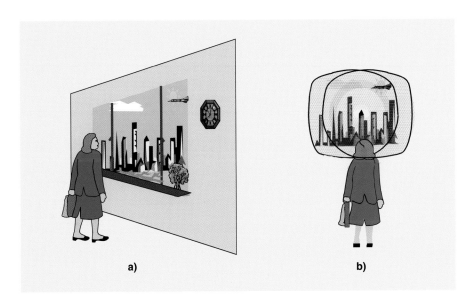

a)   b)

Figure 12.30 The concept of global vision. (a) The subject views a distant scene and fixates the triangular roof of the distant skyscraper (note there is an aircraft crossing in front of the sun). (b) The subject, fixating the triangular roof of the distant skyscraper, is aware of the movement of the aircraft near the edge of the field of vision (despite its image being blurred), since it lies within the field of vision, even though the aircraft's image falls on a peripheral portion of the retina

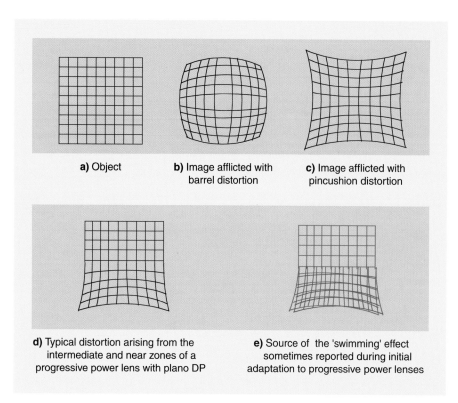

a) Object   **b)** Image afflicted with barrel distortion   **c)** Image afflicted with pincushion distortion

d) Typical distortion arising from the intermediate and near zones of a progressive power lens with plano DP

e) Source of the 'swimming' effect sometimes reported during initial adaptation to progressive power lenses

Figure 12.31   Distortion and its application to progressive power lenses. The object shown in (a) for the study of distortion can be superimposed on the visual scene and the positions of the images corresponding to each intersection of the 'net' calculated by ray tracing through the lens. The method is used to compare the positions of the images obtained by the right and left eyes and, thus, calculate the swim caused by the lenses

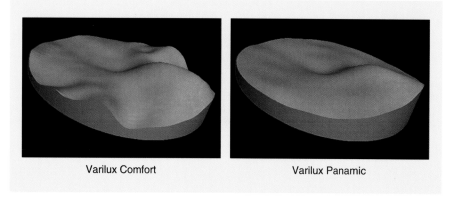

Varilux Comfort   Varilux Panamic

Figure 12.32   Comparison of the surface topography of Varilux *Comfort* and Varilux *Panamic*. Note the smooth change in power with the Panamic design at the periphery of the intermediate portion

tracing through the lens. The positions of the images produced by the right and left lenses are calculated and, by superimposing the two images, an indication is obtained of the relative speed difference between the movements of the right and left images in the peripheral field when the eyes rotate to view various parts of the scene (Figure 12.31e).

The effect can be visualized from Figure 12.31e, in which the field obtained with one eye through the progression and near zones is drawn in green and the field obtained with the other eye in red. Ideally, as the eye rotates behind the lens the two fields should correspond exactly to form the binocular image. If the fields do not coincide, as depicted in Figure 12.31e, and worse, if the separation increases and decreases as the eyes roam to use different zones of the lens, the scene appears to swim.

The real breakthrough achieved in the *Panamic* design is the reduction of the swim effects in progressive power lenses, obtained by ensuring that the power increases steadily from the progression zone to the near zone, particularly in the peripheral portions of the lens. The smoothing of the surface is clearly visible in Figure 12.32, which compares the surface topography of

the Varilux *Comfort* design on the left, with that of the *Panamic* design on the right.

The new design has been subjected to critical wearer tests, which combined objective measurements, subjective measurements and wearer feedback from those who wore the new design in everyday life. In a Pan-European wearer test carried out between June and November 1999, the results reported by the 631 presbyopic subjects showed that 95% of Varilux *Panamic* wearers were satisfied with their new lenses, claiming wide fields of vision at all distances, and speedy adaptation to the new design.[7] As the previous benchmark was the *Comfort* design, it was natural to compare *Panamic* with *Comfort*; this specific wearer test was carried out on a sample of 93 wearers with prescriptions between −4.00D and +3.00D, with additions varying between +0.75D and +2.75D (Figure 12.33). The various criteria shown in Figure 12.33 were noted on a scale between 0 and 10, and it is seen that no criterion scored less than seven on this scale (which starts at six in Figure 12.33). On all the chosen criteria, the results obtained by *Panamic* are superior to those for *Comfort*, with the most significant improvement in the criterion of global vision. The most

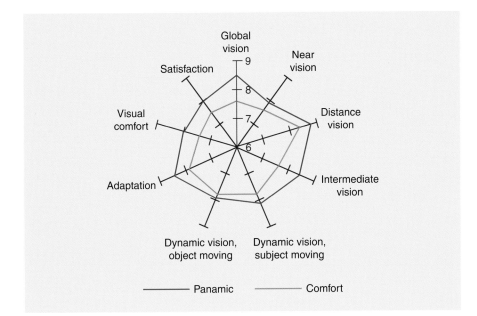

Figure 12.33 Results of wearer tests to compare Varilux *Panamic* and Varilux *Comfort* designs. The criteria used were noted on a scale between 0 and 10. On the graph, notation axes begin at six in the centre and end at nine at the outer edges

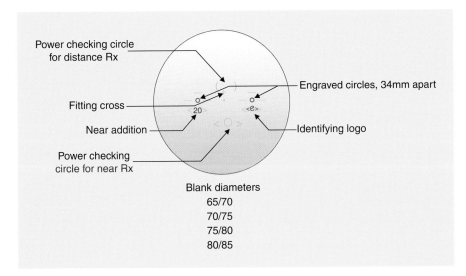

Figure 12.34 Markings on Varilux *Panamic* designs in the current range offered in the UK. The yellow markings are painted on the lenses and removed after final dispensing has taken place

important reason why subjects preferred the new design was the wider field of vision.

Integrating the binocular prismatic effects with the individual insetting required for different base curves and near additions resulted in 72 different surface designs to cover the range. Currently the *Panamic* design is being offered in both plastics and glass materials (Figure 12.34):

- *Orma* – 1.5
- *Airwear* – 1.586
- *Stylis* – 1.67
- *Lineis* – 1.74
- *Glass* – 1.60
- *Glass* – 1.80

Other recent designs

The latest generation of progressive lens designs from other manufacturers combine atoroidal concave surfaces with low-base aspherical progressive power surfaces, to offer optimal performance from the designs when the prescription incorporates a cylinder. For example, the *Multigressiv* design from Rodenstock has an atoroidal concave surface, designed to provide optimum correction, not just for the prescribed cylinder power, but, in combination with the aspherical progressive surface, to improve the optical performance of each zone of the lens.

Seiko P-1SY progressive lens

Until the end of the 20th century, with the exception of the Essel *Variplas* design of the 1960s, the progressive power was generally incorporated on the convex surface of the lens. This enabled the finishing laboratory to work any cylinder on the concave side using their normal surfacing machinery and without the need for a large range of plus base toric tools with compensated cylinder powers. In 1996, a patent[8] was applied for by H. Mukaiyama and K. Kato of the Seiko Epson Corporation of Japan (the US Patent was granted in 2000) for a progressive lens which had a concave surface which incorporated both the progression and any correction for astigmatism. The convex surface of the lens was a simple spherical or aspherical surface and the concave surface was either a progressive power surface in the case of spherical prescriptions or a progressive surface of atoroidal form in the case of astigmatic prescriptions (Figure 12.35).

A typical concave progressive surface was described in the patent by its x, y, z coordinates (Figure 12.35) and, in theory, the surface could be manufactured by programming the CNC generator to reproduce these points. However, the representation in Figure 12.35 gives x and y in 5mm intervals and in practice, the intervals may need to be as close as 0.25mm! Since the surface is described by its x, y, z coordinates rather than by a mathematical equation, it is described as a *freeform* surface.

Seiko market this lens as their *P-1SY* progressive design but have now made the software available to any company to buy and produce their own freeform surfaces.

Rodenstock Multigressiv [ILT]

Rodenstock introduced their original *Multigressiv* design in 1995. With *Multigressiv* 2 came on-line optimization of the concave surface with an aspherical surface being applied to spherical prescriptions and an atoroidal surface being used when the prescription calls for a cylindrical correction. Manufacture of the concave surface of the lens can only begin when all the prescription data is to hand, since the form of the atoroidal surface depends not only on the base curve, but also on the cylinder power, axis direction and the inset required for the lens. This technology required the development of special software for rapid computation of the second side.

The *Multigressiv[ILT]* applies Individual Lens Technology (ILT) to the design, which enables the optimum progressive power surface to be computed individually for each lens from knowledge of the prescription data and base curve of the lens. With this new design, the progressive surface has been switched from the front to the back surface of the lens, which, in the case of astigmatic prescriptions, also incorporates the cylindrical correction. The front surface of the lens is a simple spherical surface, with the near addition and necessary aspheric correction for the form built into the concave surface. With astigmatic prescriptions, the concave surface is an atoroidal progressive one (Figure 12.36). One advantage of this method of construction is that the geometrical inset is no longer dependent on the convex surface geometry, when the inset is fixed by the progressive surface geometry, but can now be calculated individually for the lens prescription. Correct positioning of the meridian line results in larger clear-vision zones for distance and near, and a wider progressive zone with smooth transition to the lens periphery.[8]

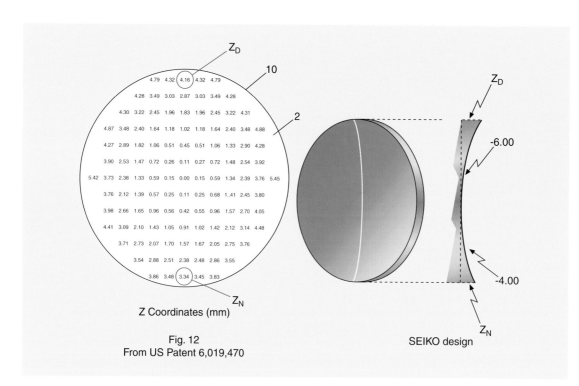

Z Coordinates (mm)

Fig. 12
From US Patent 6,019,470

SEIKO design

Figure 12.35   Freeform description of a concave atoroidal progressive power surface of the type found on the Seiko *P-1SY Progressive lens* design

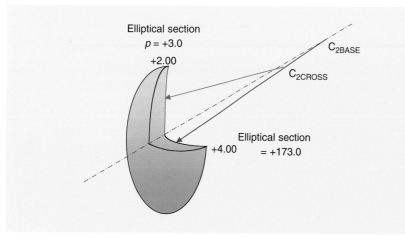

Figure 12.36   Atoroidal surface that incorporates the cylindrical correction and possesses different asphericities along each meridian of the surface. This type of surface is employed by Rodenstock for their *Multigressiv* design and by Zeiss (optimum surface design) for their *Gradal* series of progressive power lenses. Simple conic sections are assumed here for the purposes of demonstration

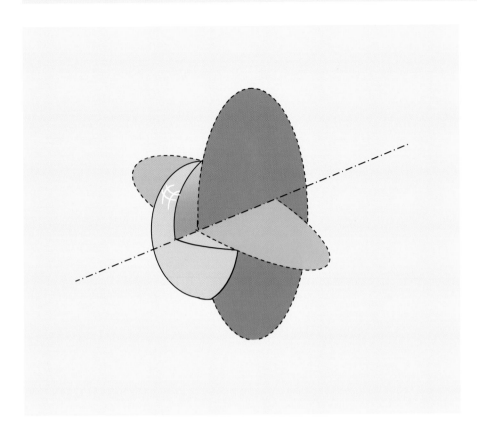

Figure 12.37 The atoral lens, a toric lens with an atoroidal surface, was introduced in 1970 by Essel Optical Company (now Essilor International) to improve the optical performance of deep plus astigmatic lenses, required for the correction of aphakia. Each principal meridian of the concave surface is of oblate elliptical cross-section, the *p*-values decreasing from a maximum along the base curve to a minimum along the cross curve. A progressive version was also made available, the Atoral *Variplas*

The geometry of this atoroidal progressive surface can be visualized as a concave toroidal surface to which asphericity is applied to form a surface of the type illustrated in Figure 12.37. The heights of each point on this atoroidal surface (the *z*-values) are then known. To provide the progressive power property to the surface, the *z*-values in the lower portion of the lens must be decreased by stipulated amounts to obtain the necessary decrease in power along each meridian to form the progression and near zones.

Figure 12.38 shows the principal curvatures at a point, P, on the concave surface of an atoroidal progressive surface. At the vertex, A_2, the principal sections are oblate ellipses, as depicted in Figure 12.38. At point P the radii of curvature of both the base curve and the cross curve are increased to produce the reading addition, and the asphericity of the elliptical sections through P are also altered to optimize the performance at this point in the NP. Traces of the altered sections through P are depicted in Figure 12.38. Effectively, each elliptical section evolves from a minimum vertex radius at A_2, with a given value for the asphericity factor, *p*, to a maximum vertex radius at P with a new value for the asphericity factor, *p'*.

In the case of a progressive lens that incorporates a cylinder power of $-1.50DC \times 180$ and a reading addition of $+2.00D$, the power of the toroidal surface for the DP may be $-6.50DC \times 90/ -8.00DC \times 180$, when the required power for the NP would be $-4.50DC \times 90/-6.00DC \times 180$. The changes in radii of curvature along one meridian (the vertical cross-curve meridian of Figures 12.38 and 12.39) are illustrated in Figure 12.39, which shows the locus of the centres of curvature for the cross-curve meridian (the evolute for the cross curve) between the points, A_2 and P.

Rodenstock Impression[ILT]

The *Impression*[ILT] lens is Rodenstock's new flagship progressive power lens design. Just like the *Multigressiv*[ILT], it has a concave progressive power surface, which is combined with the cylinder in the case of astigmatic lenses, but can also incorporate the precise

positioning of the lens in its design. In addition to the individual CDs and progression heights, practitioners can submit the vertex distance, pantoscopic angle and the dihedral (face form) angle of the front. The dihedral angle takes into account the bow of the front of the frame and may be defined as the angle between a vertical tangent plane to the front surface of the frame and the vertical plane tangential to the front surface of the lens (Figure 12.40). Note that the dihedral angle could differ for each lens!

The computer software allows input of all the different fitting parameters as variables in deciding the optimum form of the concave surface, so the resultant lens is custom designed for the individual fitting of the frame to the face.

Zeiss Gradal Individual

The *Gradal HS* and *Gradal Top* progressive designs are enhanced versions of the Zeiss *Gradal 3* design that offer optimum surface design (OSD), in which the concave toroidal surface combines both the astigmatic power with aspheric corrections along each principal meridian of the lens.

In 2000 a new, custom-designed progressive power lens was launched by Zeiss, based upon the *Gradal* design. With the new Zeiss lens, a convex progressive surface is employed and the lens completed by incorporating an aspherical or atoroidal concave surface as the prescription demands. This method of construction used to be employed for the earlier *Gradal OSD* lens, but the new aspect of the *Gradal Individual* design is the ability to incorporate precise positioning of the lens in the design. Again, in addition to the individual CDs and fitting-point heights, practitioners can submit the vertex distance and pantoscopic angle relating to the frame fitting, which Zeiss then incorporate in the design of the progressive power surface.[9]

Effectively, the design process first determines the parameters of the concave surface, assuming a given progressive surface

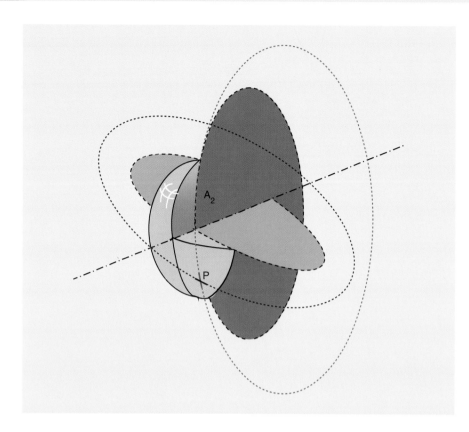

Figure 12.38 Atoroidal progressive surface showing principal sections through the back vertex, A_2, and through a point, P, in the near portion. At the back vertex, A_2, the principal curvatures are the same as those depicted for the single vision atoral design shown in Figure 12.37. The curvature of the surface decreases through the progression zone by the value of the reading addition, and the asphericity of the principal section also changes as necessary to optimize the optical performance. Note the principal sections may not be the simple conics illustrated here

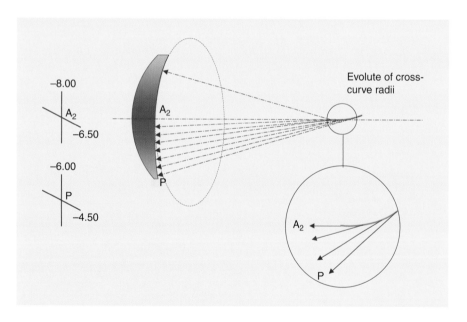

Figure 12.39 Evolute of the cross-curve radii for the vertical section of the lens depicted in Figure 12.38. The evolute is the locus of the instantaneous tangential centres of curvature of the surface between A_2 and P. To obtain an addition of +2.00D the cross-curve power must decrease from −8.00D in the distance portion to −6.00D in the near portion. If the cylinder power is −1.50D, the base-curve power at right angles to the cross curve changes from −6.50D to −4.50D

design, and then recomputes the progressive surface to take into account the individual fitting values supplied by the practitioner. New algorithms have been developed that allow the progressive surface to be designed in about 20 seconds, instead of the former 2 to 3 hours of interactive work with the computer.

Individually designed progressive power lenses should remove the uncertainties of what happens when the progressive surface is combined with a strong cylinder power, perhaps with an oblique axis. Widening the zones in which the inherent surface astigmatism might be a problem must be of particular benefit to first-time wearers and may prove to be the solution for those subjects who have not been able to adapt to progressive lenses in the past.

Hoyalux iD

Described as an integrated double surface design, the *Hoyalux iD* lens had its near addition incorporated partly on the convex surface and partly on the concave surface. In the design of the lens Hoya have incorporated the progressive component that gives rise to a vertical change in power on the convex surface of the lens and the progressive component that gives rise to the horizontal change in power on the concave surface. A simple simulation of how this results in a spherical increase in power in the near portion is obtained by considering the magnification effects of two plano-cylinders that have been combined at right angles to one another.

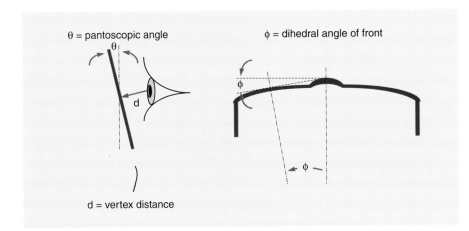

Figure 12.40 Pantoscopic and dihedral angles of the spectacle front. The dihedral angle is defined as the angle between a vertical tangent plane to the front surface of the frame and the vertical plane tangential to the front surface of the lens

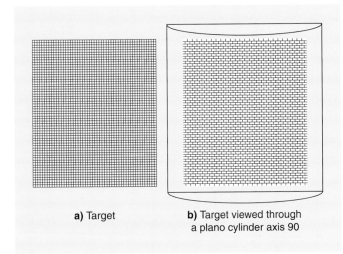

a) Target

b) Target viewed through a plano cylinder axis 90

Figure 12.41 (a) The target (b) Meridional magnification by a plano-cylinder axis 90. This element can be considered to represent the horizontal progressive power component.

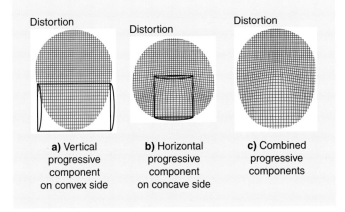

a) Vertical progressive component on convex side

b) Horizontal progressive component on concave side

c) Combined progressive components

Figure 12.42 (a) The vertical progressive component on the convex side. (b) The horizontal progressive component on the concave side. (c) The vertical and horizontal progressive power components combine to produce the progression zone and near portion.

Figure 12.41a illustrates a target in the form of graph paper, which is viewed through a plano-convex cylinder with its axis vertical (Figure 12.41b). Since the cylinder has power only at right angles to its axis, the squares are magnified in the horizontal meridian only and when viewed through the cylinder, appear as horizontal rectangles.

In Figure 12.42a, the target is shown with a plano-convex cylinder placed with its axis horizontal over the progression area to represent the vertical progression components whilst in Figure 12.42b the plano-convex cylinder has been placed with its axis vertical over the progression area to represent the horizontal progression components.

The result is shown in Figure 12.42c; the magnifications combine to produce images which are the same shape as the object over most of the central field.

If the magnification produced by the lens in the peripheral field is irregular, due to rapid changes in the shape of the surface, peripheral objects will appear to change direction. This is the 'swimming' effect reported by new wearers of progressive lenses, as images viewed through peripheral portions of the right and left lenses apparently move at different speeds.

The swimming effect is a combination of distortion produced by the increasing power between the distance and near portions and changes which take place in surface topography as the result of trying to achieve the correct blend between the various zones

of the lens. The effect is particularly troublesome to the new progressive lens wearer especially when looking at the floor, or walking down stairs, when the visual system is attempting to process information which is arriving from oblique sight directions.

Hoya have considered this problem in some detail and derived a method whereby they can control the deformation using the concept of a *point deformation index*. They represent each point in object space as a small circle and calculate, by ray tracing through the lens, the spectacle magnification throughout the progression zone and near portion of the lens. If the spectacle magnification is the same in every direction, then the circles which describe the object points will be imaged as circles and apart from the magnification itself, there will be no deformation produced by the lens for each point.

Spectacle magnification (the ratio of the retinal image size in the corrected eye to that in the uncorrected eye) can be expressed in terms of the two angles, ω' and ω as shown in Figure 12.43. The object point, Q, is represented by the circle of radius q and the image formed by the lens is seen to be drawn out into an ellipse of semi-major axis, a, and semi-minor axis b. The spectacle magnification for each of the meridians a and b is expressed as:

$$SM_a = a/q$$

and

$$SM_b = b/q.$$

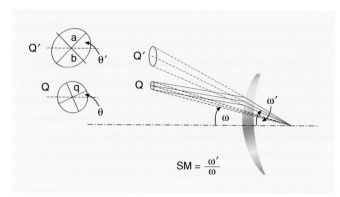

Figure 12.43 Spectacle magnification is the ratio of retinal image size in the corrected eye to that in the corrected eye. SM can be shown to be the ratio of the angle subtended by the image, ω', at the eye's entrance pupil, E, to the angle subtended by the object, ω, at the entrance pupil. Note that in the case of the lens illustrated, an infinitely small object point Q, represented by a circle, is drawn out into an ellipse whose major axis might be tilted out of the azimuth of the object meridian under consideration.

The figure illustrates a severe case of deformation where it can be seen that not only are the two spectacle magnifications different, but the azimuth of *a* differs from the azimuth of *q* (θ' is greater than θ).

The point deformation index, *P*, is defined as:

$$P = (a - b)/b$$

and depends only upon the shape of the spectacle magnification ellipse. It does not describe its orientation. It is immediately apparent from Figure 12.44 that when the spectacle magnification ellipse has its major axis vertical or horizontal it does not trouble the wearer as much as when the major axis lies obliquely. The ellipses drawn alongside each view show the orientation of the major axis of the ellipse.

The normal point deformation index, P_N, is at a maximum when $\theta_b = 0°$ or when $\theta_b = 90°$ and represents the deformation component along the horizontal and the vertical meridians respectively.

The skew point deformation index, P_S, is at a maximum when $\theta_b = 45°$ or when $\theta_b = 135°$ and represents the deformation component along the 45 and 135 meridians respectively. It is the skew

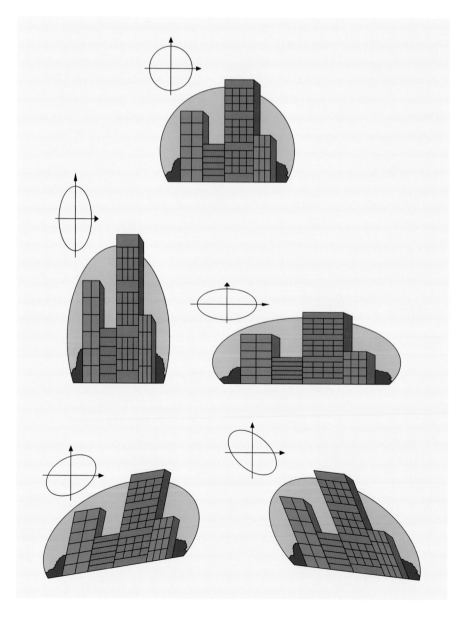

Figure 12.44 The effect of different orientations of the spectacle magnification ellipse. An oblique deformation is far more disturbing than when the deformation is simply vertical or horizontal.

deformation index, P_S, that gives rise to the most objectionable feeling of deformation and the swimming effect.

The total point deformation index, P, and the skew point deformation index, P_S, are evaluated for a large number of points in object space and plotted as shown in Figure 12.45 to provide the designer with an indication of the areas of the lens where the wearer is not likely to experience spatial distortion. As a result, the apparent curvature of objects is reduced to levels where it is barely perceptible.

The double aspheric *Hoyalux iD* lens is offered with two different progressive lengths, 14mm and 11mm, the shorter length being designed for shallow-eye frames. Hoya recommend that the 14mm design should be fitted in a frame which provides a minimum height of 18mm from the bottom rim of the frame to the pupil centre and a minimum distance of 10mm from the pupil centre to the upper edge of the lens or to the bottom edge of the upper frame rim. The compact 11mm design should be fitted in a frame which provides a minimum height of 14mm from the bottom rim of the frame to the pupil centre and a minimum distance of 10mm from the pupil centre to the upper edge of the lens or to the bottom edge of the upper frame rim. The fitting point is designed to be mounted in front of the centre of the pupil.

Varilux Ipseo

A new design from Essilor takes into account the actual degree of head and eye rotation which the wearer employs when viewing through the intermediate and near zones of the lens. Research[11] had shown that each individual has a specific head and eye behaviour, which can be measured and the progressive surface then designed to incorporate the wearer behaviour. This principle has been incorporated into the personalized progressive design from Essilor, the *Varilux Ipseo*.

Figure 12.46 illustrates the visual point positions on the lens for two successful progressive lens wearers, denoted A and B. The positions of the visual points were measured when the wearers were asked to identify targets which appeared at random in the intermediate field of view. Wearer A is quite clearly an 'eye-turner' who perceives objects quite clearly over a wide zone of the lens. Such a wearer would claim that the width of their intermediate field was as wide as the lens itself.

Wearer B, on the other hand, tends to 'point the nose' at objects in the intermediate field and for whatever reason, prefers not to view through peripheral parts of the lens. The experimental set up is shown in Figure 12.47, the relative movement of the head is

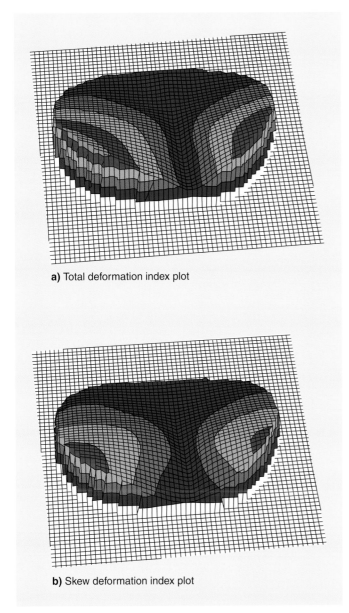

a) Total deformation index plot

b) Skew deformation index plot

Figure 12.45 Distribution of deformation indices, P and P_S. Hoya plot the distribution of the deformation indices for the design to obtain an idea of which zones of the lens are likely to provide comfortable undistorted vision.

Figure 12.46 Visual point positions for a subject who (a) mainly turns the eyes, (b) mainly turns the head.

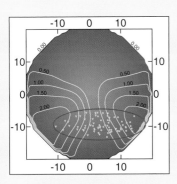

a) Wearer A eye turner

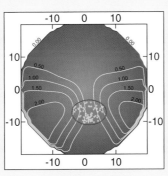

b) Wearer B head turner

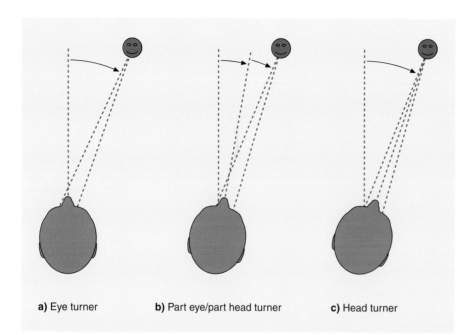

Figure 12.47 Eye turners and head turners.

a) Eye turner   **b)** Part eye/part head turner   **c)** Head turner

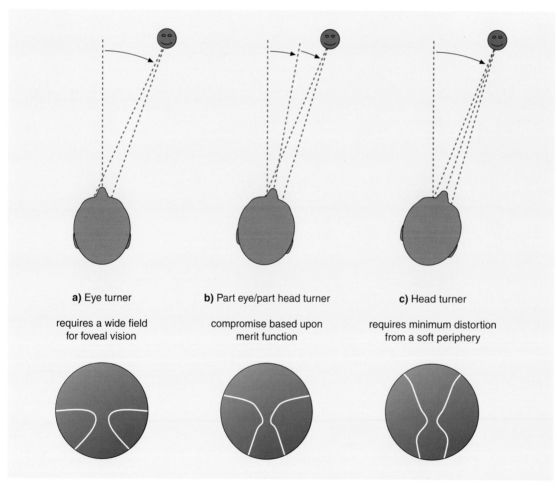

Figure 12.48 Progressive designs for eye turners and head turners.

a) Eye turner

requires a wide field
for foveal vision

b) Part eye/part head turner

compromise based upon
merit function

c) Head turner

requires minimum distortion
from a soft periphery

detected by sensors attached to the head when the subject is asked to view an object in the temporal portion of the field. Knowledge of this characteristic can help the practitioner to choose the best progressive design for an individual wearer (Figure 12.48).

A new instrument has been produced to determine eye/head movement for a specific individual, the *VisionPrint System* (Figure 12.49), the results of which can be incorporated into the progressive surface. Essentially, the *VisionPrint System* consists of three lamps, the central lamp is viewed at 40cm from the centre of the subject's forehead, with two separate lamps, 40cm on either side of the central lamp. The subject is directed to look at the lamp which is illuminated and the movement of the head recorded by an ultrasonic signal which is emitted by the system and reflected by a transponder attached to the special trial frame

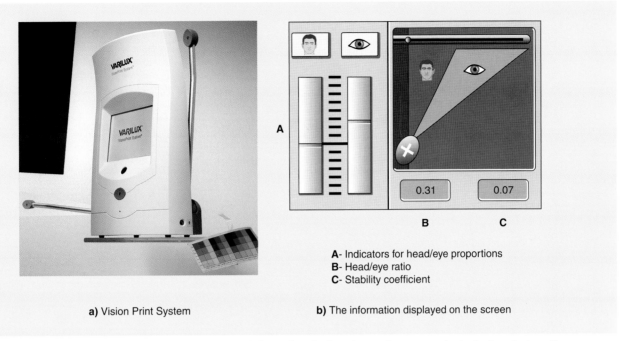

a) Vision Print System

b) The information displayed on the screen

A- Indicators for head/eye proportions
B- Head/eye ratio
C- Stability coefficient

Figure 12.49   (a) The *VisionPrint System* from Essilor. (b) The information displayed upon the screen. A – indicators for head/eye; B – 0.31 signifies that the subject is majority eye movement (0 = eye mover, 1 = head mover); C – stability coefficient (confidence factor with 0 meaning no variation)

being worn by the subject. As far as the subject is concerned, the lamps are illuminated at random and following a short cycle to familiarize the subject, the test sequence is repeated some 20 times to enable the system to calculate and display the eye/head ratio, along with a consistency factor, referred to as the stability coefficient.

In order to quantify the relative eye/head movement, a variable is used which is called the Gain and is equal to the ratio of the angular movement of the head to the total angle of the target:

Gain = head angle/target angle

Thus if the target angle is 45° and the head rotates 15° to view the target the Gain is 0.33. Clearly a Gain of zero would indicate that the subject was an eye turner whereas a Gain of 1.0 would indicate that the subject was a head turner.

People who tend to turn mainly their heads when viewing lateral objects will benefit from a design which provides optimum central acuity, i.e. a softer design, whereas people who tend to turn mainly their eyes, will benefit from a design which provides good acuity over a wider field, i.e. a harder design. The *Vision-Print* system enables the practitioner to determine the wearer profile of the individual quickly and accurately and provides a method for communicating the information to the laboratory for incorporation in the design of the surface. Thus each *Varilux Ipseo* lens is designed for the individual wearer, manufactured by freeform technology and, in recognition of its individual nature, micro-engraved with the wearer's initials.

Varilux Physio

Essilor's constant desire to perfect the *Varilux* lens has led to a new design which retains all the best features of previous generations and applies the very latest technology to both the design and method of manufacture of the lens. This enables the design to address the comfort of the field of vision and provide a significant improvement in the overall effect of the lens in wear.[12]

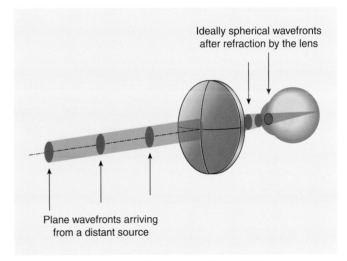

Ideally spherical wavefronts after refraction by the lens

Plane wavefronts arriving from a distant source

Figure 12.50   *Wavefront Management System*™ The wavefronts in the pencil arriving from a distant source are plane. The refracted wavefront will be free from aberration if the form of the wavefronts all along the refracted pencil are spherical, with a common centre at the second principal focus of the lens.

Ophthalmic lens design is normally concerned only with foveal vision, where the visual acuity is at its maximum and the resolution is, therefore, highest. The criterion for a best form spectacle lens is that it should produce a good quality image on the fovea. Since the pupil diameter is small, it is usual to consider the effect of the lens only upon single rays of light which meet the lens at a point.

At night time, however the pupil may increase its diameter several times and the new analysis method employed for the *Physio* design has assumed a finite pupil diameter of 6mm. At this diameter, the light emanating from the lens is not just a single ray but, instead, a narrow pencil of light within which, for an ideal spherical lens, the emergent wavefront should be spherical (Figure 12.50). For distance vision, the wavefront aberration in the

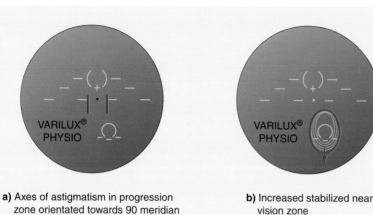

a) Axes of astigmatism in progression zone orientated towards 90 meridian

b) Increased stabilized near vision zone

Figure 12.51   (a) Astigmatism is directed towards the vertical in the lateral regions of the progression zone. Wearers report that the intermediate field appears wider when viewed through this region of the lens. (b) Extended near zone. The *Wavefront Management System*™ has enabled Essilor to stabilize the power over a larger region of the near zone.

refracted pencil is defined as any departure from a spherical surface concentric with the second principal focus of the lens. Owing to the peculiar nature of a progressive surface, the refracted pencil is not strictly spherical but any deformation can be corrected by adjustment of the concave surface of the lens. This is the principle of Essilor's new *Wavefront Management System*™ which sets out to provide the optimum acuity for distance vision. In the case of a spherical distance correction, the shape of the wavefront is calculated after emergence from the lens and any departure from a sphere is corrected by suitable adjustment of the form of the concave surface. In the case of an astigmatic distance correction, the form of the pencil should be toroidal with the centre of each of the two principal circular wavefronts coinciding with the point where the line focus intersects the optical axis.

Needless to say, only the shape of the wavefront as it leaves the lens can be considered. Its form after refraction by the cornea, of course, is unknown. However, if the prescription in the distance portion of the lens is designed to fully correct the subject's ametropia, the wavefront leaving the posterior surface of the crystalline lens should be spherical and concentric with the fovea.

The intermediate zone of a progressive lens, within which the power increases from distance to near, inevitably suffers from astigmatism which increases as the eye roams further in a horizontal direction from the meridian line which runs down the centre of the progressive surface. It is well known that in the presence of uncorrected astigmatism, the eye will find it easier to discern the proper shape of an object if the axis of the astigmatism is orientated vertically or horizontally. Acuity is generally poorest when the axis is oblique. This is particularly true when the subject is viewing text which tends to be recognized, mainly, from the vertical strokes of the individual letters.

The importance of the axis direction of the residual aberrational astigmatism was recognized by the designers of Varilux *Physio* who used the *Wavefront Management System* both to reduce the amount of unwanted astigmatism and to direct its axis towards the vertical meridian (Figure 12.51a). That lateral vision in the intermediate zone is improved, is clearly indicated by the wearer tests where subjects obtain a wider field of perception in this region of the lens. This is just one of the gains which were reported by the wearer tests to which the new design was subjected in direct comparison with Essilor's previously most popular design, the *Varilux Comfort* lens.

The importance of providing a deep and wide near zone in which the wearer can obtain the benefit of the full near addition was also a major consideration in the design of *Physio*. By means of the newly introduced *Wavefront Management System*

Table 12.1 Progressive power lens series	
Manufacturer	**Current series**
General purpose series	
American Optical/Sola/Zeiss	PRO; b'Active, Percepta; SOLAOne; Gradal 3; Top; HS
BBGR	Visa; Selective; Evolis; Anateo
Essilor	Liberty; Comfort; Panamic; Physio
Hoya	Hoyalux; Hoyalux Wide; Hoyalux Summit PRO
Kodak	Navigator; Progressive Elegance; Progressive; Precise
Nikon	Presio i; Presio X; Presio W
Pentax	AF; HIX 1.6; A-PRO
Rodenstock	Progressiv R; S; life 2; Start; Multigressiv
Rupp & Hubrach	Selectal; Sentoris
Seiko	P-1W; P-1SY
Shamir	Genesis; Panorama
Younger	Image
Short corridor designs	
American Optical/Sola/Zeiss	Compact; Brevis
Essilor	Ellipse
Hoya	Summit CD
Kodak	Concise
Nikon	Presio i-13
Pentax	Mini AF
Rodenstock	Progressiv life XS
Shamir	Piccolo
Personalized designs	
American Optical/Sola/Zeiss	SOLAOne Ego
Essilor	Ipseo
Hoya	Hoyalux iD
Pentax	Super Atoric F
Rodenstock	Impression[ILT]; Impression XS[ILT]; Impression[ILT]; Impression Hyperop[ILT]; Impression Hyperop XS[ILT]
Rupp & Hubrach	Ysis
Shamir	Autograph; Insight
Occupational designs	
American Optical/Sola/Zeiss	Technica; Access; Gradal RD; Business
Essilor	Interview; Anti-fatigue; Computer 2V and 3V
Hoya	Hoyalux Office
Nikon	O*nline*
Rodenstock	Cosmolit Office; Nexyma
Shamir	Shamir Office

the designers were able to stabilize the optical characteristics of the design over a larger region of the near zone (Figure 12.51b).

Production of the new lens design was made possible by modern surfacing methods employing computer numerically controlled (freeform) grinding and polishing technology.

Freeform is the term used to describe a surface, not by a mathematical equation, but by stating its *x*, *y*, *z* coordinates over the entire surface (see Chapter 17). Normally, freeform surfaces cannot be specified by means of an algebraic equation but instead, are described numerically by listing the *x*, *y*, *z* coordinates for thousands of points on the surface. As many as 30 000 data points may need to be specified and the method enables non-rotationally symmetrical surfaces to be described in such a fashion that they can be both analyzed and manufactured accurately.

For the production of *Physio*, Essilor have introduced *Twin Rx Technology*™ where the refraction is analyzed at each point on the back surface through which the chief ray of the pencil passes, and the convex progressive surface adjusted to ensure that optimum performance is obtained for all directions of gaze. Sophisticated computing software has been developed to carry out this *Point by Point Twinning*™ of the convex and concave surfaces in order to determine the complementary surface to manufacture to ensure that the required optical performance is obtained. Thus, instead of only one power for each base curve having the ideal optical performance, this method of advanced digital surfacing enables each lens to be manufactured individually to provide the optimum performance.

Table 12.1 lists most of the progressive power lens series currently available from the major lens manufacturers in the UK. In addition, many companies still stock previous generations of progressive power lenses.

References

1. Davis J K, Fernald H G 1976 US Patent 3960442 Ophthalmic Lens Series
2. Essilor International. Personal communication. In-house analysis of wearer rejection of progressive lenses, 1997
3. Sullivan C M and Fowler C W 1990 Investigation of progressive addition lens patient tolerance to dispensing anomalies. Ophthal Physiol Opt 10:16
4. Winthrop J T 1989 US Patent 4861153 Progressive Addition Spectacle Lens.
5. Tunnacliffe A H 1995 Ophthalmic lens data SC. Hardy & Co, Wadhurst
6. Bourdoncle B 2000 Varilux Panamic: the design process. Points de vue 42. Essilor, Paris
7. Meslin D 2000 How wide is Varilux Panamic Near? Essilor of America Inc, St Petersburg
8. Mukaiyama H, Kato K 2000 US Patent 6019470 Progressive multifocal lens and manufacturing method of eyeglass lens and progressive multifocal lens
9. Rodenstock 2000 Rodenstock Impression[ILT] und Multigressiv[ILT] Die Zukunft im Gleitsichtglasbereich. Rodenstock, Munchen
10. Zeiss 2000 Aus einer Vision wurde ein Gleitsichtglas. Gradal Individual von Carl Zeiss. Zeiss, Aalen
11. Simonet P et al 2003 Eye–head coordination in presbyopes. Points de vue 49. Essilor, Paris
12. Allione P, Bourdoncle B, Marin G and Padiou J M 2006 Varilux Physio: cutting-edge eyecare technologies. Points de vue 54. Essilor, Paris

Dispensing in aphakia

Removal of the crystalline lens from the eye results in the condition known as aphakia. If the eye was emmetropic before surgery, it is left with a high degree of hypermetropia, and requires a lens of power of +10.00 to +12.00D to correct it for distance vision. The aphakic eye has no mechanism for accommodation and requires separate corrections for intermediate and near vision. It is also in need of protection from ultraviolet (UV) radiation, since it was the crystalline lens that governed the lower limit of transmission of radiant energy by the ocular media. Today, the first choice for the correction of aphakia is the intraocular lens, which is implanted into either the anterior or the posterior chamber of the eye and is usually inserted at the same time as the cataract extraction. Notwithstanding the surgical correction of aphakia, a large number of people still remain who wear strong plus post-cataract spectacle lenses.

The dispensing of lenses for hypermetropia is considered in detail in Chapter 9, in which it is pointed out that, ideally, strong plus lenses should be surfaced individually to provide the required edge thickness for the finished diameter when full details of the prescription, decentration and frame size are known. In this chapter the optical and mechanical problems encountered with the very strong plus lenses normally required for the spectacle correction of aphakia are considered.

As discussed in Chapter 9, the wearers of plus lenses suffer a loss in field of view at the edge of their lenses and, in addition, must put up with the annoying *jack-in-the-box* effect. Recent cataract lens designs have done much to address these field problems and it is useful to look again at these effects before describing how the designers of post-cataract lenses have tried to eliminate them.

Field of view

Figure 13.1 shows that wearers of plus lenses suffer a loss in their real field of view in the object space. For example, in Figure 13.1 an apparent angular field of 73° for a +12.00D lens at 40mm diameter corresponds to a real angular field of only 53°. It can be seen in Figure 13.1 that there is an area surrounding the edge of the lens from which no light can enter the eye. With the example illustrated, the angular extent of this ring scotoma is 10°, which is one-half the difference between the real and apparent fields. Since 10° is very nearly equal to 18Δ, the linear extent of this ring scotoma on a Bjerrum screen mounted 1m in front of the subject is 18cm. Or, 10m away, the loss is 180cm, enough to obscure the view of two or three people standing in a group! These figures ignore both the thickness of the rim of the frame and spherical aberration, the effects of each of which are to increase the size of the scotoma. The ring scotoma is stationary while the head remains stationary. When the head is turned the ring scotoma also turns, roaming around the field of vision and, for obvious reasons, this phenomenon is referred to as a *roving ring scotoma*.

A secondary problem for the wearers of strong plus lenses is the sudden disappearance and reappearance of objects as they pass through the ring scotoma, a phenomenon known as the *jack-in-the-box* effect.

The characteristic head swing evident in many corrected aphakic subjects, when they wish to view laterally placed objects, obviously is developed to minimize the effects of the roving ring scotoma.

The real macular field of view of a spectacle lens of power, F, and diameter, $2y$, mounted 27mm in front of the eye's centre of rotation is given by:[1]

$$\tan \theta = y(37 - F)/1000$$

where θ is half the field of view. Hence, a +10.00D lens edged 40mm round has a real angular field of view of 57° and a +12.00D lens made in lenticular form with a 32mm round aperture has a real field of view of just 44°.

To obtain the maximum field, whatever size the aperture might be, the correcting lens should be fitted as close to the eyes as the lashes permit. In cases of aphakia, a close fit has the added advantage of reducing the retinal image size, and the magnification of the eye and surroundings viewed through the lens.

Lens form

Spectacle lens powers over about +7.00D cannot be made free from oblique astigmatism when confined to the use of spherical surfaces. This is neatly demonstrated by Tscherning's Ellipse for distance vision point-focal lenses, described in detail in Chapter 2.

For example, the field diagram illustrated in Figure 13.2 shows the off-axis performance of a +12.00D lens made with spherical surfaces. The increase in tangential power of the lens and the large amount of aberrational astigmatism can be read from the diagram. When the eye views through the optical centre, the vergence in the refracted pencil that leaves the lens is the prescribed value, +12.00D.

When the eye begins to rotate through 10°, 20° and 30° from the optical axis there is a dramatic change in the vergence of the refracted pencil that leaves the lens. This is indicated by the curves shown as F'_T and F'_S in the field diagram, which represent the tangential and sagittal oblique vertex sphere powers of the lens; in other words, the real off-axis effect of the lens upon the eye.

The sagittal power remains about +12.00D, but the tangential power can be seen to increase, reaching about +14.00D at 35° from the optical axis. This ocular rotation corresponds to an eye that views through a point about 17mm from the optical centre of the lens. At 35°, the real effect of this lens form that employs spherical surfaces is +11.91 with a +2.00 cylinder, not

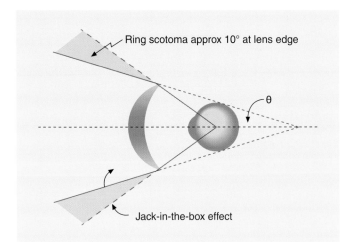

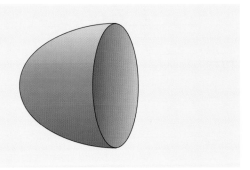

Figure 13.3   Aspherical surface – the prolate ellipsoid. A convex prolate ellipsoidal surface introduces negative surface astigmatism to neutralize the positive astigmatism of oblique incidence

Figure 13.1   Decreased field of view of a plus lens. Note the area that forms the ring scotoma and causes the jack-in-the-box effect at the edge of lens. θ is the semi-angular real field of view

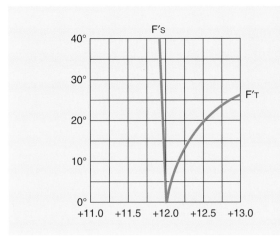

Figure 13.2   Field diagram for +12.00D lens made with spherical surfaces: $n = 1.498$, $F_2 = -3.00$, $t = 10$mm, centre of rotation distance (CRD) = 25mm. Note that for a 20° rotation of the eye, the effective Rx is +12.00/+0.50 and at 30°, the effective Rx is +11.93/+1.37

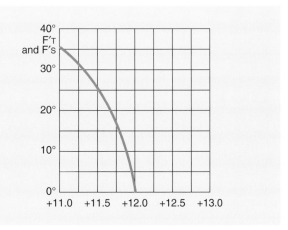

Figure 13.4   Field diagram for +12.00D lens made with convex prolate ellipsoidal surface: $p = +0.65$, $n = 1.498$, $F_2 = -3.00$, $t = 10$mm, CRD = 25mm. Note that for a 20° rotation of the eye, the effective Rx is +11.68DS and at 30°, the effective Rx is +11.31DS

the +12.00 sphere intended. At this point, the lens exhibits 2.00D of unwanted astigmatism.

Ideally, the oblique vertex sphere powers should remain +12.00 for all zones of the lens. Clearly, if the subject's distance prescription is +12.00, when wearing this spherical lens form, maximum visual acuity is obtained only in a small zone around the optical axis. The aberrations impose a limit on the field in which the subject obtains optimum vision.

When the designer is not limited to the use of spherical surfaces, oblique astigmatism can be eliminated to provide a massive increase in the field of useful vision. This is achieved by employing a surface that is, itself, astigmatic, the surface astigmatism varying in just the right way to counteract the astigmatism of oblique incidence. One such surface is the convex prolate ellipsoid illustrated in Figure 13.3, the essential features of which are described in detail in Chapter 4.

Aspheric lenses of the type needed for the correction of aphakia usually employ a convex prolate ellipsoidal surface to eliminate aberrational astigmatism in the post-cataract range of prescriptions.

The improvement in off-axis performance can be judged from the field diagram illustrated in Figure 13.4, which shows the zonal variation in oblique vertex sphere powers for a point-focal +12.00D lens made with a –3.00D back curve and a properly chosen ellipsoidal front surface with p-value +0.65. It is seen for this design that the tangential and sagittal oblique vertex sphere powers remain the same for all zones out to 40°.

It is also seen that the lens performance is by no means perfect. The mean oblique power (MOP), which is now the same as the tangential and sagittal oblique vertex sphere powers, drops rapidly as the eye rotates away from the optical axis of the lens. This loss in power, the mean oblique error (MOE), amounts to almost 1.00D at 35° from the optical axis, but at least the error in off-axis performance is a spherical one. Ideally, of course, the designer would like to be able to increase the marginal power of the aspheric design to provide a constant correction for all zones of the lens.

This large drop in tangential power does provide one advantage for lens powers in this range: there is a reduction in distortion compared with the spherical design. The aberration distortion causes a change in shape of the image produced by an optical system. Typically, a plus spectacle lens with spherical surfaces causes the image of a square object viewed through the lens to take on a characteristic pincushion shape.

In the adaptation to a spectacle correction, newly operated aphakic subjects have to cope with an enormous change in prescription, usually an addition of some +11.00D to +12.00D to any previous correction before surgery. One of the most disturbing effects from the large amount of pincushion distortion is the apparent narrowing of a doorway as the subject walks towards it. The pincushion effect increases as the apparent size of the object increases (i.e. as the subject approaches the doorway), since the light passes through more remote sections of the lens. The apparent curvature of the doorway increases to such an extent, and the disorientation is so great, that the subject begins to doubt whether he or she will be able to squeeze through the door! This is one more effect peculiar to post-cataract spectacle lenses.

The use of an aspherical surface reduces the amount of pincushion distortion that the wearer experiences. The reduction in distortion occurs because there is a significant reduction in the tangential power of the deep convex surface when the eye rotates away from the vertex of the curve. In the case of a convex spherical surface, the tangential surface power increases as the eye uses zones of the lens further and further from its optical centre. This is because the angles of incidence and refraction, and thus the deviation produced, increase as the ocular rotation increases.

The tangential surface power of the front surface of a lens is given by the relationship:[1]

$$F_{1T} = n\sin(i - i')/r_{1T}\cos^2 i'$$

where i and i' are the angles of incidence and refraction at the front surface and r_{1T} is the tangential radius of curvature of the surface at the point in question. Table 13.1 lists the tangential front surface powers and the distortion for +12.00D post-cataract lenses.

Inspection of Table 13.1 shows quite clearly that, for the spherical lens, the tangential surface power increases quite significantly as the eye uses zones further from the optical axis and that this increase is accompanied by a large increase in distortion. For the aspheric lens, the tangential power of the convex prolate ellipsoidal surface decreases as the surface flattens away from the vertex of the curve. The surface is still undercorrected for spherical aberration, which indicates that it remains afflicted with pincushion distortion, but the distortion is considerably reduced when compared with the spherical surface.

When aspheric lenses are prescribed for near vision, the loss in power caused by near vision effectivity errors (NVEEs) is exacerbated by the loss in mean oblique image vergence (MOIV) when the eye uses extra-axial zones of the lens. Figure 13.5 illustrates the off-axis performance of +15.00D lenses used for near vision at 33.3cm from the lens. In the case of the +15.00D lens made with spherical surfaces (Figure 13.5a), there is a gain in MOIV as the eye rotates away from the optical centre of the lens. In effect, the aberrations put back the loss in NVEE. However, in the case of the aspheric design illustrated in Figure 13.5b, the loss from NVEE is increased by the drop in MOIV. About 1.00D is lost in

the case of this aspheric design with a convex prolate ellipsoidal surface.

Obviously, the aphakic eye has no mechanism to compensate for this loss in power in near vision and it is to the subject's advantage to increase the prescribed reading addition, by an amount that depends, like the change in NVEE, upon the form of the trial lens used during refraction (see below).

CD-ROM

Lens form is considered in more detail on the CD-ROM

Lens material

The lower limit of transmission of radiant energy in the eye is governed by the crystalline lens. A young lens absorbs UV radiation below about 310nm and, with increasing age, this lower limit rises to about 375nm, which encompasses most of the UV spectrum. In cases of incipient cataract, further absorption and scattering by the cloudy crystalline lens might also prevent the short-wavelength blue portion of the spectrum from reaching the retina. In the absence of the crystalline lens as a result of cataract surgery, this UV-filtering mechanism is removed and needs to be replaced by UV attenuation by the spectacle lens. All post-cataract lenses should absorb, or reflect away, UV radiation.

Today, spectacle lenses for aphakia are invariably made from plastics materials. There are two very good reasons for this. Firstly, as we have just seen, good off-axis performance for the lens powers involved is only possible with aspherical surfaces, which can be reproduced far more cheaply in plastics. Furthermore, it is easy to 'dope' CR39 monomer to provide absorption of all radiation below 400nm.

Secondly, the use of glass for full-aperture, post-cataract lenses makes the final spectacles uncomfortably heavy. Typically, a +12.00D lens made in crown glass and edged 40mm in diameter weighs 16 grams; in CR39 the lens weighs just 9 grams. In the days before plastics materials became the norm for spectacle lenses, several types of glass post-cataract lenticular lenses were listed in the lens catalogues. The current Norville catalogue now lists just two glass lenticular designs, both solid convex lenticulars, with 34mm aperture diameters. When the small field of view of this lens is taken into account, it is clear that such a design is really only suitable for use in near vision. Even then the spherical aperture curve leaves much to be desired in terms of off-axis performance of the lens. In most parts of the world plastics lenses have become the first choice for spectacles, and these glass lens forms are obsolescent.

Table 13.1   Comparison of tangential front surface powers and distortion for +12.00D lenses made in spherical and aspheric forms. Each lens has a –3.00D base curve and a front surface power at the vertex of +13.63D. The p-value of the aspherical surface is +0.65

Lens zone (°)	Spherical lens		Aspheric lens	
	F_{1T}	Distortion (%)	F_{1T}	Distortion (%)
40	+14.21	20.84	+11.63	14.45
30	+13.88	10.22	+12.42	7.18
20	+13.73	4.15	+13.06	2.93
10	+13.65	0.99	+13.49	0.70
0	+13.63	0.00	+13.63	0.00

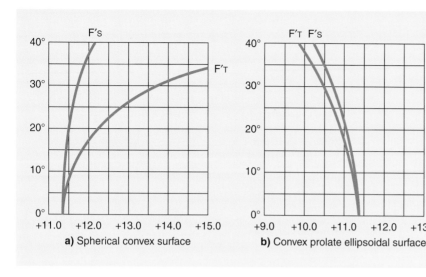

Figure 13.5 Comparison of near vision performance of +15.00D lenses made with spherical and aspherical surfaces: (a) +15.00D lens with spherical convex surface used for near vision at 33.3cm ($n = 1.498$, $F_2 = -3.00$, $t = 10$mm, CRD = 25mm). Note that for a 20° rotation of the eye, the effective Rx is +11.50/+0.75. (b) +15.00D lens convex prolate ellipsoidal surface used for near vision at 33.3cm ($p = +0.646$, $n = 1.498$, $F_2 = -3.00$, $t = 10$mm, CRD = 25 mm). Note that for a 20° rotation of the eye, the effective Rx is +11.00/−0.12

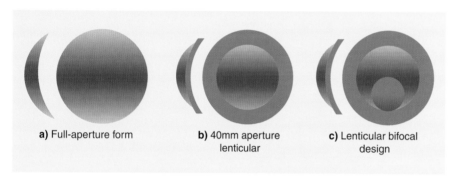

Figure 13.6 Modern cataract lens designs with convex prolate ellipsoidal surfaces

Cataract lens designs

Most of the major lens manufacturers offer CR39 aspheric lenses with convex prolate ellipsoidal surfaces. These series are available in both full-aperture and lenticular form, usually with a 40mm aperture diameter (Figure 13.6). They are also available in bifocal form with round or D-shape segments. However, the segment surface itself is normally not aspherical and, since it is cast on the ellipsoidal DP surface, the segment tends to be oval in shape rather than circular.

During the 1970s a new lens design appeared with an optical performance deliberately compromised towards the edge of the field to produce lenses with improved mechanical characteristics. The mechanical advantages and optical disadvantages of these blended lenticular designs are understood most easily by considering the principles of ordinary lenticular lenses. The usual lenticular lens for the correction of aphakia has a central aperture that incorporates the optical correction, surrounded by a carrier or margin, which is of lower power, or may even be afocal.

Naturally, sharp foveal vision is only possible when the wearer views through the aperture and, in the case of a deep plus lens that has a spherical aperture surface, when the visual axis is close to the optical axis of the lens. Off-axis there are severe aberrations if spherical surfaces are used, which further limit the useful field of view.

The carrier, however, which may be afocal, does permit some awareness of objects and movement, provided these lie outside the ring scotoma that occurs at the dividing line. Obviously, peripheral vision is important and an essential part of the normal visual function.

During the 1970s, several workers in the field of cataract lens design asked the question, 'Is the dividing line between the aperture and the margin really necessary?' Its removal would not only improve the appearance of the lens, but should also increase the field of vision by removing the ring scotoma associated with the abrupt change in power at the edge of the aperture.

The performance of these designs can be understood by considering the female glass mould used for the convex aperture side of a plastics lenticular (Figure 13.7). It can be seen that a concave annulus with its centre of curvature at C_B blends the aperture curve and marginal curve to produce a continuous surface on the mould. The blending tool must be arranged so that its centre of curvature rotates about Q, through a circle of radius QC_B, which is concentric with the aperture.

Smoothing and polishing of the blended annulus can be achieved with a floating pad system in which the pads follow the generated curve. The necessary radius of curvature of the blending curve depends upon the width of the blended zone ($y_M - y_A$) and the radii of curvature of the aperture and marginal curves.[1] If the width of the blended zone is made too narrow, then the blending curve on the mould needs to be convex and the corresponding curve on the cast lens becomes concave, which is undesirable.

The blended zone is of the same form as a barrel-form toroidal surface and, as such, is indeed highly astigmatic. In general, the blended region of the lens cannot provide good vision, which is restricted to the central zone of the design – just as in the case of a normal lenticular lens.

These blended lenticular designs have been described as *zonal aspherics*, and they are simply lenticular lenses without a visible dividing line. They have a central power some 3.00D to 6.00D

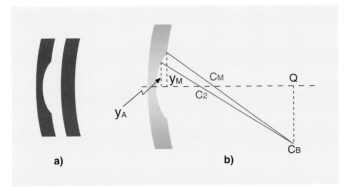

Figure 13.7   Blending the dividing line of a mould for a convex lenticular

greater than their marginal power. For example, a +10.00D blended lenticular may have a marginal power of just +6.00D, so the design has a power of +10.00, but the centre thickness is the same as a lens of power +6.00, and the field of view is the same as a +6.00D lens without the ring scotoma that occurs at the normal lenticular dividing line. Furthermore, at the edge of the lens, where the ring scotoma does occur, it is smaller than would be the case if the central power was maintained to the edge of the lens.

Against these undoubted merits must be offset the obvious disadvantage that the wearer obtains the optimum correction only in the central zone of the lens and must learn to turn the head to view laterally placed objects.

The first zonal aspheric, or blended lenticular, design was introduced in the early 1970s by Dr Robert Welsh, who was one of the first people to recognize the advantages of thinner full-aperture lenses for the correction of aphakia. Known originally as the *Welsh 4-drop Aspheric*, since the zones dropped in power by 4.00D from centre to edge, it is now available in several forms, such as the Signet *Hyperaspheric*, the Sola *Hi-drop* and the *Thi-Aspheric* in glass of high refractive index from Hoya.

With the advent of computer-assisted design and computer numerically controlled grinding techniques, it became possible to design and manufacture surfaces of higher order than the conicoids, and during the 1970s designs with convex polynomial surfaces appeared (Figure 13.8). The term *polynomial* is used because the equation to the convex surface is of polynomial form, involving powers of *y* up to the tenth or twelfth degree, for example:

$$x = ay^2 + by^4 + cy^6 + dy^8 + ey^{10} \ldots$$

If the zone AA′ in Figure 13.8 is a convex prolate ellipsoid, this zone of the lens enjoys the same optical properties as a traditional aspheric lens that employs an ellipsoidal surface. Zone AA′ is then free from aberrational astigmatism and exhibits less distortion, since the tangential surface power within this zone decreases as the eye rotates away from the optical axis. Zone A′M is seen to be concave in its tangential section. The surface flexes backwards in this region. Since the surface is continuous, however, no annular scotoma occurs between the central ellipsoidal zone and the margin. Zone MM′ has the same purpose as the margin of a lenticular design. It supports the central aperture. If the polynomial surface becomes parallel with the back surface in this region, the margin is virtually afocal.

The polynomial surface acts in much the same way as the blending process described earlier – but with two very important differences. Firstly, the aspheric optical zone has excellent properties. It does not have the aberrational astigmatism associated

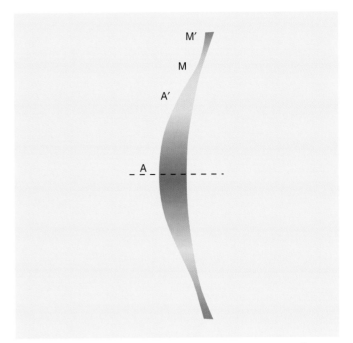

Figure 13.8   A post-cataract lens design with a convex polynomial surface

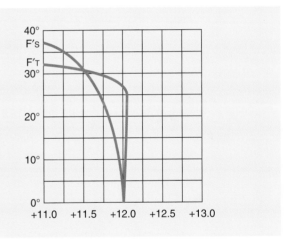

Figure 13.9   Field diagram for a +12.00D lens made with a convex polynomial surface. Note that for a 20° rotation of the eye, the effective Rx is about +11.75/+0.25 and at 30° the effective Rx is +11.50DS

with spherical surfaces. Secondly, the blending is concave. It can be imagined that the region between the aspheric aperture and spherical margin of a traditional lenticular has been filled with material to eliminate the dividing line. The result of this is to eliminate the ring scotoma that exists at the edge of every plus lens and the accompanying *jack-in-the-box* effect, which is so annoying to wearers of deep plus lenses.

The optical performance of a post-cataract lens that employs a convex polynomial surface can be judged from the field diagram illustrated in Figure 13.9, which shows the variation in tangential and sagittal oblique vertex sphere powers for a +12.00D lens used for distance vision. The lens is designed to provide an optical zone of 40mm diameter within which the tangential error is negligible out to 25° and the aberrational astigmatism very well corrected out to 30°, which is about 20mm from the optical axis. Beyond

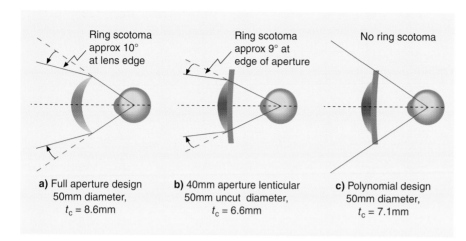

Ring scotoma
approx 10°
at lens edge

Ring scotoma
approx 9° at
edge of aperture

No ring scotoma

a) Full aperture design
50mm diameter,
t_c = 8.6mm

b) 40mm aperture lenticular
50mm uncut diameter,
t_c = 6.6mm

c) Polynomial design
50mm diameter,
t_c = 7.1mm

Figure 13.10   Comparison of fields of view of aspheric post-cataract lenses of power +12.00D; (a) full aperture aspheric lens with a convex prolate ellipsoidal surface; (b) aspheric lenticular with a 40mm aperture and convex ellipsoidal aperture curve; (c) aspheric lens with convex polynomial surface

the optical zone the tangential power falls off rapidly as the surface begins to change direction.

The first ophthalmic lens design to employ this type of convex polynomial surface was the *Ful-Vue Aspheric* cataract lens introduced by the American Optical Corporation in 1978. It is available in both single-vision and bifocal form, the bifocal version incorporating a 22mm diameter segment on the convex surface.

Other manufacturers followed suit in the subsequent few years; for example, Essilor with their *Omega Aspheric* design in 1981. The convex surface of the *Omega* is a figured ellipsoid that has an optical zone of 43mm diameter (zone AA′ in Figure 13.8) and is indistinguishable from the ellipsoidal surface used for their traditional aspheric lenticular lens. Such a surface could be produced by blending the ellipsoidal aperture curve with a spherical margin. The *blending* zone, A′M, is about 10mm in width and is designed to blend the aperture curve with the peripheral zone, MM′, which forms the margin of the design. A bifocal version is also available with a 22mm diameter segment incorporated on the polynomial surface.

Similar designs are available from Zeiss, the *Clarlet Aphal*, and Rodenstock, the *Perfastar*, which is also available in bifocal form, the *Perfastar Bifo*, with a 22mm diameter segment.

Polynomial lens designs combine the advantages of both lenticular lenses and full-aperture lens designs (Figure 13.10). The lenses are thinner and lighter than full-aperture designs for just the same reasons as a lenticular lens, but there is no visible dividing line between the aperture and the margin. This is of particular benefit when strong plus lenses must be dispensed in a frame with a large eye size. The wearer obtains a wide central field within which the aberrations, which are normally severe in the case of post-cataract lenses, are exceptionally well corrected, together with a useful peripheral field with no ring scotoma between them.

Prescription translation in aphakia

The high powers of the lenses mean that spectacle fitting in aphakia requires the greatest skill in ophthalmic dispensing, and co-operation between the refractionist and the dispensing optician is essential to ensure that the trial frame prescription is reproduced accurately. It has been suggested that in cases of aphakia, for which it is known at the outset that a spectacle correction is to be given, the final frame that the subject is to wear should be chosen and fitted before refraction takes place. This ensures

that the trial frame, which is fully adjustable, is set up to match the characteristics of the final frame rather than attempting the reverse process.

If the trial frame is set up to match the details of the final frame, the final prescription that is dispensed then depends upon the form, pantoscopic angle and the vertex distance of the trial lenses. Since the form of plus trial case lenses does not usually match the form of the final lens, there may be particular difficulties during the sight-testing procedure if the trial frame is not carefully set up in front of the eyes. If the subject's visual axis does not coincide with the optical axis of the trial lens, the real effect of the lens will not be the same as the marked power of the lens. Proper attention must be paid to the angle of side of the trial frame, since this governs the pantoscopic angle of the lens. If the optical centre is lowered to compensate for the pantoscopic angle, to satisfy the centre of rotation condition, the actual effect of the trial lens will not be its marked power, but the off-axis performance at 10° or even 15° from the optical axis. Table 13.2 indicates the 5°, 10° and 15° performance of the most common forms of spherical trial lenses of powers +10.00, +12.00, +14.00 and +16.00D. The values shown are the sagittal oblique vertex sphere powers, F_S and the oblique astigmatic errors (OAEs). The other off-axis data, F_T, MOP and MOE, can be deduced from these two values, as described in the section on best-form lenses in Chapter 2. If the lenses are angled in front of the eyes so that they occupy the usual plane, the axis direction of the OAE is 180°.

Trial lens type A is a reduced-aperture lens with the curved surface designed to face the eye, and is the most common form of trial lens in use in the UK. It is obviously unsuitable for obtaining an accurate estimate of the refraction when used as intended, unless it is mounted at right-angles to the visual axis. It is becoming the usual practice when employing this type of trial lens to turn it back-to-front for deep plus powers. The effect of this on the off-axis powers is seen to be greatly beneficial, a much better indication of the effect of the lens being obtained. Naturally, the paraxial power of the reversed trial lens is the front vertex power, and not that marked on the trial lens rim.

Trial lens B is a full-aperture symmetrical form. Its off-axis performance begins to differ significantly from its marked power just 5° from the optical axis.

Type C is a curved trial lens form, and is assumed to have been made with a –3.00D base curve. The values given are also typical of the performance of the final lens, assuming this to be made with spherical surfaces. If the final lens is obtained from the same

Table 13.2 Off-axis performance of different forms of modern trial lenses

Type	Angle (°)	Actual effects of various trial lens forms			
		+10.00	+12.00	+14.00	+16.00
A	0	+10.00	+12.00	+14.00	+16.00
	5	+10.07/+0.18	+12.10/+0.25	+14.14/+0.33	+16.18/+0.42
	10	+10.30/+0.77	+12.43/+1.08	+14.59/+1.45	+16.77/+1.90
	15	+10.72/+1.99	+13.03/+2.85	+15.42/+3.95	+17.91/+5.37
A reversed	0	+10.20	+12.34	+14.48	+16.67
	5	+10.20/+0.05	+12.35/+0.05	+14.49/+0.07	+16.68/+0.08
	10	+10.23/+0.19	+12.37/+0.22	+14.52/+0.27	+16.72/+0.33
	15	+10.26/+0.43	+12.42/+0.51	+14.59/+0.63	+16.84/+0.78
B	0	+10.00	+12.00	+14.00	+16.00
	5	+10.04/+0.10	+12.05/+0.13	+14.06/+0.16	+16.08/+0.19
	10	+10.14/+0.41	+12.19/+0.53	+14.24/+0.67	+16.30/+0.82
	15	+10.32/+1.00	+12.43/+1.30	+14.55/+1.65	+16.71/+2.06
C	0	+10.00	+12.00	+14.00	+16.00
	5	+10.00/+0.02	+12.00/+0.03	+14.00/+0.05	+16.01/+0.07
	10	+9.99/+0.10	+11.99/+0.14	+14.01/+0.20	+16.05/+0.28
	15	+9.97/+0.22	+11.99/+0.32	+14.02/+0.46	+16.11/+0.66

manufacturer as that of the trial lens, then the effect of the final lens should be identical with that of the trial lens. The superior performance of these lenses for deep plus powers is self-evident.

Many of the problems associated with prescription translation in cases of aphakia can be understood from the information presented in Table 13.2. For example, if a trial lens of type A, with a marked power of +12.00, is used during refraction and the subject views through the 10° zone of the lens, its actual effect is +12.50/+1.00 × 180. If a +12.00D sphere is ordered and dispensed with a – 3.00D back surface power, its effect is only about +12.00/+0.12 × 180, even when the vertex distance, pantoscopic angle and horizontal centration are duplicated accurately. It is, perhaps, fortunate that intraocular lens implants have almost entirely superseded spectacle correction in aphakia!

Clearly, the vertex distance of the rearmost lens in the trial frame should be measured carefully and, where possible, reproduced by the final lens. If a change in vertex distance occurs, then the effective power of the final lens should be computed so that it reproduces the effect of the trial lens system. If a number of lenses are employed in the trial frame, the back vertex power of the trial lens system may not be simply the sum of the marked powers on the trial lens rims. If any doubt exists, it is easy to ascertain the back vertex power of a system of trial lenses by means of the focimeter.

Near vision effectivity errors with post-cataract lenses

As pointed out in Chapter 9, the back vertex power of a lens represents the vergence that leaves the lens when the light originates from a distant object. In near vision, the light originates from a point that lies at a finite distance in front of the lens and the

vergence that leaves the back surface now depends not just on the back vertex power, but also on the form and thickness of the lens. With strong plus lenses, the axial thickness of which cannot be ignored when considering the lens power, vertex power notation does not give a good indication of the performance of the lens in near vision.

The vergence that leaves the back surface of the lens, L'_2, which arrives from a near object lying at L_1 dioptres in front of the lens, is given by:[1]

$$L'_2 = (L_1 + F_1)/\left[1 - t/n(L_1 + F_1)\right] + F_2$$

When L_1 is zero, this expression reduces to the expression given in Chapter 9 for the back vertex power of the lens, as would be expected.

The difference between the vergence that leaves a lens when the light originates from a near object, L'_2, and the anticipated vergence obtained from the sum of the incident vergence and the back vertex power, $L_1 + F'_V$, is the NVEE of the lens.

It can be shown that the NVEE is given by the approximate relationship:

$$\text{NVEE} = (t/n)L_1(L_1 + 2F_1)$$

NVEE is a problem in the case of high-power plus lenses. Its significance is that lenses of the same back vertex power, but of different forms, are not interchangeable in near vision. Typically, trial case lenses are either plano-convex in form, with the curved surface designed to face the eye, or they may be symmetrical, equi-convex in the case of plus lenses. However, the final lens eventually dispensed is certain to be curved in form with its concave surface facing the eye. For a trial lens of power +15.00 used to obtain a correction for near vision at 33.3cm, the trial lens being symmetrical in form with a front surface of +7.37 and axial thickness of 7.0mm, the NVEE is (given by the above relationship):

$$NVEE = 7/1523 \times -3 \times (-3 + 14.75) = -0.16D$$

If the final lens is made in aspheric form with a +16.00D front curve and axial thickness of 10mm, the NVEE would be:

$$NVEE = 10/1498 \times -3 \times (-3 + 32) = -0.58D$$

It can be seen that the back vertex power of the final curved-form lens that the subject is dispensed needs to be increased by about +0.50D from that of the flat-form trial lens. Some manufacturers include tables in their technical literature that detail the errors likely to be found in trial lenses and in their own lens series. As a rule, they propose a correction factor that can be added to the back vertex correction to ensure the final lens duplicates the effect of the trial lens.

At present, the great majority of refraction and dispensing of lenses for aphakic subjects takes place in the ophthalmology department of a general hospital or in an eye hospital. It is common sense that, to avoid poor correction or cases of non-tolerance, the lens dispensing actually needs to begin both before and within the consulting room.

CD-ROM

Near vision effectivity errors are also considered in detail on the CD-ROM

Reference

1. Jalie M 1984 Principles of ophthalmic lenses. ABDO, London

Safety lenses

Richard Earlam, BSc MCOptom FBDO

Filter lenses that protect the eyes from harmful radiation are considered in Chapter 7. It may also be necessary to protect the eyes against mechanical injury from dust, flying particles and sports injuries, such as those encountered in racquet sports (squash, cricket, etc.).

Legislation is now in place to protect the eyes, both in the work environment and in certain sports such as squash (see Chapter 16), and protection may need to be provided whether the lenses include a refractive correction or not.

Safety and safe practice in industry are defined in the Health and Safety at Work Act (1974) and the Personal Protective Equipment Regulations (1992). It is stated quite clearly that it is the legal responsibility of the employer to supply the approved safety appliances, and the legal obligation of the employee to wear them in an environment where there is a foreseeable risk from flying particles, harmful liquids, fumes and gases or radiation. Companies generally police these regulations quite vigorously, as they are responsible for the welfare of their workforce and those people who will not wear the approved appliances usually face job loss.

In the home and garden (Figure 14.1), however, the situation is completely different. There are many people who routinely expose themselves to the dangers of playing sport, or who work at their favourite hobby without taking the precautions that would be expected of them if they were in an industrial environment. Indeed, the rules of many sports do not require any safety appliances to be worn and little guidance has been offered to help people to understand the risks they take. This situation, however, is now changing and there are the beginnings of greater public awareness of the dangers of everyday life. Indeed, people are starting to understand the need to protect themselves.

Safety appliances are now readily available. They can be bought from the local sports shop or DIY store with plano-lenses, but if the patient has a prescription, they may choose instead to visit their optician. Optometrists and dispensing opticians receive training in occupational vision and safety and are well qualified to offer advice, and supply the appropriate aids.

Some of the patients who visit the practice ask for professional advice regarding safety. To advise correctly, and in doing so demonstrate the duty of care we owe to others, it is vital to understand the dangers present in the various sporting or hobby activities. Also in this respect, it is an advantage to understand the materials and tools used, and to know the safety appliances available.

To illustrate this further, consider, for example, the appliance you feel would be ideal for your patients who repair the body of their cars with fibreglass. The questions you need to answer are:

- What level of impact resistance should you recommend to give adequate protection from the flying particles produced by hammering, grinding or chiselling the damaged areas to make way for the car reconstruction?
- What do you know of fibreglass? Do you know that fibreglass has many small spicules that can impale the skin and be inhaled into the lungs? Should you also recommend a face mask?
- Fibreglass resins are softened by the solvent acetone, so it is usually suggested that the immediate area surrounding the repair be cleaned prior to applying new material. Will you recommend a metal or plastics frame, and what lens material would you choose?
- Can you also imagine that in this environment there will be a very real danger of flying particles driven by a small explosion? It is well known that solvents have very low flash points, but they have become so commonplace that the danger of an explosion is generally forgotten. Forgotten, that is, until the explosion occurs with all the characteristics of a flame-thrower.

This short list of questions and facts demonstrates the diverse nature of a work environment and illustrates the difficulty of choosing an 'ideal' appliance. A totally safe area, one that is free from any potential hazard, in which every eventuality has been considered, is most unlikely to exist, but the provision of safety spectacles is a very important feature of professional responsibility; it must always be said that 'we did our best'.

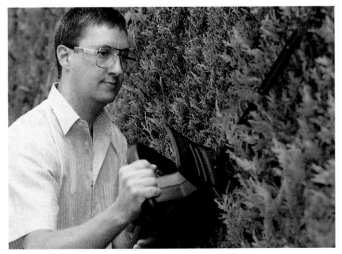

Figure 14.1 Safety eyewear, such as these polycarbonate safety spectacles from Norville, should be worn in a wide range of activities. Gardening accidents are a common source of eye injury

Outline of the history and development of safety materials

The first reference relating to safety was of a presentation given by Prince Rupert* to the Royal Society in 1655. He described the production of what are now known as Prince Rupert's Drops, tear-shaped pieces of soda glass with a bubble at the centre. He described how these pieces of glass were strong enough to withstand heavy blows with a hammer, but would explode if the tail was broken off. Breaking the tail destabilized the internal stress and released the tension within. They were made easily by melting the end of a bar of soda glass into a bucket of water. Even the smallest drops were quite dangerous, and it was suggested that they be handled with great respect. When made they were collected with care, wrapped up in cotton wool and stored in a box. Eye protection was absolutely essential for this procedure. His observations and the techniques he described form the basis of the manufacture of the heat-toughened safety lenses used today.

In 1897, François Bastie carried out experiments in which he immersed samples of glass, heated to just below melting point, into a mixture of linseed oil and tallow. In this way he hoped to produce heat-tempered glass with more stable characteristics than those produced by the more aggressive chilling in water. Unfortunately, his experiments in heat-toughened glass were not totally successful and, in spite of many attempts, little headway was made for some years. Heat-toughened lenses did not develop because the true nature of the process was not understood fully. It was believed that in some way the surfaces became harder. In this same era, however, research was developing that ultimately would lead to chemically toughened lenses. In 1890 the *Annals of Physical Chemistry* reported some experiments that looked at the electrical conductivity of glass and rock crystal after it had been exposed to molten potassium and lithium. This was a doping process very similar to that used today to produce chemical toughened lenses. This was the first description of research in this field. The work of Burt (1924)[2] further extended the boundaries of this knowledge. He carried out experiments to toughen glass chemically by an ionic exchange of sodium for potassium and lithium. By 1924 the technology for producing chemical toughening of glass was available.

In 1891, Otto Schott[3] produced a German patent that described a method of making boiler-gauge tubes by fusing two tubes, one inside the other. One tube was made of high thermal expansion glass and the other of low thermal expansion glass. This method of construction produced a compression layer within the tube that could resist the strains imposed from within a boiler. While this approach was a success, it took many more years to explain satisfactorily why toughened glass was able to withstand more impact than untreated glass. In 1917, however, Twyman described the optical and mechanical properties of glass and showed, for the first time, the nature of the compression envelope.

In 1920 Griffiths studied the phenomena of rupture and flow in solids and, together with Preston in 1933,[4,5] looked at the strength of glass under load. Later, the implications of the known variations in the strength through surface flaws that gave rise to variable results was researched and presented by Hampton and Gould in 1934.[6]

The first reference to the impact testing of toughened glass was made in 1933 when Meikle[7] tested the plate glass windows used for ships by applying hydraulic loads. This was very important research, as large waves have sufficient energy to break the windows of a ship and allow the sea to enter. The testing and development of toughened glass progressed slowly, but in 1957 Hood and Stookey obtained the first US patent of Chemical Toughened Lenses. The science that surrounds glass safety lenses was complete by 1945, in the era of the Second World War.

By 1950 researchers were turning their interests towards testing the various lens materials available to find out how they performed in an industrial situation. This trend was continued into the 1970s by researchers such as Wigglesworth, and others, who published many articles on the assessment of materials for eye protectors. This research was carried out at the time when new materials were coming onto the market and their performance and their ability to provide safety demonstrated.

Research into aspects of safety is still being carried out today, but we find that the research effort is now directed towards patient care; many articles assess the number of eye injuries that require hospital treatment. This work records the occupations of the people involved and identifies the industries and sporting pursuits in which people are most at risk. With this in mind, it is interesting to note that De la Hunty & Sprivulis[8] found that 63% of their sample of 51 patients sustained eye injuries while wearing inappropriate appliances.

Industrial workplaces are commonly regarded as having a large potential for eye injury, a fact supported by the findings of Fong & Taouk,[9] who showed that metal workers who drill, hammer and grind, together with car mechanics and building workers, are among those who are very much at risk. Many of those in their study had serious penetrating injuries. Industrial injuries, however, are not limited to the workplace, as there are many hobby-related hazardous situations in the home environment. These are reported in a European accident surveillance document,[10] compiled from the records of five hospitals, that isolates drilling (Figure 14.2), grinding and welding as being sources of eye injury.

Sporting activities also have a reputation for eye injury. Fong[11] records the dangers of squash and badminton in that

---

* Prince Rupert (1619–1682), third son of Frederick V, Elector Palatine (1596–1632), and nephew of King Charles I of England, was born in Prague. After a year and a half at the English court, he fought (1637–1638) against the imperialists during the Thirty Years' War. In 1648 he commanded the portion of the English Fleet that remained loyal to the King during the wars of the English Revolution.[1]

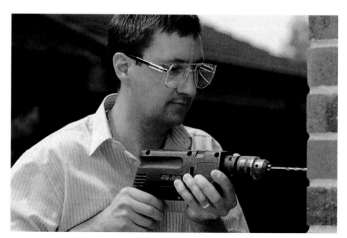

Figure 14.2   Particles flying up from drilling can cause serious eye injury. This do-it-yourself enthusiast wears Norville polycarbonate lenses to protect himself

there is a potential for both hyphaema and ruptured globes. His work is supported by Ariel,[12] who states, 'If patients play squash at any level it is the duty of the optometrist to advise safety goggles'. Those who regulate the sport in the UK have made the wearing of safety appliances mandatory for Juniors only and not for all players, as in Canada and the USA. It is estimated that a squash ball can travel at a velocity of 140 miles/hour and that a badminton shuttlecock can reach a speed of 162 miles/hour.

From the description above, it is very easy to imagine that the need for eye protection relates only to adults and, in doing so, tend to forget that many children are also at risk. Eye protection is recommended for monocular children by Drack et al.,[13] who state that safety glasses saved the good eye in 15 of 33 cases and recommended the use of polycarbonate lenses.

Tables 14.1 and 14.2, extracted from research data, show how the need for eye protection is spread over most of our daily activities and identify many areas of concern.

Types of lenses used for safety and how they are made

Laminated glass safety lenses

Laminated glass safety lenses have not been produced for many years and are now only found as museum examples of the technique. They were made initially by cementing together two pieces of glass with materials such as cellulose acetate. Materials that bonded better to the glass surfaces, like polyvinyl butyrate, were used later, and were therefore less likely to delaminate when in use. These lenses were not very strong, but were able to withstand significantly more impact than a standard glass lens. When broken, however, they tended to remain intact as the particles generally adhered to the centre plastic layer. By modern standards,

these lenses could hardly be described as safe, as not all the particles adhered to the centre layer. The broken glass pieces were usually shaped like scalpel blades, sharp and potentially very destructive.

The technique of laminating glass is still used today in the manufacture of car windscreens, but the outer components are made stronger by toughening. It is usually accepted that these screens perform much better than those that are toughened only, and are the screens of choice.

Laminated lenses were not regarded highly by the technicians who had to cut them, as it was difficult to keep the strain needed to hold the lenses in the frame away from the interlayer between the two layers of glass. Pressure on this plastics layer frequently caused the lens to delaminate. When these lenses were cut using a diamond glass cutter, the cut had to be made on both sides and the lens shanked from the uncut. When cut by a glazing machine, the plastics interlayer formed a coil that frequently blocked the drain from the machine. Care was also needed during the surfacing process, as the heat generated could damage the plastics centre layer. These lenses were used extensively, and were marketed under the trade name of *Salvoc*.

Polarized laminated lenses are available today, but are not designed to provide safety. These lenses are supplied by Norville Optical Company and made by sandwiching a piece of polarizing material between two pieces of glass.

Heat toughened safety lenses

The production of heat-toughened lenses begins by surfacing a somewhat thick glass lens. A heat-toughened 'safety' lens needs to be made thicker than a standard stock lens to ensure that it withstands the final test impact. These lenses must be glazed before they are toughened, as edging them afterwards upsets the strains imparted during the toughening process and the lens may crumble. To assess the length of time the lens needs to be in the toughening oven, the cut lens is weighed to find its volume and the process time is read from a table. The lens is mounted in a holder and placed in the oven, the temperature of which is raised to the lens' softening point, just below the melting point of the glass at 650°C. When the lens has been in the oven for the correct length of time, and the correct temperature reached, it is removed and cooled rapidly by jets of air. These blow on to the lens surfaces from both sides simultaneously. The lens can be withdrawn from the oven mechanically or manually, depending on the level of sophistication required. If an operator works more than one machine a mechanical device is preferable, as this helps to reduce the number of warped lenses caused by overheating. Heat-treating lenses in this way sets up strains inside the lens that result in the outside of the lens being put

Table 14.1	Environments in which eye injuries occur[14]
Causes	Percentage
Children at play/sport	38.8
Road traffic accidents	19.3
Industrial accidents	15.4
Civil disturbances	9.1
Home accidents	6.8
Assault	6.8
Adult sport	4.8
Farm	4.0

Table 14.2	Occupation and type of eye injury[15]			
Occupation	Burn	Contusion	Foreign body	Corneal abrasion
Press/machine tool operators	13	13	425	64
Motor vehicle/aircraft mechanic	10	7	111	18
Metalworker	7	4	111	27
Construction	16	6	82	37
Sheet metalworker	3	3	108	12
Electrician	5	3	77	24
General labourer	6	5	79	34
Welder	9	3	72	18
Bus/coach/lorry driver	4	5	46	23
Processing	4	1	23	8
Painter and decorator	7	1	23	17

into compression, so forming what is called the compression envelope (see Figure 6.13). If this envelope is irregular and thin, the lens is not able to resist impact very well and fails the final impact test (see Figure 6.14).

The heat-toughened method of producing 'safety' lenses is attractive to the manufacturer as it typically takes only a few minutes to heat a lens to the correct temperature and toughen it by cooling. It is not a difficult process to understand and therefore requires only a short time to show someone how to carry out the procedure. No special training programme is required. The machine used in a prescription workshop is based on a small electric oven with an attachment to withdraw the lens at the correct time. The equipment is compact and need not occupy much bench space. Heat toughening is also an ideal process for a prescription workshop with a relatively low production output that provides a tailor-made service to optical practices. The apparatus is very simple to operate and the process times can be modified to accommodate the many various shapes and sizes required by the individual nature of a prescription order.

Although the lenses used for heat toughening are of increased substance, breakage is common and jobs are often returned to the surfacing department for replacement lenses. As the process requires the lenses to be heated virtually to the melting point of the glass, some warping of the lens surfaces may occur, similar to that found, for example, when measuring the power in the segment area of a fused bifocal that has a wavy contact surface through heat distortion.

This process is quite unsuitable for photochromic glass, because it much reduces the activity of the photochromic salts and darkens the lenses. If heat-toughened photochromic lenses have to be used, they must be annealed slightly after the toughening process is complete to restore some of the photochromic activity. This secondary heat treatment consists of heating the lens to 260°C and then cooling it at the rate of 6°C/min. This may, of course, slightly weaken the lens.[16] In general, it is much better to avoid photochromic glass completely when heat-toughened lenses are ordered.

Heat-toughened lenses can be identified reliably by viewing the lens through a polarizing strain viewer in which a Maltese cross with or without a surrounding ring can be seen. This pattern is unique to these lenses, but varies slightly in shape depending on the size of nozzle used to direct the air to cool the lens (see Figure 6.15).

Heat-toughened lenses are often said to be 'safe' because the broken pieces are described as being shaped like cubes and relatively blunt. Not all the fragments are blunt, however, and in testing these lenses it has been found that there are, consistently, splinters sharp enough to cut the fingers.

Special heat-toughened safety lenses

Special heat-toughened lenses became widely available around 1970. The technology involved was developed by Chance Pilkington and is currently the property of Norville Optical Co. The lenses are heated in the same way as air-quenched lenses, but then cooled by immersion in oil, in much the same way as was proposed by Bastie at the end of the 19th century. These lenses are somewhat thinner than the usual heat-toughened variety, and can be identified with a polarizing strain viewer, in which a 'worm-like' pattern, not unlike that of burr walnut seen in furniture, can be observed. This strain pattern is obviously very different to that found in the conventional heat-toughened lens and the two types can hardly be confused.

Chemically toughened safety lenses

In the chemical-toughening process, developed in the USA, large batches of cut lenses are first preheated and then immersed in a bath of molten potassium nitrate at a temperature of 440°C (see Figure 6.16). They are left in the bath for 16 hours, during which time ion-exchange occurs, with potassium ions replacing smaller sodium ions at the surface of the glass. This causes a fairly thin, but extremely regular, compression envelope to form and gives a reasonably strong lens.

This method of producing a glass-toughened lens is probably the most successful if large-volume production is required, as all the lenses, regardless of their power and thickness, are treated in the same way. Lenses of increased thickness are not required, so stock substance lenses can be used and, because the temperatures are much lower than those used in the heat-toughening process, warping does not occur.

As with heat-toughened lenses, lenses toughened by the chemical process should not be edged after they have been toughened, as this disturbs the forces and equilibrium within the lens body. Unfortunately, such lenses are difficult to identify as a polarizing strain viewer does not reveal a characteristic strain pattern. The method is ideal for photochromic lenses, since it does not darken or reduce the photochromic activity.

The process is fully automated, because the chemicals used are both hot and dangerous, and the equipment extremely expensive, as it must be made of materials that do not react with the chemicals used.

CR39

This material was introduced by the Columbia Chemical Division of the Pittsburg Plate Glass Company in 1941 and first became available as a spectacle lens material in the 1950s (Jalie 1984).[17] It is a thermosetting material used during World War II to seal the fuel tanks of damaged B17 bombers.[18]

CR39 produces good-quality lenses and has become the material of choice for in-house glazing, as it is very easy to cut with standard diamond-edging wheels. It has a reputation as a safety material because it is supposed to break into large, non-sharp pieces. This, however, is not always the case and it has been found that many of these lenses broken by means of the drop-ball test or by ballistic methods result in broken pieces that are quite sharp and often have a characteristic hook on the end, which resembles a craft-knife blade. In general, it is also observed that lenses of this material break quite easily.

The performance in relation to other materials is shown in Table 14.3, but remember that the application of anti-reflection and hard coats significantly reduces the already less than ideal impact performance. This material has now been ranked correctly as a low-impact material by the new EN standards.[19]

Polycarbonate

Polycarbonate material was first produced in the late 1950s, since when there has been a steady increase in its quality and use. It was used widely to manufacture goods such as drinking glasses, luminaires for lighting in public areas and as screens to protect bank staff from shotgun blasts. It has also been used for the front panels of tanks in which snakes are kept, as it absorbs well in the ultraviolet (UV) end of the spectrum (the reptiles require UV to remain healthy) and is strong. Initially, the ophthalmic use of this material was restricted to industrial safety lenses because it was quite grey in appearance and not of sufficient quality to be used for everyday, cosmetically appealing, ophthalmic lenses.

Table 14.3 Impact test standards (modified from EN 166[19])

Name of standard	Test standard	Energy (J)	Symbol
Increased robustness	22mm steel ball of weight 43g strikes the lens at a velocity of 5.1m/s	0.56	S
Low-energy impact	6mm steel ball of weight 0.86g strikes the lens at a velocity of 45m/s	0.87	F
Medium-energy impact (applies to goggles and face shields only)	6mm steel ball of weight 0.86g strikes the lens at a velocity of 120m/s	6.19	B
High-energy impact (applies to face shields only)	6mm steel ball of weight 0.86g strikes the lens at a velocity of 190m/s	15.52	A

Since the 1950s much research and development has taken place, as a result of which polycarbonate lenses are now readily available, not only as safety lenses, but also as high-quality spectacle lenses for dress wear. These can be coated more reliably with both hard and multilayer anti-reflection coatings. This development is in some part because of the advances made in the production of compact discs.

Properties of polycarbonate

Polycarbonate material has a resistance to distortion by heat, is quite transparent and has electrical insulating properties. It is also very tough, and is widely used to make eye protectors.[20] It is a thermoplastic polymer that melts at a fairly low temperature and can be moulded and remoulded easily by a process of heating and cooling. When the strength of polycarbonate is compared to that of metals, the mechanical strength is fairly low, but it is very light and, as a spectacle lens material, very strong.[21] Lenses can be produced by both moulding and surfacing techniques. Both methods of production produce good-quality impact-resistant lenses (Figure 14.3).

Polycarbonate crazes when hit. The crazed areas that surround the point of impact can be seen easily by the way in which light is scattered through the lens. The amount of crazing produced is dependent on the time period of the load and the temperature of the material. When the temperature is low, the material crazes more readily and fracture by a small high velocity particle occurs at a lower velocity.[21] Greenberg et al.[22] state that 'as polycarbonate has almost a limitless capacity to withstand massive blows from a hammer, a more realistic test would use a small particle directed against the lens at high velocity'. This is supported by Wigglesworth,[23,24] who states, 'The drop-ball test [stimulates a] blunt trauma from large missiles'. As a result, it is not appropriate to use the drop-ball test to establish the fracture resistance of polycarbonate, as the test is unlikely to break the material. (The author has never managed to break a polycarbonate lens by means of the drop-ball test, even when testing from quite extreme heights.)

Polycarbonate is a fairly good material for the production of spectacle lenses. It has a refractive index of 1.586, Abbe number 30 and density 1.2. It also absorbs UV radiation below 380nm. Inspection of this data shows that the material has many good qualities, but the Abbe number is rather low. However, experience has shown that correctly centred lenses do not cause patients any visual problems. It is therefore possible to produce lightweight lenses that are of good optical quality, and very strong.

Polycarbonate lenses are more difficult to glaze than those made of CR39. Machines dedicated to this material are fitted with special edging wheels, as it is very difficult to cut using the standard diamond-edging wheels. It seems to fight back by clogging the wheels, which reduces the cut to a very slow pace, and by

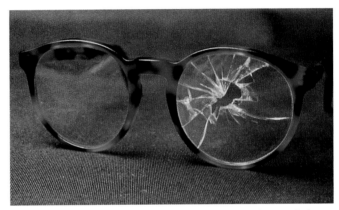

Figure 14.3 Result of a drop-ball test showing a shattered glass lens and intact polycarbonate lens (courtesy of Safety Eyeware)

producing long, thin cuttings that matt together to obstruct the waterways that supply the coolant.

Results of surface coatings on polycarbonate

The surface of polycarbonate is fairly soft and, in wear, scratches very easily. To overcome this problem the usual practice now is to hard-coat polycarbonate lenses to protect the surfaces, but polysiloxane coating also reduces the fracture resistance of the lens. This reduced impact resistance occurs when both CR39 and polycarbonate lenses are hard-coated or anti-reflection coated.

Note that solvents such as acetone also severely reduce the ability of polycarbonate to resist impact. This is of great importance to people who work with solvents. There are two usual methods to test a surface for its abrasion resistance in the laboratory:

- Calibrated amounts of carborundum are dropped onto the surface, inclined at 45°, and the gloss of the surface in that area is compared to gloss on the rest of the sample.
- Taber Abrader – the sample is mounted on a table and revolved, and the surface then abraded by an abrasive wheel that travels at a different speed. The quantity of abrasion is measured optically or expressed as the loss of weight following a specific number of revolutions.[25]

Elasticity and glazing

When an object hits the surface of a lens it imparts kinetic energy to the lens. If this exchange is complete, the object ceases movement at the lens surface and the lens absorbs all the energy. This is demonstrated neatly by Newton's Cradle, in which a swinging ball impacts another that then begins to swing under the impact. If the lens is unable to move or flex, all this energy is imparted to the body of the lens and, if the energy is too great, the lens breaks. However, if the lens is made of an elastic material it is able to

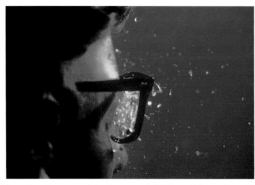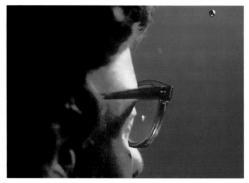

Figure 14.4   Ball-bearing tests on (a) glass $n = 1.523$ and (b) polycarbonate $n = 1.59$. The steel ball travelled at over 100mph. The glass shatters but the polycarbonate, although marked, remains intact (courtesy of Norville Optical)

Table 14.4 A comparison of the impact resistance of materials	
Lens material	6.5mm ball (m/s)
Glass	
Toughened glass	18
Untoughened glass	12
Laminated glass	12
Plastic	
CR39	49
PMMA	34
Polycarbonate coated	152
Polycarbonate uncoated	244

Data obtained from 3mm thick samples (Wigglesworth[24])

move, take on board the energy and give some back in the form of a ricochet. Polycarbonate, unlike glass, is a fairly elastic material and provides a good example of this mechanism.

Lenses are, in general, made in meniscus form with the convex surface facing forwards. The effect of a body hitting the front surface is to try to move it backwards, which results in the lens attempting to spread and increase in diameter. If the lens is contained by a rim it is unable to flex and repel some of the energy, and will fracture much more easily. This was demonstrated by Storey,[26] who held polycarbonate lenses by their edges in an inflatable ring support that mimicked the rim of a spectacle frame. The edge pressure applied to the lens could be varied by adjusting the air pressure within the ring. In his experiments he tested the fracture resistance of polycarbonate lenses by firing a steel ball 6.5mm in diameter at the front surface at many different velocities. He found that the maximum edge pressure allowable for a polycarbonate lens to pass even the low-energy impact was 7psi and that, as this pressure was released, the lenses were able to withstand progressively more impact. This work is supported by observations made during routine ballistic testing of many prescription safety spectacles (Figure 14.4).

This work has a considerable bearing on the way in which polycarbonate lenses are glazed, as it shows quite clearly that to attain the maximum level of safety from the lenses, they should be glazed slightly loose in the frame. However, this exposes the need to define the ideal tightness of a rim for safety spectacles and the need to find methods to measure it, as there is the obvious duty to ensure that injuries do not occur through the lens being driven out of the frame. A rim tightness device, which twists the rim under a specific weight, is available, but it was designed for routine prescription work and not specifically for testing safety lenses. While there is no immediate solution to this conundrum, it may support

the manufacturers who increase the back edge of the groove in the spectacle frame to provide a ridge for the lens to press against.

Cellulose acetate

This material has not been used to manufacture ophthalmic lenses as it is far too soft to hold its shape accurately. However, it is used to make both frames and side-shields and to make covers to protect the surfaces of lenses.

Comparison of materials and the test standards

The standards that now apply to impact resistant lenses are defined in the EN Standards 166, 167 and 168.[19] These have now completely replaced the old BS 2092 Standard. These standards are somewhat more demanding as the impact velocities recommended for impact-resistant lenses are increased significantly. All lenses used for safety have to pass a basic level, referred to as 'increased robustness', which distinguishes these lenses from those that do not pretend to embody any safety feature. All appliances that have impact-resistance features are classified as able to pass either low-, medium- or high-energy impact. All these are marked with a symbol to indicate the level of safety they offer, as shown in Table 14.3.

Note that the increased robustness, low-energy impact and medium-energy impact are very similar to the old BS 2092 Standard, but the high-energy impact is a new, much more severe test.

From the data available, the best material for the production of impact-resistant safety spectacles is, without doubt, polycarbonate (Table 14.4). Spectacles of this material easily pass the general robustness and low-energy impact test defined by the EN 166. They need to be glazed correctly and ideally in a plastics frame that will, to some extent, allow for movement of the lens in the rim. Their use depends on the environment in which they will be employed. If it is felt that a higher level of safety is needed than that provided by safety spectacles, goggles or shields should be suggested. Shields would also be the appliance of choice if a dust mask is being used, as they tend to suffer less from condensation.

It is important that great care be exercised when recommending an appliance to ensure that all the relevant facts are understood and that the person who makes the purchase understands its limitations.

The PPG Trivex™ material was specifically developed to be as strong as, if not stronger than, polycarbonate, and the new revised US Z87 Standard is certain to permit not just the use of polycarbonate, but also the new Trivex™ material surfaced down to 2.0mm thickness for industrial safety use. At present the Standard still requires prescription polycarbonate lenses to be a minimum of 3.0mm thick for industrial safety eyewear, but the addition of this second impact-resistant lens material with favourable optical properties will contribute to a continued improvement of eye safety among spectacle wearers.

Practitioner's guide

1. Always use appliances of appropriate EN Standard:
   - Check to ensure the task is clearly understood
   - Check that both frames and lenses are marked
   - Check that there is a manufacturer's identification
   - Identify the manufacturer
   - Check that the appropriate symbols are present.
2. Examine every eye protector supplied for faults. Check the side-shields and the security of lenses in the rim. Side-shields should not displace under pressure.
3. Ascertain that spectacles with side-shields provide sufficient protection.
4. Make sure you have a copy of EN 166/167.
5. Keep an accurate record of all transactions.
6. Remember that you must know of and approve of the appliance being supplied and as such are legally responsible.

Both Trivex and polycarbonate are strong lens materials and routinely used for fashion eyewear and to make safety appliances for eye protection. Unlike fashion eyewear, all eye protectors are tested to the appropriate EN standard and, although neither material shows the same impact resistance when hard or anti-reflection coated, they pass the tests and are 'safe' for the purpose for which they were intended.

It would be easy to suggest that a lens is 'safe' just because it is made of plastics. Fashionable glasses are not supplied for combat and are not impact tested. Lightweight, cosmetically appealing, expensive eyewear is not manufactured to provide sufficient eye protection for pursuits like playing squash, but is ideal for dress wear and going to work.

References

1. Microsoft 1994 Encarta CD-ROM. Microsoft, Redmond
2. Burt R C 1924 Sodium by electrolysis through glass. J Opt Soc Am 11:87–91
3. Schott O 1891 German patent 61573
4. Preston F W 1933 Surface strength of glass and other materials. J Soc Glass Tech 17:5–8
5. Preston F W 1933 Glass as a structural and stress resistant material. J Am Ceram Soc 16:163–186
6. Hampton W M, Gould C E 1934 Some implications of the known variables in the strength of glass. J Soc Glass Tech 18:194–200
7. Meikle J 1933 Some notes on toughened plate glass. J Soc Glass Tech 17:149
8. De la Hunty D, Sprivulis P 1994 Safety goggles should be worn by Australian workers. Aust NZ J Ophthalmol 22:49–52
9. Fong L P, Taouk Y 1995 The role of eye protection in work related eye injuries. Aust NZ J Ophthalmol 23:101–106
10. Holmich L R, Holmich P, Lohman R F 1995 (Translated) Eye injuries during hobby-work using machine tools. Ugeskrift fur Laeger 157:2131–2134
11. Fong L P 1994 Sports related eye injuries. Med J Aust 160:743–747
12. Ariel B R 1997 The importance of sports vision in clinical practice. Br J Optom Dispens 5:93
13. Drack A, Kutschke P J, Stair S, Scott W E 1994 Compliance with safety glasses wear in monocular children. J Ophthal Nursing Technol 13:77–82
14. Canavan Y M, O'Flaherty J, Archer D B, Elwood J H 1980 A ten year survey of eye injuries in Northern Ireland 1967–76. Br J Ophthalmol 64:618–625
15. Chiapella A P, Rosenthal A R 1985 One year in an eye casualty clinic. Br J Ophthalmol 69:865–870
16. Woodcock F R 1982 Lens toughening up to date: pros & cons of thermal and chemical processes Part 1. Thermo-tempering. Manufacturing Optics International Dec/Jan:19–24
17. Jalie M 1984 The principles of ophthalmic lenses. 4th edn. ABDO, London
18. Crundall E J 1980 CR39 Special – How it all started – the story of Armorlite. Manufacturing Optics International
19. European Standards EN 166, 167, 168 (1994–2001) Various titles. BSI, London
20. Freitag D, Grigo U, Nouvertine W Polycarbonates. In: Mark H F, Bikales N M, Overberger C G, Menges G, Kroschwitz J I, (eds) Encyclopaedia of polymer science and engineering, John Wiley, New York
21. Young R J 1981 Introduction to polymers. Chapman and Hall, London
22. Greenberg I, Chace G, Lamarre D 1985 Statistical protocol for impact testing prescription polycarbonate lenses. Optical World 14:7–8
23. Wigglesworth E C 1971 The impact resistance of eye protector lens materials. Am J Optom Arch Am Acad Optom 48:245–261
24. Wigglesworth E C 1971 A ballistic assessment of eye protector lens materials. Invest Ophthalmol 10:958–991
25. Golding B 1959 Polymers and resins. Van Nostrand, New York
26. Storey C 1979 How can polycarbonate lenses be processed to ensure maximum safety? Undergraduate thesis

Special lenses

So far, we have considered the various types of spectacle lenses in regular use in modern dispensing practice. In this chapter we consider lenses prescribed only rarely, either to provide magnification or for vocational purposes.

Iseikonic lenses

Spectacle lenses are sometimes used to alter the size of the retinal image without changing its position. This is usually required in the condition known as *aniseikonia*, in which an inequality in the size or shape of the retinal images prevents comfortable binocular vision.[1] Aniseikonia may arise as a result of anisometropia between the eyes or it could be induced by a pair of lenses of equal power, but of different forms and thicknesses.

Lenses specifically designed to alter the size or shape of the retinal image are called *iseikonic lenses*. They usually include a refractive correction, but they may be afocal. They are also known as *size lenses*, since they alter the size but not the position of the retinal image.

The magnification of a spectacle lens arises partly from its form and partly from its power.[2] The magnification from the form of the lens is known as the *shape factor*, S, since it depends upon the degree of bending, expressed in terms of the front surface power, F_1, and the thickness, t, of the lens. The shape factor is given by:

$$S = \left[1 - (t/n)F_1\right]^{-1}$$

The magnification from the power of the lens is known as the *power factor*, P, and is a function of the position of the lens with respect to the eye's entrance pupil, d, and the back vertex power of the lens, F'_v. The power factor is given by:

$$P = \left(1 - dF'_v\right)^{-1}$$

The total spectacle magnification, SM, of the lens is the product of these two magnification factors:

$$SM = S \times P$$

In general, in the design of an iseikonic lens, the power factor is determined by the prescription and the designer alters the shape factor to produce the required spectacle magnification. Increasing the bending of the lens, or increasing its thickness, produces an increase in magnification.

By way of example, consider the +4.00D lens shown in Figure 15.1. Suppose the lens is made in a material of refractive index 1.5 and mounted 15mm in front of the eye's entrance pupil. The total spectacle magnification of the lens is the product of its shape and power factors:

$$S = \left[1 - (t/n)F_1\right]^{-1}$$
$$= \left[1 - (0.006/1.5) \times 10\right]^{-1}$$
$$= 1.042$$

which could also be expressed as 4.2%.

$$P = \left(1 - dF'_v\right)^{-1}$$
$$= (1 - 0.015 \times 4)^{-1}$$
$$= 1.0638$$

which could be expressed as 6.38%. The total spectacle magnification, $SM = S \times P = 1.042 \times 1.0638 = 1.1085$ or 10.85%.

Suppose it is found that the magnification of this lens needs to be increased by 1.0%. This might have been determined, for example, by the addition of a 1% afocal trial lens to the subject's existing lens. The power factor, of course, is fixed by the prescription, and assuming no change in vertex distance, the change in magnification must be effected by increasing the shape factor of the lens.

The new total magnification required is the original magnification, 1.1085, multiplied by 1.01 (the additional magnification of 1%), so the new spectacle magnification = 1.1196. Since the contribution from the power factor is 1.0638, the shape factor that is required must be:

$$1.1196/1.0638 = 1.0524$$

This can be obtained either by increasing the bending of the lens or by increasing the lens thickness. If it is decided to increase the lens thickness, substitution into the expression for the shape factor of the lens leads to:

$$S = \left[1 - (t/n)F_1\right]^{-1}$$

so:

$$1.0524 = \left[1 - (t/1.5) \times 10\right]^{-1}$$

from which:

$$t = 0.007469\text{m or } 7.47\text{mm}$$

This example embodies the principles of the design of iseikonic lenses.

The total spectacle magnification is made up partly by the shape factor and partly by the power factor. Usually, the power factor

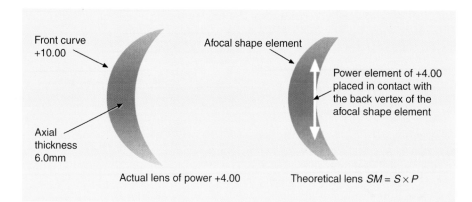

Figure 15.1 Derivation of shape and power factors of a spectacle lens

of the lens is fixed by the prescriber, that is, the prescription and vertex distance of the lens are to remain unaltered. Generally, two possibilities should be considered. The designer could be asked to produce a lens that incorporates a specified spectacle magnification or to produce a pair of lenses that have identical spectacle magnifications irrespective of differences in their powers.

In the first case, the prescriber gives details of the subject's existing lens and the percentage increase to be incorporated in the lens. This information must include the form and thickness of the lens and its vertex distance, in addition to the back vertex power. From this information, the designer can deduce the spectacle magnification of the original lens and incorporate with this the additional spectacle magnification required. The resultant lens might be called a pure iseikonic lens.

In the second case, the prescriber simply gives the back vertex powers of the right and left lenses together with their vertex distances, and asks that the final lenses have equal spectacle magnifications. Here, the designer must calculate the power factor of each lens and, if these are different, arrange for any difference to be eliminated by modifying the shape factors of each lens.

Plano-size lenses

The magnification of an afocal iseikonic lens (plano-size lens) is due to the shape factor alone, since the power factor is unity. The shape factor of an afocal iseikonic lens can be expressed in the more convenient form:

$$\Delta = -tF_2/10n$$

where Δ is the required magnification expressed as a percentage increase and t is the axial thickness of the lens as before. For example, a 1% afocal iseikonic lens made in a material of refractive index 1.5, with an axial thickness of 3.0mm, would need a back curve of −5.00D and a front curve, by accurate transposition, of +4.95D.

Meridional magnification can be provided by means of bi-cylindrical or bi-toric construction.

For anisometropia, it has been suggested,[3] especially for those cases in which the refractive error is known to be refractive in origin, that the magnification of the weaker lens should be increased to match that of the stronger, so the effect of any aniseikonia that might be induced by the prescription is eliminated. A pair of lenses with the same spectacle magnification, despite a difference in the powers of each lens, is called an *isogonal* pair. The design of isogonal lenses follows the outline given above. In general, a stock lens is chosen, where possible, for the higher plus prescription (or weaker minus lens) of the pair, and the spectacle magnification of this lens computed from the

relationship given above. The power factor of the other lens is then determined, as detailed above, and the shape factor of the second lens found from:

$$S = (SM \text{ of 1st lens}) / (P \text{ of 2nd lens})$$

When the required shape factor for the second lens is known, the design method follows the same sequence as that detailed above.

In cases of astigmatism, one lens of the pair needs to incorporate a meridional correction and is of bi-toric construction.

Low-vision appliances

From the theoretical point of view, low-vision appliances (LVAs) can be classified into the following groups:

- *Spectacle magnifiers*, which consist essentially of a plus lens or lens combination mounted close to the eye. As far as its optical properties are concerned, this group includes similar appliances held in the hand at the same short distance from the eye.
- *Binocular magnifiers* are also part of this group, and comprise a pair of magnifiers designed to allow binocular viewing of a near object. Usually, a binocular magnifier incorporates base-in prism in each lens to relieve convergence. Prismatic half-eye spectacles have proved to be a very popular form of binocular magnifier.
- *Hand-held or stand magnifiers*, which are differentiated from the previous group in that they are held close to an object at a normal near-work viewing distance from the eye.
- *Telescopic spectacles*, which are the only type of device that caters for distance or intermediate vision, but may also be adapted for near vision. They are normally in the form of a Galilean telescopic system. This has the enormous advantage of enabling an erect image to be formed from a compact system.
- *Low-power projectors and closed-circuit television systems* enable the printed page to be projected onto a screen and viewed by the subject under varying amounts of magnification. The design principles for these devices are not considered here.

Spectacle magnifiers

Spectacle magnifiers are essentially high-powered plus lenses (or lens systems) mounted close to the eye and are usually restricted to monocular use. The magnification of a spectacle magnifier, M, is given by the relationship:

$$M = qL/(1 - dL')$$

where L and L' are the object and image distances, respectively, expressed in dioptres, and q is the least distance of distinct vision, usually taken to be -25cm.

When the object coincides with the anterior principal focus of the magnifier, the magnification (so-called nominal magnification) of the device is simply $-qF$, where F is the *equivalent* power of the lens or lens system. In the following discussion it is assumed that q is the conventional -0.25m, so the magnification ascribed to a device is simply $F/4$.

The most serious defects of high-powered spherical lenses when used as spectacle magnifiers are transverse chromatism, oblique astigmatism and distortion. Without using compound elements, little can be done to combat chromatism, so spectacle magnifiers tend to be restricted to single high-power plus lenses with just a single variable, the form of the lens surfaces.

When restricted to the use of spherical surfaces it is possible to bend the magnifier into a form that exhibits minimum oblique astigmatism, but the use of an aspherical surface also enables distortion to be corrected.

Perhaps the best-known series of aspheric magnifiers is the *Hyperocular* series of spectacle magnifiers (Figure 15.2) from Combined Optical Industries Ltd (COIL), which were introduced as long ago as 1956. Details of the current range of *Hyperocular* lenses are given in Table 15.1. These lenses are employed in several different forms of magnifying devices.

Compound spectacle magnifiers

The field-of-view of strong spectacle magnifiers, over about 8×, can be increased significantly by means of a compound system such as illustrated in Figure 15.3. This system is akin to a Ramsden Eyepiece, except that the second surface of the front plastics element is aspherical. The rear meniscus component could be made of glass or plastics material.

The magnification of a compound system depends on its equivalent power, which may be appreciably less than the sum of the two component powers because of the separation of their principal points.

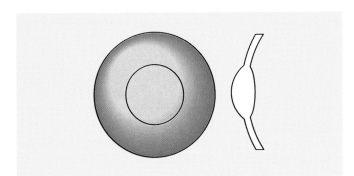

Figure 15.2   6× *Hyperocular* spectacle magnifier

Spectacle magnifiers of Galilean type

The chief drawback of the spectacle magnifier – its very short working distance – can be overcome to some extent by employing a Galilean system. As with an ordinary spectacle magnifier, the object is held in, or just inside, the anterior focal plane, in which case the magnification is given by the same formula, $M = F/4$. F is the equivalent power of the system, as before.

The advantage of the Galilean system lies in the fact that the combination of a positive and a negative lens shifts the first principal focus, F, forwards, as shown in Figure 15.4. Since the equivalent focal lengths (f') of the two systems are the same, their equivalent powers, and hence the magnification of each system, is the same.

The principle of the Galilean magnifier can be deduced as follows. The equivalent power of the system, F, is given by:

$$F = 4M = F_1 + F_2 - dF_1F_2$$

from which:

$$F_2 = (4M - F_1)/(1 - dF_1)$$

Also, since the object is placed at the anterior focus of the system, the emergent pencil of light is parallel, that is:

$$(L_1 + F_1)/\left[1 - d(L_1 + F_1)\right] + F_2 = 0$$

which can be simplified to:

$$L_1 + F - dL_1F_2 = 0$$

from which:

$$F_2 = (L_1 + F)/dL_1$$

Equating these last two expressions for F_2, we have:

$$(4M - F_1)/(1 - dF_1) = (L_1 + F)/dL_1$$

from which:

$$F_1 = \left[L_1(1 - dF) + F\right]/dF$$

By making aspherical the deep convex surface of the objective and the deep concave surface of the eyepiece, acceptable optical performance can be obtained from such a system, both oblique astigmatism and distortion being reduced to low levels.

Binocular spectacle magnifiers

The very short working distance of spectacle magnifiers, with the object being held at, or just inside, the anterior focal plane, means a large effort of convergence is required by the eyes to view

Table 15.1	The *Hyperocular* lens series					
Magnification	**Equivalent power**	**Type of conicoid**	F_2	t	**Effective aperture**	**Uncut diameters**
4×	+16.00	Ellipsoid	+1.00	7.5	40	50 and 65
5×	+20.00	Ellipsoid	+3.00	8.5	38	50 and 65
6×	+24.00	Paraboloid	+4.00	9.5	36	50 and 65
8×	+32.00	Hyperboloid	+11.00	10.5	34	50 and 65
10×	+40.00	Hyperboloid	+12.00	11.3	32	65
12×	+48.00	Hyperboloid	+16.00	12.0	30	65

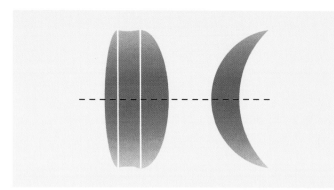

Figure 15.3 Compound spectacle magnifier

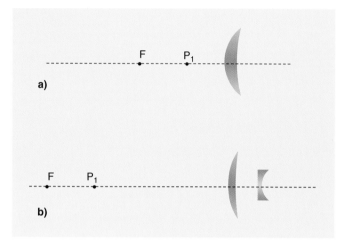

Figure 15.4 Galilean spectacle magnifier: (a) short working distance of single plus lens; (b) telephoto system moves first principal focus well forward, providing far greater working distance

Table 15.2 Typical series of aspheric–prismatic half-eye spectacles	
Power	Prism (each lens)
+4.00	6Δ base in
+6.00	8Δ base in
+8.00	10Δ base in
+10.00	12Δ base in
+12.00	14Δ base in
+14.00	16Δ base in

the image binocularly. It is usual to relieve the effort of convergence by incorporating base-in prism in the lenses. Obviously, the greater the amount of prism included in the lenses, the less becomes the effort of convergence, but at the same time the worse becomes the optical performance of the lenses.

The amount of prism that is incorporated depends upon the power of the lenses. One suggestion is that there should be the same number of prism dioptres as the dioptric power of the lens. Hence, a +8.00D lens would have 8Δ base-in included, that is, 16Δ base-in for the pair. A rule that seems to be preferred in America is that the prism should be 2Δ more than the power of the lenses, so a +8.00 would have 10Δ base-in each eye, that is, 20Δ base-in for the pair.

Making aspherical the convex surface of the lenses reduces both oblique astigmatism and distortion and, at the same time, enables somewhat thinner lenses to be produced, in particular enabling a reduction in the thickness of the lenses on their nasal edges.

A typical series of aspheric-prismatic half-eye spectacles (available from COIL) is given in Table 15.2.

Hand-held magnifiers

When a strong plus lens is used as a magnifying glass held close to the eye, the pupil of the eye acts as the aperture stop and the lens itself acts as the field stop. Since the pupil limits the bundles of rays that arrive at the eye from the virtual image in front of the lens, it is also the exit pupil of the system. When the eye lies

between the lens and its second principal focus, the entrance pupil is the virtual image of the pupil of the eye and lies on the same side of the lens as the eye.

In the case of the rotating eye, we assume the aperture stop to coincide with the eye's centre of rotation, so the entrance pupil is the image of an imaginary pupil placed at the eye's centre of rotation. If the centre of rotation lies between the lens and its second principal focus, the entrance pupil still lies on the same side of the lens as the eye.

Under these circumstances, the spherical aberration between the entrance and exit pupils will be much smaller when the steeper convex surface of the magnifier faces the object. If the lens is plano-convex, for example, the spherical aberration between the pupils, and therefore the distortion, will be much smaller when the plane surface faces the eye.

Different circumstances arise when the lens is held at some distance from the eye, as is the case when the object is at the usual viewing distance of, say, 33.3cm. The pupil of the eye still acts as the exit pupil of the system, but its image, the entrance pupil, now lies on the opposite side of the lens beyond the object. Under these circumstances, the spherical aberration between the entrance and exit pupils will be much smaller when the steeper convex surface of the magnifier faces the eye, that is, the lens is reversed with respect to its position when held close to the eye.

If the lens is plano-convex, the spherical aberration between the pupils, and therefore the distortion, will be much smaller when the plane surface faces the object. This is confirmed easily by viewing a square-grid object through a strong plano-convex lens, held with the plane surface initially close to the eye and then moved steadily away, together with the object and the object distance remaining fixed with respect to the lens. The quality of the image deteriorates rapidly, the distortion in particular becoming quite objectionable.

When this experiment is repeated with the lens turned back-to-front, so that the convex surface faces the eye, the distortion is objectionable when the lens is held in the spectacle plane, but improves rapidly as the object and lens are moved away from the eye. When the lens is at 33.3cm from the eye with the plane surface facing the object, the optical performance is much improved, as already noted above.

Thus, the design requirements for a hand-held magnifier are just the reverse of those for a spectacle magnifier designed to be mounted close to the eye. As a general rule, the shallower curve of a hand-held magnifier is designed to face the object and the steeper convex surface faces the eye. Obviously, if the lens is symmetrical, it is immaterial which way round it is held.

As with spectacle magnifiers, replacing the steeper convex curve with an aspherical surface produces a considerable reduction in pincushion distortion.

The focusing distance is critical with a strong hand-held magnifier, so it is often mounted on a stand to ensure it is positioned

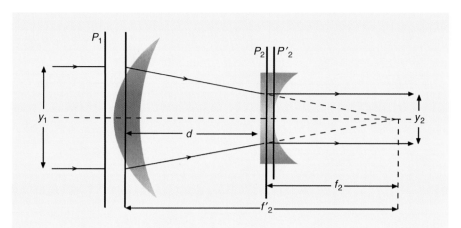

Figure 15.5　Galilean telescopic system in normal adjustment

correctly at a fixed distance from the object. Stand magnifiers have the added advantage that they leave the user's hands free, which is very useful to elderly people who might not otherwise be able to hold the lens still.

Telescopic spectacles

When magnification is required for distance or intermediate vision, it must be provided in the form of a telescopic system. These telescopic systems must be lightweight and compact so that they can be worn for long periods in the spectacle plane. The Galilean system is usually employed, since it provides an erect image without the necessity for inverting lenses or prisms and, as it consists essentially of just two elements, a positive objective and a negative eyepiece, can be very compact, provided it is not made too powerful. Normally, no more than about 2× magnification is prescribed.

A Galilean system is depicted in Figure 15.5. When parallel light both enters and leaves the system it is said to be in normal adjustment. When used in normal adjustment a distant object is seen in sharp focus by an unaccommodated emmetropic eye.

The magnification of the system is given by:

$$M = y_1/y_2 = -F_2/F_1 = 1/(1 - dF_1)$$

The paraxial design of a telescopic system is very simple. A 2× unit, for example, might be made from a +20.00D objective and a –40.00D eye lens separated by 25mm.

The Galilean system illustrated in Figure 15.5 is afocal and assumes an emmetropic observer. Any necessary distance correction may be incorporated in the eye lens or in a special cell mounted directly behind the eye lens.

A telescopic unit designed for distance vision cannot be used alone for near vision because the accommodative demand is much greater than with a single spectacle lens. Consider the afocal 2× unit described above. For near vision at 33.3cm, the vergence that leaves the eye lens when the incident vergence upon the objective is –3.00 will be –10.43. Hence, the accommodative demand measured in the spectacle plane is almost 10.50D.

Similarly, for intermediate vision at 80cm, the accommodative demand in the spectacle plane is 4.71D. The distance unit can be converted to near vision use, quite simply, by adding a reading cap to the objective lens; the cap incorporates a plus lens with dioptric power the same as the required dioptric reading distance. Thus, for near vision at 33.3cm, a +3.00D cap is required; for intermediate vision at –50cm, a +2.00D cap is required and so on.

The magnification of the unit adapted for near vision by the addition of a cap of power, F_N, is simply:

$$M = F_N/4 \times M_{distance}$$

Thus, the 2× unit described above adapted for use at 33.3cm by the addition of a +3.00D cap has a magnification for near vision of:

$$M = 3/4 \times 2 = 1.5×$$

The advantage of a telescopic near vision unit is its greatly increased working distance. A +6.00D spectacle magnifier, which offers the same magnification of 1.5×, requires the shorter working distance of just 16.67cm.

The design of telescopic units is complicated by the criteria that the unit must be both compact and light in weight, which imply the use of high-power components. However, the designer does have two elements and, therefore, four surfaces to work with. By making aspherical the steeper curves, excellent results can be obtained, since it is possible to combat chromatism, oblique astigmatism and distortion.

Transverse chromatism can be reduced by the choice of suitable media. For the 2× telescope described above, the Abbe numbers of the objective and eye lens should be in the ratio 2:1. PMMA (Perspex), for example, for which $V = 58$, and polycarbonate, for which $V = 30$, produce a lightweight all-plastics unit. Alternatively, a high-index glass, such as a 1.700 index glass with an Abbe number of 30, may be used for the eye lens, combined with a PMMA or CR39 objective.

A typical 2× telescopic system is illustrated in Figure 15.6. The 40mm diameter objective is made in PMMA and is biconvex in form, with a convex prolate ellipsoidal front surface and a rear surface of power +1.00. The eye lens is made from polystyrene, in biconcave form, with a –1.00 front surface and a deep concave ellipsoidal rear curve. The separation of the components is 40mm.

Fresnel lenses

Among the many works of the French mathematician, engineer and physicist Augustin Jean Fresnel (1788–1827), was the invention of flat, weight-saving lenses for use in lighthouses. Today, Fresnel lenses and prisms are thin discs of polyvinyl chloride precision-cut on one surface to form prismatic elements that refract the light in the same way as a lens or prism. The principle can be deduced from Figure 15.7, which compares a normal prism with a Fresnel prism. The latter can be imagined to consist of a large number of strips of the small prismatic element taken from the normal prism and laid side by side on a thin flexible membrane.

The membrane can be cut to any desired shape and size and attached to a plano-carrier lens to form a single-vision lens, or to a prescription single-vision lens to form a bifocal and so on. The membrane is attached by hydrostatic force, simply by pressing the plane surface of the thin membrane against the carrier lens surface under clean running water to exclude air bubbles at the interface.

Current availability of these Fresnel press-on lenses is as follows:

Spheres:

Plus	+0.50 to +4.00 in 0.50D steps
	+5.00 to +8.00 in 1.00D steps
	+10.00 to +16.00 in 2.00D steps
Minus	−1.00 to −14.00 in 1.00D steps

Prisms:

1Δ to 8Δ in 1Δ steps and
10Δ, 12Δ, 15Δ, 20Δ, 25Δ and 30Δ

Flat-top D25 segments:

+1.00 to +3.00 in 0.50D steps and
+4.00 to +6.00 in 1.00D steps

The discrete nature of the zones and the imperfect optical surfaces of the PVC sheet mean a drop in visual acuity is to be expected when compared with a conventional lens. However, this disadvantage may be outweighed by the convenience and the thinner, lighter and neater lens form that results from the process. Perhaps the most important use in practice is to produce a temporary correction or an experimental bifocal or trifocal lens that can be made later in a permanent, more conventional form if the temporary correction proves to be successful.

Corning photochromic filters

Concern has been expressed in recent years about the possible ocular hazards that may arise from exposure to long-wave ultraviolet radiation (waveband UVA) and the blue range of the visible spectrum. Corning photochromic filters (CPFs) are glass filters that comprise a series of photochromic contrast filters specially developed to absorb UVA and the shorter visible waveband, to provide relief from glare and dazzle conditions that might be met, for example, on the ski slopes or on the beach in strong sunlight. Four different filters are available; the code number given indicates the shortest wavelength transmitted by the filter, that is, the cut-off value at the blue end of the spectrum. The characteristics of the filters are given in Table 15.3.

Corning's research indicates that the CPF series is of benefit both in conditions of extreme sunlight and in providing some relief in certain pathological conditions, such as incipient cataract, aphakia, retinopathy, corneal dystrophy, etc.

CPF prescription lenses are available from the Norville Group in three different forms: single-vision lenses, D28 flat-top bifocals and *Graduate* progressive power lenses.

Special multifocal designs

Occasionally, prescriptions occur that need different cylinder powers and/or axes for distance and near. Such specifications are met easily by dispensing two separate pairs of spectacles for distance and near, but it is also possible to provide the prescription in bifocal form. The most obvious bifocal design for these unusual specifications is the split bifocal, in which the distance and near portions are made up from two separate lenses. Each portion may have any power and prism specification, the lenses cut in half and the two elements combined in one eye of the frame.

Different cylinder powers and/or axes for distance and near can also be produced in cemented bifocal form, by incorporating

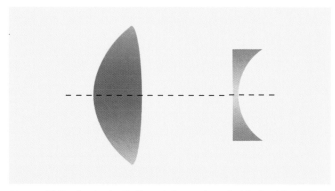

Figure 15.6   Aspheric Galilean telescopic unit, *M* = 2×. The PMMA objective has a convex ellipsoidal surface. The polystyrene eye lens has a concave ellipsoidal surface

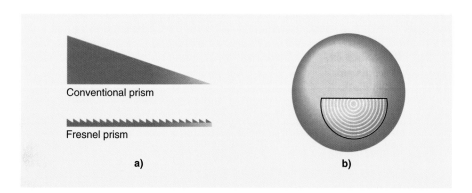

Conventional prism

Fresnel prism

a)

b)

Figure 15.7   Fresnel press-on lenses: (a) Fresnel prism – the PVC film is cut with parallel grooves, each element of which can be considered to be a tiny prism and, in a Fresnel lens, are arranged concentrically; (b) bifocal lens made by attaching a flat-top D25 press-on segment to a single-vision lens

Table 15.3 Corning photochromic filters

Filter	Cut-off (nm)	Transmittance (%)		UV filtering (%)		Tint	
		Unactivated	Exposed	UVB	UVA	Unactivated	Exposed
CPF 450	450	73	18	100	97	Yellow	Brown
CPF 511-S	511	47	12	100	99	Yellow–amber	Brown
CPF 527	527	34	9	100	98	Orange–amber	Brown
CPF 550-S	550	20	5	100	99	Orange–red	Brown

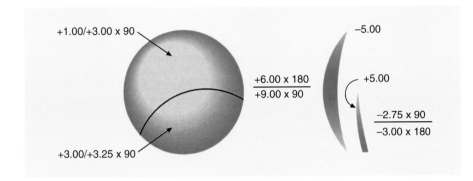

Figure 15.8 Cemented bifocal design for the prescription DV +1.00/+3.00 × 90, NV +3.00/+3.25 × 90. The contact surface is ±3.00D. In practice, the two components would be bonded together, but are separated here for clarity

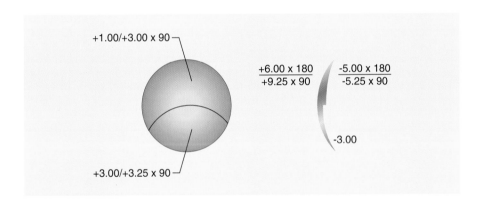

Figure 15.9 Solid visible bifocal design for the prescription DV +1.00/+3.00 × 90, NV +3.00/+3.25 × 90. The segment surface is –5.00D. The curve worked on the distance-portion surface is not operative in the near portion

a toroidal surface on the back surface of the segment. Consider the prescription:

DV   R + 1.00/+ 3.00 × 90

NV   R + 3.00/+ 3.25 × 90

in which the addition for near is +2.00/+0.25 × 90, and the cylinder power needs to be increased to correct fully the ocular astigmatism at near.[1,2]

Figure 15.8 illustrates the nominal surface powers for this specification made as a cemented bifocal with a ±5.00D contact surface. In practice, the two components are bonded together to produce a permanent design.

Such complex prescription requirements can also be produced in solid bifocal form by using a visible design with a segment surface depressed below the level of the distance-portion surface. The curves worked on the distance-portion surface are then not operative in the near portion, the power of which is controlled by the curves on the front surface and the spherical reading-portion surface. Figure 15.9 illustrates the nominal curves used for a solid visible bifocal made to the prescription given above, assuming that the reading-portion curve is –5.00DS.

These lenses are currently available from Rodenstock, who can produce such requirements with their visible solid no-jump bifocal

designs, the *Ardis* downcurve bifocal and their E-Style *Excellent* design. The lenses are surfaced in Germany, but are available here to special order.

Different cylinder powers and/or axes for distance and near can also be produced in fused bifocal form, by grinding a toroidal depression surface. Figure 15.10 illustrates the nominal curves that could be worked to produce the above specification, assuming the use of a pair of glasses with a blank ratio of 4:1 (e.g. 1.523 and 1.654). This specification, made in fused bifocal form, is available from Zeiss in their *Duopal C25* design (Figure 15.10).

Occupational progressive-power lenses are considered in detail in Chapter 12. These are designed to provide intermediate and near vision for use at the desk or at a computer workstation. The *Perfalit Prosectal* design from Rodenstock is a progressive lens designed for use in half-eye spectacles by emmetropic presbyopes in cases for which no prescription is needed, or worn for distance vision. In cases of uncorrected hypermetropia, Rodenstock ask that the distance correction and near addition also be supplied.

The wearers of downcurve bifocal designs and progressive power lenses suffer the inconvenience of not having an intermediate or near correction to view objects situated overhead. Vocational trifocal designs that have an intermediate or near portion in the upper portion of the lens are discussed in Chapter 11.

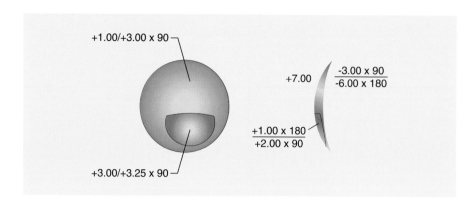

Figure 15.10   Fused bifocal design for the prescription DV +1.00/+3.00×90, NV +3.00/+3.25×90. The spherical front surface produces a near addition of +1.75 and the toroidal depression curve, −1.00/−1.00×90, produces an add of +0.25 in the vertical meridian and +0.50 in the horizontal meridian

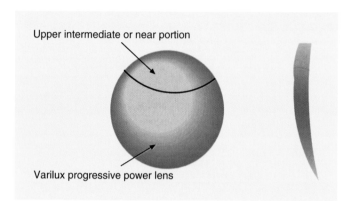

Figure 15.11   The Essilor *Varilux Pilot* lens

Progressive-power lens wearers who could benefit from an intermediate portion in the upper portion of their lenses are also catered for by Essilor, who offer their *Varilux Pilot* design, which is a CR39 Varilux lens with an upcurve segment bonded to the upper portion of the lens (Figure 15.11). As the name suggests, it was designed for use by airline pilots who need to have a clear view of their overhead instrument panels, but will be found useful in many other vocational situations.

Sola Optical offer a bifocal design in which the segment has progressive power. The distance portion of the Sola *Smart-Seg* bifocal has no blended regions, so it performs in the same way as other bifocal designs. The 30×23 flat-top segment, however, has a progressive addition, which provides some add power at the segment top with the full near addition being reached 12mm below the segment top. The current range of near additions is +1.00 to +3.00 and the addition at the segment ledge varies with the near addition as shown in Table 15.4.

Table 15.4   Change of segment length addition with near addition

Ledge power	Full addition
0.75	1.00
0.75	1.25
1.00	1.50
1.00	1.75
1.00	2.00
1.00	2.25
1.00	2.50
1.25	2.75
1.25	3.00

References

1. Bennett A G, Rabbetts R B 1989 Clinical visual optics. Butterworths, London
2. Jalie M 1984 Principles of ophthalmic lenses. ABDO, London
3. Halass S 1959 Aniseikonic lenses of improved design and their application. Aust J Optom 42:387–393

Lenses for sport

Spectacles which are designed for use in sport must offer a wide field of undistorted vision and at the same time, be lightweight and offer eye protection by being robust, shatterproof and resistant to abrasion. Modern tough, low density, plastics materials, such as polycarbonate and Trivex™, possess these mechanical properties and in hard-coated form offer excellent resistance to abrasion. Early spectacle lens shapes for sport were typically upswept with deep lower temporal corners as illustrated in Figure 16.1 to provide the wearer with a large field of view.

Spectacle frames designed for active sports are usually made from plastics materials, often with a thick cushioned bridge, for maximum safety and comfort and, today, are generally of wrap-round style allowing them to follow closely the facial contour (Figure 16.2). Various recommendations are made to assist in the choice of frame for use in sport. In order to cushion the lens adequately, the frame should have a continuous solid rim that is formed wholly of the frame front without any element of the side or temple forming part of the rim. The groove should have an angle of some 135° and be accessible from both sides of the front so that the entire frame rim can accommodate lenses with thicker edge substances. The deeper the groove, the better – with a minimum recommended depth of 0.5mm.

Eye injuries often result from people who play racket sports, so eye protection should be used. This is especially important when playing squash because of the size of the ball and the speed at which it travels. The Squash Rackets Association Ltd (http://www.englandsquash.com), which is the sport's governing body, has guidelines and rules for the use of eye protectors in their sport. Since 2000, all Junior events require the use of certified eye protection and use of eye protection is now recommended for all Doubles games. There is a British Standard which gives details of the requirements for eye protection suitable for playing squash (BS 7930[1]).

At present, no recommendations are made for tennis, badminton or other racket sports although there are Standards relating to personal eye protection for ski-goggles for downhill skiing (BS EN 174:2001) and for snowmobile users (BS EN 13178:2000).

Spectacles for use under water

Many ametropes simply wear their normal spectacles when they swim and put up with the nuisance of water-splashed lenses. However, normal spectacles do not help when clear vision is required under water and for this activity a special pair of swimming spectacles is advisable. Swimming spectacles can be provided in one of two forms, either as swimming goggles with two separate individual lenses mounted before the eyes (Figure 16.3) or in the form of a single face plate to which the lenses are bonded on the inside of a diving mask. When the surface of a lens is in contact with air, no compensation is required to the surface power to provide the correct effect. However, if the surface is in contact with water, its power needs to be modified to take into account the different refractive index of water.

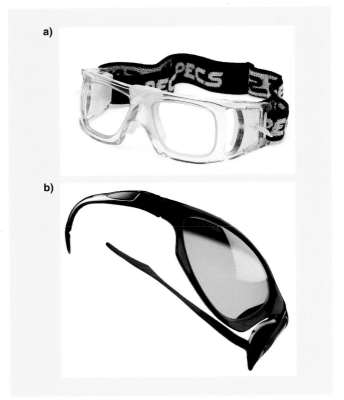

a)

b)

Figure 16.2 Wrap-round sports spectacles

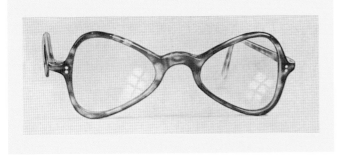

Figure 16.1 An early form of sports spectacles designed to maximize the field of view

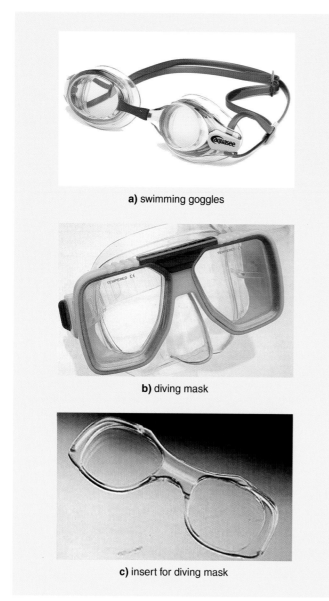

a) swimming goggles

b) diving mask

c) insert for diving mask

Figure 16.3   Swimming goggles and diving mask showing insert for a typical full faceplate mask. (a) Swimming goggles: each eye can be glazed to individual prescription. The outer surface of each lens must be plane so that when in use, the water has no effect upon the power of the lens. (b) Diving mask: lenses may be bonded to the inside surface of the mask, or an insert may be used as shown in (c). (c) Prescription lenses can be glazed into this insert which is designed to be worn inside a mask

The power of a lens, F, can be expressed in terms of its refractive index, n', and surface curvatures, R_1 and R_2, by the Lensmaker's Equation[2]:

$$F = (n' - n)(R_1 - R_2)$$

where n is the refractive index of the medium surrounding the lens.

Thus, when a lens made in CR39 material ($n' = 1.498$) is placed under water ($n = 1.333$), its power reduces to one-third of its power in air. This follows since the power in air is given by:

$$F_{air} = 0.498\ (R_1 - R_2)$$

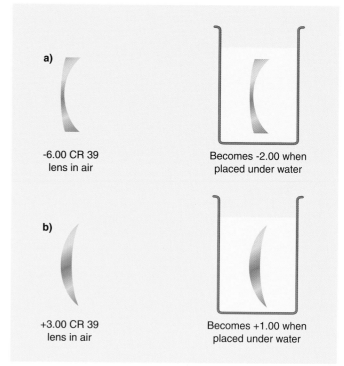

a)

-6.00 CR 39
lens in air

Becomes -2.00 when
placed under water

b)

+3.00 CR 39
lens in air

Becomes +1.00 when
placed under water

Figure 16.4   Comparison of the power of CR39 lenses in air and when placed under water

whereas the power under water is given by:

$$F_{water} = 0.165\ (R_1 - R_2).$$

Hence,

$$F_{water} = 0.165\ F_{air} / 0.498\ = F_{air}/3\ \text{(Figure 16.4)}.$$

If a CR39 lens, whose power in air is −6.00D, is placed under water, its power in water would reduce to −2.00D and the power of a +3.00D CR39 lens, in air, if placed under water, would reduce to +1.00D (Figure 16.4).

This 3:1 ratio between the power of a CR39 lens in air to its power under water, applies not only to the total power of the lens but also to either surface when the surface is in contact with water.

Thus if a CR39 lens of power −2.00 is made with a −7.00D concave surface and mounted in a swimming goggle where the concave surface is used with air between the lens and the eye, but the convex surface is in contact with water, then the convex surface power must be made +15.00D (three times its required power in air which is +5.00D).

The lens will have the desired power of −2.00 when used under water, but when worn in air, has a power in excess of +8.00D (depending upon its thickness). This latter power, of course, is not of much help to the 2.00D myope when leaving the water!

This problem can be overcome by ensuring that the front surface of the lens mounted in the swimming goggle is always plane, all the power being provided on the rear surface of the lens which is used in air within the goggle between the lens and the eye. Thus all minus lenses intended for use when swimming under water are normally made plano-concave in form and if they incorporate a cylindrical component, as minus base torics, whereas all plus lenses are normally made plano-convex in form and if they incorporate a cylindrical component, as plus base torics, with the convex surfaces of the lenses facing the eye. Needless to say, the optical performance of the plus lenses, in particular, leaves much to be desired.

In the case of a diving mask which has a single flat plate, the lenses can be bonded to the inner surface of the plate, however, a better optical result is obtained by glazing the lenses to an insert which is designed to be worn inside the mask. Care should be taken to ensure that the lenses are correctly centred and, in the case of strong minus lenses, the edges of the lens are well clear of the subject's nose, brows and cheeks.

The lens position in swimming goggles or the plate of a diving mask is often some 10–15mm further from the eyes than the usual spectacle plane and it is normally necessary to modify the wearer's spectacle prescription to compensate for the increased vertex distance. Minus lenses need to be made stronger and plus lenses weaker, when the vertex distance is increased. The vertex distance should always be ascertained as accurately as possible and any necessary compensation to the prescription due to the altered vertex distance should be made (see Table 1.1).

Since, when in use, no water is supposed to seep around the edges of the goggle or mask, they are usually quite air tight and the user should be advised to use an anti-misting agent to keep the inner surfaces of the lens/mask assembly clean and thus reduce any fogging due to condensation in wear.

Billiard spectacles

Billiard (or snooker) spectacles are frames with angling joints which allow the lenses to be swivelled about the horizontal axis to enable the player to apply the necessary reversed pantoscopic angle in order to obtain a clearer view of the table and ball when in the cueing position (Figure 16.5). Lens centration for a pair of billiard spectacles is usually a compromise. If the lenses are single vision, they should be centred assuming that the frame has zero pantoscopic angle so that the optical centres lie in front of the centre of the pupil when the head is in the primary position. Then, when the pantoscopic angle is adjusted to its normal value (say 10°) the off-axis performance is the same as when a reverse dihedral angle of 10° is applied. During play, the wearer will no doubt adjust the front to obtain the clearest view of the ball.

Wrap-round sports lenses

In recent years, sports frames with large wrap-round lenses have become very popular. They frequently employ curl sides, or sides which are capable of being secured to the head by means of a headband. The spectacle lenses that are mounted in these frames tend to have a large horizontal box dimension in order to provide a wide field of view and may need to be steeply curved to follow the wrap-round style of the frame. The visual axes are thus not normal to the lenses when the eyes are in the straight-ahead position, the lenses are tilted about both their horizontal axis (pantoscopic angle) and their vertical axes (dihedral angle as shown in Figure 12.39).

Compensation for the tilt can be made by increasing the curvature of the lenses (Wollaston form lenses) or by suitably decentring the lenses (or working prism) or by a combination of these two expedients if it is suspected that horizontal differential prism might cause difficulties in a specific case.

Compensation can also be provided by modifying the prescription to neutralize the astigmatism introduced by tilting the lens. However, as explained later, this causes an alteration in the magnitude of the cylinder power and axis as the eye rotates around the field, and this effect may give rise to blurred vision in certain positions of gaze.

Decentration to compensate for dihedral angle

When a lens is tilted in front of the eye, compensation for the tilt can be provided by decentring the lens. This is the basis, for example, of the centre of rotation condition where downward decentration is provided to compensate for the pantoscopic tilt of the front (Figure 16.6). Typically, the necessary decentration is 0.5mm for each 1° of pantoscopic tilt so that, if the pantoscopic tilt is 8°, then the optical centres would be decentred downwards by some 4mm. Note in Figure 16.6 that when a plus lens is decentred downwards before the eye it introduces base down prism and the eye must now rotate upwards in order to view a distant object. The ocular rotation, θ, for a distant object is given in prism dioptres by:

$$\theta = yF\left[Z/(Z-F)\right]$$

where y is the decentration in centimetres, Z is the distance from the lens to the eye's centre of rotation, expressed in dioptres, and F is the power of the lens. Thus, a +4.00D lens which is mounted

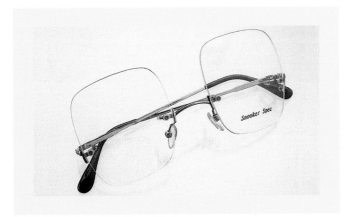

Figure 16.5   Billiard (Snooker) spectacles

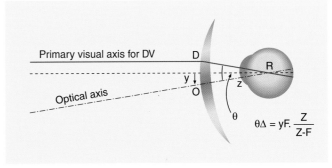

Figure 16.6   Decentration to compensate for pantoscopic and dihedral angles

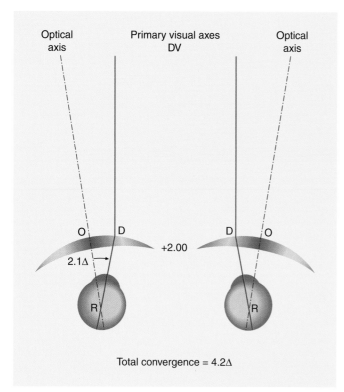

Figure 16.7   Plan view of a pair of eyes viewing a distant object behind lenses of power +2.00D which have been decentred 10mm outwards in order to compensate for a lens dihedral angle of 20°. O is the optical centre of the lens and D is the visual point when the eyes are viewing straight ahead

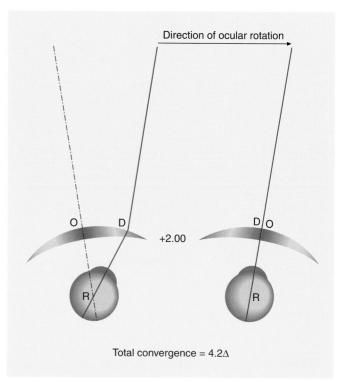

Figure 16.8   The eyes depicted in Figure 16.7 have now rotated to the right so that the right visual axis passes through the optical centre of the lens (D now coincides with O for the right lens). Note that the horizontal differential prism remains 4.2Δ base out between the eyes

27mm in front of the eye's centre of rotation and decentred 5mm downwards, will cause the eye to rotate

$$0.5 \times 4\left[37/(37-4)\right] = 2.2\Delta \text{ upwards.}$$

In the same way, and assuming orthophoria, it is possible to compensate for the dihedral angle by an outward decentration of the lens. Of course, the effect of outward horizontal decentration of each lens is to induce horizontal differential prismatic effect before the eyes. If the dihedral tilt is 20° then the outward decentration which is necessary is 10mm per eye. In the case of a +2.00D hypermetrope, 10mm of outward decentration would induce 4.2Δ base out horizontal differential prismatic effect before the eyes for distance vision. This prism would cause convergence which may induce accommodation and therefore slight blurring for distance. The effect is shown in Figure 16.7, which represents a plan view of the eyes viewing a distant object through a pair of +2.00D lenses.

Note that as the eyes roam about the field, the visual axes will lie further from or closer to the optical centre of each lens. For example in Figure 16.8, which represents the same pair of eyes which were depicted in Figure 16.7 which have now rotated to the right to follow the object which previously lay on the eye's primary axis. It can be seen that the right eye is now viewing through the optical centre of the lens and the left eye has converged further to maintain single vision of the object of regard. Note that the total convergence between the axes remains 4.2Δ.

In the case of a −2.00D myope, 10mm outward decentration would induce horizontal differential prismatic effect of 3.8Δ base in before the eyes. This prism would cause divergence which may not be acceptable (Figure 16.9).

Table 16.1 shows the horizontal differential prismatic effect for various lens powers to which a dihedral angle of 20° has been applied. Note that for low powers the expedient of decentring the lenses to compensate for dihedral angle produces only small amounts of horizontal differential prismatic effect. However, the subject's fusional reserves should always be fully investigated before compensation by decentration is undertaken.

Wollaston form lenses

Over 200 years ago, Wollaston[3] suggested that spectacle lenses whose curvatures were such that the surfaces were virtually concentric with the eye's centres of rotation (average curvature around ±20.00D) would provide excellent peripheral vision, free from aberrational astigmatism which arises from oblique incidence. He named them *periscopic* (looking about) lenses. In view of the steep curvature of the lenses, they were difficult to produce and were never to become successful. However, recently, lenses of Wollaston form have been introduced by Sola Optical USA under the trade name *Enigma*™ (Figure 16.10). The exclusive frames, specifically designed by Sàfilo, enable the steeply curved form lenses to be securely mounted. Initially available in the USA, in the range +1.00D to −5.00D spheres with cylinders to −1.00DC, and spheres only up to −6.00D, the lenses are made from polycarbonate with a dual layer anti-abrasion coating and specially designed anti-reflective coating. Five different frame designs are available, two in metal and three rimless mounts, and although not promoted specifically as sports spectacles, in view of their close fitting to the facial contour, could certainly be used as

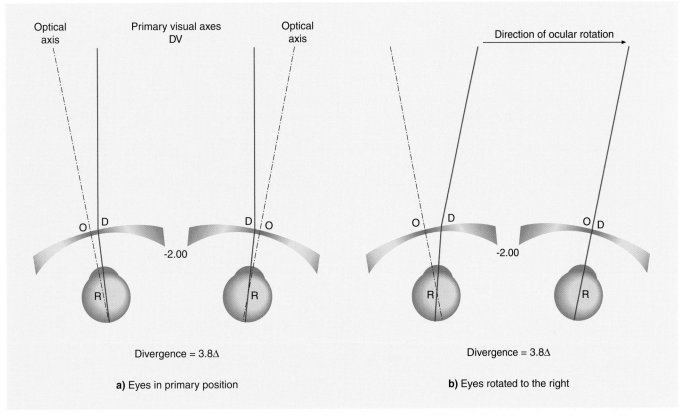

a) Eyes in primary position

b) Eyes rotated to the right

Figure 16.9   Plan view of a pair of eyes viewing a distant object behind lenses of power –2.00D which have been decentred 10mm outwards in order to compensate for a lens dihedral angle of 20°. (a) Object lies straight ahead, (b) Object has moved to the right. Note that the horizontal differential prism remains 3.8Δ base in between the eyes

Table 16.1   Horizontal differential prismatic effect between the eyes for various lens powers, when 10mm outwards decentration is applied to compensate for 20° dihedral angle

Plus lens powers		Minus lens powers	
Power	Convergence	Power	Divergence
+1.00	2.1Δ	–1.00	1.9Δ
+2.00	4.2Δ	–2.00	3.8Δ
+3.00	6.6Δ	–3.00	5.6Δ
+4.00	9.0Δ	–4.00	7.2Δ
+5.00	11.6Δ	–5.00	8.8Δ
+6.00	14.3Δ	–6.00	10.3Δ

such for non-contact sporting activities which require a large field of view.

The vision benefits claimed for the lenses are:

- Up to 40% wider field of view compared with ordinary lenses
- Less distortion of object shape and size
- Correct location of objects viewed through the periphery
- Up to 65% less chromatic aberration compared with polycarbonate lenses made with regular base curves.

The optical performance of –3.00D lenses made in both regular and in Wollaston forms in polycarbonate material is compared in Figure 16.11. The vertex distance for the regular +5.00D base curve lens depicted in Figure 16.11a was assumed to be 13mm and the vertex distance for the *Enigma* lens with +17.85D base curve was assumed to be 19mm (Figure 16.11b). Note the smaller amounts of chromatic aberration and distortion from these steeply curved forms.

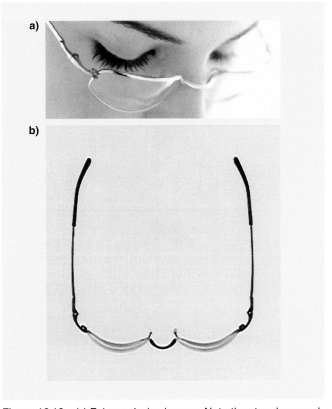

Figure 16.10   (a) Enigma design in wear. Note the steeply curved form of the lenses. (b) Plan view of pair of Enigma rimless spectacles (model Delta in gunmetal)

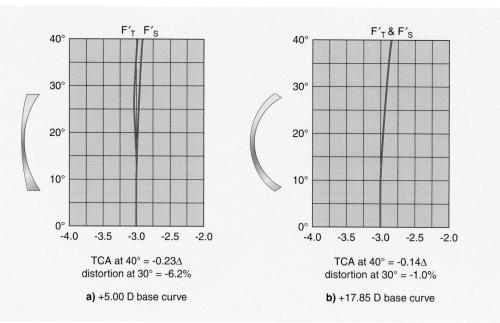

F′$_T$ F′$_S$

TCA at 40° = -0.23Δ
distortion at 30° = -6.2%

a) +5.00 D base curve

F′$_T$ & F′$_S$

TCA at 40° = -0.14Δ
distortion at 30° = -1.0%

b) +17.85 D base curve

Figure 16.11 Field diagrams for –3.00D lenses made in regular and Wollaston forms. (a) –3.00D lens made with +5.00D base curve, (b) –3.00D lens made in Wollaston form with +17.85D base curve

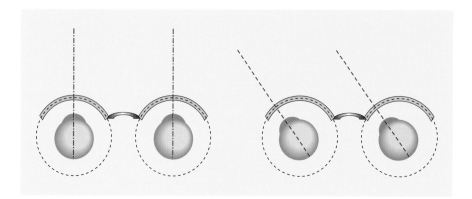

Figure 16.12 Concentric nature of Contour Optics Wollaston form lenses

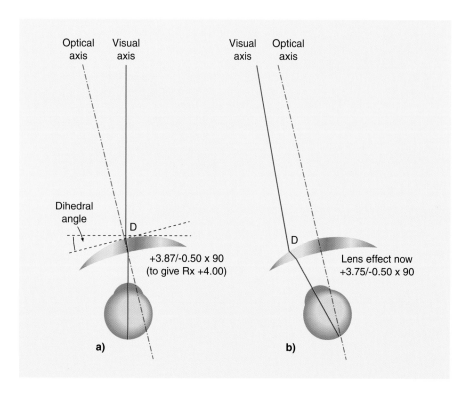

Optical axis   Visual axis

Visual axis   Optical axis

Dihedral angle

D

+3.87/-0.50 x 90
(to give Rx +4.00)

D

Lens effect now
+3.75/-0.50 x 90

a)

b)

Figure 16.13 Effect of modifying the prescription to compensate for the dihedral angle. (a) The required effect of the lens is +4.00D sphere. In order to produce this, the power of the lens worn at a dihedral angle of 20° must be +3.87/–0.50 × 90. When the eye looks straight ahead through point D on this lens, the effect is then +4.00D sphere. (b) When the eye rotates to the left behind the lens, the cylindrical effect of the lens changes and its effect tends towards the compensated power, +3.87/–0.50 × 90. The actual spherical value of +3.75 arises from the mean oblique error exhibited by the lens

As can be seen in Figure 16.12, in the case of the Wollaston form lenses, the lens surfaces are virtually concentric with the eye's centres of rotation.

Power compensation for dihedral angle

Some lens manufacturers offer to compensate the lens prescription to take into account the large dihedral angle which is to be found on some wrap-round frames. They also supply a slightly deeper lens form (+7.00D, +8.00D or +9.00D front curves) to follow the steeper bow of the frame. The front or back curve of the lens is then aspherized as necessary to maintain the off-axis performance of the lens (Figure 16.13).

The general problem of power compensation for dihedral angle can be deduced from Figure 16.9. It is seen that the effect of the dihedral angle is to tilt the lenses around the 90° axis before the eyes. If the optical centres of the lenses are placed in the usual position, at D, the effect of this tilt is to introduce astigmatism with its axis at 90, which could result in an alteration of the final power and cylinder axis direction of the lens. In the case of low power lenses it is possible to compensate for the tilt as described earlier, simply by decentring the lenses outwards. For lenses of medium to high power the differential prism induced by decentration would probably be excessive and compensation might be provided by modifying the prescription.

Suppose a +4.00D correction is required with the lens being worn at a dihedral angle of 20° (Figure 16.13). The lens which when tilted through 20° about a vertical axis actually produces an effect of +4.00D sphere is +3.87/−0.50×90. If the manufacturer were to produce this prescription, information would be

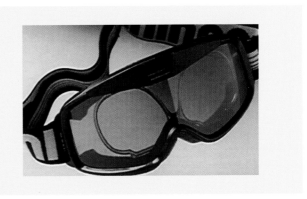

Figure 16.14   Use of an insert to enable the normal spectacle prescription to be worn inside a wrap-round front

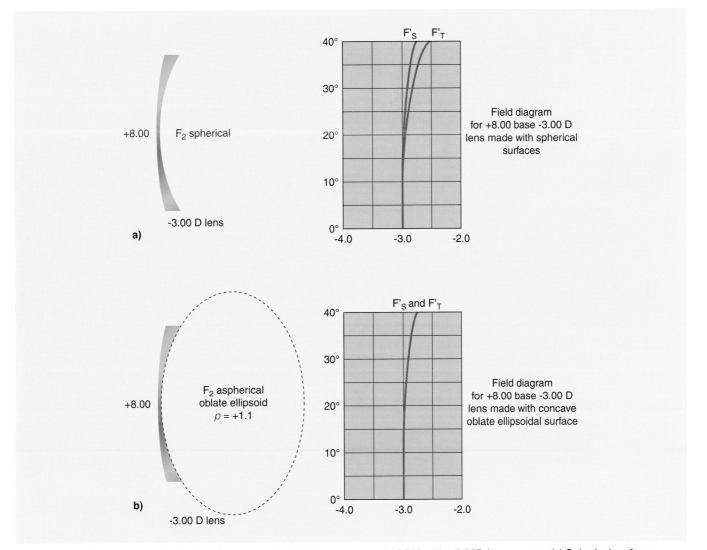

Figure 16.15   Comparison of optical performance of −3.00D lenses made in CR39 with +8.00D base curves. (a) Spherical surfaces, (b) Essilor *Open View* design with concave oblate ellipsoidal surface

correction × 90 is no longer valid for this direction of gaze. Clearly, the effective dihedral angle in the horizontal meridian depends upon the direction of gaze.

There can be no doubt that in the majority of sports, the wearer needs to be able to obtain a wide horizontal field of vision, for example to be able to judge accurately the flight of an incoming squash or tennis ball. The eyes often execute frequent rotation in the horizontal meridian. As the eyes rotate horizontally, the dihedral angle alters with the direction of gaze.

A more satisfactory method of ensuring that the optimum prescription is provided over a wide field is to mount the lenses into an insert which fits inside a plano-glazed, wrap-round, goggle-style front (Figure 16.14).

Despite the uncertainties related to the precise effect obtained in different directions of gaze with compensated prescriptions, several manufacturers offer a range of lenses for sport which incorporate prescription compensation for dihedral tilt. These include *Open View* from Essilor, available in both single vision (Figure 16.15) and Varilux form, *Sport Lenses* from Rodenstock and *Sports Lenses* from Rupp & Hubrach.

Rupp & Hubrach have introduced a special rule which can be used to measure the dihedral angle of the frame (Figure 16.16). When sent this information they will calculate the compensation required to the sphere, cylinder, axis direction and centration to minimize the effect of the dihedral tilt.

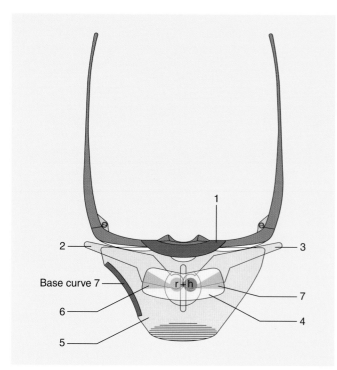

Figure 16.16 Rule for measuring dihedral angle of front (courtesy of Rupp & Hubrach)

provided that when checking the power of this lens in the focimeter, it would read +3.87/−0.50 × 90 but that the 'as-worn' power is +4.00D as had been ordered (Figure 16.13a).

In Figure 16.13b, the eyes have rotated to the left behind the lens, effectively reducing the dihedral angle and its need for correction, and it will be realized that the −0.50D cylindrical

References

1. BS 7930 1998 Eye protectors for racket sports. Part 1 – Squash. BSI, London
2. Jalie M 1984 Principles of ophthalmic lenses. ABDO, London
3. Wollaston W H 1812 On a periscopic camera obscura and microscope. Phil Trans R Soc Lond 102:370

Lens manufacture – single vision lens surfaces

Modern spectacle lenses are no longer made by simple rotating machinery. Generators may be single-point cutters, with the position of the cutting point in space being controlled by a computer program. Smoothing and polishing may be by flexible pads that float over the surface of the lens, following the surface shape, rather than trying to form the surface shape, as in the older type of smoothing and polishing equipment.

Plastics lenses do not even need to be produced by a grinding process; they can be cast finished in glass moulds or moulded by compression- or injection-moulding techniques. Casting processes have become so sophisticated that casting units are small enough to be situated easily in a high-street practice.

Surfacing instruction

When a prescription laboratory receives a specification for a lens that has to be surfaced, the first operation is to determine which blank must be used to obtain the specification and what thickness and curves are necessary to produce the lens. Most modern ophthalmic blanks are supplied in semi-finished form, with the convex surface completed by the blank manufacturer. Some designs, notably solid bifocals and deep plus flats, are finished on the back surface, but the great majority of blanks require the surfacing department to work the concave side to provide the prescription. Blank selection and determination of the other surface power and the thickness of the finished lens is known as surfacing instruction. The various stages that the prescription order must undergo during the surfacing instruction routine, starting with the optician's written prescription, are as follows:

- blank selection
- checking the curves
- determination of any prism to cut
- deciding the minimum thickness of the lens
- calculating the necessary centre thickness
- finding the back surface power of the lens (taking lens thickness into account)
- selecting the smoothing and polishing tools, either by curve or by coding
- selecting the generator settings to provide the correct curves and axes or prism base settings
- selecting the prism ring, or setting that will provide the correct prism
- providing the blocking instructions.

Without doubt, the most complicated steps in the surfacing instruction procedure concern the determination of the thickness of the lens. Today, the equations used to evaluate the thickness are solved by computer programs. It is not always appreciated that the calculation of the thickness of spectacle lenses is a very sophisticated mathematical process that involves the solution of equations of the second, third and, for prismatic lenses, fourth degree. Before the advent of the computer all specially surfaced lenses were designed by hand from information provided in surfacing tables; one can only marvel at the ingenuity of the prescription technicians who could manipulate the information in the tables to achieve the desired results. Even so, making spectacle lenses was often a trial and error affair, particularly with plus lenses, which, in the main, were designed from their centre thickness rather than from their edge thickness. Since the exact mathematical methods involve the solution of a quadratic equation when the front curve is unknown and a cubic equation when the back curve is unknown, it was not practical to attempt to solve the equations for individual lenses.

With the arrival of the microcomputer some 25 years ago, laboratories were provided with the means whereby individual prescriptions could be considered. The various mathematical sequences are programmed and stored in the computer memory, which enables unskilled operators to key in the prescription and other data relevant to the blank and frame that are to be used. The calculation proceeds automatically and the solution is printed out on a workshop ticket.

In addition to providing surfacing tickets, the computer systems in current use may also be linked to stock-control systems, invoicing and progress chasing, and to electronic edging equipment in the glazing department.

To provide a flavour of the routines the computer must consider, the various stages are described here in more detail.

Blank selection

The great majority of modern spectacle lenses that pass through the surfacing workshop are semi-finished blanks, of which the convex surface has been completed by the blank manufacturer and the prescription required obtained by completing the concave side. Various manufacturers provide their own different ranges of base curves, but in the main they are not far removed from the series: plano, +2.00, +4.00, +6.00, +8.00, +10.00, +12.00 and so on.

Assuming the use of CR39 material, the convex semi-finished curve that would be selected for a given power can be determined from the rule:[1]

front curve = half lens power + 6.00

So, for a +4.00D lens the required front curve is +8.00D. In practice, the nearest curve to this is selected, which might range from +8.25 to +7.87.

In the case of astigmatic prescriptions, the blank selection rule is applied to the spherical component of the minus cylinder transposition. Thus, in the case of the prescription:

−6.00/+1.00×90

the front curve required is:

$$(-5.00/2) + 6.00 = +3.50D$$

It is usual, when the blank has been removed from its packet, to check the power of the curve with a sag gauge to ensure that the correct information about the curve is fed into the computer.

Prism-to-cut

As stated earlier, the most difficult mathematical sequences in surfacing instruction involve calculations for the thickness of the lens. The problem of the correct thickness is aggravated by the incorporation of prism, which is often required for today's large lenses to obtain the desired centration. The amount and base direction of prism to cut depends upon the required decentration, the sphere and cylinder powers, and the axis direction of the cylinder.

By way of example, consider the specification illustrated in Figure 17.1, in which 5mm of inward decentration is required to move the optical centre to the correct position. Table 17.1 shows the prism and its base direction necessary to move the optical centre 5mm inwards for the given prescriptions. The astigmatic prescriptions chosen are all special cases in which the sphere is half the power of the cylinder and opposite in sign. The general rule for this specification is that the amount of prism is a function of the sphere alone and the base direction is always double the cylinder axis direction. However, this is a special case and, as a general rule, calculation of prism-to-cut cannot be performed mentally!

In general, the mathematical sequence to determine the amount of prism, P_R, and its base direction, ϕ, necessary to move the optical centre $y$cm vertically and $x$cm horizontally for the prescription $S/C \times \theta$ is:[2]

$$P_V = yS + C \cos\theta \ (x \sin\theta + y \cos\theta)$$

$$P_H = xS + C \cos\theta \ (x \sin\theta + y \cos\theta)$$

$$P_R = \sqrt{(P^2_V + P^2_H)}$$

$$\tan\phi = P_V/P_H$$

This sequence of equations is programmed easily for the computer, which outputs the required prism-to-cut and the base direction on the workshop ticket.

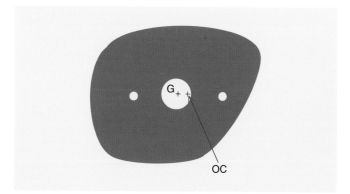

Figure 17.1   Prism-to-cut: the specification includes a distance between centres of 74mm and a required centration distance of 64mm. An inward decentration of 5mm is required. G is the box centre of the former and OC the desired position of the optical centre

Table 17.1 Prism-to-cut	
Prescription	Prism and base direction
R, −2.00	1Δ base 180 (out)
R, −2.00/+4.00 × 180	1Δ base 180 (out)
R, −2.00/+4.00 × 90	1Δ base 360 (in)
R, −2.00/+4.00 × 30	1Δ base 240 (down at 60)
R, −2.00/+4.00 × 45	1Δ base 270 (down)
R, −2.00/+4.00 × 60	1Δ base 300 (down at 120)

Minimum lens thickness

The thinnest point on a minus lens lies at its optical centre and for glass lenses can be determined from the rule:

$$t_c = 2 + 0.2F$$

where F is the power of the spherical element of the lens in minus cylinder transposition. The minimum permissible centre thickness, t_c, is about 1.0mm, a value that would be applied to minus lenses stronger than −5.00D. This rule can also be applied to plastics lenses made from rigid polyurethane materials, but CR39 lenses are not normally surfaced to a centre thickness less than 2.0mm for danger of them flexing in the mount if they are overglazed to a fully rimmed frame.

An adjustment is made for fixed tinted and photochromic glass lenses to ensure there is sufficient material at the centre of the lens. Lenses made in these materials are not normally allowed to have a centre thickness less than about 1.6mm.

In the case of prismatic minus lenses, the thinnest point of the lens still lies at the optical centre of the lens, but this does not coincide with the geometric centre of the blank. Compensation must be made so that the thickness fed to the generator ensures that the minimum thickness does not fall below the desired amount.

The optimum thickness for a plus lens depends on its power and the type of mount into which it will be edged (see 'Edge thickness of plus lenses' in Chapter 9). For lenses that have a large variation in thickness between their centre and edges, usually lenses over the power of +2.00D, the optimum edge thickness for mounting in a plastics frame varies from about 1.0mm to 2.0mm, depending upon the power of the lens. For example, a +2.00D lens to be mounted in a plastics frame requires an edge thickness of about 1.5mm, whereas a +10.00D lens only needs an edge thickness of 1.0mm at its thinnest point. When the lens is to be mounted in a metal frame, or needs to be drilled for a rimless mount, the edge thickness must be increased to prevent it from flaking under pressure from the rim or a rimless screw.

The thinnest point on a plus lens lies somewhere round the edge of the lens. In the case of circular lenses, for spherical lenses the thinnest point on the edge of the lens lies at the furthest point from the optical centre. If the lens is not decentred (or incorporates no prism), the edge thickness is the same all around the edge of the circular lens (Figure 17.2a).

For circular plus astigmatic lenses, the edge thickness is greatest along the minimum power meridian (i.e. along the plus axis meridian) and least along the maximum power meridian (along the minus axis meridian). It is, therefore, the minus axis meridian that controls the thickness of the lens. This can be seen in Figure 17.2b, which illustrates a plano-convex cylinder with a plus axis at 90° and thin-edge substance (at 180) of zero (i.e. the cylinder is supposed to be knife-edged). Clearly, when a spherical element is combined with the cylindrical element, the positions of the minimum and maximum thickness on the edge of a circular lens do not change.

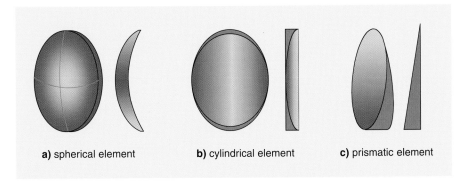

Figure 17.2 Variation in edge thickness of circular lenses: (a) Centred spherical component, in which the edge thickness is the same all round the periphery; (b) Plus cylinder with vertical axis, in which the thinnest points on the edge of the lens lie at the extremities of the power meridian, at 180; (c) Base down prism, in which the thinnest point on the edge coincides with the prism apex

a) spherical element   b) cylindrical element   c) prismatic element

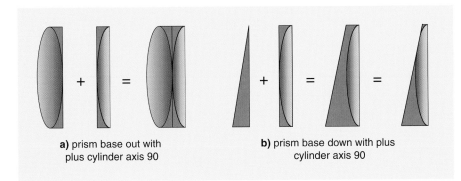

Figure 17.3 Astigmatic prisms. (a) When the prism is combined with the cylinder so that the prism apex coincides exactly with the minus axis meridian of the cylinder, the necessary centre thickness is the sum of the centre thicknesses of each component. (b) When the prism is combined such that the prism apex coincides with the plus axis meridian, the edge thickness of the combination is no longer zero. A considerable amount of material can be surfaced from the lens to obtain a knife-edge at the periphery

a) prism base out with plus cylinder axis 90

b) prism base down with plus cylinder axis 90

In the case of circular prisms, the minimum edge thickness corresponds with the prism apex and the maximum edge thickness with the prism base, which is shown base down in Figure 17.2c. When a cylindrical element is combined with a prismatic element, the position of the minimum edge thickness varies with the angle between the cylinder axis and the base setting of the prism. This should be obvious from Figure 17.3, which compares the results of combining a prism with a cylinder in two different ways.

In Figure 17.3a, the plus cylinder axis is vertical and the prismatic element is added with its base at 180 (i.e. base out for the right eye). Since both the cylindrical element and the prismatic element have zero edge thickness at their thinnest points on the edge, the combination also has zero edge thickness at 0°, on the nasal edge of the lens. The centre thickness of this astigmatic prism is the sum of the centre thicknesses of the individual components.

In Figure 17.3b, the base direction of the prism has been rotated through 90°, so the base now lies at 270 and the edge thickness of the combination is no longer zero.

It is clear from Figure 17.3b that a significant amount of material can be removed from this combination to obtain zero edge thickness, and that when this is done by further surfacing of one component, the thinnest point on the edge of the astigmatic element no longer lies along the 180 meridian. To calculate the thickness of this combination it is first necessary to determine the position on the edge of the lens at which the minimum substance occurs. The solution to this is found using a quartic equation, so it is easy to appreciate why the computer is employed to solve this everyday problem!

The discussion so far has been restricted to circular uncuts. In the case of shaped lenses, the computer calculates the contribution of any cylinder and prism to different meridians of the lens in turn, rotating around the periphery in, say, 5° intervals. The lens dimensions along these meridians are obtained from digitized measurements supplied by the frame tracer, which measures the

aperture of the frame, or a scanned shape drawn round a former along the different meridians. The computer simply compares the variation in edge thickness all round the lens periphery until it finds the point of minimum thickness, and thus the meridian for the shape and prescription in hand, which controls the thickness of the lens.

In the case of aspherical and progressive power surfaces, the calculations would be impossible without the assistance of the computer!

Calculating the necessary centre thickness

Above, attention is drawn to some of the variables that influence the centre thickness of the finished lens. In the case of minus lenses, the centre thickness is simply the sum of the minimum thickness required at the optical centre and any allowance that must be made for the worked prism at the geometrical centre of the blank.

In the case of plus lenses, the minimum edge thickness is determined from the type of mounting and the position of the thinnest point on the edge, calculated from knowledge of the prism and cylinder components and their axis directions.

This information can be fed into the equations that determine the centre thickness of the lens. When the front surface power is given, as is usually the case, the equation for the centre thickness of the lens is cubic in form, but adequate results can be obtained from a simplified quadratic solution.

The problem can be visualized from Figure 17.4, which, for simplicity, illustrates a plano-convex lens form of given power, diameter and edge thickness, e, and for which it is required to determine the centre thickness, t_c. It shows quite clearly that the centre thickness is made up from the sum of the edge thickness and the sag of the front curve, s_1, at the finished diameter. Unfortunately, the front curve is not yet known. What is known is that the front curve will be less than the nominal curve by an amount (known as the vertex power allowance) that depends on the centre

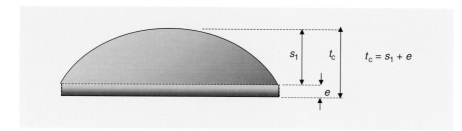

Figure 17.4 Thickness of a strong plano-convex lens. The front curve must be compensated for the thickness of the lens. The compensation required, however, depends upon the thickness. Neither the front curve nor the thickness is known

thickness of the lens. Thus, at the outset, both the thickness and the curve are unknown, each depending upon the other. This impasse can be solved by means of a simultaneous equation[2] that produces both the required centre thickness for the lens and the unknown front curve. The ability to specify the edge thickness of the lens at a given diameter is one of the most important routines to be provided by the computer software.

In the case of fused bifocals, the computer program must also check that the centre thickness suggested is large enough to ensure that the back surface of the lens does not break into the depression curve of the segment.

Determination of the back surface power

When the centre thickness of the finished lens is known, calculation of the compensated back-surface power is relatively straightforward. If the back vertex power of the lens is denoted by F'_V, the individual surface powers by F_1 and F_2, the centre thickness of the lens by t_c and the refractive index of the lens material by n, then the compensated back surface power is given by:

$$F_2 = F'_V - F_1/\left(1 - t_c F_1/n\right)$$

The resultant curve is the true power of the back surface. If the refractive index for which the tools are calibrated is not the same as the lens material, then the back surface power must be converted into the tool index.

In the case of astigmatic lenses, which are made as minus-base torics, once the compensation for thickness has been determined for the base curve, the same allowance can be applied to the cross curve.

In the working of plus-base torics, such as solid bifocals that have the segment incorporated on the concave surface of the lens, the compensation for the base curve is different from that for the cross curve and the computer must find both vertex power allowances for the convex surface.

Tool selection

Most surfacing workshops now carry tool ranges in which the base curves step in 0.12D intervals and the nearest 0.12 tool is selected. Cylinder powers, of course, are ordered in 0.25D intervals so the cross curves need only step in 0.25D intervals. If the tool index differs from that of the lens material, it is usually possible to select a sphere tool that will produce a spherical power to within the current British Standard tolerance on lens power. However, the cylinder power on the tool is usually not correct for other indices and a further calculation needs to be made to determine whether it is necessary to cut a special tool for the job in hand to produce the correct cylinder power. As a rule, most surfacing laboratories stock a range of tools for working glass that have been calibrated for refractive index 1.523, and a range of tools for working plastics materials that have been calibrated for refractive index 1.498.

Table 17.2 Typical series of tool codes

Base	Sphere	Cylinder powers			
		0.25	0.50	0.75	1.00
-6.00	9200	9201	9202	9203	9204
-6.12	9225	9226	9227	9228	9229
-6.25	9250	9251	9252	9253	9254
-6.37	9275	9276	9277	9278	9279
-6.50	9300	9301	9302	9303	9304

If it is necessary to produce the curves -10.00/-10.50 on a plastics material of refractive index 1.60, using tools calibrated for CR39, the required tool curves are:

$$0.498/0.60 \times -10.00 = -8.30$$

and

$$0.498/0.60 \times -10.50 = -8.72$$

The CR39 tool, -8.25/-8.75, would be selected and actually produces surface powers on 1.60 index material of -9.94 and -10.54. If all other parameters of the lens are correct, the spherical component of the finished lens will be 0.06D weak and the cylinder component 0.10D strong.

Some laboratories now code their tools with a code number rather than the actual tool power. For example, the tool -6.00/-6.50 might be known simply as tool 9202, the principle being that the technician is less likely to pick the wrong tool if given a single number than a pair of numbers to find. Table 17.2 lists a series of tool codes for tools in the range -6.00 to -6.50 with cylinders up to 1.00D. Tool ranges usually extend up to 6.00D of cylinder power.

Generator settings

When the curves and centre thickness are known for a given job, the information is used to set up the generator. This is often performed electronically, the information from the layout computer being relayed to the onboard computer, which translates it into generator settings.

The settings on the generator usually need to be modified to ensure that the curves produced match exactly the face of the smoothing tool. Compensation may be needed to one curve for the so-called elliptical error that results from a mismatch in the path followed by the cutting head as it traverses the blank. The amount of compensation varies with the lens diameter, the value of the cylinder and whether the base curve is blocked in the same direction or at right angles to the sweep of the head.

The prism that needs to be blocked, either by the addition of a prism ring or by building prism into the alloy block itself, also depends upon the power of the convex surface in contact with the block face. This can be deduced from Figure 17.5, which illustrates semi-finished blanks of different base curves placed in contact with their alloy blocks and that incorporate prism in the block. In Figure 17.5a, the base curve of the semi-finished blank is plano and the angle through which the blank rotates when presented to the generator wheel is exactly the same as the angle between the two faces of the block. Thus, to produce a prism with an apical angle of, say, 3°, the angle that must be incorporated into the metal block is also 3°.

In Figure 17.5b, the base is a deep convex curve and the effect of blocking prism is to move the pole of the convex surface from the position it would occupy if no prism had been included in the block. The shift in the position of the pole effectively reduces the angle between the axes of revolution of the convex surface and the concave surface of the blank. If no compensation is made the generator does not produce enough prism, which, of course, is checked at the point on the concave surface of the finished lens through which the generator axis passes.

Symmetrical blocking

It is usual these days to block lenses on the centre of the blank and to shift the optical centre, when necessary, by working prism on the lens. Another way to simplify the blocking procedure in the case of round or crescent segments is to produce segment inset-ting by rotation of the blank, swinging the segment to its desired position.

Consider the bifocal specification:

R +5.00/−1.00×90 Add +2.00

Segment 24×2 below ×2 in

for which it is also required to decentre the distance optical centre inwards by 5mm to achieve the correct centration and segment position. The traditional method of blocking this lens is illustrated in Figure 17.6a, which represents a front view of the blank with the button shown behind. The blank has been blocked asymmetrically with the required position of the distance optical centre, O, marked 5mm to the nasal side of the geometrical centre of the blank, G. The segment has been inset a further 2mm from O so that the total inset of the segment from G is 7mm. It was usual to crib the blank on its temporal side after blocking to prevent problems from overhang during the generating process.

The usual blocking method today, made possible because computer programs calculate the details, is to block the lens symmetrically with no decentration or inset of the segment; the prism is worked to push the optical to the correct position, and the angle through which the blank must rotate to position the segment correctly after surfacing is calculated. For the specification detailed above, it is necessary to work 2Δ of base-in prism to push the optical centre of the lens 5mm inwards.

Symmetrical blocking could, therefore, be accomplished by rotating the segment inwards by 7mm and working 2Δ of prism to obtain the correct position of the optical centre (Figure 17.6b). The cylinder axis is marked at 90° and the symmetrical blocking here overcomes the need to crib the blank to reduce the risk of breakage from overhang.

However, the computer can simplify the blocking process even further by eliminating the need to inset the segment at the blocking stage. It can calculate the angle through which the blank must rotate to obtain the required position of the distance optical centre and the segment. It then specifies the directions of the cylinder

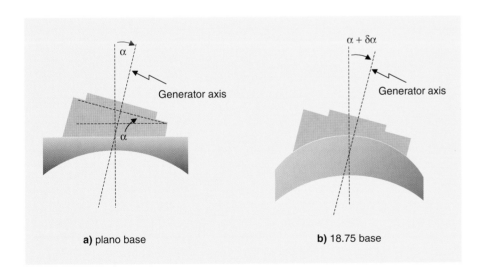

a) plano base   **b) 18.75 base**

Figure 17.5 Blocked prism and generated prism. (a) When the semi-finished blank has a plano-base curve, the amount of generated prism is the same as the blocked prism, and the angle α between the faces of the block is the same as the apical angle of the prism. (b) When the semi-finished blank has a convex face in contact with the alloy, it is necessary to increase the blocked prism to end up with the correct amount of prism in the lens. The angle α must be increased by $\delta\alpha$ to compensate for the tilt of the convex surface

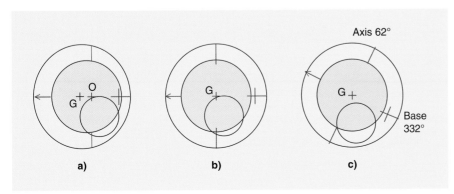

a)   **b)**   **c)**

Figure 17.6 Symmetrical blocking: (a) asymmetric blocking without prism; (b) symmetrical blocking with prism-to-cut of 2Δ base in; (c) symmetrical blocking with compensated axis and prism base settings

axis and base setting for the prism, allowing for the rotation, and the blank can be blocked symmetrically with zero segment inset. At the blocking stage, the operator need only adjust the position of the blank in the vertical meridian to obtain the required segment drop and totally ignore the inset. In the example under consideration, the blank needs to be rotated 27° anti-clockwise to allow for compensated symmetrical blocking. The computer outputs the blocking instructions (Figure 17.6c):

> Set cylinder axis at 62°
> Set prism base at 332°

if the blocking height is 2mm.

When the lens is deblocked and the axis rotated to 90, the distance optical centre lies 5mm inwards and the segment is inset a further 2mm.

Obviously, segments that have straight dividing lines, such as flat top and E-style segments, cannot be rotated during the blocking process. For these, especially with decentred blanks, prism is worked to shift the distance optical centre to its prescribed position.

Spherical surface

Geometry

A spherical surface is formed by the locus of a point in three dimensions moving at a fixed distance from a fixed point[3] (Figure 17.7). Assuming the origin to lie at the vertex, A, of the surface, the equation to a spherical surface is:

$$x^2 + y^2 + z^2 - 2rz = 0$$

Note in Figure 17.7 that the axes have been chosen such that z is the optical axis of the surface and the sag of the curve for the point P on the surface is z.

A spherical surface can be imagined to have been produced by the rotation of a circle about its diameter and, indeed, because the surface is symmetrical, can be produced by ordinary rotating machinery. The lapping process by which the surface to be produced is rotated against a tool of equal (but opposite) curvature has probably been in use for 3000 years, although the first written evidence does not appear until the 16th century.[4]

Since the surface is symmetrical, it is very convenient to describe its form in a single plane by putting x equal to zero,

when the well-known quadratic solution for the depth (or sag) of the curve is given by:

$$y^2 + z^2 - 2rz = 0$$

from which:

$$z = r - \sqrt{(r^2 - y^2)}$$

or the more useful form:

$$z = y^2 / \left[r + \sqrt{(r^2 - y^2)} \right]$$

The use of these expressions is illustrated in the sections below on computer numerically controlled (CNC) machining and testing of spherical surfaces.

Single surface working

Although the great majority of modern spectacle lenses are made from plastics materials, the working procedures for completing the prescription of the lens are exactly the same as those used for glass lens surfacing. Naturally, there are differences in the cutting tools, grinding materials, smoothing and polishing pads and temperatures involved, but, in the main, surfacing equipment designed for glass lens production is equally at home with most plastics lens materials. An enormous advantage with surfacing plastics materials is that the processing times are much quicker and the wear and tear on the machinery is usually less.

The various stages in the grinding of spherical surfaces, to be seen in every prescription laboratory, are as follows:

- Lens marking (blank layout): marking of a lens blank to control centration, axis direction, segment setting, etc.
- Blocking or sticking on: the mounting of one or more blanks on a holder in preparation for surfacing.
- Generating: the preparation of a curved surface with a form that depends on the predetermined relation between the motions of the material and the tool.
- Roughing: grinding to the approximate form and thickness with a coarse abrasive. This process has been universally replaced by surface generating.
- Truing: the second stage of grinding, following the roughing process, in which the surface is brought close to the desired curvature.
- Smoothing: the last stages of grinding prior to polishing.

Figure 17.7 The spherical surface. C is the centre of curvature of the surface and r the radius of curvature. The equation to the surface is $x^2 + y^2 + z^2 - 2rz = 0$

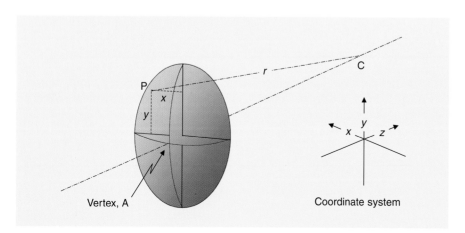

P
x
y
Vertex, A

C

x y z
Coordinate system

- Polishing: the final stage of the surfacing process, which results in a smooth surface that exhibits specular instead of diffuse reflection and regular instead of random transmission.
- Deblocking: the releasing of lenses from their holders by tapping the lens, or *freezing off* by chilling the block to facilitate removal of the lens from the holder.
- Inspection and verification: ensure that the surface is free from defects, such as greyness or waves, and ensure that the prescription characteristics of the lens are correct.

Lens marking, or marking and setting for the surfacing laboratory, is usually performed by mechanical layout markers. These enable the blank to be centred and marked, simply by laying it over an illuminated graticule, adjusting the blank by hand to the desired position and operating a lever that stamps the finished surface of the blank neatly with ink markings. The magnified viewing screens allow accurate placement of the cylinder axis, prism-base setting and segment top.

Lens blocking has changed greatly from the days when separate metal buttons were attached to the blank by means of pitch. The old-style button used when surfacing spherical surfaces usually had one central depressed hole into which fitted the pin that drove the lens across the tool. The curve to be produced being spherical, it does not matter if the lens revolves under the pin, but the old-style button had the drawback that the single depressed hole at the centre of the button was removed from the plane of the tool. Today, single lens blocking is almost exclusively by means of low-melting point alloys (between 55°C and 80°C). These not only act as a holder for the lens, but also allow the button to be gripped by the chuck of the machine and thus do away with wear in the button hole.

Metal blocking has three advantages over the old-style pitch. The temperature differential between the solid and fluid form is quite small and easy to achieve. The alloy is far cleaner in use than pitch or wax. Lenses can be removed very easily with a small tap, or a short period in a chiller, without risk of damaging the lens or the need for freezing.

The metal alloy, however, has a high initial and subsequent replacement cost, since in daily use some metal is wasted and,

with continuous use, oxidization of the metal may occur and calls for special treatment.

In the case of glass lenses, adhesion is ensured by first varnishing the finished surface to which the button is to adhere. In the case of plastics lenses a surface saver tape is applied to the plastics lens surface to be blocked, to both protect and insulate the surface against the heat of the button. Saver tapes have also been developed for glass lens surfaces. Surface saver applicators often use a vacuum to ensure an even adhesion of the tape to the surface.

The initial form of a spherical surface may be produced by roughing or by generating. The older roughing process is rarely used today; most spherical surfaces in the prescription industry are produced by generating the curve. Modern toric generators are quite capable of producing good spherical surfaces, free from form error, even though the lens does not rotate during the generating process. In the production of a convex spherical surface, as is required for the front surface of a semi-finished blank or the convex curve on a mould, dedicated spherical generators are employed.

The principle of the spherical generator is illustrated in Figure 17.8. The sintered cup tool has a diamond-impregnated cutting edge, the diamonds being bonded to a bronze or copper base that allows the blunt diamonds to detach themselves as the tool wears.

Different tilts of the cup tool produce curves of different radii; the curve shape depends on the tool diameter, the radius of the cutting edge and the angle through which the tool is tilted.

Figure 17.8a shows a cross-sectional view of the cup tool resting on a plane surface parallel with the line that joins the tool edges. In this situation, if the tool and surface rotate, a plane surface is generated.

In Figure 17.8b, the tool is rotated through an angle, α, and now generates a convex surface. If the diameter of the tool is $2y_T$ and the radius of the cutting edge of the tool is r_T, then the radius of curvature of the generated surface, r, is given by:

$$r = y_T \csc \alpha - r_T$$

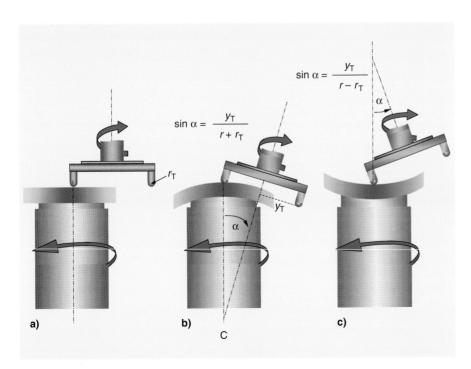

Figure 17.8   Principle of the spherical generator. (a) When the axis of the generator tool is parallel with the axis of rotation of the lens, the generated surface is plane. (b) Tilting the generator tool through the angle α produces a convex surface. The centre of curvature of the generated curve lies at C. (c) Tilting the generator tool in the opposite direction produces a concave surface

$$\sin \alpha = \frac{y_T}{r + r_T}$$

$$\sin \alpha = \frac{y_T}{r - r_T}$$

a)   b)   c)

C

In Figure 17.8c, the tool rotates in the opposite direction and now generates a concave surface of radius:

$$r = y_T \csc \alpha + r_T$$

Usually, the cutting head of the generator is designed to tilt in one direction only and is moved laterally over the workpiece to place the opposite edge of the cutting tool over the centre of the blank.

In many prescription laboratories spherical surfaces are produced with a toric generator, the base curve being set to the same value as the cross curve. This is indicated in Figure 17.9, which represents a plan view of the workpiece held in the chuck of the generator. The curve in one meridian is obtained by tilting the generator head, just as in the case of the spherical generator, but the curve at right angles is obtained by swinging the tool around the point C_T. If the radius of the 'base curve' is set the same as the radius of the 'cross curve', the generator cuts a spherical surface.

When surfaces were produced on glass lenses by the roughing process, they were only of approximate form and needed three or four truing and smoothing stages before being ready for polishing. The process of truing reduces the surface to its proper curvature by using a finer grade abrasive, and the smoothing stages bring the lens to its final thickness and prepare the surface for polishing. Smoothing of glass lenses is rarely performed on the tool face these days; either a pad is first attached to the tool face (Figure 17.10a) or diamond tools are used.

Two forms of diamond lapping tools are used. For long runs of the same curve, as needed for the mass production of semi-finished blanks, the entire tool face may be diamond impregnated. For short runs the tool has several small round diamond-impregnated pellets stuck over the face of a metal holder with a suitable radius of curvature (Figure 17.10b).

Figure 17.10a illustrates a cross-sectional and plan view of a smoothing tool to which a pad has been attached. Modern pads are self-adhesive and easily applied to the tool face by small, dedicated pneumatic (or manually operated) pad applicators that press the pad evenly onto the tool to ensure it remains wrinkle-free. The use of pads has reduced greatly the fining times for plastics lenses. The pads can be impregnated and they ensure the smoothing slurry is evenly distributed over the surface. When they wear out, the pads can be stripped off the tool and replaced very easily. Since wear takes place on the pad face rather than on the tool face, the use of pads has made it possible to make tools

from lightweight alloys or rigid plastics materials, rather than the traditional cast iron, which is both heavy and difficult to cut.

Use of diamond-smoothing tools, such as that illustrated in Figure 17.10b, reduces the smoothing time enormously and produces a surface ready for polishing. The small pellets can be used to produce a tool of any curvature at short notice. Adjustment of diamond concentration can be achieved simply by varying the number of pellets used in a given area. Machine cycles for diamond smoothing depend on several factors, including the coarseness of the surface produced by the generator, but are generally in the range of 10–30 seconds.

With plastics lenses, smoothing or fining of the surface produced by the generator rarely needs more than two stages of abrasive. The pads are usually abrasive and the radius of the pad face is the same as that required on the finished lens surface.

Polishing of the lens surface, which brings the surface to its final stage of transparency, is the final surfacing process before inspection and verification. The process is similar to smoothing, but softer pads and finer abrasives are employed. Polishing pads are usually made from polyurethane impregnated with zirconium oxide and are available in several thicknesses and different grades of hardness for working different materials. Typically, the polishing cycle may take as little as 90 seconds if the smoothed surface is reasonably fine.

It is important to maintain both the mechanical and chemical actions of the slurry during the smoothing and polishing processes, so concentration, temperature and pH values are monitored constantly to ensure that the slurries are working optimally.

Deblocking from alloy buttons is relatively simple and the polished lens surface is usually inspected for quality and freedom from sleeks and scratches before removal from the button by placing the lens in a reclaim tank, which enables the metal alloy to be recycled.

Computer numerically controlled machining

Single-point diamond turning has been employed in the precision optical industry for at least 30 years to improve the finish of the generated surface and speed smoothing and polishing times on glass lenses.[5] A diamond burr is illustrated in Figure 17.11a. It consists of a relatively soft graphite core surrounded by a hard shell impregnated with 5000-grit diamond dust. The graphite core ensures that the tool is rigid, but is soft enough not to harm the surface being generated when the bond of the burr starts to

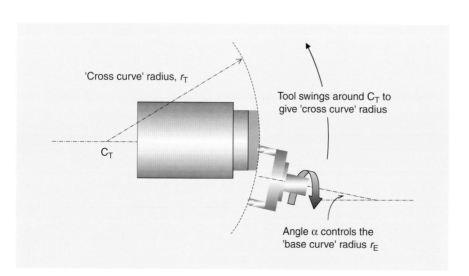

'Cross curve' radius, r_T

Tool swings around C_T to give 'cross curve' radius

C_T

Angle α controls the 'base curve' radius r_E

Figure 17.9 Machining a spherical surface with a toric generator. A plan view of the workpiece is shown with the 'base curve' blocked at right angles to the plane of the page. The 'base-curve' radius is controlled by the tilt of the generator head, just as in Figure 17.8, and the 'cross-curve' radius is obtained by swinging the head of the generator around C_T. (When the base curve and the cross curve are the same, the surface is spherical)

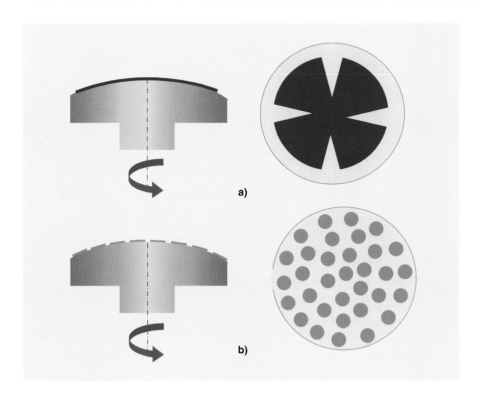

Figure 17.10 Smoothing tools. (a) A smoothing tool to which a pad has been attached to prevent wear on the tool face and to improve the abrasion to the surface. (b) A diamond-smoothing tool with sintered diamond pellets attached to a holder. Diamond smoothing dramatically reduces smoothing times and provides a fine surface for polishing

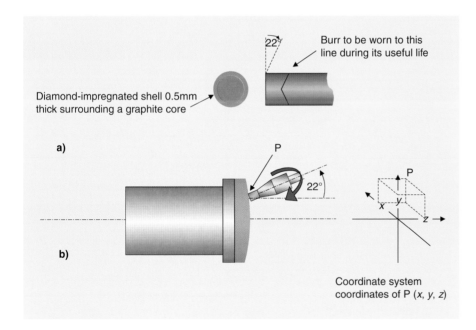

Figure 17.11 The principle of single-point diamond turning. (a) The diamond burr. (b) CNC machining. The position of the cutting point P at any moment in time is numerically controlled by the onboard computer (or a tape or disk), which controls the machine. Typically, the computer has been programmed to move the cutting point in a vertical sweep, along the y axis

wear away. The overall diameter of the burr is about 10mm, but the thickness of the diamond shell is only some 0.50mm. The burr illustrated in Figure 17.11a is designed for presentation to the workpiece at an angle of 22°. It rotates at high speed, in excess of 30 000rpm.

In Figure 17.11b, the burr is shown making a single-point contact with the workpiece at P, the position of which is given by the computer in geometrical form by means of the three coordinates (x, y, z). In the insert to Figure 17.11b, which shows the origin of the coordinate system, P has been positioned at $(+10, +10, +10)$, that is, it lies 10mm above the origin, 10mm to its left and 10mm behind. The sign convention follows from the fact that the surface is supposed to be viewed from behind.

Figure 17.12 shows a CR39 blank in the process of having a +6.00 convex curve machined by a single-point diamond cutter. The machine lines are visible on the left-hand side of the surface and the cutter is about to make a sweep down the 90 meridian of the lens. The current information in the computer memory for the first 10 points on this meridian is shown in Table 17.3.

The data are obtained as follows (schematic of the computer software is given in the caption to Figure 17.12):

- In line 1 the refractive index of the lens material is fed into the software, and the value of 1.498 is assigned to n.
- In line 2 the desired power of the surface is given either as an input or a data statement.

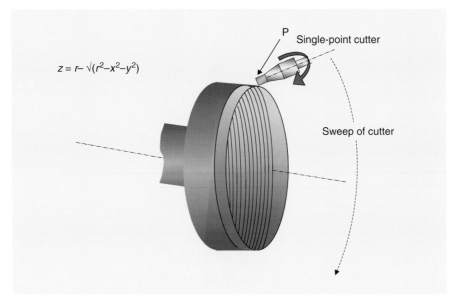

$$z = r - \sqrt{(r^2 - x^2 - y^2)}$$

P Single-point cutter

Sweep of cutter

Figure 17.12 CNC machining of ophthalmic blank. The computer program obtains the value of *r* and, using the equation to the sphere, calculates the correct position of the single-point diamond for an 80mm diameter workpiece. The CNC is programmed to cut the lens in vertical sweeps, starting at point (+40.00, +40.00, +22.26), the coordinates being calculated from the equation shown. Assuming that the machine is exactly halfway through its program, and is about to begin its sweep along the 90 meridian of the lens, the cutting point now lies at (0.00, +40.00, +10.27).

Machining software:

1   $n = 1.498$
2   $F = 6$
3   $r = 1000 \times (n - 1)/F$
4   For $x = 40$ to -40
5   For $y = +40$ to -40
6   $z = r - \sqrt{\left(r^2 - x^2 - y^2\right)}$
7   Point P(x, y, z)
8   Next y
9   Next x

Table 17.3 Machining data for 90 meridian of +6.00D curve on an 80mm diameter blank		
x coordinate	y coordinate	z coordinate
0.00	+40.00	+10.27
0.00	+39.00	+9.73
0.00	+38.00	+9.21
0.00	+37.00	+8.70
0.00	+36.00	+8.21
0.00	+35.00	+7.74
0.00	+34.00	+7.28
0.00	+33.00	+6.84
0.00	+32.00	+6.42
0.00	+31.00	+6.01

- In line 3 the software computes the radius of the curve, from the usual surface power relationship of $r = 1000(n - 1)/F$. For the values given, the radius is found to be 83.0mm.
- In line 4 the computer is instructed to start with a value of +40 for x and the for/next loop performs the instructions that follow from line 5 to line 9, which is the end of the subroutine. The program then returns to line 4 and assigns a new value of +39 to x and repeats the routine and so on until a value of -40 is reached, when the program jumps out of the loop.
- In line 5 the computer initially assigns a value of +40 to y and decrements this value in its own for/next loop until it reaches -40.

- In line 6 the value of z is calculated from the current values for r, x and y. The current value for x is zero, the current value for y is +40 and the value for r is 83.0.
- Hence, since $z = r - \sqrt{(r^2 - x^2 - y^2)}$ the software calculates the value of +10.27 and in line 7 positions the cutter at the coordinates (0.00, +40.00, +10.27). At the moment in time depicted in Figure 17.12, x has decremented to zero, y has been assigned the value of +40 and the cutter head is poised at (0.00, +40.00, +10.27).
- In line 8, the software returns to line 5 to assign the next value for y, which is +39 for the for/next loop as written, decrements by one, and recalculates the value of z, which is now 9.73.
- Line 7 repositions the cutter at (0.00, +39.00, +9.73), and so on.

In the late 1980s, the well-known optical machinery company, Coburn Optical International Inc. revolutionized the processing industry for plastics lenses with the introduction of single-point precision turning technology for ophthalmic lenses. The Coburn IQ CNC Lensmaker series of generators provides a finish that is precise and much smoother than that obtained from conventional generating techniques. The cool-cutting technique generates no heat during the cutting cycle, which reduces the possibility of waviness on the lens surface as a result of warpage through heat. The new breed of generator was designed to decrease production time while providing a lens with precise curves and a very finely ground surface that needs just one smoothing operation and final polishing. The cutter is a single-point diamond that produces surfaces in the range +7.00 to –20.00 on blanks up to 90mm diameter and cylinder and prism powers up to 10D. The largest machine in the range, the Lensmaker XRT, also allows the operator to produce precision curves on plastics lap tools within the range plano to 17.00D, which allows the surfacing laboratory to produce accurate curves on all refractive index materials.

Other CNC machines that employ single-point precision turning mechanisms, such as the Gerber generator, quickly followed. The Gerber cutting head is a small metal ball fitted with sharp cutting blades. When the ball rotates at high speed, only one point on the spherical cutter is in contact with the workpiece. Such equipment is able to cut plastics materials in the dry state without the use of cooling lubricant. However, vacuum suction must be employed to remove the material dust and the work area must be well ventilated for the comfort of the machine operator.

Freeform surfaces

The advent of computer numerically controlled grinding methods has enabled surfaces to be described and produced not by a mathematical equation but instead by giving the z-coordinates of the surface for closely spaced values of x and y (see, for example, Figure 12.37). This numeric description of the surface allows not only its optical characteristics to be determined but also enables the surface to be manufactured by a single point cutter whose path is directed in the x-, y- and z-meridians by the software controlling the position of the cutting head (computer numerically controlled machining). Surfaces which are described in this fashion have come to be known by the term *freeform surfaces*. A freeform surface may be an ordinary spherical, toroidal or rotationally symmetrical, aspherical surface which is simply described by its x-, y- and z-coordinates, rather than by the equations given in this Chapter. However, the real advance which freeform technology has provided is the ability to describe and manufacture any surface (such as an atoroidal or progressive surface) which need not be rotationally symmetrical, i.e. surfaces of revolution. Furthermore, aspects of the design which could not previously be altered at the grinding stage (such as modifications to the curves to take into account individual fitting characteristics of the wearer) can now be computed upon receipt of the prescription order and incorporated in the final lens by the software controlling the grinding process.

Testing spherical surfaces

In the precision lens-making industry, optical surfaces are tested by both optical and mechanical methods. In ophthalmic lens work, optical methods are normally reserved for moulds, particularly those that possess aspherical and progressive power surfaces.

The usual method for checking the accuracy of a curve in the surfacing laboratory is by means of a sag gauge or sagometer. The read-out may be with dial gauges similar to those found on the simple lens measure, or the read-out may be digital, in which case it can be converted into a surface-power reading and then converted into a curve for any refractive index at the touch of a button. Normally, the sag gauge simply reads the sag height of the curve under test and the value of the curve is then read from a set of tables.

The principle of the sag gauge is illustrated in Figure 17.13. The rim of the bell gauge is placed in contact with the surface under test and the spring-loaded central rod is pressed gently onto the surface under test. Notice that, in the case of a convex surface under test, the inner edge of the bell is in contact with the curve, whereas in the case of a concave surface, the outer edge of the bell is in contact with the curve. Either two different gauges can be used with one set of tables, or a single gauge can be used with two sets of tables. The former is the rule in practice, since it reduces the length of travel that must be undertaken by the central leg. The bell often has a cut-out section so that the distance-portion curve can be read in the case of solid bifocals, which have raised segment portions.

If the sag of the curve, z, is read from the gauge it can be converted into the surface power, F, by the expression:

$$F = 2000(n-1)z/(y^2 + z^2)$$

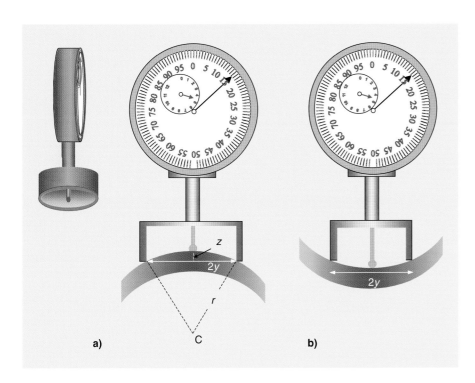

Figure 17.13 Principle of the sagometer. (a) Measurement of a convex surface. The instrument reads the height of the central leg above a fixed chord. The centre of curvature of the surface under test lies at C and the relationship between the height, z, the chord length, $2y$, and the radius of curvature of the surface, r, is:

$$z = r - \sqrt{(r^2 - y^2)}$$

Note that the chord is measured across the inside diameter of the bell. (b) For a concave surface, the chord is measured across the outside diameter of the bell

Digital sagometers use a knife-edge bell to obtain the same values for the bell diameter for both convex and concave surfaces.

Toroidal surface

Geometry

Essentially, a toroidal surface can be looked upon as a cylindrical surface that has been curved so that the axis meridian of the cylinder is no longer plane (Figure 17.14). Hence, a toroidal surface has two different principal powers, neither of which is zero. The lower power is referred to as the base curve of the surface and the higher power as the cross curve. In the simple cylindrical surface shown in Figure 17.14a, the base-curve power along the axis is zero and the cross-curve power is simply the power of the cylindrical surface.

In the case of the toroidal surface (Figure 17.14b), the 'axis meridian' is curved and the cylindrical power of the surface is the difference between the cross curve and the base curve.

A toroidal surface is formed by the rotation of an arc of a circle about an axis in the plane of the circle, but lying outside it.[3] Toroidal surfaces now exist for which the generator is not a circular arc; such atoroidal surfaces are described later in this chapter. Three quite distinct forms of the surface have been used in ophthalmic work (illustrated in Figure 1.32). They take their names from their obvious similarity to a car tyre's inner tube, a barrel and a capstan.

It can be seen from Figure 1.32 that each form of the surface has two principal radii of curvature corresponding to its two principal meridians. The generator in each form is the arc DD′ and the centre of curvature of the generating arc is C_T, with the locus around the axis of revolution, YY′, indicated. The axis of revolution meets the axis of symmetry that passes through the vertex of the surface, A, at C_E, which represents the equatorial centre of curvature of the surface. C_T represents the transverse centre of curvature of the surface and the distance AC_T represents the transverse radius of curvature, r_T. The distance AC_E is the equatorial radius of the surface r_E.

In the tyre-formation toroidal surface illustrated in Figure 1.32a, which is the most common form of the surface in practice, r_E is the base-curve radius and r_T is the cross-curve radius. The tyre-form surface results when the centre of curvature of the generating arc, C_T, lies between the pole of the surface, A, and the axis of revolution, YY′.

In the case of the barrel-formation toroidal surface illustrated in Figure 1.32b, r_E is the cross-curve radius and r_T is the base-curve radius. The barrel form of the surface results when the centre of curvature of the generating arc, C_T, lies on the other side of the axis of revolution, YY′, from the pole of the surface, A.

The rarely encountered capstan formation surface, illustrated in Figure 1.32c, is concave in one meridian and convex in the other. In this form, the surface lies between the centre of curvature of the generating arc, C_T, and the axis of revolution, YY′. It is conventional in this form of surface to describe the convex curve as the base curve, whatever the numerical value of the concave curve happens to be.

If each principal meridian is considered to be circular, then the equation to each meridian reduces to the well-known quadratic solution for the depth (or sag) of the curve and is given by (Figure 17.15):

$$y^2 + z^2 - 2rz = 0$$

from which:

$$z = r - \sqrt{(r^2 - y^2)}$$

or, using the alternative form given earlier:

$$z = y^2 / \left[r + \sqrt{(r^2 - y^2)} \right]$$

In these expressions, the semi-chord value, x, for the other principal meridian simply replaces the value for y.

The tyre-formation toroidal surface is the usual form of surface to be found on stock-range toric lenses, since it lends itself well to mass production. The barrel-form surface is hardly ever used for mass production, as fewer lenses can be produced from a single toric block. From an optical point of view, the barrel-form surface does possess certain advantages, in that it improves the off-axis performance of the usual range of low-power toric lenses. Some toric generators are able to cut a toroidal surface in either tyre or barrel form.

The difference in geometry between the tyre- and barrel-form surfaces can be deduced from Figure 17.16, which illustrates the use of a lap gauge of the type that might be employed in the surfacing workshop to check the accuracy of the tool face.

Figure 17.16a shows a lap gauge of the correct curvature (6.00D) applied to the base-curve meridian of a toric lap that has

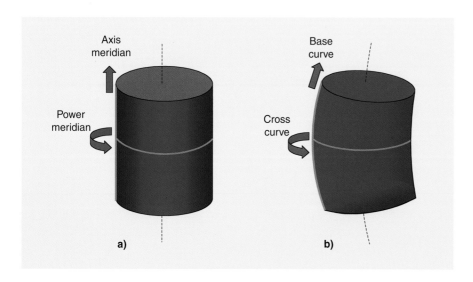

Figure 17.14   Comparison of the cylindrical and toroidal surface. (a) The cylindrical surface has a plane axis meridian and circular power meridian. (b) The toroidal surface can be imagined to be a cylindrical surface whose 'axis' meridian is not plane

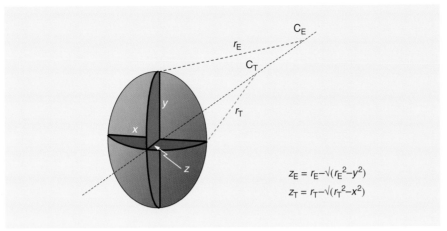

Figure 17.15 The sag equations for the principal meridians of the surface. The base curve lies in the vertical meridian, so:

$$z_E = r_E - \sqrt{\left(r_E^2 - y^2\right)} \text{ and } z_T = r_T - \sqrt{\left(r_T^2 - x^2\right)}$$

Note that here z_E and z_T are equal, which means that the lens shape must be an oval with the vertical meridian longer than the horizontal meridian

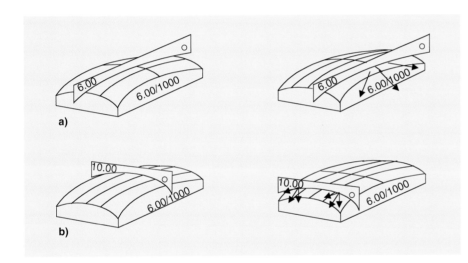

a)

b)

Figure 17.16 Lap gauge used to determine the form of a toroidal surface with curves of –6.00/–10.00. (a) Tyre-form toric tool – base-curve meridian under test. When the lap gauge is held parallel to the base-curve meridian and slid along the cross curve, daylight is seen to escape beneath the centre of the gauge. The curve has become too shallow. (b) Barrel-form toric tool – cross-curve meridian under test. When the lap gauge is held parallel to the cross-curve meridian and slid along the base curve, daylight is seen to escape beneath the edges of the gauge. The curve has become too steep.

This test provides an easy method to determine whether the tool has been cut in tyre form or barrel form

a 6.00D base curve and a 10.00D cross curve. The lap has been cut in tyre form. The gauge is held along the equator of the tool and can be seen to fit the tool perfectly along the equator.

When the gauge is moved to some other position along the base-curve meridian, still held parallel with the equator of the tool, the curvature of the tyre-form surface is seen to decrease. The centre of the gauge no longer makes contact with the tool face and daylight is seen beneath the centre of the gauge.

A 10.00D gauge held at right angles to the equator of the tool, along the cross-curve meridian, is seen to fit the cross curve no matter where it is placed on the tool. If the cylindrical power of the tool is small, the change in curvature may be seen more easily with a sagometer of the type described below for the measurement of toroidal surfaces.

If the tool had been cut in barrel form (Figure 17.16b), the 6.00D gauge is seen to make contact with the base-curve meridian in any position on the tool, provided it is held parallel with the base-curve meridian.

When the 10.00D gauge is used to check the cross-curve meridian, it makes perfect contact along the equator of the cross curve, but is seen to be too shallow when moved to a new position, parallel with the equator, but near the edge of the tool

(Figure 17.16b). Daylight is now seen beneath the gauge, near each edge of it.

The variation in surface power of these two forms of the toroidal surface is illustrated in Figure 17.17. This shows that, in the case of the tyre-form surface (Figure 17.17a), the cross-curve power remains constant at 10.00D, but the base-curve power decreases as we move away from the equator, along the cross-curve meridian.

For the barrel-form surface (Figure 17.17b), the base-curve power remains constant at 6.00D, but the cross-curve power increases as we move away from the equator along the base-curve meridian.

This is seen to be the case from Figure 17.18, which illustrates a barrel-form toroidal surface with vertex power that is supposed to be +6.00/+10.00. The +6.00D power lies in the vertical meridian. Imagine a lens measure placed at point A with its legs lying along the horizontal meridian, AQ. This is the equatorial meridian and the power recorded by the lens measure is the power of the cross curve, +10.00. If the lens measure is now slid along the cross curve so that its centre leg lies at Q, the lens measure continues to read +10.00. If the lens measure is now rotated through 90° on the surface at Q, the reading is reduced to +6.00, as we

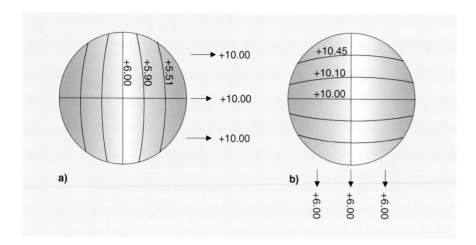

Figure 17.17   Variation in curvature of tyre-form and barrel-form toroidal surfaces. (a) In the tyre-form surface, the base-curve powers decrease away from the principal meridian. (b) In the barrel-form surface, the cross-curve powers increase away from the principal meridian

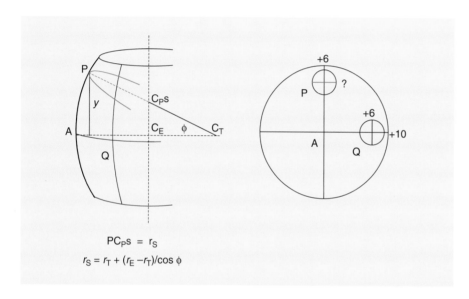

Figure 17.18   Sagittal radius of curvature of the toroidal surface. The curvatures of the principal meridians at Q are exactly the same as the curvatures at A. The tangential power at P is the same as that at the vertex, A, but the sagittal power has increased from the equatorial power at A

should expect, since the meridian is parallel with the base-curve meridian AP.

If the lens measure is again placed at the vertex with its centre leg at A, along the cross-curve, AQ, the instrument should read +10.00. If the lens measure is now slid along the base-curve meridian so that its centre leg lies at P, the reading on the dial increases. The sagittal radius of curvature at point P has decreased and the sagittal centre now lies at C_{PS}, where the normal to the surface crosses the axis of revolution of the surface.

If the height of P is known (y), then the sagittal radius of curvature, r_S, is given by:

$$r_S = r_T + (r_E - r_T) / \cos \phi$$

where $\sin \phi = y / r_T$. This expression applies equally to tyre-formation surfaces.

By way of example, suppose that a barrel-form toroidal surface of power +6.00/+10.00 is worked on a material of refractive index 1.523. The radii of curvature of the two principal meridians are given by:

$$r = 1000 (n - 1) / F$$

For the 6.00D meridian the radius is found to be 87.17mm and for the 10.00D meridian it is found to be 52.3mm. Since the surface is

of barrel form, the transverse radius of curvature, r_T, is 87.17mm and the equatorial radius, r_E, is 52.3mm. At a point 15mm from the pole of the surface (point P in Figure 17.18), angle ϕ is given by:

$$\sin \phi = 15/87.17$$

from which angle ϕ is found to be 9.91°. The sagittal radius of curvature at P is given by:

$$r_S = r_T + (r_E - r_T) / \cos \phi$$

so

$$r_S = 87.17 + (52.3 - 87.17) / \cos 9.91 = 51.77 \text{mm}$$

The sagittal power of the surface at P is 523/51.77 = +10.10D, which is the value indicated for this meridian in Figure 17.17b.

Clearly, the form of the smoothing and polishing tools must match the form of the generated surface. Toroidal surfaces that have been generated, say, in tyre form cannot be smoothed and polished with tools that have been cut in barrel form!

Production of the toroidal surface

For the mass production of glass toric lenses the toroidal surface is produced on a toric wheel block (Figure 17.19). Blanks are attached to the outside of a wheel block to produce convex toroidal

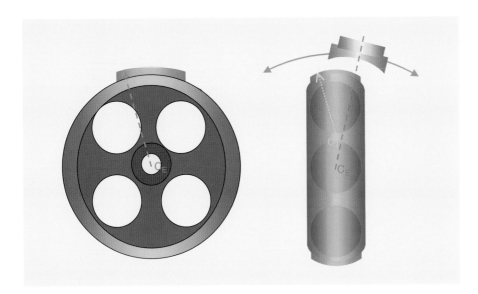

Figure 17.19   Toric block showing trans-verse and equatorial radii of curvature

surfaces, or to the inside of the block for concave toroidal surfaces.[5,6] The value of the base-curve radius determines the number of blanks that can be blocked on a single wheel. The blanks are secured rigidly to the blocks by means of a sophisticated casting system that uses an alloy of low melting point.

Surfacing the blocks follows the usual generating, smoothing and polishing operations described earlier for spherical surfaces.

Generating is carried out on a machine that works to a precise toroidal geometry. The high-speed peripheral diamond tool produces true toroidal curves with no trace of, so-called, elliptical error (see below). Rigid construction of the machines ensures accurate curves with minimum cycle times. The radius of curvature of the base curve is simply the distance from the centre of the block to the outer surfaces of the blanks being worked. The cross-curve power can be adjusted by varying the position of the slides that control the position of the transverse centre of curvature (C_T in Figure 17.19).

Since continuous grinding of the toroidal surface on the wheel gradually reduces the value of the base curves radius, it is necessary to rough the toric block slightly oversize to allow for the glass removed during the smoothing process, generally some 0.4 to 0.5mm.

Smoothing is carried out in a two-step operation performed on one double-headed machine, which allows two diamond-smoothing tools, with diamond particles of different size, to smooth and fine the surfaces in sequence.

Polishing is performed on machines with the same geometry as the smoothing machine. Twin polyurethane-covered pads act simultaneously on the lenses as the wheels rotate at varying speeds. Frequent spindle-direction changes combined with carefully designed polishing-tool oscillation ensures accurate and distortion-free polishing.

At the end of the polishing cycle and before removal of the lenses from the block, one lens is subjected to critical inspection to ensure that there are no polishing defects or obvious errors of form.

When checked and passed, the lenses are de-blocked by immersing the wheel in a large tank of hot water from which the alloy can be retrieved.

Single surface working

In the surfacing laboratory, the final prescription is usually obtained by working the concave surface of a semi-finished blank of which the convex surface has been finished with a spherical curve. When the prescription contains a cylindrical component, the concave surface must be toroidal.

The various stages in the grinding of a single toroidal surface are the same as those for spherical lenses detailed earlier, from lens marking (blank layout) to final inspection and verification. Most of the individual processes are exactly the same for both spherical and toroidal surfaces.

When generating a toroidal surface, the base-curve setting and cross-curve setting differ. This is indicated in Figure 17.20, which represents a plan view of the workpiece held in the chuck of the generator. The curve in one meridian is obtained by tilting the generator head, in the same way as for spherical surfaces, but the curve at right angles is obtained by swinging the tool around the point C_T. As the actual contact of the generator tool with the surface at any instant in time is a straight line, this procedure results in an error of form of the surface, known as elliptical error. This error of form produces a mismatch between the generated surface and the form of the surface of the smoothing tool, and results in a dramatic increase in the necessary smoothing and polishing times. The smoothed surface is, invariably, poorly finished and, usually, wavy with grey areas at the extremities of the curve at right angles to the sweep of the head.

Clearly, if the base curve is blocked vertically, so that the sweep of the generator cuts the cross curve of the toroidal surface, the elliptical error will occur in the base-curve meridian. If the base curve is blocked horizontally, compensation for elliptical error must be applied to the cross curve of the surface.

Compensation for elliptical error is provided by increasing the value of the curve by an amount that depends on the powers of the two curves and the diameter of the blank. If the correct amount of compensation is provided, the shape of the surface corresponds almost exactly with that of the smoothing tool.

Computer numerically controlled machining of toroidal surfaces

With the advent of CNC machining, it has become possible to generate toroidal surfaces that are completely free of elliptical error. Single-point diamond turning,[5] as described earlier, improves the finish of the generated surface and speeds smoothing and polishing times on glass lenses.

The Gerber and Coburn generators mentioned earlier produce toroidal surfaces, as does the Norville toric generator, which also

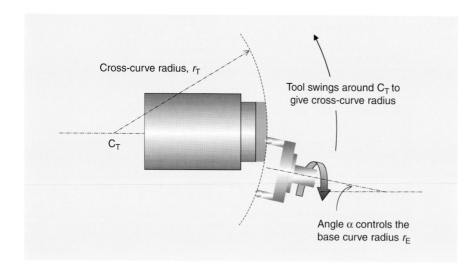

Cross-curve radius, r_T

Tool swings around C_T to give cross-curve radius

C_T

Angle α controls the base curve radius r_E

Figure 17.20   Machining a toroidal surface by toric generator. A plan view of the workpiece and the base curve, blocked at right angles to the plane of the paper. The base-curve radius is controlled by the tilt of the generator head and the cross-curve radius is obtained by swinging the head of the generator around C_T. As the contact of the generator tool with the surface at any instant in time is a straight line, this procedure results in an error of form of the surface, known as elliptical error

employs a single-point diamond-cutting tool and leaves the generated surface completely free from elliptical error.

Smoothing and polishing of singly worked toroidal surfaces is accomplished by specially developed machinery, usually twin-spindle units, which carry the smoothing or polishing tools. There must be no rotation of the surfaces of the tool and the blanks relative to each other, so, essentially, the tool motion is in two straight lines, one along the base-curve meridian and one along the cross-curve meridian. Provided that these essential motions are maintained, the tool and blank may rotate together to distribute the slurry evenly between the surfaces. A typical smoothing and polishing machine is illustrated in Figure 17.21.

Testing toroidal surfaces

The sag gauge described for spherical surfaces can also be used for toroidal surfaces, but a bell gauge cannot be used since the surface power varies between the base curve and the cross curve. Instead, the three legs of the sagometer are arranged to lie in a straight line that can be placed along either the base-curve or the cross-curve meridians (Figure 17.22). Just as with the bell gauge sagometer, the spring-loaded central rod is pressed gently onto the surface under test.

To minimize the risk of damaging the surface when taking readings on plastics lenses, the feet of the instrument may be made spherical, in which case the chord value over which the gauge measures varies with the curvature of the surface under test. Notice in Figure 17.22 that, in the case of a convex surface under test, the inner edges of the balls are in contact with the curve, whereas in the case of concave surfaces, the outer edges of the balls are in contact with the curve.

The relationship between the chord diameter of the instrument, y', and the chord diameter of the surface under test, y, is a function of the radii of the surface and the balls on the feet of the instrument.[7] It is obvious from Figure 17.22c that:

$$y = y'r/(r \pm r_B)$$

where r is the radius of the surface under test and r_B is the radius of the ball on the foot of the sagometer.

If the sag of the curve is read from the gauge it can be converted into the surface power, F, using the expression:

$$F = 2000(n-1)z/(y^2+z^2)$$

just as for spherical surfaces.

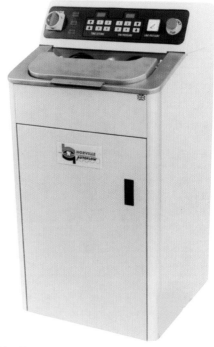

Figure 17.21   Typical smoothing and polishing machine for working toroidal surfaces (courtesy of Norville Optical)

Digital sagometers may use single-point contact to obtain the same values for the gauge diameter for both convex and concave surfaces.

Geometry of the conicoidal surface

In Chapter 4 it is shown that the simplest aspherical surfaces are those produced by rotation of the conic sections about their z-axis of revolution. The conic sections are all described by the single equation:

$$y^2 = 2r_0z - pz^2$$

where r_0 is the radius of curvature of the surface at the vertex, and the type of conic depends upon the value of p, as indicated in Figure 4.3.

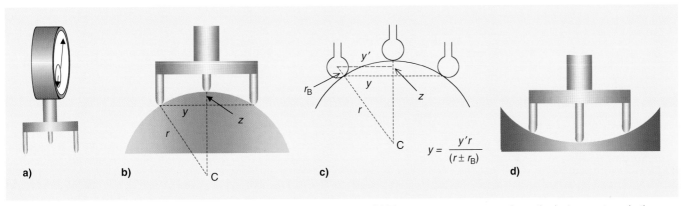

a) b) c) $y = \dfrac{y'r}{(r \pm r_\mathrm{B})}$ d)

Figure 17.22 Principle of the sagometer. (a) The three-legged sagometer. (b) To measure a convex surface, the instrument reads the height of the central leg above a fixed chord. The centre of curvature of the surface under test lies at C and the relationship between the height, z, the chord length, $2y$, and the radius of curvature of the surface, r, is:

$$z = r - \sqrt{\left(r^2 - y^2\right)}$$

Note that the balls on the feet of the legs make contact with the surface at their inside edges. (c) The relationship between the chord of contact of the gauge with the surface, y, and the chord value of the sagometer, y'. (d) Measurement of a concave surface (note that the balls on the feet of the legs make contact with the surface at their outside edges)

When the conic sections are rotated about their z-axes, the solid figures generated are known as conicoids, which comprise a group of rotationally symmetrical quadric surfaces.[3] Note that the z-axis is taken as the optical axis of the surface in Figure 17.23.

A circle rotated about its z-axis produces the solid of revolution known as the sphere. The sphere is the best-known spectacle lens surface and its great advantage over other members of the family is that it is easy to produce, and to reproduce, with simple rotating machinery.

An ellipse rotated about its major axis produces an ellipsoid. If the major axis of the ellipse is horizontal, the solid is referred to as a prolate ellipsoid. If the minor axis is horizontal, the solid is referred to as an oblate ellipsoid.

When a parabola is rotated about the z-axis it generates a paraboloid and a hyperbola generates a hyperboloid.

Assuming the origin to lie at the vertex, A, of the surface, the equation to a conicoidal surface is:

$$x^2 + y^2 + pz^2 - 2rz = 0$$

When $p = 1$, this expression reduces to the equation for a spherical surface given earlier.

The advantages that the other conicoids confer when compared with a spherical surface are three-fold. Firstly, their tangential power changes as the point under consideration on the surface moves away from the vertex of the curve. This can be understood most easily by imagining how the reading given by a lens measure varies as the instrument slides over the surface. For example, it is easy to see, in the case of the prolate ellipsoidal surface illustrated in Figure 17.23, that the maximum curvature of the surface lies at the vertex and that the tangential surface power decreases as the curve departs from the vertex.

Secondly, at every point on the surface, except at the vertex, there is surface astigmatism that can be used to counteract the aberrational astigmatism of oblique incidence.

Thirdly, in the case of conicoids with a p-value less than unity, the sag, z, of the curve is smaller than that of a spherical surface for the same diameter. This enables thinner spectacle lenses to be produced.

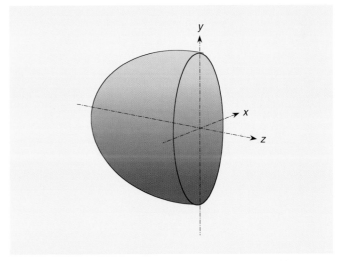

Figure 17.23 Aspherical surface of a prolate ellipsoid. Note the coordinate system employed, with the optical axis taken as the z-axis of the system

Although the three-dimensional form of this equation is required to set up the CNC software, it is helpful, for discussion purposes, to consider its two-dimensional form only. This is obtained by putting x equal to zero, in which case the sag, z, of a conicoid over a chord diameter $2y$ is given by the expression:

$$z = y^2 / \left[r_0 + \sqrt{\left(r_0^2 - py^2\right)} \right]$$

For example, a convex spherical curve of power +5.00D on CR39 material with refractive index taken to be exactly 1.5 has a radius of curvature of $500/5 = 100$mm and a sag, z, of 6.33mm at 70mm diameter. This value can be found from the above expression, substituting the value of 1.0 for p, since the surface in this case is spherical.

If the spherical surface is replaced by a convex hyperboloid with a p-value of –3.5, but otherwise of the same power at the vertex, then the radius of curvature at the vertex, r_0, remains 100mm and the sag reduces to 5.58mm over a diameter of

70mm. A trace of this surface is described by the relatively simple equation:

$$y^2 = 200z + 3.5z^2$$

In the design of spectacle lenses we are concerned with the aberrations that occur when the eye, rotating behind the lens, views through extra-axial points on the lens, that is, points removed from the optical centre. The most significant aberration in the case of the spectacle lens is oblique astigmatism.

The 5.00D hyperboloidal surface, just considered, could be used to produce a +4.00D aspheric lens without any appreciable oblique astigmatism (i.e. in point-focal form). Figure 17.24 illustrates a cross-sectional view of such a design, together with a field diagram to show its excellent off-axis performance. The axial thickness of the design is 3.8mm.

Polynomial aspherical surfaces

In Chapter 4 it is shown that surfaces of higher order than the conicoids are also used in the manufacture of modern spectacle lenses. These aspheric designs were described as ophthalmic lenses with polynomial surfaces. The term polynomial is used because the equation to the convex surface is of polynomial form, involving powers of y up to the tenth or twelfth degree, for example:

$$z = Ay^2 + By^4 + Cy^6 + Dy^8 + Ey^{10} \dots$$

The polynomial forms and values of A, B, C, etc., may be derived as follows. The equation to the sag of a conic section is given by:

$$z = y^2 / \left[r_0 + \surd \left(r_0^2 - py^2 \right) \right]$$

Binomial expansion gives rise to the power series:

$$z = \frac{y^2}{2r_0} + \frac{py^4}{2^2 2! r_0^3} + \frac{3p^2 y^6}{2^3 3! r_0^5} + \frac{15p^3 y^8}{2^4 4! r_0^7}$$

For convenience, this expansion is written in the form:

$$z = Ay^2 + By^4 + Cy^6 + Dy^8 + \dots$$

where

$$A = \frac{1}{2r_0}, \quad B = \frac{p}{2^2 2! r_0^3}, \quad C = \frac{3p^2}{2^3 3! r_0^5}, \text{ etc.}$$

Clearly, if the quantities A, B, C, etc., are altered slightly from the values given above, the surfaces depart from true conicoids to forms that the author has described as deformed conicoids.[2]

Consider the +5.00D hyperboloidal surface with vertex radius 100mm and p-value −3.5, described above. In its simplest form the surface is defined by the equation:

$$y^2 = 200z + 3.5z^2$$

The surface can also be defined in polynomial form by:

$$z = Ay^2 + By^4 + Cy^6 + Dy^8 + Ey^{10} + \dots$$

where $A = +5.00000 \times 10^{-3}$, $B = -4.37500 \times 10^{-7}$, $C = +7.65625 \times 10^{-11}$, $D = -1.67481 \times 10^{-15}$ and $E = +4.10327 \times 10^{-19}$.

Further terms could be added, but it is not actually necessary since the first five terms reproduce the hyperboloid to within 1 micrometre ($1\mu m = 10^{-3}$mm) over a diameter of 65mm. Over a diameter of 55mm, just the first four terms will reproduce the hyperboloid to an accuracy of $1\mu m$.

The designer can fine-tune any or all of these terms to produce a deformed conicoid. For example, suppose we produce a +4.00D lens with a convex surface defined by the series:

$$z = Ay^2 + By^4 + Cy^6$$

where $A = +5.0 \times 10^{-3}$, $B = -4.4 \times 10^{-7}$ and $C = +7.7 \times 10^{-11}$.

The performance of this design is illustrated in Figure 17.25, which shows that, despite a departure from the true hyperboloidal form, this design provides the same off-axis performance as the design with a pure hyperboloidal convex surface with the performance illustrated in Figure 17.24. A comparison of the profile of this surface with the hyperboloidal surface from which it was

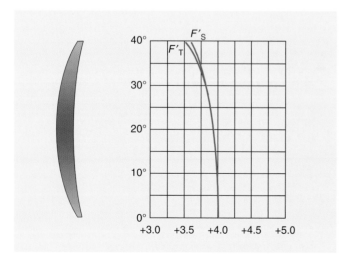

Figure 17.24   +4.00D lens made with convex hyperboloidal surface. The field diagram indicates that the design is point focal, the tangential and sagittal oblique vertex sphere powers being the same out to 35° ($n = 1.50$, $F_1 = +5.00$, $p = -3.5$, $t = 3.8$mm, centre of rotation distance = 27mm). Note that at 35°, the effective Rx is +3.73

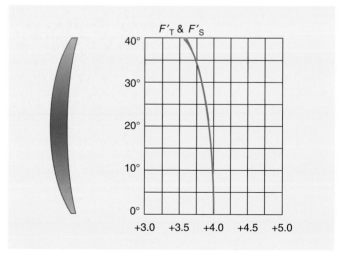

Figure 17.25   Field diagram for a +4.00D design with convex surface defined by equation $z = Ay^2 + By^4 + Cy^6$ where $A = 5.0 \times 10^{-3}$, $B = -4.4 \times 10^{-7}$ and $C = 7.7 \times 10^{-11}$

derived is given in Table 17.4, which lists the sags of the two surfaces for various diameters.

Comparing these two surfaces, it can be seen that over a diameter of 45mm they are indistinguishable to an accuracy of 1μm (0.001mm), and even at 70mm diameter they differ by only 26μm. Surfaces of this nature are used by several manufacturers to produce a series of low-power aspheric lenses.

Polynomial surfaces can be chosen to reproduce conicoids or they can be deformed even further to enable even thinner lenses to be made. For example, the patent application[8] for Essilor's *Hyperal* design describes a polynomial surface that flexes backwards in the peripheral region of the lens.

The surface is defined by a polynomial series, but with a central conicoid, in the form:

$$z = Ay^2 + By^4 + Cy^6 + Dy^8 + Ey^{10}$$

the *A* term being given by

$$\left[r_0 + \sqrt{\left(r_0^2 - py^2 \right)} \right]^{-1}$$

(In the patent application, the coefficients *B*, *C*, *D* and *E* are given as *A*, *B*, *C* and *D*.)

The second and successive terms of the polynomial give the deformation of the surface from the central conicoid. From the

information given in the original patent application, a +4.00D lens design employs a surface of power +6.06 ($r_0 = 82.518$mm) with $p = +0.1216$. A cross-sectional view of the lens, together with a field diagram for the design, is illustrated in Figure 17.26. The design is virtually point-focal over the central area and the tangential power begins to drop away from the central area, as we would expect from the shape of the surface.

As shown in Chapter 4, surfaces of this nature have also found an important application with very strong plus lenses, such as those required in the post-cataract range. Such a design is illustrated in Figure 4.8 and lenses of this form are available from several different manufacturers. By way of example, the Rodenstock patent literature[9] for their *Perfastar* design reveals that the equation to the surface includes odd polynomial terms of the form:

$$z = Ay^2 + By^3 + Cy^4 + Dy^5 + Ey^6$$

This lens is exceptionally well corrected for astigmatism over its central optical aperture.

These lens designs with polynomial surfaces combine the advantages of both lenticular lenses and full-aperture lenses. They are thinner and lighter than full-aperture designs for just the same reasons as a lenticular lens, but there is no visible dividing line between the aperture and the margin. This is of particular benefit when it is required to dispense strong plus lenses in a frame with a large eye size. The wearer obtains a wide central field within which the aberrations, which are normally severe in the case of post-cataract lenses, are exceptionally well corrected, together with a useful peripheral field with no ring scotoma between them.

Non-rotationally symmetrical surfaces

As pointed out, an aspherical surface can be considered to be a deformed conicoid. Bearing in mind that, at the vertex, all surfaces are considered to be spherical, we can consider that an aspherical surface deforms first to another type of conicoid and then may deform to an aspherical surface of higher order.

This concept is illustrated in Figure 17.27, which compares the trace of a spherical surface with traces of another conicoid, in this case a prolate ellipsoid of the type used in early forms of

Table 17.4	Comparison of the profiles of +5.00D surfaces	
Diameter (mm)	Hyperboloid	Deformed curve
20	0.496	0.496
25	0.771	0.771
30	1.104	1.104
35	1.492	1.492
40	1.935	1.935
45	2.428	2.428
50	2.971	2.972
55	3.560	3.563
60	4.192	4.200
65	4.867	4.881
70	5.580	5.606

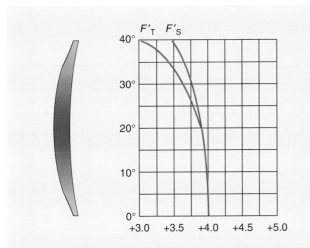

Figure 17.26   +4.00 *Hyperal* lens design (Essilor). Note that the design is virtually point-focal out to about 30°, whereupon the tangential and sagittal powers begin to fall. The tangential power actually reaches zero near the edge of the lens

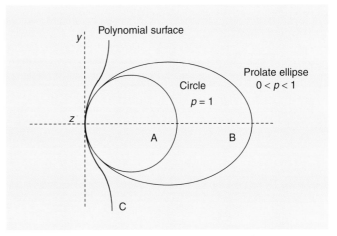

Figure 17.27   Comparison of three surfaces that share the same curvature, and hence power, at the vertex. Surface A is spherical, B is a prolate ellipsoid and C is a polynomial surface. Note the coordinate system employed, in which the optical axis is taken as the z-axis of the system

post-cataract lenses, and with a polynomial surface of the type used in modern forms of post-cataract lens designs. These surfaces all share the property that they are rotationally symmetrical, that is, the surface can be produced by the rotation of a plane curve around its axis of symmetry.

Modern ophthalmic lenses may employ surfaces that are not rotationally symmetrical. Such surfaces can be grouped broadly into three different types, two of which are used to produce single vision lenses and a third type, the progressive surface, is used to produce progressive power lenses for the correction of presbyopia.

The first group is essentially spherical at the vertex with different asphericities along different meridians of the surface. A surface of this type was employed on the convex surface of the original Zeiss *Hypal* design. It may help the reader to consider that the term asphericity here means, simply, the departure from a circular section along the meridian in question.

The second group is essentially toroidal at the vertex, but with different asphericities along its two principal meridians, the asphericity varying from a minimum along one principal meridian to a maximum along the second principal meridian of the surface. These surfaces are often described as atoroidal surfaces, since they are, essentially, aspheric toroidal surfaces. Surfaces of this type are employed on the concave surfaces of the Rodenstock *Multigressiv* design and the Zeiss *Gradal OSD* design for prescriptions that incorporate a cylindrical component.

The third group of non-rotationally symmetrical surfaces is perhaps the most familiar; it comprises progressive power surfaces, the asphericities of which are designed to produce a prescribed increase in power from the distance portion of the surface to the near portion of the surface. These surfaces are available from all the major lens producers. Progressive power surfaces are considered in Chapter 18.

Geometry of non-rotationally symmetrical aspherical surfaces

A non-rotationally symmetrical aspherical surface with principal powers the same along each of its maximum and minimum meridians, such that it is, therefore, spherical at the vertex of the surface, was originally employed on the Zeiss *Hypal* single vision lens design.

The rationale of this type of surface is as follows. Modern lenses are made flatter in form to enable them to be thinner, lighter and less bulbous in appearance (i.e. to have a smaller plate height). Flattening the lens makes the off-axis performance of the lens unacceptable. In the case of spherical prescriptions, the off-axis performance of the lens can be restored by employing an aspherical surface designed to neutralize the astigmatism of oblique incidence. For example, an ellipsoid such as that illustrated in Figure 17.27 provides the correct amount of neutralizing astigmatism for many powers, provided the chosen asphericity is suitable. As spherical lenses have the same power in every meridian, rotationally symmetrical aspherical surfaces that also have the same properties in every meridian provide excellent imaging properties for any lens power.

In the case of astigmatic prescriptions, the asphericity of, say, a conicoidal surface can only be correct for one principal meridian of the lens. The other principal meridian, of different power, requires a different eccentricity, or different *p*-value if the trace of the surface is a conic, for the power along this other meridian.

For example, in the case of the prescription +2.00/+2.00 × 90, which is made using a +5.00D front curve, the principal meridians of the lens have powers of +4.00D along 180 and +2.00D

along 90. The principal powers of this lens are made up by means of a concave toroidal surface of nominal powers:

$$-1.00 \times 90 / -3.00 \times 180$$

We have seen that, for a spherical lens of power +4.00 with a front surface power of +5.00, the lens is point-focal if the front curve has a hyperbolic section with a *p*-value of −3.5. In the case of the prescription +2.00/+2.00 × 90, along the 180 meridian the front curve should also have a hyperbolic section with a *p*-value of −3.5.

Accurate trigonometric ray-tracing shows that along the 90 meridian, for which the power of the lens is +2.00, the section of the front curve should also be hyperbolic, but, as we might expect, of different eccentricity from the section in the horizontal meridian. In the vertical meridian the section needs to be hyperbolic with a *p*-value of −0.1 if we wish this meridian to remain free from aberrational astigmatism for the 35° zone of the lens. Such a surface is depicted in Figure 17.28, which illustrates a convex 'atoroidal' surface for which the 'toricity' arises through a change in asphericity from one meridian to a second meridian at 90° to the first. It should be understood that the surface illustrated in Figure 17.28 has no cylindrical power, since the curvatures of the surface at the vertex along the two principal meridians are identical. The cylindrical component of the lens is provided in the usual way by grinding a toroidal surface on the back of the lens. As the surface has the same power along every meridian, the term atoroidal is not really a good description for this type of surface and a better definition for it might be the term used as the heading for this section, a non-rotationally symmetrical aspherical surface. However, it must be said that, strictly, this term also describes many other forms of surface, including progressive power surfaces, and the term atoroidal appears to have entered the literature without adverse comment from the profession!

As mentioned earlier, this type of surface was originally employed for the Zeiss *Hypal* series of lenses when they were produced for astigmatic prescriptions. For spherical prescriptions the convex surface is simply an aspherical surface, virtually indistinguishable from a true conicoid.

A general equation to any meridian of such a surface inclined at θ to the principal meridian, which is parallel to the concave base-curve meridian (on the other surface of the lens), the convex surface having a power, F_0, at its vertex and asphericity, p_B, along the base-curve meridian can be written in the form:

$$z = Ay^2 + By^4 + Cy^6 + Dy^8 + \ldots$$

where

$$A = F_0 / \left[N + \sqrt{(N^2 - PF_0^2 y^2)} \right]$$
$$N = 10^3 \times (n - 1)$$
$$P = p_B - (p_B - p_C)\theta/90$$

The values of *B*, *C*, *D*, etc., and the value of p_C, which is the value of the asphericity for the section of the convex surface parallel with the cross curve worked on the concave surface of the lens, are determined by accurate trigonometric ray tracing.

Table 17.5 compares typical values for *P*, *A* and *z* for different meridians of the +5.00D surface described above, when *y* is taken to be 25mm. The various sections of the surface are assumed to be pure conic sections, without deformation from their hyperbolic forms. The terms *B*, *C*, *D*, etc., in the polynomial expression given above for *z* are, therefore, all zero. The values of *P* remain constant along each meridian but, naturally, the values of *A* and *z* alter with different values of *y*.

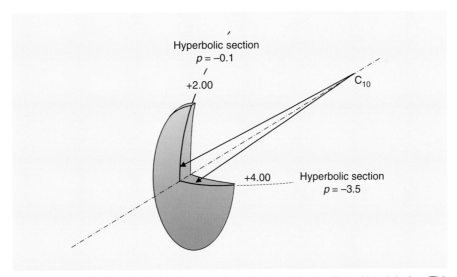

Figure 17.28 Non-rotationally symmetrical aspherical surface, such as that used for the Zeiss *Hypal* design. This convex aspherical surface was introduced by Carl Zeiss in 1986 for the *Hypal* lens, the first low-power aspheric design on the UK market (1987). In the case of spherical prescriptions, the convex surface is simply aspherical (i.e. rotationally symmetrical) and virtually indistinguishable from a hyperboloid. For astigmatic prescriptions, however, the principal meridians of the convex surface have different asphericities, each one apposite for the principal power in question. In the case of the lens illustrated here, the asphericity is greater in the horizontal meridian (lens power +4.00) than in the vertical meridian (lens power +2.00). The surface does not contain a cylindrical element for the correction of astigmatism – the cylinder is incorporated on the concave surface in the form of a minus-base toric

Table 17.5 Coefficients and sags of a +5.00D non-rotationally symmetrical aspherical surface				
Meridian	P	A	z	e
0	−3.50	$+4.753 \times 10^{-3}$	2.97	0.50
15	−2.93	$+4.790 \times 10^{-3}$	2.99	0.56
30	−2.37	$+4.828 \times 10^{-3}$	3.02	0.76
45	−1.80	$+4.867 \times 10^{-3}$	3.04	1.05
60	−1.23	$+4.907 \times 10^{-3}$	3.07	1.34
75	−0.67	$+4.949 \times 10^{-3}$	3.09	1.55
90	−0.10	$+4.992 \times 10^{-3}$	3.12	1.61

Table 17.6 Coefficients and sags of a $-1.05 \times 180/-3.05 \times 90$ toroidal surface					
Meridian	P	Q	A	z	e
0	+173.0	1.05	$+1.219 \times 10^{-3}$	0.76	0.50
15	+144.7	1.18	$+1.385 \times 10^{-3}$	0.87	0.58
30	+116.3	1.55	$+2.001 \times 10^{-3}$	1.25	0.81
45	+88.0	2.05	$+3.216 \times 10^{-3}$	2.01	1.12
60	+59.7	2.55	$+4.347 \times 10^{-3}$	2.72	1.44
75	+31.3	2.92	$+3.705 \times 10^{-3}$	2.32	1.67
90	+3.0	3.05	$+3.105 \times 10^{-3}$	1.94	1.76

These designs are symmetrical around the principal meridians, so the 105 meridian matches the 75 meridian and the 120 meridian matches the 60 meridian and so on.

The last column in the Table 17.5 gives the edge thickness of the +2.00/+2.00 × 90 lens for the stated meridians, assuming that it has been produced as a 50mm diameter round lens with the usual concave toroidal back surface. The thin-edge substance of the lens is 0.5mm. This variation in edge thickness should be compared with that given in Table 17.6 for the same specification, but made with an atoroidal surface that also incorporates the cylindrical component of the lens.

Note that a +5.00D spherical surface with a diameter of 50mm has a sag, z, of 3.18mm. The departure of the non-rotationally symmetrical surface (description given in Table 17.5) from a spherical surface of power +5.00 worked on a material of refractive index 1.50 is quite small along the 90 meridian, which is the meridian of lower asphericity. Furthermore, the difference between the two principal meridians of the surface is only 0.15mm (150μm). This form of non-rotationally symmetrical surface is illustrated in Figure 17.28.

The improvement obtained in the optical performance of the lens can be judged from Figure 17.29, which compares the residual aberrational astigmatism between the +2.00/+2.00 × 90 lenses made in a shallow curved form with an aspherical convex surface

(Figure 17.29a) and a non-rotationally symmetrical aspherical surface (Figure 17.29b).

In Figure 17.29a, the aspherical surface is chosen to optimize the performance in the stronger principal meridian (+4.00) and it is seen that along 180 the aberrational astigmatism does not exceed 0.25D. The vertical meridian, however, is not so well corrected. The design in Figure 17.29b employs a non-rotationally symmetrical aspherical surface of the type illustrated in Figure 17.28 and results in a design in which the aberrational astigmatism nowhere exceeds 0.25D.

Geometry of atoroidal surfaces

A true atoroidal surface with principal vertex curvatures that differ by the required cylindrical component, in addition to a variation in asphericity for the two principal meridians, is also employed on modern spectacle lens forms, mainly on progressive power lenses. For example, two current designs that employ atoroidal surfaces are the *Multigressiv* design from Rodenstock and the *Gradal* designs with Optimum Surface Design (OSD) from Zeiss. These two designs are both flatter in form than the traditional progressive power lenses and have asphericity built into the progressive surfaces to compensate for their flatter form, in the same way as low-power aspheric single vision lenses. Zeiss now use this method of construction for their *Hypal* single vision design.

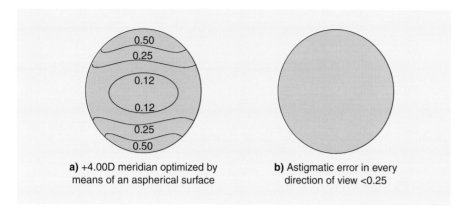

a) +4.00D meridian optimized by means of an aspherical surface

b) Astigmatic error in every direction of view <0.25

Figure 17.29   Optimization of the astigmatic prescription +2.00/+2.00 × 90 by means of a non-rotationally symmetrical aspherical surface such as that used by the Zeiss *Hypal* design. (a) The lens is made in a shallow curved form with a convex aspherical surface (such as a hyperboloid) optimized for the stronger meridian of the lens. There is residual aberrational astigmatism along the weaker meridian of the lens (90 meridian). (b) A non-rotationally symmetrical aspherical surface results in a design of which the residual aberrational astigmatism nowhere exceeds 0.25D

A proposal for how such atoroidal surfaces might be generated mathematically is disclosed in US Patent 5083859, granted to the author in 1991.[10] The equation to any meridian of the atoroidal surface, inclined at θ to the base curve meridian, which is expressed by its absolute power, F_B, and asphericity, p_B, is given by:

$$z = Ay^2 + By^4 + Cy^6 + Dy^8 + \ldots$$

where:

$$A = Q/\left[N = \surd\left(N^2 - PQ^2y^2\right)\right]$$
$$Q = F_B \cos^2 \theta + F_C \sin^2 \theta$$

N and P have the same meanings as before. Again, the values of B, C, D, etc., and the value of p_C, which is now the value of the asphericity for the absolute value of the cross curve, F_C, are determined by accurate trigonometric ray tracing.

An atoroidal surface of this nature is illustrated in Figure 17.30. For purposes of illustration, the surface has oblate ellipsoidal sections along every meridian, but differs from the surface depicted in Figure 17.28 in that not only does the asphericity vary along each meridian, but also the curvature of each section varies at the vertex of the surface.

Consider the prescription given earlier, +2.00/+2.00 × 90, which is now to be made with a +5.00D spherical front curve and

a concave atoroidal surface that is to incorporate not only the necessary asphericity to provide good off-axis performance, but also the cylindrical correction for the astigmatism. As before, the principal meridians of the lens are +4.00D along 180 and +2.00D along 90. Looking first at the +4.00D meridian, when the front surface power is +5.00 this meridian would offer an excellent off-axis performance if the back curve along the 180 meridian had an elliptical section with a *p*-value of +173.

Accurate trigonometric ray tracing shows that along the 90 meridian, where the power of the lens is +2.00, the section of the back curve should also be elliptical, but with a *p*-value of +3.0 if this meridian is to provide the same off-axis performance for the 35° zone of the lens. The surface depicted in Figure 17.30 is of this nature. It is atoroidal in the real sense that it is a concave toroidal surface that also has variable asphericities from one meridian to a second meridian at 90° to the first.

Table 17.6 compares typical values for P, Q, a and z for different meridians of the concave toroidal surface that would be employed for the prescription given above, when y is taken to be 25mm. Again, the various sections of the surface are assumed to be pure conic sections, without deformation from their elliptical forms. In practice, the terms B, C, D, etc., in the polynomial expression given above for z may not be zero. The values of P and Q remain constant along each meridian, but, naturally, the values of a and z vary with different values of y. As before, the 105 meridian matches the 75 meridian, the 120 meridian matches the 60 meridian and so on round to the 180 (zero) meridian.

The last column in Table 17.6 gives the edge thickness of the +2.00/+2.00 × 90 lens for the stated meridians, assuming that it has been produced as a 50mm diameter round lens with a +5.00D convex spherical surface and an atoroidal back surface. The thin-edge substance of the lens is 0.5mm. The variation in edge thickness should be compared with that given in Table 17.5 for the same specification, but made with a non-rotationally symmetrical surface that has different asphericities along each meridian. As a result of the different surface geometry, the variation in edge thickness of the two forms is quite different. In particular, the thick-edge substance of the design with the atoroidal surface is some 0.15mm greater than that in the design with the details given in Table 17.5.

Although atoroidal surfaces of this nature have become available for the Rodenstock and Zeiss designs mentioned above, to complement the front surfaces of their aspheric progressive power lenses, interestingly, they are not the first in the ophthalmic field.

Using their CNC machinery, originally developed for the production of *Varilux* progressive addition lenses, Essel Optical Company (now Essilor International) introduced a design in 1970 that minimized aberrational astigmatism along each principal meridian of a toric lens for the correction of aphakia. This *Atoral*

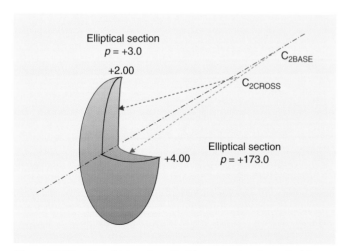

Elliptical section
p = +3.0
+2.00

C_{2BASE}

C_{2CROSS}

Elliptical section
+4.00   p = +173.0

Figure 17.30   Atoroidal surface that incorporates the cylindrical correction and possesses different asphericities along each meridian of the surface. This type of surface is employed by Rodenstock for their *Multigressiv* design and Zeiss OSD with their *Gradal* series of progressive power lenses

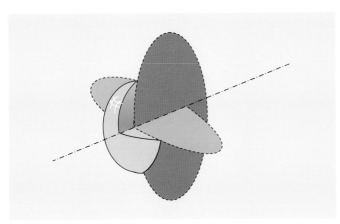

Figure 17.31 The *Atoral* lens, a toric lens with an atoroidal surface, was introduced in 1970 by Essel Optical Company (now Essilor International) to improve the optical performance of deep plus astigmatic lenses, required for the correction of aphakia. Each principal meridian of the concave surface has an oblate elliptical cross-section, for which the *p*-values decrease from a maximum along the base curve to a minimum along the cross curve

single vision lens also employed a non-rotationally symmetrical surface for which the principal sections were oblate ellipses of different eccentricities along each principal meridian. Between the two principal meridians the eccentricities varied from a minimum along one power meridian to a maximum along the other power meridian (Figure 17.31). The surface was also employed in the *Atoral Variplas* design, a progressive power lens for the correction of aphakia.

Production of aspherical surfaces

Unlike the usual forms of spherical and toroidal surfaces, aspherical surfaces cannot be produced with simple rotating machinery, so special manufacturing methods are employed to ensure accuracy of form and reproducibility of the surfaces.

Most aspheric lenses are made in plastics materials and are produced by moulding the plastics material. Both compression-moulding and injection-moulding techniques are used for the thermoplastics materials polymethylmethacrylate (PMMA) and polycarbonate. The moulds may be made from highly polished metal dies or from glass, but in either case production of the aspherical surface involves CNC machining of the mould.

Lenses made from thermosetting resins (CR39 and polyurethane) are produced by casting the monomer between two glass moulds and, again, CNC machining is employed to produce the aspheric glass mould.

In theory, aspherical surfaces on optical elements could be produced by one of the following methods:[5]

- shaping the surface by pressing
- shaping the surface by heat and pressure
- modifying the surface by applying an additional layer of material by vacuum deposition or other method of coating
- eroding the surface by removing material with an ion beam
- forming the surface by heat and sagging (slumping)
- shaping the surface by grinding and polishing.

The first of these methods, shaping the surface by pressing, has been applied successfully to plastics lenses, notably in the ophthalmic field by Combined Optical Industries Ltd (COIL), who produced PMMA lenses by means of compression moulding between two highly polished stainless-steel dies. Originally, the aspheric steel dies were hand figured, but eventually CNC turning was introduced to produce high-quality aspheric dies. The lenses were produced by first trepanning a plastics preform from a flat sheet of PMMA, the volume of which had to correspond exactly with that of the finished lens. The preform was placed between the dies and heated until it softened when the dies were forced together. The resultant aspherical surface was a mirror image of the surface on the die. Today, COIL produces its PMMA aspheric elements by a high-quality injection moulding process, the material being supplied in granular form.

In theory, an aspherical surface could be produced on a glass element by pressing, in the same way that ophthalmic pressings are produced (Figure 17.32), but in practice the fire-polished

Figure 17.32 Hot pressing process to provide a pressing ready to surface prior to slumping. A carefully measured drop of molten glass is cut by shears as it leaves the delivery tube and falls into the mould. The mould is closed and a force applied to produce the pressing. The pressing now passes into the annealing lehr, where it is cooled at a controlled rate to provide the finished pressing

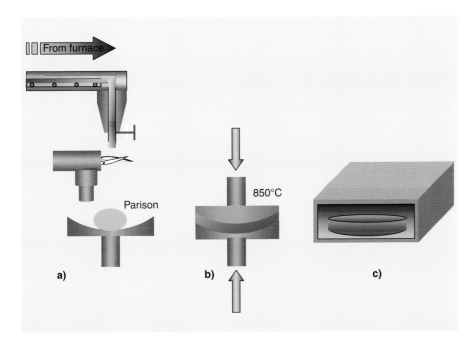

surface would not be sufficiently accurate in form after the relatively slow annealing period has occurred.

The second method, shaping the surface by applying heat and pressure to the end of a glass rod, can be applied to produce glass elements when high quality is not a paramount requirement. The glass rod is heated at one end to soften it and reshaped by pressing. This production method has the advantage that only the minimum amount of heat is required to make the glass sufficiently malleable to shape. More accurate figure and better-quality surface finish are possible than can be achieved by pressing alone.

The surface finish on the moulding depends upon the finish of the press tool and also on the surface of the glass rod. The lower the temperature, the better the surface finish of a fire-polished blank, but the greater is the force needed to shape the surface.

The third method, to modify the surface by applying an additional layer of material by vacuum deposition or other method of coating, has so far been applied only to mirror surfaces to obtain aspherical reflectors. In theory, this method could be applied to plastics lens surfaces to deposit material, the effect of which would be to make the surface aspherical. The surface would be figured by the controlled deposition of material in high vacuum. Although the departure from a sphere is often quite small, it is necessary to be able to load the chamber with sufficient material to cover the relatively broad area of an ophthalmic lens surface in a single coating operation.

The increased demand for low-cost aspherical lenses led to the investigation of technology used in atomic energy experiments in relation to ion implantation and the production of semiconductors for the microcircuit industry. Research in these fields led to the development of powerful ion accelerators that produce controlled ion beams, which can be used to chip material from a glass surface, atom by atom. As the surface fracture is on the nanometric level, the surface is left with a high degree of polish. This technology has been used to develop controlled ion-beam polishing of aspherical surfaces, but at the present time has not been applied to the production of ophthalmic lenses.

Of the possible ways to produce aspherical surfaces listed above, the final two, forming the surfaces by heat and sagging (slumping) or shaping the surfaces by direct CNC grinding and polishing, have been employed in the ophthalmic lens industry for the production of aspheric and progressive power lenses.

Slumping aspherical surfaces

The slumping or sagging process to form an aspherical surface involves heating a carefully prepared blank of glass on a ceramic mould until the glass softens and takes up the shape that the mould is designed to impart. The slumped surface on the blank that results from the process might be the finished convex surface of a glass progressive power lens or the concave surface of a glass mould from which plastics lenses are eventually cast.

Each stage of the slumping process has to be rehearsed carefully to maintain both the figure of the surface and ensure freedom from surface contamination, which might arise during the high-temperature slumping process.

The important stages of the production process involve:

- blank preparation
- mould preparation
- mould assembly
- slumping
- inspection
- engraving (in the case of progressive lenses)

- toughening (in the case of moulds for the casting of plastics lenses).

Blank preparation

Careful preparation of the blank prior to the slumping operation is critical to ensure that the lens or mould has the desired characteristics. The glass blank is produced by a hot pressing process, summarized in Figure 17.32. A carefully measured drop of molten glass, known as a parison, is cut by shears as it leaves the delivery tube and allowed to fall into a metal mould, into which the parison is pressed into a blank of given volume, known as a pressing. At this stage, the resultant surfaces of the annealed pressing have a fire-polished finish and the pressing must now be surfaced carefully to provide a blank ready for slumping.

Both sides of the pressing are generated, smoothed and polished to predetermined spherical curves and to provide a blank of a given thickness. Each individual stage of the surfacing process must be undertaken very carefully, since any surface waviness prevents the slumped blank from having the correct surface form. The thickness is also critical, since the blank must sag to a precise geometry.

Inspection of the surfaces is undertaken, both by shadowgraph and scanning focimeter, to detect any waviness or deformation from the desired spherical curves.

Preparation of the mould

The mould upon which the glass blank sits during the slumping process is made from a carefully chosen ceramic material that must have the desired refractory properties, provide a smooth surface finish after CNC machining and possess the desired porosity for successful slumping of the blank.

The aspherical surface of the mould to be transferred to the glass blank is produced by single-point turning with the cutter under numerical control of the onboard computer on the CNC grinding machine. The principle of single-point turning is illustrated in Figure 17.33, which shows the cutting burr in contact with the workpiece, with the cutter making horizontal sweeps across the surface (along the x-axis in Figure 17.33).

Since the rotating cutter takes on a spherical form, it makes point contact with the surface it is cutting. The cutter is positioned at point P (x, y, z) by the controlling computer program. Note that the workpiece, which is the ceramic mould, has been rotated about a 'fourth axis', parallel with the y-axis, through the angle ϕ. This extra facility enables the tool to meet the surface at the desired angle and gives rise to the term 'four-axis generating'.

Figure 17.34 shows a general view of the CNC machine during the process of cutting an aspherical surface on the convex surface of a mould. A close-up of the revolving burr in contact with the mould is shown in Figure 17.35.

During the slumping process, when the blank sags, the surface of the glass blank in contact with the mould mirrors the surface on the mould. If the mould surface is convex, as shown in the figures, the concave surface of the blank slumps to a curvature identical to that on the mould. The convex surface of the glass blank, which, for example, could be the progressive surface of a glass progressive power lens, then slumps to a form similar in topography to that on the mould face. However, it is not exactly identical in form, because of the different thickness of the blank across its diameter. An important part of the design sequence for the mould surface is to use mathematical modelling to account for the flow of the glass during the sagging process.

The calculations for the precise form of the surface required to be machined must take into account the geometry of the surface, the

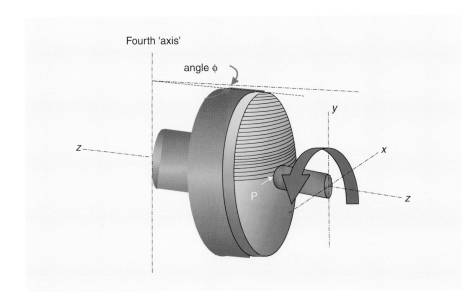

Fourth 'axis'

angle φ

Figure 17.33 The principle of single-point diamond turning with CNC machining. The position of the cutting point P at any moment in time is numerically controlled by the onboard computer, or a tape or disk, which controls the machine. Since the rotating cutter has a spherical form it makes a point contact with the surface it is cutting. The cutter is positioned at point (x, y, z) by the controlling computer program. Here, the computer has been programmed to move the cutting point in a horizontal sweep, along the x-axis. Note that the workpiece, which is the ceramic mould, is also rotated about an axis, through the angle ϕ, which gives rise to the term 'four-axis generating'

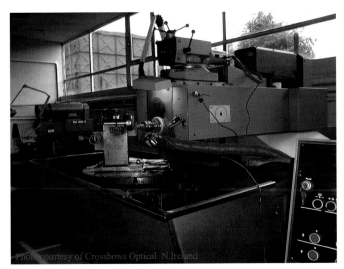

Figure 17.34 CNC machining of ceramic mould (courtesy of Crossbows Optical Ltd)

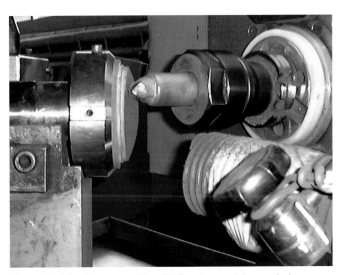

Figure 17.35 Close-up of the CNC cutter and the workpiece (courtesy of Crossbows Optical Ltd)

variation in thickness of the blank, the desired finished surface geometry and the rate of flow of the glass during the slumping cycle.

Mould assembly

When the blanks are placed into the furnace for the slumping operation they sit centrally on the ceramic mould and are covered by a ceramic cup that provides an airtight seal to ensure contamination of the surface is not possible. Assembly takes place in clean-air surroundings, the mould being brushed to clear any dust particles, and the carefully washed blanks are placed centrally in position on top of the mould. It is essential that no dust particles are present beneath the cup, since these would be burnt into the surface at the slumping temperature.

The components are shown schematically in Figure 17.36. The ceramic cup is placed over the blank and is seated on a circular flange that ensures it does not come into contact with the glass blank during the firing process. Figure 17.36a shows the separate ceramic cup, glass blank and ceramic mould. In Figure 17.36b the cup is shown resting on the circular flange, which the CNC cutter has cut at the edge of the mould. Note the geometry of the mould ensures the blank is not in contact with the ceramic cup.

Figure 17.37 shows the actual assembly station, with the components about to be put together ready for the furnace.

Slumping

The heating cycle that the assembled moulds must undergo is critical for successful slumping, so the furnace temperature is controlled electronically and monitored carefully throughout the operation. The furnaces may be of the static box variety, as in Figure 17.38, or of the belt type, similar to those used for the production of fused bifocals, in which the assembled moulds pass along a slow-moving conveyor belt into the furnace at a controlled rate. After an initial pre-heating period, the temperature in the furnace is raised to about 700°C, at which temperature the glass softens and sags to its desired form. The slumping can be assisted by applying a vacuum beneath the ceramic blocks, which are sufficiently porous to enable the blank to be sucked into firm contact with the block. Figure 17.38 shows a number of prepared moulds in position in a static box furnace at the beginning of the slumping cycle.

The temperature profile within the furnace must be known precisely to ensure success of the process. It is essential that

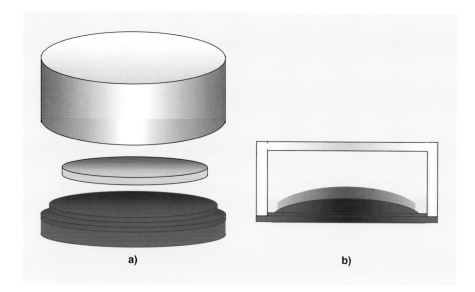

Figure 17.36   The mould components during mould assembly

a)   b)

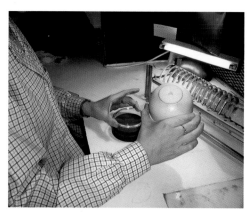

Figure 17.37   The mould assembly (courtesy of Crossbows Optical Ltd)

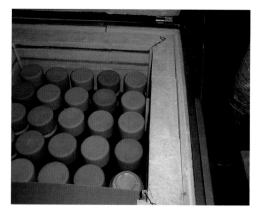

Figure 17.38   Static box furnace for slumping glass blanks. The furnace lid has been opened to provide a view of the assembled moulds arranged in rows on the floor of the furnace (courtesy of Crossbows Optical Ltd)

the temperature in the box furnace does not vary in different zones, as the glass may then not slump uniformly throughout the furnace.

At the end of the cycle, the glass blanks must be annealed carefully by reducing the temperature in the furnace at a controlled rate. The glass is held at about 400°C during the annealing cycle to ensure that the physical properties of the glass are maintained precisely and to reduce stress caused by too rapid cooling. The annealing process ensures that any stresses are distributed uniformly throughout the glass.

In the case of photochromic glasses, the heating cycle must also initiate the photochromic performance of the material. A precise heating cycle, regulated carefully to within a single degree Celsius, is required to ensure the development of the silver halide crystals in a finely determined number and size, to give the glass its photochromic properties.

At the end of the slumping cycle, the moulds and ceramic cups are returned to the assembly area for the next batch of blanks and saver tape applied to the slumped surfaces.

The surface of the glass blank that was in contact with the ceramic mould now has the same finish as that on the mould face. Generally, the glass surface is stippled and bears the impression of any markings that were inscribed deliberately on the mould face. For example, lines might have been cut on the mould face to simplify location of the progression zone of progressive power lenses. These markings can be transferred to the edge of the blank to provide a permanent record of their location before the surface is reworked to remove the ceramic surface finish.

For a glass mould from which plastics progressive lenses will eventually be cast, it may be necessary to grind, smooth and polish a flat margin round the edge of the mould to ensure a tight seal with the gasket when the casting mould is assembled.

Inspection

Inspection of the slumped surface takes place when the second side of the blank has been reworked to enable an optical check of the surface characteristics to be made. The surface is first subjected to a careful cosmetic inspection for overall finish and freedom from blemishes. Any contamination of the surface during assembly will be evident on the surface and, if very visible, will cause rejection of the blank. In the case of moulds for plastics lens casting, it is absolutely essential to ensure that the surface is completely free from defects that would otherwise be reproduced on the cast lens surfaces.

The optical characteristics of the surface are checked on the production line by means of a scanning focimeter, with any deviation from the expected pattern causing rejection of the blank. Sampling of blanks for interferometric analysis of the surface or comparison by deflectometry also occurs on a regular basis to ensure that the surface geometry faithfully reproduces the original design.

Engraving

The finished surface of a glass progressive power lens is inscribed with marks to locate the major reference point, and give the reading addition and the manufacturer's identification mark. Also, the moulds from which plastics lenses are to be cast may need to be engraved with progressive surface details or the base curve of the surface.

To ensure that these markings are positioned accurately, a transfer is applied to the surface and located in the correct position by means of the information transferred to the edge of the lens from the stippled surface prior to reworking of the surface.

When the transfer is in position, the necessary markings are engraved on the surface with a small CNC diamond point that is allowed to indent the surface polish just enough to provide visible markings on the surface. The depth of the markings must be just sufficient to enable them to be found and read by an experienced observer, but not so deep that they are sufficiently obvious to cause comment by the eventual wearer of the lens!

The CNC engraving of a progressive power surface is illustrated in Figure 17.39, which shows the cutter in the process of marking the circles to locate the major reference point of a progressive power lens.

Toughening of moulds

The high forces exerted during the polymerization of plastics lenses and, in particular, when prising open the mould to remove the lens, necessitate toughening of the glass moulds that are used to cast plastics lenses. Chemical toughening is employed, since the traditional air-quenching method for toughening glass lenses involves heating the glass to just below its softening point and is, therefore, unsuitable for aspheric moulds, since there is a danger of surface deformation.

The compressive envelope produced in the chemical process is obtained by an ion exchange near the glass surface that results from a hot dip of the finished lens in a salt bath. Potassium ions in the bath are exchanged for sodium or lithium ions in the glass. The smaller sodium or lithium ions near the glass surface are replaced by larger potassium ions, which squeeze their way into the glass surface and induce compressive stress. The usual bath composition is 99.5% potassium nitrate and 0.5% silicic acid heated to 470°C. The temperature must be controlled carefully and the length of stay in the bath is critical. The ion-exchange process is quite lengthy, as the lenses need to remain in the bath for 16 hours.

Production of aspherical surfaces by machining

As pointed out in Chapter 4, an aspherical surface is inherently astigmatic, a surface astigmatism that may be used to counteract the aberrational astigmatism that arises when light passes obliquely through a lens. This fact has been known for over 100 years and was applied successfully by Carl Zeiss of Jena at the beginning of the 20th century to produce best-form high-power plus lenses over about +8.00D, in the range used, typically, for the correction of aphakia. These high plus powers lie outside the range of Tscherning's Ellipse,[2] which indicates, broadly, the range of lens powers that can be corrected for oblique astigmatism when the designer is restricted to spherical surfaces.

The Zeiss *Katral* lens (Figure 17.40) employed a surface that was hand figured to match a concave oblate ellipsoid. This form of lens was suggested to Zeiss by Dr A Gullstrand, who was anxious to introduce an improved lens form for the correction of aphakia,[12] so the lens was known, in-house, as the Gullstrand Cataract Lens.

The *Katral* lens was made in crown glass and the aspherical surface produced by the highly skilled art of hand figuring. The asphericity of the surface was checked by means of test plates as the work progressed, to ensure the high degree of accuracy necessary to obtain the desired curve. A cross-sectional view of the lens is given in Figure 17.40a, and indicates that the surface becomes steeper as it moves away from the optical axis. It can be imagined that material is being added to the surface at an ever-increasing rate as it moves away from the vertex.

Although no precise details of the concave surface were made available, the off-axis data published by Zeiss that relates to the +12.00D *Katral* lens would be duplicated by the use of a concave oblate ellipsoidal surface of vertex radius 94.55mm and a *p*-value of +5.36. The other lens data assumed are that the lens is made from glass of refractive index 1.52, with an axial thickness 5.0mm and a centre of rotation distance of 25mm.

A field diagram showing the excellent off-axis performance of the *Katral* design is given in Figure 17.40b, which illustrates that the design is point-focal at about 30°. Like all aspheric designs, the lens is by no means perfect; the mean oblique power of the lens is seen to decrease as the eye rotates away from the optical axis and suffers a mean oblique error of some 0.50D for this zone of the lens.

The method of hand figuring continued to be used by the optical instrument industry for many years to produce individual aspheric elements and Schmidt corrector plates. The surfaces were produced either by patient hand lapping, using flexible laps with graduated facets, or by means of cam-guided grinding machines. The finely ground lens or corrector plate thus produced then had to be polished and figured again, by means of flexible laps that consisted of pitch, or pitch and felt facing on sorbo rubber. From a commercial point of view, this is a difficult and uneconomical process that involves careful optical testing

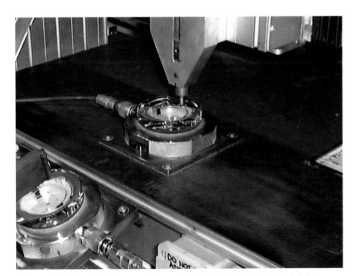

Figure 17.39   CNC engraving machine to provide the visible markings on progressive power surfaces or on moulds for plastics lenses (courtesy of Crossbows Optical Ltd)

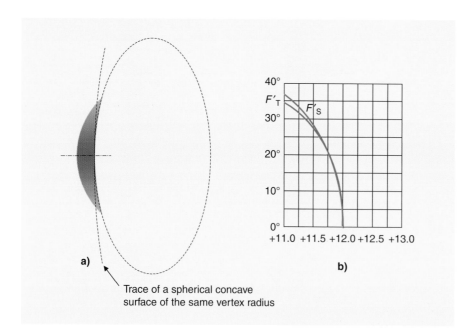

a)

Trace of a spherical concave
surface of the same vertex radius

b)

Figure 17.40 The Zeiss *Katral* Lens. (a) The hand-figured concave surface is akin to an oblate ellipsoid in which, effectively, material has been added to the base spherical surface towards the edge of the curve. (b) Field diagram for a +12.00D *Katral* lens of a form that closely matches the original configuration. Note that the design is point-focal at about 30° and suffers from a mean oblique error of some 0.50D at this point, as would be expected from an aspheric post-cataract design

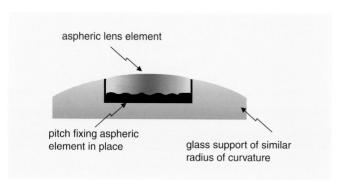

aspheric lens element

pitch fixing aspheric
element in place

glass support of similar
radius of curvature

Figure 17.41 Polishing holder for aspheric lens

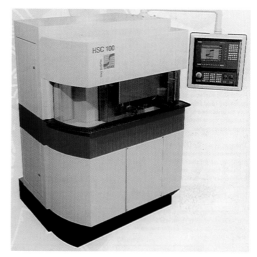

Figure 17.42 High Speed Cutting HSC 100 CNC machine (courtesy of Schneider Opticmachines)

and repeated re-figuring of the aspherical surface. The machining of aspherical surfaces in the quantities required for ophthalmic purposes and in a production time similar to that in which a spherical surface could be made requires costly machinery of extreme accuracy.

One of the leading manufacturers of precision CNC grinding equipment is Rank Taylor Hobson (RTH) Ltd, with many years experience in producing aspheric elements for use in 35mm ciné camera and TV zoom objectives. The machines have spindles of extreme accuracy with optically polished thrust and radial bearings. To avoid any bias, the spindles are driven without direct mechanical contact, through magnetic drive units. The workpiece is centred accurately in chucks and, while the spindle rotates at high speed, the single-point diamond-cutting tool traverses the lens surface in such a manner that the required aspheric profile can be produced to an accuracy of less than 0.8μm (0.0008mm).

To be able to work to this degree of accuracy, very careful design is required of all slideways and pivots on the generating machinery and constant temperatures must be maintained in the air-conditioned workshops in which the machines are used.

The CNC data, usually in the form of rectangular coordinates, are transmitted to the moving elements in the machine to superimpose the required asphericity onto a circular or a straight-line movement of the diamond tool holder. The asphericity is often defined simply as the departure from the best-fitting sphere, or

(in the case of a Schmidt plate) as the departure from a plane surface.

The machined surface produced by the generator is of sufficiently fine texture to permit direct polishing without any intermediate smoothing. Under light pressures, the polishing is not a figuring process, so inspection of the aspheric form should not be needed during polishing. The aspheric blanks may be polished singly or in blocks, but before polishing must be mounted accurately in a glass surround to ensure that there is no rounding at the edge of the surface, which would spoil the figure of the surface.

Figure 17.41 illustrates the method of locating an aspheric lens in a glass recess; the convex surface of the glass surround has a spherical curve that is substantially an extension of the surface to be polished. After location, the jig is warmed to a suitable temperature to allow pitch or wax to be applied to stick the aspheric lens to the glass block. After cooling, the jig can be removed and the block surface cleaned prior to polishing.

The polisher consists of a flexible nylon diaphragm covered with a thin flexible layer of pitch, which is maintained in contact

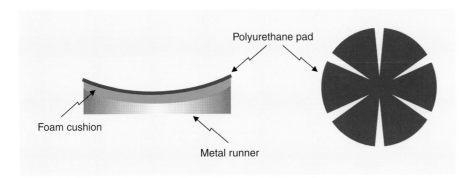

Figure 17.43   The components of a floating polishing runner. The runner is made from three components, a metal tool to which a foam pad is attached to provide the necessary floating action and finally a polyurethane pad. The face of the runner is designed to match the surface to be polished as closely as possible

Polyurethane pad

Foam cushion

Metal runner

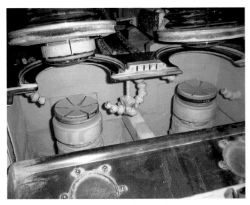

Figure 17.44   Polishing aspherical and atoroidal surfaces (courtesy of Carl Zeiss)

with the aspherical surface by means of pneumatic pressure. Specially designed polishing machines are used that ensure the minimum change in figure during the process. The procedure is to accept that some change of figure will occur, but to control the polishing process with sufficient accuracy for this change always to be constant from one lens or block to the next.

When the first lens in a production batch of aspheric lenses has been polished, it is replaced on the spindle of the generator, again with great care taken to centre it accurately. An electronic transducer is mounted in place of the diamond tool, with the stylus of the transducer in contact with the polished glass surface. The stylus is traversed across the aspherical surface and any error from the specified aspheric profile is recorded. The error is then applied as a correction to the original computing data in such a manner that less material is removed, say, from the edge of the surface if the stylus reveals that too much glass has been removed by the polishing process. All future surfaces are polished with this corrected data and, provided the polishing process is controlled so that it repeats a constant cycle with exactly the same stroke, pressure and slurry feed, the aspherical surfaces that result from the process should be of the correct profile and have constant figure.

The latest ultra-precision machining systems to be offered by RTH's sister company, Precitech, is the Nanoform 300 aspheric grinding system. This is a multi-axis, CNC diamond turning and grinding machine. When fitted with a single-crystal diamond-cutting tool it machines finished components directly in a wide variety of non-ferrous metals, crystals and polymers. Fitted with one of the optional grinding systems, the Nanoform 300 is transformed into a precision CNC grinder for the production of aspherical surfaces on glass lenses. The smooth finish that the machine can produce on glass workpieces can be achieved in a

single-step polishing operation. Subsurface damage is limited by the use of air-bearing spindles with extremely low levels of vibration. The Nanoform 300 claims a feedback resolution of 2.5 nanometres, which contributes to its ability to machine optical surfaces directly on plastics materials, which in many cases need no subsequent polishing. This has found an important application in the manufacture of contact lenses.

Polishing aspherical surfaces

The latest high-speed CNC machines produce generated surfaces that are so fine they can be polished without any further smoothing or fining of the surface.

The High Speed Cutting HSC 100 CNC machine from Schneider Opticmachines (Figure 17.42) produces surfaces capable of immediate polishing in a single cycle, and that also allows edging and chamfering of the blank without unclamping the workpiece.

Several new technologies are being applied to polish the generated surface. It is possible to use traditional polishing methods with carefully designed polishing pads that float on the surface to ensure that the pad follows the surface form without altering the curve. Here, the face of the polishing pad should match the surface to be polished as closely as possible and to this end it is necessary to maintain a large range of polishing tools to which the polishing pads are attached.

The polishing runner is made from three components, a metal block with a predetermined concave surface, to which is attached a preformed foam pad of known curvature; on top of the foam pad is the polishing face itself, which takes the form of a polyurethane pad (Figure 17.43).

There is a large range of metal tools, from which the computer makes a selection depending upon the surface that is to be polished, having taken into account the details of the curve and the diameter of the lens. The preformed foam pads provide the flexibility required to ensure that the pad remains in contact with the lens surface during the polishing cycle, and the firmness of the pad needs to be checked regularly to make sure that it retains the correct degree of resilience. Typically, the foam pads may be re-used some 20 times before they no longer have the correct resilience and must be discarded.

A view of a twin-spindle polishing machine is given in Figure 17.44. The lenses are held in pneumatically controlled chucks and are about to be lowered on to the polishing runners seen in the bowl of the machine. Two nozzles deliver the cerium oxide slurry, the concentration, temperature and pH value of which are monitored and controlled constantly.

In the case of plastics lenses, photopolymerization of lacquer coated onto the finely generated surface is a new method of applying a polished finish to the surface, and is showing great

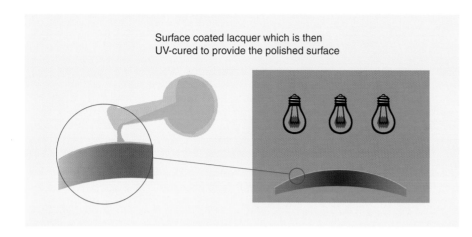

Surface coated lacquer which is then
UV-cured to provide the polished surface

Figure 17.45   Polishing a plastics lens surface by means of photopolymerization. The fine, diamond-generated surface is coated with hardener that fills in the micropores of the surface

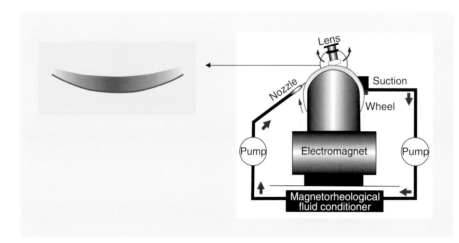

Figure 17.46   Principle of magnetorheological finishing

promise as a future technique for lens polishing. The hard lacquer is applied to the fine diamond-generated surface, which fills in the micropores of the surface. The lacquered surface is cured by exposure to ultraviolet radiation (Figure 17.45).

A completely new polishing process, known as magnetorheological finishing (MRF) has been developed in the USA by QED Technologies of Rochester. The basis of this new process is a substance called magnetorheological (MR) fluid, which was developed about 15 years ago in what is now Belarus. It sprang from work with intelligent fluids for clutches, shock absorbers and vibration isolators.

MR fluid is a suspension of non-colloidal magnetic particles and finishing abrasives. This viscous liquid becomes a solid when a magnetic field is applied to it; the viscosity is directly proportional to field strength. The MR fluid can be thought of as a compliant replacement for the conventional rigid lap in the traditional loose, abrasive grinding and finishing process. A magnetic field applied to the fluid creates a temporary finishing surface, which can be controlled in real time by varying the field's strength and direction.

In the MRF process, a convex, flat or concave workpiece is positioned above a reference surface. An MR fluid ribbon is deposited on the rotating wheel rim. The fluid is transported through the gap defined by the distance of the lens from the surface of the wheel rim. By applying a magnetic field at the gap, the stiffened region forms a transient work zone or finishing spot. Surface smoothing, removal of subsurface damage and figure cor-

rection are accomplished by rotating the lens on a spindle at a constant speed while sweeping the lens about its radius of curvature through the stiffened finishing zone.

With the standard MR fluid, MRF reduces the surface microroughness of fused silica and other optical materials to less than 10 angstroms root mean square. The time required to do this varies from 5 to 60 minutes, depending on the material and its initial roughness. A fundamental advantage of MRF over traditional technologies is that fresh abrasive is delivered constantly to the finishing zone, and finishing debris and heat are removed continuously. The principle is illustrated in Figure 17.46. A workpiece is installed at a fixed distance from a moving spherical wheel. An electromagnet located below the wheel surface generates a gradient magnetic field in the gap between the wheel and workpiece. When the MR fluid is delivered to the wheel, it is pulled against the wheel surface by the magnetic field gradient. The fluid acquires the wheel velocity, develops high stresses and becomes a subaperture polishing tool. A sophisticated computer program determines a schedule for varying the position of the rotating workpiece through the polishing zone.

References

1. Jalie M 1972 Design of spherical spectacle lenses by one-and-a-half order theory. Transactions of the International Ophthalmology Congress 1970. BOA. London

2. Jalie M 1984 Principles of ophthalmic lenses. ABDO, London
3. Selkirk K 1991 Longman mathematics handbook. Longman, Harlow
4. Twyman F 1951 Prism and lens making. Hilger (Adam) Ltd, London
5. Horne D F 1972 Optical production technology. Hilger (Adam) Ltd, London
6. Jalie M 1989 Minus-base toric lenses. Optician 198:12–14
7. Jalie M, Wray L 1990 Practical ophthalmic lenses. ABDO, London
8. Cornu D, Harsigny C, Thiebaut J 1988 Lentille ophtalmique de puissance positive et de grand diamètre. French patent application no. 2 638 (on behalf of Essilor International)
9. Optische Werke G Rodenstock 1983 Brillenglas höher positiver Brechkraft. German patent G81 19 984.8
10. US Patent 5083859 1992 Aspheric lenses
11. Henker O 1924 Introduction to the theory of spectacles. School of Optics, Jena

Lens manufacture – multifocal surfaces

Chapter 17 considers the production methods used for single vision lenses. In this chapter we look in more detail at the production of the segment side of bifocal, trifocal and progressive power lenses. Chapters 10 and 11 show that modern bifocal and trifocal designs may be made in either fused or solid form. The technology required for each of these two methods of production is quite different and we consider first the most common glass bifocal design, the fused bifocal.

Production of fused bifocals

In countries in which glass lenses still represent a sizeable section of the market, the fused bifocal remains the most common form of bifocal design in general use. The round segment version is still in production for some markets, but, without doubt, the segment most commonly used today is the D-shaped flat top or the C-shape curved top designs illustrated in Figure 18.1. From this it is seen that, as a general rule, the segment is fused into the convex surface of the lens.

The reading addition of a fused bifocal is obtained from a glass button of high refractive index that is fused to a depression curve worked on the crown glass major portion, which forms the distance portion (DP) of the lens.[1] A curve of given radius of curvature produces a higher power on a material of higher refractive index, so an increase in power is obtained in the segment area of the lens. The principle is illustrated in Figure 18.2, which assumes that a round segment design is to be made.

Preparation of the components

Figure 18.2a shows a cross-sectional view of the components that are to be fused together to form the bifocal lens. The crown major portion is made from close-tolerance crown glass, that is crown glass with optical properties that have been controlled very carefully to ensure it is thermally compatible with the flint glass that makes up the segment button. In particular, the coefficients of thermal expansion of the two glasses must match to ensure that they contract at the same rate after fusion, during the annealing process. The concave surface of the crown blank matches the curvature of a carborundum block upon which it will sit during the fusing process and a depression curve with a predetermined radius is generated, smoothed and very carefully polished on the convex surface. The crown-glass mouldings are blocked together, usually four at a time, so that a depression is ground in the lower portion of each moulding. Typically, the depression curves are opened out to a diameter of some 28mm during the roughing or generating stage and then smoothed on a bowl machine with very fine emery until the depression is about 30mm in diameter.

The block is then polished, at which stage great care must be taken to ensure that the surface is polished sufficiently well to withstand the temperature cycle during the fusing process. A plain hard polisher is employed to help keep the surface open to ensure that it does not break out into holes when heated. The power of the depression curve is marked on the blank so that it can be identified during subsequent operations.

The segment button is made from flint glass of high refractive index, usually a dense barium flint with a higher Abbe number than the older style glasses. Several glasses of different refractive indices may be employed to obtain different reading additions. If the fire polish finish of the glass strip from which the button is obtained is good enough, the front surface of the button is simply left and a predetermined contact surface worked on the rear surface of the button to match the curve on the crown blank. The quality of the contact surface after fusing is inspected through the front surface of the button; to facilitate this later inspection, it may be necessary to grind the front surface flat and then to brighten it by semi-polishing the surface.

Buttons may be blocked together, the number on the blocks depending upon the curve to be worked, and must be surfaced with the same care as the depression curves on the crown glass majors. The curve on the contact surface of the button is deliberately made some 0.25D to 0.50D steeper than the depression curve on the corresponding crown blanks so that, initially, contact is only made at the centre of the curves.

Assembly of the components

The flint buttons and crown glass majors are thoroughly cleaned before passing into an air-conditioned room for assembly. The assembly room is kept as free from dust as possible by blowing filtered air through it. The operator has to assemble the components, ready for the fusing oven, and ensure that no dust or dirt is between the two surfaces. This is done in a carefully illuminated inspection booth by placing the crown blank on the worktop, picking up the flint button and brushing the surface of each component with a soft brush. The flint button is laid carefully over the depression curve and, because the curve on the flint is a little steeper than that on the crown, an interference spot is visible at the point of contact.

The operator now gently presses down on the top surface of the button, close to the edge, with a pair of tweezers and, if all is well, the interference spot moves in a straight line to the edge of the depression curve. If some dust is between the surfaces, the spot is deflected and is seen to travel in a curved path round the particle. If this occurs the flint has to be picked up and the surfaces carefully brushed again before replacing the flint on the depression curve and repeating the sequence. This operation is repeated in a number of positions round the flint button until no deflection of the spot occurs in any meridian. The operator then places two short pieces of wire, first dipped in gum, about 1cm apart to support the flint button at the bottom of the moulding.

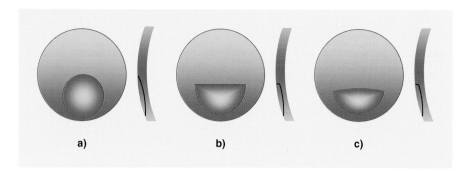

Figure 18.1   Fused bifocal designs: (a) round segment design; (b) D-segment flat top design; (c) C-segment curved top design

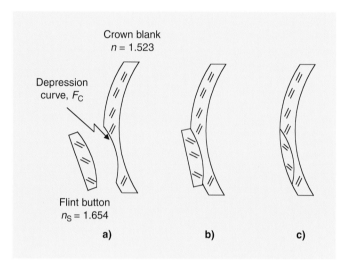

Figure 18.2   Construction of the fused bifocal: (a) components prior to fusing; (b) rough fused blank; (c) semi-finished fused blank

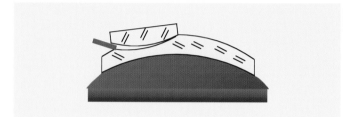

Figure 18.3   Mould components during mould assembly. The button is supported at the base of the depression curve by wire feelers. When the button softens and sags it expels air towards the feelers

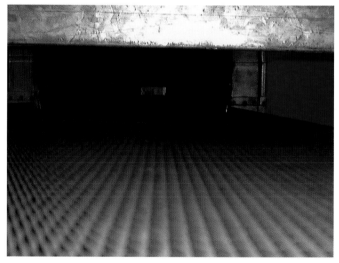

Figure 18.4   Fusing oven, looking down the conveyor belt. The hottest part of the furnace is near the centre of the oven (courtesy of Crossbows Optical Ltd)

Specially designed feelers may be used in place of the wire. The support must be sufficiently thick to cause the interference spot to disappear at the top edge of the button.

The assembled components are then placed on a carborundum block, the surface of which has been moulded to match the curve on the back of the crown glass major (Figure 18.3), and the blocks transferred to the travelling belt that takes them into the furnace. Batches of these prepared blocks travel at a regulated speed through the combined furnace and annealing lehr (Figure 18.4). After a preheating period the blanks are brought to 640°C, at which temperature the glasses fuse. At this temperature the button softens and sags under its own weight, gradually expelling air towards the wire feeler. The steeper curve on the button aids this procedure by tending to unroll the depression curve towards the feeler. Eventually, the whole surface of the button is in contact with the depression curve, except for two very small areas around the supporting wires. As the belt travels onwards the temperature in the furnace gradually reduces, annealing the glasses; the belt eventually emerges from the furnace at about 100°C. The whole operation is controlled precisely to ensure that temperature and rate of travel through the furnace are maintained correctly.

Upon emergence from the furnace, the blanks are allowed to cool and the wire feelers pulled out before checking the blanks for strain. Matching the crown and flint glasses for expansion is very important, because any serious difference causes the crown to flaw. Some tolerance is permissible in that, if the expansions are such that the flint is in compression, the crown is unlikely to fracture.

The resultant fused blanks are then subjected to a rigorous inspection of the contact surface. If by any chance some dust has remained between the surfaces, a bubble forms, which may result in rejection of the blank.

The quality of the surfacing of the depression curve and the contact surface of the flint are confirmed during this inspection. Incomplete surfacing becomes evident because the high temperatures involved in fusing the glasses can cause the surface to break open, which leaves a mass of tiny bubbles and scratches visible on the contact surface. It is a peculiar effect, in that marks such as sleeks visible before fusing seem to flow and disappear during the process, whereas two surfaces that appear to be perfect under the most rigorous examination may be so bad after fusion that they are fit only for scrap. Fusion faults can be minimized only by paying great attention to the smoothing and polishing materials and by allowing ample machine cycles for these operations.

When the blanks have passed inspection they are ground, smoothed and polished on the front surface to remove the flint button that stands proud from the surface; they can then be put into stock for sale as semi-finished fused blanks. Segment-side finishing is described below for composite buttons. Since the front curve is continuous over the distance and near portions (NPs), the dividing line of a fused bifocal segment cannot be felt.

It will be appreciated from Figure 18.2c that the diameter of a fused bifocal segment reduces as the segment-side surface is ground away and fairly close control is essential to end up with segment diameters of a given size. Typically, segment diameters of 24mm and 25mm are the norm today. The rate of reduction in the segment diameter during segment-side grinding depends upon the thickness of the segment, which depends, in turn, upon the reading addition and the convex curve on the segment side. Low reading additions and steep convex curves tend to result in the thinnest segments and the segment diameter reduces very rapidly when the convex side is surfaced.

What controls the centre thickness of the finished bifocal segment and just how thin they may turn out to be can be deduced from Figure 18.5. Figure 18.5a illustrates a semi-finished fused bifocal blank with a plano-DP curve and a –12.00D depression curve. The reading addition provided by these curves is +3.00D. If the segment diameter is 24mm, the centre thickness of the segment would be 1.69mm. If the segment diameter needs to be reduced to 22mm by reworking the front surface, then 0.28mm of glass must be removed from the front surface to obtain this smaller diameter. As a general rule, when the front curve is shallow and the reading addition is high, the segment has a reasonable thickness and it is very easy to control the segment diameter.

Figure 18.5b illustrates a semi-finished fused bifocal blank with a +8.00D DP curve and a +4.00D depression curve. The reading addition provided by these curves is +1.00D. If the segment diameter is 24mm, the centre thickness of the segment would be just 0.56mm. If the segment diameter now needs to be reduced to 22mm by reworking the front surface, only 0.09mm of glass would need to be removed from the front surface to obtain this smaller diameter. Clearly, when the front curve is steep and the reading addition is low, the segment is very thin and it is more difficult to control the final segment diameter. In particular, any distortion on the contact surface may cause the finished segment to appear somewhat oval in shape.

Composite buttons

Shaped fused bifocals are produced by means of a composite button, made up from two or three different pieces of glass. For a bifocal lens, one of the glasses is of high refractive index and the other is composed of crown glass. In the case of a fused trifocal design, two different glasses of higher refractive index are employed, together with a crown glass component.

Four different multifocal designs are illustrated in Figure 18.6, together with the composite buttons from which each segment is formed. Figure 18.6a illustrates the most common form of shaped fused bifocal, the D-segment flat top design. The button consists of a crown component and a larger flint glass component, which makes up the NP of the design. The crown glass employed for the composite button must have exactly the same refractive index as the crown glass major to which it is to be fused. Any slight difference in index is readily seen in the form of a circular ring between the two glasses. This necessitates a refractive index tolerance of

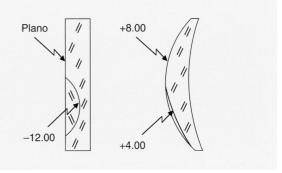

Figure 18.5 Variation in thickness of segment with front curve and depression curve. (a) Semi-finished fused bifocal blank with plano-DP curve and –12.00D depression curve. The reading addition provided by these curves is +3.00. At a segment diameter of 24mm the centre thickness of the segment is 1.69mm; to reduce the diameter to 22mm would need 0.28mm of glass to be removed from the front surface. (b) Semi-finished fused bifocal blank with +8.00D DP curve and +4.00D depression curve. The reading addition provided by these curves is +1.00. At a segment diameter of 24mm the centre thickness of the segment is 0.56mm; to reduce the diameter to 22mm would need 0.09mm of glass to be removed from the front surface

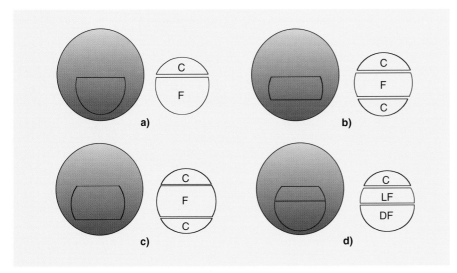

Figure 18.6 Composite buttons for different multifocal designs (C, crown glass component; F, flint glass component): (a) D-segment flat top bifocal; (b) B-segment ribbon segment; (c) R-segment flat top bifocal; (d) trifocal design with three different glasses for the composite button (LF, light flint glass component forms the intermediate portion; DF, dense flint glass component forms the near portion)

just ±0.0003 for crown glasses used for all forms of fused bifocal that require fusing of crown-to-crown components.

The button is produced by grinding and smoothing the contact surfaces along the straight edges, the two pieces of glass are cleaned carefully and then clamped together with an asbestos strip to hold the components in place while they pass through the furnace to fuse the two elements together. The other designs illustrated in Figure 18.6 consist of three pieces of glass, two crown glass components and one flint in the case of the B-segment and the R-segment designs, and one crown and two different flints in the case of the trifocal design. The components are prepared in the same fashion described for the D-segment. They are ground and smoothed along their contact edges before being fused together to form the composite button. Some manufacturers deliberately angle the two flat contact faces to deflect the reflections that occur at the dividing line; these reflections give rise to streaks of light that run down from the segment edge, and cause annoyance to the wearer under certain circumstances.[1] They may, in addition, coat the contact faces to reduce the intensity of the reflection at the line.

When the button has been fused, it is ground flat and semi-polished on one side, and then ground smooth and very carefully polished on the other side to the required curve. Subsequent operations to fuse the composite button to the depression curve on the crown component follow the sequence for round segments, except that a slightly higher temperature of 680°C is required to fuse the crown glasses together.

The position of the straight line in relation to the depression curve affects the ratio of the segment diameter to its depth. When roughing the segment to remove the excess flint with a diamond generator, it is usual to reduce the segment to some 3–4mm larger than the required finished diameter. The diamond-smoothing cycle for the fused round segment can then be determined to ensure that, after smoothing, the round segment finishes at the required diameter. In the case of shaped segments, however, the shape of the segment must first be checked and if necessary corrected so that it has the required segment diameter and segment depth. This is achieved by grinding a small amount of vertical prism relative to the segment side surface. The amount is quite critical; for instance, an angle of about 10 minutes of arc alters the diameter:depth ratio by 0.5mm in the case of a low addition. When the proportion has been corrected, the segments are measured and diamond smoothed to their final diameter.

To avoid blocking complications, the segment sides of the smoothed bifocal surfaces are polished individually. The polishing material selected is important because unsuitable characteristics of the slurry may cause different rates of polishing of the crown and flint glasses. In some cases the flint may wear away at a faster rate than the crown, which results in a ridge at the dividing line that can actually be felt! A combination of high-grade cerium compounds and hard wax or pitch polishers generally produces the best results.[2]

Reading addition of a fused bifocal

From Figure 18.7 the total reading addition, A, of a fused bifocal is made up partly from the addition due to the front surface and partly from the contact surface in situ, F_{CON}. The addition due to the front surface is, simply, how much stronger the convex curve is on the glass of higher refractive index n_S, than it is on the crown glass of the main lens, of refractive index n.

The addition from the front surface is $F_3 - F_1$, so the total addition is given by:

$$A = F_3 - F_1 + F_{CON}$$

Now the quantity $F_3 - F_1$ can be shown to be equal to $F_1(n_S - n)/(n-1)$ and F_{CON} can be shown to be equal to $-F_C(n_S - n)/(n-1)$, where F_C is the power of the depression curve in air, that is, the curve worked on the crown major into which the button of high refractive index is fused. The quantity $(n-1)/(n_S-n)$ is defined as the fused bifocal blank ratio, denoted by the symbol k. Hence, the reading addition of a fused bifocal is given by:

$$A = (F_1 - F_C)/k$$

Typical glasses in use in Europe use crown glass of refractive index 1.523 and a segment glass of refractive index 1.654. When these glasses are used their blank ratio is $k = 0.523/0.131$, which is very nearly equal to 4.

It is very convenient to think of the reading addition of a fused bifocal in terms of the blank ratio of the glasses, since the addition is then a simple function of the blank ratio. For example, assuming a blank ratio of 4:1, a fused bifocal of front curve +6.00D and depression curve –4.00D would have a reading addition of +2.50D. This follows because the addition from the front surface is 6.00/4 = +1.50D and the addition from the contact surface is 4.00/4 = +1.00D.

A blank ratio of 4:1 was assumed for the glasses used for the bifocal lenses illustrated in Figure 18.5, where it is stated that the lens shown in Figure 18.5a has a near addition of +3.00 and the lens shown in Figure 18.5b has a near addition of +1.00.

Compatible flint series

Although it is possible to obtain a full range of reading additions with one high-refractive glass and varying the depression curves, as has just been described, it is becoming usual to employ glasses of different high refractive index for different reading additions.

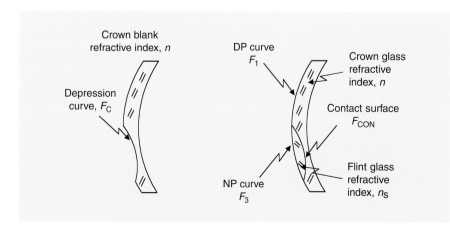

Crown blank refractive index, n

Depression curve, F_C

DP curve F_1

NP curve F_3

Crown glass refractive index, n

Contact surface F_{CON}

Flint glass refractive index, n_S

Figure 18.7 Calculation of the near addition of a fused bifocal. The depression curve to which the button of high refractive index is fused has a power in air of F_C. When the button is fused to the depression curve the power of the contact surface in situ is F_{CON}, which forms part of the total addition. When the segment side is surfaced, the power of the curve on the DP is F_1, but its power over the segment area, F_3, is greater owing to the higher index glass of the segment. The addition from the front surface is $F_3 - F_1$. The total near addition, A, is the sum of these two components

This has the advantage for the bifocal surface manufacturer that fewer depression curve powers need to be worked. In theory, it would be possible to employ just one depression curve and use a different glass for each reading addition, and some bifocal manufacturers have switched their production method entirely to compatible flint systems. Others use just three or four different glasses and a reduced number of depression curves.

To determine the refractive index of the flint glass required to produce a given near addition, A, the expression, $F_C = F_1 - Ak$, derived earlier, can be written in the form:

$$k = (F_1 - F_C)/A$$

and, since $k = (n-1)/(n_S - n)$, the refractive index of the segment glass is given by:

$$n_S = n + A(n-1)/(F_1 - F_C)$$

It is easy to arrange for the term $(F_1 - F_C)$ to be constant throughout the range by suitable choices of front curve and depression curve. For example, to produce a range of reading additions from +0.75 to +3.00 we might choose the combinations of front curves and depression curves in Table 18.1. The quantity $(F_1 - F_C)$ is seen to equal +10.00 in each case and, assuming the refractive index of the crown glass to be 1.523, the necessary flint glasses are given by $n_S = 1.523 + 0.0523A$.

The required series of glasses would be:

Add	n_S	Add	n_S
+0.75	1.562	+2.00	1.628
+1.00	1.575	+2.25	1.641
+1.25	1.588	+2.50	1.654
+1.50	1.601	+2.75	1.667
+1.75	1.614	+3.00	1.680

The advantage to the bifocal manufacturer of being able to produce a complete range of reading additions from just four different depression curves is self-evident.

Intermediate addition of a fused trifocal

The intermediate and near portions (IPs and NPs) of fused trifocals are constructed from a button that is normally made up from three different glasses, a crown glass of exactly the same material as the main lens and two glasses of high refractive index, chosen to provide the correct IP/NP ratio (Figure 18.6d). After completion of the segment side, the segment surface, which is continuous over the DP, IP and NP, produces different powers on each surface. The reading additions, A_I and A_N, obtained depend upon the power of the DP surface, F_1, the power of the original depression curve, F_C, and the fused bifocal blank ratios for the two glasses used. If the refractive index of the crown glass main lens is denoted by n_1, the refractive index of the light flint glass used for the IP by n_2 and that of the glass of higher refractive index used for the NP by n_3, then the IP/NP ratio is given by:

$$\text{IP/NP ratio} = (n_2 - n_1)/(n_3 - n_1) \times 100\%$$

Typical segment glasses used in Europe are $n_1 = 1.523$, $n_2 = 1.606$ and $n_3 = 1.654$. Since the IP/NP ratios of these designs depend upon the glasses used, they are fixed by the manufacturer, usually at 50%, but some designs are available with the IP addition at 40%, 60% or 70% of the near addition.

Table 18.1 Combinations of front curves and depression curves for reading additions from +0.75 to +3.00

DP curve	Depression curve
+7.75	−2.25
+5.87	−4.12
+4.00	−6.00
+1.50	−8.50

Production of solid bifocals

Without doubt, the popularity of the fused design is simply because its method of manufacture lends itself well to the production of shaped segments. With a composite button, it is possible to make flat and curved top segments that provide reduced jump at the segment dividing line and less prismatic effect in the near visual zone of the segment. It is quite apparent that in the richer countries, and certainly in the UK, the increased use of plastics lenses has resulted in the virtual disappearance of the round segment fused bifocal.

Despite its popularity, the flat-top fused bifocal suffers from two drawbacks, inherent in its method of construction. The first is the increased chromatism found near the edge of the segment, which arises from the use of high-refractive glass, with a low Abbe number, to form the segment. Some improvement has been made in recent years in the level of chromatism in the segment area, with the introduction of dense barium crown-segment glasses, which have the necessary high refractive index together with a higher Abbe number. Despite these new glasses, chromatism might still give rise to complaints in the fused bifocal design.

The second problem concerns the integrity of the contact surface, which should remain spherical and free from waves, despite the high temperatures to which the blank is subjected during the fusing process. Proof that some distortion of the contact surface has taken place during the heat process is found when checking the power of the reading addition with a focimeter. An image of the target less sharp than that found when the DP is under test is usually evidence of distortion of the contact surface.

Both these drawbacks are overcome by the use of the solid bifocal made from one piece of glass, so the material used for the NP is the same as that used for the DP, normally spectacle crown glass. Also, the method of construction generally ensures that the NP can be produced without distortion of the surfaces. Indeed, optical engineers have long considered that the production of the solid bifocal surface is one of the most significant achievements of the ophthalmic optical industry. No mere microscope or camera lens requires the precision grinding techniques necessary to ensure that a sharp, invisible dividing line is formed between the distance and near portions.[2]

Geometry of the solid bifocal surface

The reading addition of a solid bifocal is obtained by raising a second curve on one surface of the lens to form the segment (Figure 18.8). Traditionally, the segment was incorporated on the concave surface of the lens. This means the prescription house that supplies the finished lens must work the convex side to complete the prescription. Today, convex-side working is undertaken only by a few comprehensive surfacing laboratories that have maintained the large range of plus-side glass tools necessary to produce the final prescription. Most of the smaller surfacing laboratories are tooled only to work concave surfaces, since the great majority of modern semi-finished blanks are supplied with the convex side finished. This situation has been addressed by the solid bifocal

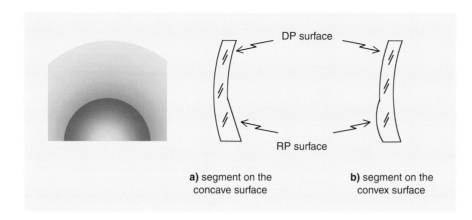

Figure 18.8   The solid bifocal in which the reading addition is the difference between the RP curve and the DP curve

a) segment on the concave surface

b) segment on the convex surface

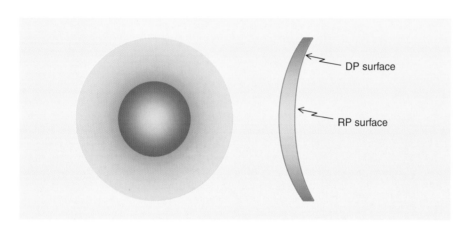

Figure 18.9   Solid bifocal saucer blank (38mm or 45mm segment)

manufacturers, who now supply 30mm and 38mm diameter segments incorporated on the convex surface of the lens.

Segment diameters currently available when the segment is situated on the concave surface of the lens are 22mm, 30mm, 38mm and 45mm. The 30mm diameter segment is also available in prism segment form.

The surface on the segment side of the lens that forms part of the DP is called the DP surface. The power of this surface is referred to as the DP curve. The raised curve on the segment side that forms the NP is called the segment surface and its power is known as the RP curve. The reading addition is the difference between the RP curve and the DP curve. Thus, if the segment is on the convex surface of the lens and the DP curve is +6.00 and the RP curve is +8.00, the reading addition would be +2.00. Alternatively, if the segment is situated on the concave surface of the lens and the DP curve is –6.00, then to produce a reading addition of +2.00D, the RP curve would need to be –4.00.

As the difference in the radius of curvature of the DP portion and the RP portion is designed to produce an increase in the power of the lens, ordinary surfacing techniques cannot be used and an entirely different method of production is required. The methods in use today follow the method of working suggested by Bentzon & Emerson in 1904, but, clearly, refined to reflect the technology of the 21st century.

Production of the solid bifocal surface

A solid bifocal moulding for a 38mm or 45mm diameter segment is depicted in Figure 18.9. Mouldings are supplied by the glass manufacturer, who presses them specifically for the purpose. The diameters of the mouldings vary from about 80mm in the case of

the 22mm diameter segment up to about 100mm in the case of the 45mm diameter segment.

It is absolutely essential that the geometry of the surface be maintained precisely during the surfacing process, so the introduction of the solid bifocal was heralded by specially designed machinery that allows the tools and blanks to rotate about their given axes without running out of true. The sequence of operations for working the bifocal surface is as follows.

- blocking
- roughing
- smoothing
- polishing
- inspection
- knocking off
- sawing the disks into semi-finished blanks.

Blocking

The blanks are attached singly to alloy blocks using a low-melting point alloy, the blocks being specially designed to allow a circular stainless steel boss to be inserted in a depression cast into the mould (Figure 18.10). The boss ensures that the blanks are located correctly on the grinding, smoothing and polishing machines. The holders have to be machined to fine limits to ensure that there is no loss of true when the holders are transferred from one machining process to another.

To ensure adhesion, the back of the glass is sprayed with three or four coats of black rubberized paint. This black coating also facilitates inspection of the bifocal surface before the lens is deblocked. It is essential to ensure that the surface is free from

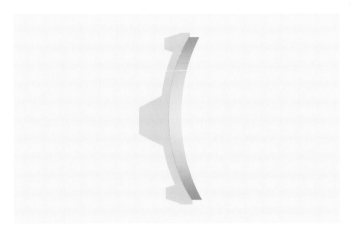

Figure 18.10   Form of blocking for a solid bifocal saucer blank

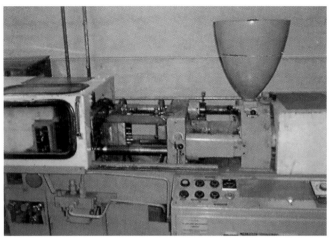

Figure 18.12   Injection moulding machine that produces smoothing and polishing buttons (courtesy of SB Optical Ltd)

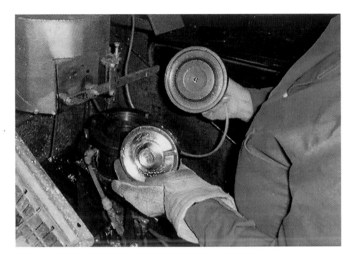

Figure 18.11   Vacuum blocking chuck with a blocked lens shown in the operator's left hand (courtesy of SB Optical Ltd)

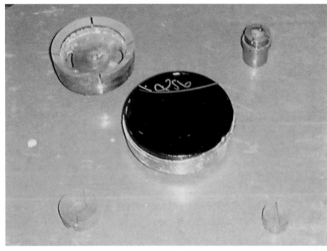

Figure 18.13   Solid bifocal tools around a blocked saucer blank (starting top left and moving clockwise): DP roughing tool, RP roughing tool, RP smoothing tool, DP smoothing tool (courtesy of SB Optical Ltd)

defects before it is removed from its holder. Once deblocked, it is most unlikely that it could be reworked, since it would need to be reblocked exactly concentric with its original axis of rotation.

To ensure that the lens is located accurately in its alloy block, the sprayed saucer blank is placed in a vacuum chuck, designed to hold the blank firmly while the alloy is distributed around the mould. Figure 18.11 shows a newly blocked saucer blank that has just been released from the chuck.

Before the grinding process takes place, the tools to be used for a given bifocal surface are selected. For roughing, diamond-impregnated ring tools are used as they leave a reasonably fine surface ready for smoothing. The smoothing and polishing tools, however, are made from specially prepared mixtures, which combine wax and wood flour with suitably selected grinding compounds. These tools are made in-house, by first mixing the components, allowing them to dry to a solid form and then granulating the mixture so that it can be injection moulded into the desired shape (Figure 18.12).

The various tools employed in the working of solid bifocal surfaces, arranged around a blocked saucer blank, are illustrated in Figure 18.13.

Roughing

The roughing machines for grinding the bifocal surface comprise a bottom rotating head on which the blocked saucer blank sits and a top grinding spindle to which the tools are mounted. The

principle is very similar to that of the spherical generator, except that a different tool is used for different surface powers. A bank of roughing machines is illustrated in Figure 18.14.

The generator slurry is a mixture of soluble oils dissolved in water and fed onto the surface during the grinding operation in a continuous stream by means of a pump.

For invisible solid bifocals, the DP surface is generated first, followed by RP generation, a sequence followed through in the subsequent smoothing and polishing operations. In the working of solid prism segment bifocals, the sequence is reversed, with RP working undertaken before DP working. The DP roughing tool is offset to rotate on the saucer blank in such a way that a raised central portion, the segment to be, remains at the centre of the blank. The DP tool, naturally, is not allowed to encroach on the central area, which is to become the RP curve.

The RP surface is ground with a smaller ring tool, set up so that it cannot make contact with the DP surface. The RP surface must be ground carefully down to the same level as the DP surface; inadequate working leaves the RP surface too proud, a defect known as 'high ridge' since the dividing line is very prominent. It is also important that the RP surface is not 'lopsided', which results in unintentional prism being incorporated in the segment.

Figure 18.15 shows the area of contact that the DP and RP roughing tools make with the surface at a given moment in the roughing operation.

Smoothing

Smoothing and polishing machines are of the same design, one that allows the tool to float, and thereby pick up its own axis in the correct plane to ensure that the surface remains truly spherical.

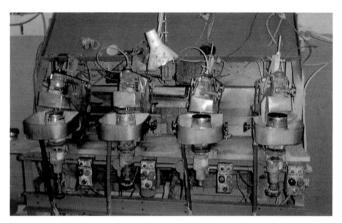

Figure 18.14 Bank of roughing machines (courtesy of SB Optical Ltd)

Again, with invisible solid bifocals, the DP surface is smoothed first followed by RP smoothing. The DP smoothing tool is set up exactly to the segment ridge and covers just the DP surface. The smoothing slurry is fed onto the surface continuously by means of a pump, in the same way as in the generating process.

After DP smoothing the RP is again left raised above the DP surface, so the RP must now be smoothed down with a small floating tool set up, again, exactly to the segment ridge. The segment surface must be ground down until it is nearly level with the DP surface once more.

It is sometimes necessary to adjust the RP curve. This can be done by setting a tilt on the top spindle, which introduces a slight bias by friction of the driving pins, to increase the pressure of the tool on the centre or edge, according to the direction of the tilt, and thus shorten or lengthen the radius slightly.

Figure 18.16 shows the area of contact that the DP and RP smoothing tools make with the surface at a given moment in the smoothing operation.

Polishing

The polishing tools used for solid bifocals have to be very hard to preserve a sharp dividing line between the DP and RP surfaces. The injection-moulded polishing tools are designed to have sharp edges to reduce waviness in the region of the ridge.

For invisible solid bifocals the DP is polished first by setting its edge to coincide with the ridge. The machine is then started, the tool being fed with the polishing lubricant until all traces of grey have disappeared. If the edge of the polisher wears down

Figure 18.15 Roughing – tool in contact with surface at any instant

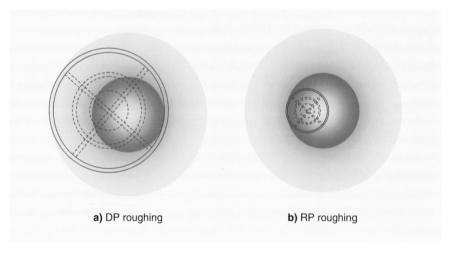

a) DP roughing   **b)** RP roughing

Figure 18.16 Smoothing – tool in contact with surface at any instant

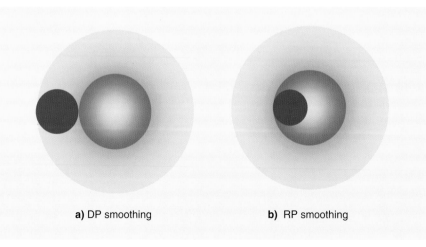

a) DP smoothing   **b)** RP smoothing

too quickly, losing its sharp edge, it leaves a narrow band around the dividing line known as aberration or 'aber'. By re-turning the polisher and running the surface again on the machine for a few minutes, with the smallest trace of polishing compound, the band of aber is polished away to leave a clean sharp ridge on the DP side. Figure 18.17 illustrates polishing the DP of a prism segment bifocal, the depressed segment ridge being clearly visible. As mentioned earlier, the RP surface of this prism segment design has already been polished.

The RP is polished in a similar manner, with a polisher approximately half the diameter of the RP. After polishing the DP, a perceptible ridge is left because material has been removed from the DP surface. The RP surface must, therefore, be polished until it is nearly level with the DP and, if necessary, run for a few minutes with very low rouge concentration to ensure that the dividing line is clean with a sharply defined edge. Figure 18.18 illustrates polishing the RP of a prism segment bifocal and, again, the segment ridge is distinguishable.

The bifocal surface is now complete, but a small pip may remain at the centre of the segment. In the case of 22mm and 30mm segments it is necessary to remove this pip by running the RP surface with a small soft wax polisher that has been moulded to the RP curve. Strictly, this action causes the curvature of the surface to alter, but as it takes only 30–45 seconds to remove the pip, the alteration to the curve is negligible.

Since the dimensions of 38mm and 45mm segment blanks are such that the pip is not included in the finished edged lens, it is ignored unless an extra-deep RP has been ordered.

Inspection and knocking off

Before deblocking, the completed bifocal surface is inspected carefully for traces of grey, pip or other defects of the DP and RP surfaces, including defects of the ridge, such as lopsidedness, high ridge, aber and so on. It is necessary at all stages in the surfacing operation to ensure that the tools and polishers are set up exactly to the ridge to obtain a clean dividing line; stringent checks at each stage of the operation do much to reduce the number of rejects at this inspection.

When the saucer blanks have passed a preliminary inspection, they are deblocked by tapping the edge of the block with a hammer (knocked off). The rubberized paint is peeled off and both the

paint film and the alloy of low melting point are recycled for use in their separate tanks. The blanks are cleaned and given a final inspection before being cut into semi-finished solid bifocal blanks ready for distribution to the prescription house (Figure 18.19).

Sawing the disks into semi-finished blanks

The characteristic shapes of solid bifocal blanks result from the way in which the saucer disks are cut to provide semi-finished blanks ready for surfacing the second side. In the case of 38mm and 45mm diameter segments it is usual to cut the blanks in half to obtain two semi-finished blanks from one saucer. Figure 18.20 illustrates how the disk is cut to obtain a pair of semi-finished blanks. The exception is when an extra-deep RP has been ordered, in which case it is only possible to obtain one semi-finished blank from the saucer disk.

For 22mm and 30mm diameter segments a single semi-finished solid blank is obtained from each saucer; Figure 18.21 illustrates how a blank with a 22mm or 30mm diameter segment would be cut.

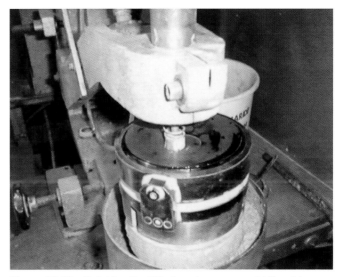

Figure 18.18   Polishing the RP of a prism segment bifocal (courtesy of SB Optical Ltd)

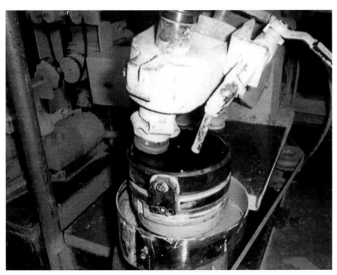

Figure 18.17   Polishing the DP of a prism segment bifocal (courtesy of SB Optical Ltd)

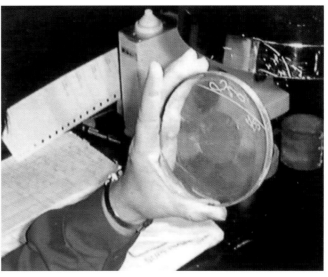

Figure 18.19   Final inspection of the surface before sawing the disk into blanks (courtesy of SB Optical Ltd)

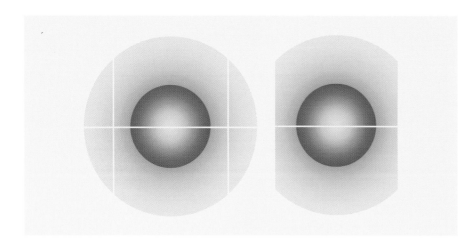

Figure 18.20   Cutting of solid bifocal disk to obtain two semi-finished 38mm or 45mm segment blanks

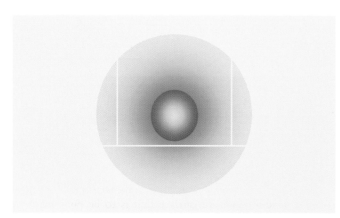

Figure 18.21   Cutting of solid bifocal disk to obtain one semi-finished 22mm or 30mm segment blank

Table 18.2   Segments on the concave surface

Segment diameters (mm)	DP curves				
22	Plano	−4.00	−6.00	−8.00	−10.00
30	Plano	−2.00	−4.00	−6.00	−8.00
38	Plano	−4.00	−6.00	−8.00	
45	Plano	−4.00	−6.00	−8.00	

Table 18.3   Prism segment solids with prism in the segment in 0.5Δ steps from 0.5Δ to 4.0Δ

Segment diameters (mm)	DP curves				
30	Plano	−2.00	−4.00	−6.00	−8.00

Prism powers over 4.0Δ are available at extra charge

The electric twin-bladed diamond saw employed to cut the blanks is set to produce two vertical cuts simultaneously down the saucer disk. A glasscutter is then used to divide the remaining part of the saucer to obtain the final semi-finished blanks. This method of cutting ensures that the depth of the crescent segments is equal to half their segment diameters, which provides maximum flexibility in the use of the blank.

Prism-controlled solid bifocals

If the segment surface of a solid bifocal saucer blank shares the same axis of revolution as the DP surface, the centration of the RP is dependent upon the segment diameter and the prescription of the lens. The segment does not incorporate a separate prismatic effect.

If the segment surface does not share the same axis of revolution as the DP, it will be angled with respect to the DP surface. As a result, the RP of the lens incorporates a separate prismatic effect, which is independent of the prescription in the DP of the lens. Bifocal designs that can incorporate independent prism in the RP only are known as prism-controlled bifocals.

In theory, if the segment surface can be rotated through any angle, it is possible to include any amount of prism in the segment, and thereby offer total control of the centration of the RP.

The dividing line of the prism-controlled segment is no longer invisible, but includes an angled step of which the maximum depth represents the position of the prism apex. It can be imagined that the segment is constructed by depressing the RP surface below the level of the DP surface and then dropping a prism into the depression. The apical angle of this prism is the same angle as that which the blank must rotate through to obtain the prescribed prism in the segment.

To provide the best cosmetic effect for the dividing line, it is usual to bring the RP surface at the position of the prism base up to the same level as that of the DP surface. This ensures that the dividing line at the position of the minimum depth of segment ridge is virtually invisible. If this does not occur, the segment surface remains depressed below the level of the DP surface and the ridge forms a step all round the edge of the segment.

If this is allowed to happen deliberately, it is possible to work a toroidal DP surface to fulfil complex prescription requirements, such as the different cylinders or cylinder axes in the DP and RP described in Chapter 15.

Current availability of solid bifocal blank

Since solid bifocals are made individually, the available range of segment side curves and diameters is restricted. Semi-finished solid bifocal blanks are currently offered in the forms shown in Tables 18.2–18.4. Many of these designs are also available in photochromic form, in either brown or grey.

Progressive power surfaces

As already discussed in Chapter 17, a progressive power surface is an aspherical surface of the non-rotationally symmetrical type, generated by means of computer numerically controlled (CNC)

Table 18.4 Segments on the convex surface			
Segment diameters (mm)		DP curves	
30	+4.25	+6.25	+8.25
38	+4.25	+6.25	+8.25

machining of either the surface itself or of the mould from which the surface may be cast or slumped.

The important stages in the production process for a progressive power surface are as follows:

- surface design and numeric description
- grinding, smoothing and polishing of the spherical DP curve
- generating the aspherical surface
- polishing the aspherical surface
- inspection.

Surface design and numeric description

Surface design and computation of the surface topography is translated into numeric data in the form of coordinates that can be fed directly into the CNC generators. Up to 50 000 numeric data points may be required for an individual surface, information that must be stored for all combinations of DP curves and reading additions.

The basic reference for the progressive surface is usually taken to be a spherical surface of curvature similar to the DP curve required. This spherical DP curve is subsequently made aspherical in accordance with the design philosophy for the lens. The spherical convex surface must be generated, smoothed and polished accurately so that its topography has precisely the known desired characteristics before regrinding occurs.

Generating the progressive surface

The principle of CNC generating is explained in Chapter 17. The blocked lens is attached to a spindle that rotates slowly about the z-axis of the surface and the workpiece can move in the x, y and z meridians as directed by the CNC grinding program (Figure 18.22a). The diamond-impregnated cutting wheel rotates about the y-axis and makes single-point contact with the surface during the grinding operation. The cutter moves in a spiral pathway over the face of the workpiece, as illustrated in Figure 18.22b. Typically, the generator cycle time is some 10 minutes for a surface of 70mm diameter.

During the grinding cycle, glass is removed from the surface up to a depth of about 1mm, depending, of course, on the base curve and reading addition of the lens; the accuracy of the cut has to be better than 2μm (0.002mm) to prepare the surface for polishing.

To obtain this order of accuracy, machining has to take place in an air-conditioned workroom in which the temperature and humidity are controlled carefully to ensure there is no fluctuation in the machine cycle through different operating conditions.

Polishing the progressive surface

The surface obtained at the end of the generating process is so finely ground that it is ready for polishing without any intermediate smoothing being necessary. Polishing methods for aspherical surfaces are described in detail in Chapter 17.

In general, when polishing a progressive power surface on a glass lens, the concave face of the polishing pad should closely match the convex surface to be polished, and so it is necessary to maintain a large range of polishing tools to which the polishing pads are attached.

The polishing runner is composed of three components, a metal block with a predetermined concave surface, to which is attached a preformed foam pad of known curvature and, on top of the foam, the polishing face itself, which takes the form of a polyurethane pad, as illustrated in Figure 17.43.

The computer makes a selection from a large range of metal tools, depending upon the surface that is to be polished, having taken into account the DP curve and reading addition of the lens. The preformed foam pads provide the flexibility required to ensure that the pad remains in contact with the lens surface during the polishing cycle. The firmness of the pad needs to be checked regularly to ensure that it retains the correct degree of resilience. Typically, the foam pads may be reused some 20 times before they no longer have the correct resilience and must be discarded.

A view of a twin-spindle polishing machine is given in Figure 17.44. The lenses are held in pneumatically controlled chucks and are about to be lowered on to the polishing runners seen in the bowl of the machine. Two nozzles deliver the cerium oxide slurry,

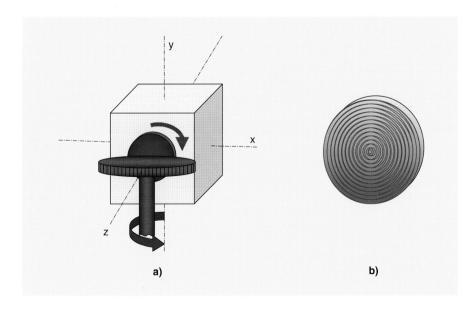

Figure 18.22   Principle of the generating process. (a) The lens blank rotates slowly around the z-axis and the diamond-impregnating cutting wheel, shown in the horizontal plane, rotates around the y-axis. Since both the workface and the tool face are convex, the tool makes contact with the surface at just one point at a time. (b) Spiral pathway of cutter across the surface

a)   b)

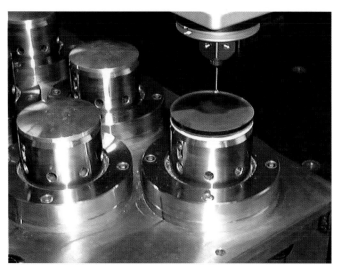

Figure 18.23 In surface measurement the ruby tip of the measuring probe is held in contact with a known point on a progressive power surface, the lens under test being mounted on a measuring block that ensures no movement of the lens under test. Typically, measurements are taken at 400 different points on the surface (courtesy of Carl Zeiss)

of which the concentration, temperature and pH value are monitored and controlled constantly.

Inspection

It is anticipated that some 25–30μm of glass is removed during the polishing process, so it is essential to ensure that the polished face faithfully follows the precise design characteristics of the surface. As with all aspherical surface production, before the final machine settings are determined for the surface, an iterative process is used to ensure that glass removal during the polishing process is controlled accurately. When a new progressive lens design is under development, at the end of the polishing process the surface characteristics of a test lens are measured carefully and any departure from the desired surface profile is fed back to the CNC generator so that it can take into account the glass removal in different zones of the surface. Typically, the surface is measured at some 400 points to provide a close comparison with the design profile. The measurements are stored in the on-board computer so that the profile of the entire surface obtained can subsequently be compared with the desired profile for the surface.

To take accurate measurements, a high-precision micrometer is used, of which the position of the measuring tip is accurately known in the x, y and z planes. The measuring tip is located precisely by the onboard computer-controlled servo-motors in the desired measuring position in the x and y planes, and the z measurement recorded by the micrometer. The integrity of the measuring tip is ensured by the use of a precious crystalline substance, such as ruby, cut in the shape of a sphere.

The measurement of one point is illustrated in Figure 18.23, which shows the ruby tip of the measuring probe in contact with a known point on a progressive power surface. The lens under test is mounted on one of the measuring blocks, which ensures no movement of the lens during measurement.

References

1. Jalie M 1984 Principles of ophthalmic lenses. ABDO, London
2. Horne D F 1972 Optical production technology. Hilger (Adam) Ltd, London

Multiple choice questions

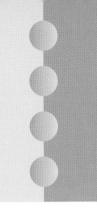

Chapter 1

1. A ray of light is incident at 40° to the normal on the surface of a parallel-sided glass block of refractive index 1.60 in air. Which of the following is the angle of refraction that the ray makes inside the block?

   A 20.5° B 22.6° C 23.7° D 24.8° E 25.0°

2. If the thickness of the block in Question 1 is 10cm, what is the displacement of the ray when it emerges from the second face?

   A 2.54cm B 3.07cm C 3.70cm D 3.95cm E 4.24cm

3. How deep does a clear pool of water (refractive index 1.333) appear to an observer looking straight down from above if the real depth of water is 120cm?

   A 75cm B 160cm C 80cm D 90cm E 120cm

4. A prism of apical angle 4° is made in glass of refractive index 1.701. What is the power of the prism in prism dioptres?

   A 4.1Δ B 4.4Δ C 4.6Δ D 4.7Δ E 4.9Δ

5. A plano-prism made in a plastics material of refractive index 1.60 has a diameter of 45mm, a thin-edge substance of 1.2mm and a thick-edge substance of 4.2mm. What is the power of the prism in dioptres?

   A 2.50Δ B 3.00Δ C 3.25Δ D 3.50Δ E 4.00Δ

6. Two plano-prisms of power 1Δ and 2Δ are placed together with a right-angle between their base settings. What single prism will replace the combination?

   A 2.25Δ B 2.50Δ C 2.75Δ D 3.00Δ E 3.25Δ

7. A concave surface of radius 80mm is ground onto the end of a glass rod of refractive index 1.56. What is the power of the surface?

   A +5.00D B −5.00D C −6.00D D +7.00D E −7.00D

8. A convex spherical surface has a sag of 3.975mm when measured over a 40mm diameter. What surface power would it have if worked on glass of refractive index 1.523?

   A +9.25 B +9.50 C +9.75 D +10.00 E +10.25

9. An object is placed 25cm in front of a thin lens of power +9.00D. Where is the image formed by the lens?

   A 25cm behind the lens   B 25cm in front of the lens
   C 20cm behind the lens   D 20cm in front of the lens
   E 15cm behind the lens

10. A lens made in CR39 material of refractive index 1.498 has surface powers of +11.00 and −3.62 and an axial thickness of 7.3mm. What is the back vertex power of the lens?

    A +7.38 B +7.62 C +8.00 D +8.12 E +8.32

11. The lens described in Question 10 is placed on a focimeter with its convex surface in contact with the lens rest. What power will the instrument read?

    A +7.25 B +7.31 C +7.37 D +7.44 E +7.50

12. A +10.00D lens is to be made with a −4.00D inside curve, in glass, n = 1.60, with an axial thickness of 8.8mm. What front curve must be used?

    A +14.00 B +13.75 C +13.50 D +13.25 E +13.00

13. A +6.00D lens is to be made with a +10.75D front curve, in glass, n = 1.52, with an axial thickness of 6.3mm. What back curve must be used?

    A −5.25 B −5.12 C −5.00 D −4.87 E −4.75

14. A subject is corrected by a −12.00D lens worn at a vertex distance of 12mm. What power lens would be required to be worn at a vertex distance of 15mm?

    A −11.50 B −11.75 C −12.00 D −12.25 E −12.50

15. A toric lens is made to the prescription −9.00/−1.00 × 45 with a +1.50 base curve. What is the power of the concave surface of the lens?

    A −10.50   B −11.00
    C −11.50   D −11.50/−12.50 × 45
    E −10.50/−11.50 × 45

16. A +8.00D lens made in a plastics material, n = 1.5, with a −6.00 back curve and axial thickness 7.5mm, is used for near vision at 25cm from the front surface. What is the vergence of the light that leaves the back surface of the lens?

    A +3.25 B +3.50 C +3.62 D +3.75 E +4.00

17. A focimeter has a standard lens of +25.00D. What is the movement of the target per dioptre of lens power under test?

    A 1.6mm B 1.8mm C 2.0mm D 2.25mm E 2.5mm

18. The two plano-cylinders, +2.00DC × 20 and +2.00DC × 140, are placed in close contact. What is the power of the resulting combination?

    A +4.00DC × 20   B +4.00DC × 140
    C +0.50/+2.50 × 80   D +1.00/+2.00 × 170
    E +1.00/+2.00 × 80

Chapter 2

1. The transverse chromatic aberration exhibited by a −6.00D lens made in plastics material with an Abbe number of 40, when the eye looks through a point 8mm below the optical centre, is which of the following?

   A 0.10Δ B 0.12Δ C 0.14Δ D 0.16Δ E 0.18Δ

2. A spectacle lens has a back vertex focal length of +200mm and a tangential oblique vertex sphere focal length of +204.08mm for the 35° zone of the lens. The sagittal focal line lies 6mm beyond the tangential focal line. Which of the following correctly describes the aberrations for this zone?

   A OAE +0.14, MOP +4.83, MOE −0.17
   B OAE 6mm, MOP +4.90, MOE 4.08mm
   C OAE −6mm, MOP +4.90, MOE −4.08mm
   D OAE −0.14, MOP +4.83, MOE +0.17
   E OAE +0.14, MOP +4.83, MOE +0.17

3 The tangential and sagittal oblique vertex sphere powers for the 30° zone of a −5.00D lens are found to be −6.00D and −5.25D, respectively. Which of the following describes the off-axis performance?

A OAE −0.75, MOE −0.75   B OAE −0.62, MOE −0.62
C OAE −0.75, MOE −0.62   D MOP −5.25, MOE −0.75
E MOP −5.62, MOE −0.75

4 A +12.00D lens is found to have OAE = +2.00 and MOE = +1.00 for the 30° zone. What are the tangential and sagittal oblique vertex sphere powers of the lens?

A +12.00 and +14.00   B +14.00 and +12.00
C +12.25 and +14.25   D +14.25 and +12.25
E +13.00 and +15.00

5 To provide very thin lenses you decide to dispense the prescription BE −8.00 in glass of refractive index 1.80. In the past, the subject has worn crown glass lenses, which have always been dispensed in plano-concave form. What would you write in the box marked FORM on the order to the prescription house for the new pair of lenses?

A flats   B plano-concave
C meniscus   D periscopic
E +1.50 base meniscus

6 The prescription −6.00/+3.00 × 90 is dispensed in toric form with a +4.00 spherical front curve. Which of the following correctly describes the form of the lens?

A +4.00 base toric   B −10.00 base toric
C −7.00 base toric   D toric lens with −7.00 cross curve
E toric lens with −10.00 cross curve

7 Which of the following is true for a glass type with n_d = 1.747?

A CVF = 0.65, reflectance = 7.2%
B CVF = 0.68, reflectance = 7.2%
C CVF = 0.70, reflectance = 7.4%
D CVF = 0.71, reflectance = 7.4%
E CVF = 0.72, reflectance = 7.6%

8 Taking only losses by surface reflectance into account (i.e. ignoring any loss of radiation by absorption), what would be the transmittance of a plastics lens made in material of refractive index 1.61, assuming no anti-reflection coating is applied?

A 94.5%   B 89.0%   C 90.4%   D 89.4%   E 88.4%

9 A −6.00D lens is made in a 1.80 index material that has a density of 3.3g/cm³. Which of the following statements best describes the weight of the lens when compared with the weight of the same power lens made in crown glass?

A much heavier   B a little heavier
C more or less the same   D a little lighter
E much lighter

10 A subject is dispensed a pair of −3.00D lenses in a material of Abbe number 42. Assuming the threshold value for TCA to be 0.1Δ, what is the diameter of the circular zone concentric with the optical centre within which TCA is unlikely to be noticed?

A 14mm   B 18mm   C 22mm   D 24mm   E 28mm

11 A lens measure calibrated for refractive index 1.523 reads +4.25 and −11.00 when applied to a lens made in a material of refractive index 1.60. What power is found for this lens when it is tested in a focimeter?

A −6.75   B −7.75   C −8.75   D −9.75   E −10.75

12 The power of a lens determined by a focimeter is +1.50 and a lens measure calibrated for CR39 material when placed on its surfaces reads +4.50 and −3.50. What is the refractive index of the lens material?

A 1.75   B 1.70   C 1.65   D 1.60   E 1.55

Chapter 3

1 The boxed centre of a lens shape lies at which of the following?

A at any point specified by the prescription house
B at any point on the HCL as specified by the prescription house
C at a point midway between the vertical tangents to the temporal and nasal edges of the lens shape
D at the point intersected by the diagonals of the rectangle that just contains the lens shape
E midway between the temporal and nasal ends of the HCL, where it intersects the lens periphery

2 A bifocal lens is edged to a 48 × 40 oval shape and has a segment of specification 38 × 18 high × 2in. Which of the following is the segment drop?

A 18mm high
B 0mm
C 3mm below the HCL
D 2mm above the HCL
E more information is necessary for it to be specified

3 When measuring the PD of a subject for distance vision with a simple rule you note that the horizontal distance between the centres of the pupils as read from the rule is 56mm. Your exact PD is 64. Which of the following would you record the PD of the subject as?

A 56.5   B 56.0   C 55.5   D 57.0   E 55.0

4 The PD of a subject is accurately given as 68. You wish to make the subject a pair of intermediate spectacles for use at a VDU where the working distance is 45cm. You assume the subject's centres of rotation to lie 28mm behind the spectacle plane. What intermediate CD would you order?

A 65.0   B 64.5   C 64.0   D 63.5   E 63.0

5 A subject whose monocular CDs for distance vision are 34/31 has the following prescription for bifocal lenses: BE +6.00 Add +2.00. Assuming you could obtain an accuracy of 0.1mm, what geometrical inset would you prescribe to bring the near fields into coincidence? (Use Table 3.2)

A 1.5 in each eye
B 2.0 in each eye
C R 3.2 in, L 2.9 in
D R 2.7 in, L 3.0 in
E R 3.0 in, L 2.7 in

6 You dispense a pair of +5.00D lenses in aspheric form to a subject whose CD is 64, in a frame that has a 46 × 40 oval shape and note that when the head is held in the primary position, the centres of the subject's pupils lie 26mm above the lower horizontal tangent to the lens periphery. The pantoscopic angle of the frame is 12.5° and the distance between centres of the frame is 68mm. Assuming the standard optical centre position to coincide with the boxed centre, which of the following specifications would you order for the lenses? (Use Table 3.3)

A decentre 6mm up
B decentre 2mm in
C decentre 6mm up and 2mm in
D OCs 20mm high and decentred 2mm in
E OCs to coincide with pupil centres

7 What is the prismatic effect at a point 8mm below and 3mm inwards from the optical centre of the lens L −3.00/−2.00 × 90?

A 2.4Δ up and 1.5Δ out
B 2.4Δ up and 1.5Δ in
C 2.4Δ down and 1.5Δ out
D 2.4Δ down and 1.5Δ in
E 1.5Δ down and 2.4Δ in

8 What is the prismatic effect at a point 10mm below the geometrical centre of the plano-cylinder L −3.00DC × 150?

A 3Δ base down
B 1.5Δ base down and 2.6Δ base in
C 2.6Δ base down and 1.5Δ base in
D 2.6Δ base up and 1.5Δ base out
E 1.5Δ base up and 2.6Δ base out

9 What is the prismatic effect produced by decentring the lens −2.00/+4.00 × 135, 10mm upwards before the right eye?

A 2Δ base up   B 2Δ base down
C 0   D 2Δ base out
E 2Δ base in

10 You are to make a new pair of spectacles for a subject whose prescription is R +2.00/−4.00 × 45, L plano. The PD of the subject is 58mm and he has selected a frame with a distance between centres of 72mm. What CD would you order?

A 58 – to avoid 1.2Δ of horizontal differential prism
B 72 – on the grounds that the L lens is plano
C 72 – on the grounds that the R lens has no power horizontally
D 72 – on the grounds that the R lens has no power horizontally and the L lens is plano
E 58 – to avoid 1.2Δ of vertical differential prism

11 The 2Δ iso-V-prism zone for the lens R −2.00/−2.00 × 180 is a band of which of the following dimensions?

A 10mm wide along 90
B 10mm wide along 180
C 10mm wide along 45
D 5mm wide along 90
E 5mm wide along 180

12 The 2Δ iso-V-differential prism zones for the prescription R −3.00/−2.00 × 90, L −4.00/−2.00 × 60 are a pair of bands of which of the following dimensions?

A 11.5mm wide lying along 30
B 11.5mm wide lying along 60
C 11.5mm wide lying along 90
D 11.5mm wide lying along 120
E 11.5mm wide lying along 150

Chapter 4

1 What name is given to the conic section obtained when a plane intersects a cone parallel to one side of the cone?

A circle   B prolate ellipse
C oblate ellipse   D parabola
E hyperbola

2 A conic section is described by the equation $y^2 = 100x + 2x^2$. Which of the following describes the surface?

A prolate ellipsoid with vertex radius 100mm
B prolate ellipsoid with vertex radius 50mm
C hyperboloid with vertex radius 100mm
D hyperboloid with vertex radius 50mm
E paraboloid with vertex radius 100mm

3 Which of the following statements best explains the improved optical performance of a strong plus lens that has one aspherical surface?

A the aspherical surface produces no aberrations
B the aspherical surface has less spherical aberration than a spherical surface
C the aspherical surface has no astigmatism
D the astigmatism of an aspherical surface is so small that it can be ignored
E the astigmatism of an aspherical surface can neutralize the astigmatism of oblique incidence

4 What is the sag of a spherical surface of radius 100mm over a chord diameter of 70mm?

A 6.3mm   B 6.6mm   C 6.9mm   D 7.2mm   E 7.5mm

5 What is the sag of a hyperboloidal surface of vertex radius 100mm and p-value −2.0, over a chord diameter of 70mm?

A 5.5mm   B 5.8mm   C 6.1mm   D 6.4mm   E 6.7mm

6 An aphakic subject is found to be corrected for near vision at 33.3cm by the addition of a +3.00 trial lens to the distance correction in the trial frame, which is +11.00/+1.00 × 175. The final spectacle lens dispensed is a 40mm aperture solid convex lenticular and there is no change in vertex distance. Which of the following reading additions is most likely to duplicate the near vision prescription in the trial frame?

A +4.50   B +4.25   C +4.00   D +3.75   E +3.50

7 Which of the following is the reason for low-power aspheric lenses being thinner and lighter than traditional best form lenses?

A they are always made from a plastics material
B they are flatter in form
C they use an aspherical surface
D they are flatter in form and use an aspherical surface
E they are flatter in form and use an aspherical surface with a sag smaller than that of a sphere with the same vertex radius

8 Which of the following claims can be made for the optical performance of low power aspheric lenses?

A it is worse than the performance of lenses made with spherical surfaces
B it is about the same as the performance of lenses made with spherical surfaces
C it is a little better than the performance of lenses made with spherical surfaces
D it is much better than the performance of lenses made with spherical surfaces
E it is far superior to the performance of lenses made with spherical surfaces

9 Which of the following statements best describes the correction of distortion in a low-power aspheric lens?

A a low-power aspheric lens has much more distortion than a best-form lens with spherical surfaces
B a low-power aspheric lens has much less distortion than a best-form lens with spherical surfaces
C a low-power aspheric lens has about the same distortion as a best-form lens with spherical surfaces
D a low-power aspheric lens has a little less distortion than a best-form lens with spherical surfaces
E a low-power aspheric lens exhibits no distortion

10 A typical front curve for a +4.00D lens made with spherical surfaces is +8.75D. What front curve would be typical for a low-power aspheric lens of this power?

A +8.00   B +7.00   C +6.00   D +5.00   E +4.00

11 What is the sag (x value) of an aspherical surface described by the power series $x = Ay^2 + By^4 + Cy^6$, where $A = +1.14 \times 10^{-3}$, $B = +1.69 \times 10^{-7}$ and $C = +5.01 \times 10^{-11}$, over a chord diameter (2y) of 70mm?

A 1.74mm   B 1.60mm   C 1.23mm   D 1.85mm   E 1.50mm

12 What is the essential difference between the atoroidal surface used on the Zeiss Hypal design and that used on the Rodenstock Multigressiv lens?

A none
B the atoroidal surface of the Multigressiv lens is convex
C the atoroidal surface of the Hypal includes the cylindrical correction
D the atoroidal surface of the Multigressiv does not include the cylindrical correction
E the atoroidal surface of the Hypal does not include the cylindrical correction

13 A subject whose distance PD is 68 (35/33) is to be dispensed a pair of lenses for near vision at 33.3cm. Which of the following NCD specifications would you order?

A 63   B 31.5/31.5   C 32/31   D 32.5/30.5   E 33/30

14 A subject whose distance PD is 60 (30/30) is to be dispensed a pair of +7.00D lenses in aspheric form for near vision at 33.3cm. The final frame is an oval-eye of box lens size 46×40, distance between centres 64 and pantoscopic angle 8°. When the final frame is fitted to the subject, whose head is held in the primary position for distance vision, it is noted that the pupil centres have a height of 24mm. Which of the following fitting specifications fully satisfies the centre of rotation condition?

A the centre of rotation cannot be fully satisfied both vertically and horizontally
B decentre lenses 4mm in for each eye from the box centre
C decentre lenses 4mm down and 4mm in for each eye from the box centre
D decentre lenses 4mm down and 4mm in for each eye from the box centre and apply a reverse dihedral angle of 4° to each lens
E decentre lenses 4mm in for each eye from the box centre and apply a reverse dihedral angle of 4° to each lens

15 The prescription +6.00 with 5Δ base in is to be dispensed as an aspheric lens to be worn 30mm in front of the eye's centre of rotation. How could you ensure that the visual axis passes through the pole of the aspherical surface when the eye is in its primary position?

A by asking for the prism to be produced by decentration
B by ensuring that the centre of rotation condition is fulfilled
C by asking for the lens to be decentred 3mm out after the prism has been surfaced
D by asking for the lens to be decentred 3mm in after the prism has been surfaced
E by asking for the lens to be decentred 3mm down after the prism has been surfaced

16 Why should an aspheric lens not be decentred to produce prismatic effect?

A because aspheric lenses cannot be decentred
B because decentration of an aspheric lens does not produce a prismatic effect
C because the decentration shifts the pole of the surface from the visual axis
D because an aspheric lens is not thick enough to accommodate prism
E because aspheric lenses are not supplied in prismatic form

17 When a ray of light is incident parallel to the optical axis and 2cm from the optical centre of a +4.00D lens, the paraxial decentration relationship tells us that the prismatic deviation of the ray will be 8Δ. Using *Table 4.3*, which of the following is the true deviation for the ray when the lens is made in spherical and aspherical forms?

A 8.4Δ and 7.35Δ   B 8.4Δ and 8Δ
C 8.4Δ and 7.91Δ   D 8.96Δ and 7.91Δ
E 8.96Δ and 8Δ

18 The spherical aberration of the +4.00D aspheric lens is listed in *Table 4.3* for an incidence height of 16mm as +12.11mm. What is the focusing distance of this ray?

A +237.89mm   B +262.11mm
C +250.00mm   D +253.89mm
E +221.89mm

Chapter 5

1 Which of the following are *not* conditions that must be satisfied for a spectacle wearer to be aware of ghost images?

A the ghost image must be bright enough to stand out in the surrounding illumination
B the vergence of the ghost image must be similar to the power of the correcting lens
C the ghost image must be superimposed upon the refracted image
D the ghost image must lie within the visual field
E there must be some illumination in the visual field

2 What is the relative intensity of ghost image 4 for a lens made in a plastics material of refractive index 1.56?

A 4.4%   B 4.5%   C 4.6%   D 4.7%   E 4.8%

3 What is the relative intensity of ghost image 1 for a lens made in a plastics material of refractive index 1.66?

A 0.33%   B 0.34%   C 0.35%   D 0.36%   E 0.37%

4 A young subject wearing the prescription −0.75DS states that she can see ghost images of oncoming car headlights which, at first, are out of focus, but which, if she makes an effort, she can see as sharp pinpoints of light. She is wearing uncoated, 1.6 index, glass spectacle lenses. What effort of accommodation is she making to bring the images into focus?

A 0.75D   B 5.25D   C 4.75D   D 4.00D   E 3.25D

5 A subject wearing the prescription −6.00, made in uncoated plastics lenses of refractive index 1.5, states that when sitting at his study desk in the evening with his table lamp at the side, he can see by reflection a sharp image of his eyelid (assumed to be 25mm behind the lens). What is the base curve of his lens?

A +1.50   B +2.00   C +2.50   D +3.00   E +3.50

6 A plano-sunlens made in glass of refractive index 1.523 has its back vertex 15mm in front of a spherical cornea of radius 7.8mm. The emmetropic wearer can see a ghost image formed by reflection at her cornea and the back surface of the lens in sharp focus without the need to exert any accommodation. What is the radius of curvature of the back surface of the lens?

A 40.0mm   B 37.8mm   C 36.5mm   D 35.0mm   E 34.4mm

7 Which of the following is the amount of light reflected by an uncoated spectacle lens made in a plastics material of refractive index 1.66?

A 10.4%   B 10.8%   C 11.2%   D 11.6%   E 12.0%

8 Which of the following is the amount of light transmitted by an uncoated spectacle lens made in glass of refractive index 1.9?

A 80.4%   B 81.6%   C 82.4%   D 83.0%   E 84.4%

9 To satisfy the amplitude condition, the refractive index of a single-layer coating to be applied to a lens of refractive index 1.56 should be:

A 1.240   B 1.249   C 1.255   D 1.262   E 1.270

10 To satisfy the path condition for light of wavelength 560nm, which of the following must be the actual thickness of a single-layer anti-reflection coating of magnesium fluoride?

A 101.4nm   B 102.4nm   C 103.4nm   D 104.4nm   E 105.4nm

11 Why is it necessary to apply a layer of titanium oxide to a plastics lens before applying a top coat of material of low refractive index?

A to provide a hard surface to the lens
B to enable the top coat to adhere to the plastics substrate
C to satisfy the path condition
D to satisfy both the path condition and the amplitude condition
E to enable the amplitude condition to be satisfied

12 Why is it necessary to achieve a vacuum of 10^{-6} millibar to vacuum coat lenses?

A to ensure the lenses have a purple tint
B to ensure that the operator does not contaminate the coating material
C to ensure that a sufficiently high temperature can be achieved within the chamber
D to ensure that the molecules of coating material can travel 1 metre
E to ensure that the mean free path of the molecules of coating material is 1 metre

Chapter 6

1 Which of the following is a property of thermoplastic materials?

A can be created by the action of heat
B cannot be created by the action of heat
C can be created by the cross-linking of molecules
D can be reformed after heating
E cannot be reformed after heating

2 The thickness of surface coatings on spectacle lenses decreases in which of the following orders?

A MAR, single-layer anti-reflection, hard coating, hydrophobic coating
B hard coating, hydrophobic coating, MAR, single-layer anti-reflection
C hydrophobic coating, single-layer anti-reflection, MAR, hard coating
D hard coating, single-layer anti-reflection, MAR, hydrophobic coating
E hard coating, MAR, single-layer anti-reflection, hydrophobic coating

3 What is the most obvious effect of a variation in thickness of a hard coat?

A the hard coat begins to show
B interference patterns become visible on the surface
C interference patterns become visible on the surface when the lens is anti-reflection coated
D interference patterns become visible on the surface when the lens is tinted
E the hard coat peels easily from the lens surface

4 Which of the following explains why hydrophobic coatings repel water?

A they have a wetting angle
B they have a low wetting angle
C they have a high wetting angle
D the coating decreases the wetting angle of the surface
E they do not have any wetting angle

5 Why are anti-reflection-coated lenses more difficult to clean?

A because the dirt shows more
B because the surface is greasy
C because they have a high wetting angle
D because they are so thin
E because a special cleaner is necessary

6 What would be the transmittance of a 2mm thick, pink 1.70 index glass lens with a luminance transmission for a 2mm thickness quoted as 83%, after the application of a multi-layer anti-reflection coating that provides 99% transmittance on a 1.5 index material?

A 83%   B 84%   C 85%   D 87%   E 90%

Chapter 7

1 Which of the following gives the specification of tints required for industrial protection?

A BS 3062   B BS 2092
C BS 169 and BS 379   D BS 2724
E BS 2738

2 A filter intended to improve contrast will absorb principally:

A at the blue end of the visible spectrum
B at the red end of the visible spectrum
C plane-polarized reflections
D in the yellow region of the visible spectrum
E evenly across the visible spectrum

3 A tint has a luminous transmittance of 0.64. Which of the following is its optical density?

A 0.36   B −3.21   C 1.45   D 1.64   E 0.19

4 A solid glass filter coloured deep green is intended to absorb mainly:

A in the green region of the visible spectrum
B plane-polarized light
C heat
D infrared radiation
E in the yellow region of the visible spectrum

5 A solid tint has a transmittance of 45% at 3mm thickness. What, approximately, will be its transmittance at 1.5mm thickness?

A 90%   B 64%   C 52%   D 34%   E 55%

6 What is the current recommendation for the CIE Standard Illuminant for determining the luminous transmittance of a sunglass filter?

A A   B B   C C   D D_{55} E D_{65}

7 Which of the following is a photochromic material with a transmission that varies from 90% to 20% classified as?

A light–medium   B light–dark
C dark–light   D medium–extra dark
E light–extra dark

8 The basic difference between the photochromic process in glass and in plastics is that in the former it is:

A photographic whereas in the latter it is physical
B reversible whereas in the latter it is fatiguing
C physical whereas in the latter it is chemical
D chemical whereas in the latter it is physical
E temperature dependent whereas in the latter it is non-temperature dependent

9 The addition of which of the following shifts the optimum activating wavelength towards a longer wavelength?

A silver   B silver chloride
C silver bromide and silver D copper
  iodide
E cerium oxide

10 The maximum size of silver halide crystal in a photochromic glass before it begins to become opalescent is:

A 400nm   B 800nm   C 1500nm   D 10000nm   E 10^8nm

11 What is the minimum recommended luminous transmittance for non-photochromic lenses for driving motor vehicles?

A 8%   B 10%   C 15%   D 20%   E 25%

12 What is the minimum acceptable value for the relative visual-attenuation quotient proposed in European Sunglass standards for the red signal lamp?

A 0.2   B 0.4   C 0.6   D 0.8   E 1.0

13 Which of the following luminous transmittances would a filter with a shade number of 2.6 have?

A 18.4%   B 20.6%   C 21.8%   D 22.5%   E 25.0%

14 Which of the following is the maximum permitted spectral transmittance value in the UVB region for general-purpose sunglasses?

A 0.01 τ_v B 0.25 τ_v C 0.5 τ_v D 0.2 τ_v E 0.1 τ_v

15 The Standard for sunglass lenses specifies that a photochromic lens should be measured at which of the following additional light intensities?

A 0 lux   B 15 000 lux (±1500)
C 15 000 lux (±750)   D 50 000 lux (±750)
E 50 000 lux (±5000)

Chapter 8

1 What surface powers would you expect to be used on an individually surfaced −8.00D lens made in CR39 material?

A Plano and −8.00   B +1.00 and −9.00
C +2.00 and −10.00   D +3.00 and −11.00
E +4.00 and −12.00

2 Which of the following is the real macular field of view of a −8.00D lens edged 40mm round and mounted 27mm in front of the eye's centre of rotation?

A 42°   B 66°   C 84°   D 106°   E 110°

3 Which choice of centre thicknesses is correct for a stock −3.50D lens made in (i) white crown glass, (ii) photochromic glass, (iii) CR39 material?

A (i) 1.2mm (ii) 1.5mm (iii) 1.9mm
B (i) 1.3mm (ii) 1.6mm (iii) 2.0mm
C (i) 1.3mm (ii) 2.0mm (iii) 2.2mm
D (i) 1.4mm (ii) 1.5mm (iii) 2.1mm
E (i) 1.4mm (ii) 1.6mm (iii) 2.0mm

4 What is the edge thickness of a −6.00D lens made in crown glass and edged 60mm in diameter?

A 5.4mm   B 5.8mm   C 6.0mm   D 6.4mm   E 7.8mm

5 What is the edge thickness of a −8.00D lens made in glass of refractive index 1.800 and edged 50mm round?

A 3.1mm   B 3.9mm   C 4.1mm   D 4.7mm   E 5.8mm

6 A lens of power −10.00/+2.00 × 90 is made in CR39 material, edged to a 54 × 45 oval shape and its optical centre coincides with its geometrical centre. The thin-edge substance is 7.3mm; what is the thick-edge substance?

A 7.5mm   B 7.6mm   C 7.7mm   D 7.8mm   E 7.9mm

7 Assuming the sag factor for a 50mm diameter lens is 0.6, what would be the edge thickness of a −10.00D lens made in crown glass if the centre thickness is 1.0mm?

A 4.9mm   B 5.7mm   C 6.6mm   D 7.0mm   E 8.0mm

8 Assuming the curve variation factor for a glass of refractive index 1.80 is 0.65, what would be the edge thickness of a −10.00D lens at 50mm diameter if it were made in 1.80 material with a centre thickness of 1.0mm?

A 4.9mm   B 5.8mm   C 6.6mm   D 7.0mm   E 8.0mm

9 A −16.00D plano-concave, uncut lens is to converted into an oval aperture lenticular of aperture size 38 × 34. What cylinder tool must be employed to produce an aperture of this dimension?

A +3.00DC   B +4.00DC   C +4.75DC   D +5.25DC   E +6.00DC

10 A −16.00D lens is to be made as a workshop-flattened lenticular with plano-flattening and a 22mm aperture diameter. If the refractive index of the lens material is increased from 1.523 to 1.700, by how many millimetres can the aperture diameter increase without causing an increase in the edge thickness of the design?

A 2mm   B 4mm   C 6mm   D 8mm   E 10mm

11 A subject whose prescription is BE −18.00 wishes to be dispensed a pair of lenticulars in a dark photochromic glass. Which is the best type of lenticular for this specification?

A solid concave lenticular   B hand-edged lenticular
C hand-edged semi lenticular   D plano-flattened lenticular
E bonded lenticular

12 A −12.00D myope who has been dispensed a pair of spectacles without the benefit of anti-reflection coated lenses complains that, when driving at night, he can see distracting ghost images of oncoming car headlamps. These reflections are likely to be formed from light that is reflected in which of the following ways?

A by the windscreen
B by dashboard instrumentation
C at both the front and back surfaces of the lens
D at the cornea and the front surface of the lens
E at the cornea and the back surface of the lens

Chapter 9

1 What is the back vertex power of a spectacle lens made in a plastics material of refractive index 1.60 with surface powers +8.75 and −3.25, and axial thickness 5.0mm?

A +5.50   B +5.62   C +5.75   D +5.87   E +6.00

2 A +6.00D lens is to be made in CR39 material with an axial thickness of 5.4mm. What back surface power must be used?

A −3.62   B −3.75   C −3.87   D −4.00   E −4.12

3 A +4.00D lens is to be made in glass of refractive index 1.8 using spherical surfaces. What front curve would you expect the lens to be given if its off-axis performance is to match that of the subject's best form CR39 lenses?

A +7.80   B +8.00   C +9.62   D +10.00   E +11.00

4 What is the real macular field of view of a +5.00D lens that is edged 47mm round and mounted 27mm in front of the eye's centre of rotation?

A 70°   B 74°   C 78°   D 82°   E 86°

5 What is the centre thickness of a +6.00D lens made in crown glass and edged 60mm in diameter?

A 5.4mm   B 5.8mm   C 6.0mm   D 6.4mm   E 7.8mm

6 What is the thick-edge substance of the lens +3.00/+2.00 × 90 made in a plastics material of refractive index 1.50 and edged to a 50 × 45 oval shape?

A 2.5mm   B 3.0mm   C 3.5mm   D 4.0mm   E 4.5mm

7 The prescription +3.00/+2.00 × 90 is made in CR39 and edged 45mm round. The thin-edge substance is 1.8mm. What is the centre thickness of the lens?

A 3.4mm   B 3.8mm   C 4.0mm   D 4.4mm   E 4.8mm

8 What is the thick-edge substance of the lens described in Question 7?

A 2.3mm   B 2.6mm   C 2.9mm   D 3.2mm   E 3.7mm

9 The prescription +4.00/+3.00 × 120 is knife-edged all round its periphery and is elliptical in shape. Along which meridian does the long axis of the ellipse lie?

A 30°   B 60°   C 90°   D 120°   E 150°

10 If the diameter of the long axis of the knife-edged uncut in Question 3 is 60mm what is the short axis diameter?

A 41mm   B 45mm   C 49mm   D 53mm   E 57mm

11 Which of the following lenses made with the specifications suggested in *Table 9.5* would be the lightest?

A +2.00 made in 1.523 glass and edged 40mm round
B +4.00 made in CR39 and edged 50mm round
C +6.00 made in 1.70 glass and edged 40mm round
D +8.00 made in 1.6 plastics material and edged 50mm round
E +8.00 made in 1.60 glass and edged 40mm round

12 A +4.00D hypermetrope sees the reflection of a window that lies 10 metres behind his head by reflection at the back surface of his lens, the ghost image being in sharp focus without need of accommodation. What is the back surface power of the lens?

A −1.00D   B −2.00D   C −3.00D   D −4.00D   E −5.00D

Chapter 10

1 A fused bifocal is constructed from glass of refractive index 1.52 for the main lens and 1.624 for the segment, with a DP curve of +5.00 and a depression curve of −7.50. What reading addition is obtained?

A +1.00   B +1.50   C +2.00   D +2.50   E +3.00

2 When a bifocal lens with the segment on the front surface is measured in a focimeter the following readings are found:

Front vertex powers   DP +3.87   NP +5.62
Back vertex powers   DP +4.00   NP +6.00

What is the correct specification for the lens?

A +3.87 Add +1.75   B +3.87 Add +2.12
C +4.00 Add +1.62   D +4.00 Add +1.75
E +4.00 Add +2.00

3 A frame of lens shape with box dimensions of 54 × 48 is selected for a subject. When the frame is correctly fitted on the subject's face, it is found that the height from the bottom edge of the lens directly beneath the centre of the subject's pupil to the point at which the segment top is to be positioned is 20mm. The optician orders bifocals with a segment height of 22mm. What segment-top position should be obtained?

A 20mm high
B 22mm high
C on the horizontal centre line
D 2mm below the horizontal centre line
E 4mm below the horizontal centre line

4 An E-style bifocal with an add of +2.00 is to be edged to a 50 × 46 eye with the dividing line positioned 2mm below the horizontal centre line. How much thinning prism would be incorporated to equalize the edge thickness at the top and bottom edges of the lens?

A 0.75Δ base down   B 0.75Δ base up
C 1.25Δ base down   D 1.25Δ base up
E 1.75Δ base down

5 A no-jump bifocal is made to the prescription −2.00 Add +2.50 with a segment drop of 2mm. What is the vertical prismatic effect at a point in the near portion 10mm below the distance optical centre of the lens?

A nil   B 0.5Δ base down
C 0.5Δ base up   D 2.0Δ base down
E 1.75Δ base down

6 A bifocal is made to the prescription +2.00 Add +1.50, with a flat-top D-shape segment of size 28 × 18. What is the jump exerted by the segment?

A nil   B 0.6Δ base down
C 1.35Δ base down   D 2.1Δ base down
E 2.7Δ base down

7 When a bifocal lens with the segment on the convex surface is measured in a focimeter the following readings are found:

Front vertex powers   DP +6.00   NP +8.25
Back vertex powers   DP +6.25   NP +8.75

What is the correct specification for the lens?
A +6.00 Add +2.25   B +6.00 Add +2.75
C +6.25 Add +200   D +6.25 Add +2.25
E +6.25 Add +2.50

8 A bifocal lens with the segment on the front surface is to be made to the Rx +6.00 Add +2.00 in CR39 with a +9.62 base curve and the finished lens is to have a centre thickness of 6.0mm. What reading addition should be ordered if a difference of 2.00D in the back vertex powers is required for the lens?

A +1.75   B +2.00   C +2.25   D +2.50   E +2.75

9 The results from an accurate trigonometric ray trace through the centre of the near portion of a flat-top fused bifocal lens with Rx −6.00 Add +2.00 are $L'_T = -6.30$ and $L'_S = -6.78$, and a paraxial trace through the near point through the DP yields the value $L'_2 = -9.02$D. What reading addition does the subject obtain for this zone of the lens?

A +2.00   B +2.24   C +2.37   D +2.48   E +2.62

10 The results from an accurate trigonometric ray trace through the centre of the near portion of a fused bifocal lens with Rx +4.00 Add +2.00 are $L'_T = +2.89$ and $L'_S = +2.80$, and a paraxial trace from the near point through the DP yields the value $L'_2 = +0.88$D. What reading addition does the subject obtain for this zone of the lens?

A +1.80   B +1.89   C +1.97   D +2.00   E +2.12

11 A subject who has worn the correction −8.00 Add +2.00 in the form of an E-style bifocal with the segment on the concave surface is dispensed new E-style bifocals to the same prescription but this time with the segment on the convex surface. What is the actual reading addition that the subject is likely to obtain with the new lenses when using a zone about 11mm below the dividing line?

A +2.50   B +2.37   C +2.25   D +2.12   E +2.00

12 A subject who has worn the correction +6.00 Add +3.00 in the form of glass solid bifocals with 22 segments on the back surface is dispensed new plastics 22 bifocals to the same prescription, but this time with the segments on the front surface. What are the old and new reading additions that the subject obtains with the lenses when using zones about 5mm below the segment centres?

A old +3.25 new +3.00   B old +3.12 new +3.12
C old +3.25 new +3.25   D old +3.00 new +3.12
E old +3.00 new +3.25

13 A subject whose monocular CDs are 34/34 and whose prescription is +6.00 Add +2.00 is dispensed a 24 round bifocal in a frame for which the lens has box dimensions of 50 × 44. A segment height of 20mm is required and the distance optical centre is to lie 1mm above the HCL. Which of the following segment specifications should be ordered for the spectacles?

A 24 × 1 up × 1.5 segment drop −1
B 24 × 1 × 1.5 segment drop 1
C 24 × 1 × 2 segment drop 2
D 24 × 2 × 3 segment drop 2
E 24 × 2 × 3 segment drop 3

14 The prescription in Question 13 is required, mainly for near vision use at a desk, by an architect, who has mentioned that the field of view should be as large as possible. You realize that chromatism should be minimized in the near portion. Which of the following bifocal types is likely to prove most successful?

A 24 fused   B 38 solid
C extra-deep 45 solid   D 35 flat-top D-segment
E E-style

15 The prescription R −4.00/−2.00 × 90 Add +2.50 is dispensed as an E-style bifocal with a segment drop of 2mm. What are the prismatic effects at a point 8mm below and 2mm inward from the distance optical centre?

A 4.7Δ base up and 1.2Δ base out
B 4.7Δ base down and 1.2Δ base in
C 1.7Δ base up and 1.2Δ base out
D 1.7Δ base down and 1.2Δ base in
E 3.3Δ base down and 0.8Δ base in

16 The prescription −2.00 Add +2.00 is dispensed as a flat-top bifocal with segment size 34 × 20. What is the jump exerted by the segment?

A 0   B 0.3Δ base up
C 0.3Δ base down   D 0.6Δ base up
E 0.6Δ base down

17 The prescription R −3.00/−2.00 × 30, L −1.00/−2.00 × 35 Add +1.50 is dispensed as 25 flat-top bifocals with segment drops of 4mm. What is the difference in the vertical prismatic effects at NVPs 8mm below and 2mm inwards from the distance optical centres?

A 2.1Δ base down R eye
B 2.1Δ base up R eye
C 2.1Δ base down L eye
D 1.7Δ base down L eye
E 3.8Δ base down R eye

18 What is the chromatism at a point 8mm below the distance optical centre and 6mm below the segment top of an E-style bifocal made to the prescription −6.00 Add +2.00 in a plastics material with an Abbe number of 60?

A −0.04Δ   B −0.06Δ   C −0.08Δ   D −0.10Δ   E −0.12Δ

19 It is required to dispense the bifocal prescription BE +2.00 Add +1.50 using invisible segments so that there is no vertical prismatic effect at NVPs situated 9mm below the distance optical centres and 7mm below the segment tops. What segment diameters should be ordered?

A 24   B 28   C 30   D 38   E 45

20 The prescription R −3.00/+1.00 × 90, L −1.00/+1.00 × 90 Add +2.50 is to be dispensed using invisible bifocal segments so that there is no vertical differential prism at NVPs situated 10mm below the distance optical centres and 7mm below the segment tops. A 22 segment is chosen for the right eye. What diameter segment must be chosen for the left eye?

A 24   B 28   C 30   D 38   E 45

21 The prescription R −4.00/+2.00 × 180 Add +2.00 is to be dispensed as a solid prism segment bifocal with a 30mm diameter and a drop of 2mm. How much prism must be incorporated in the segment to eliminate all prismatic effect at a point 8mm below and 2mm inward from the distance optical centre?

A 1.5Δ base up at 117
B 1.5Δ base down at 117
C 1.5Δ base up
D 3.5Δ base down at 103
E 3.5Δ base up at 103

22 The prescription R −2.00/−1.00 × 90, L −4.00/−2.00 × 165 Add +2.25 is to be dispensed as 28 D-segment fused bifocals and, to secure no vertical differential prism at NVPs 8mm below and 2mm inwards from the distance optical centres, one lens is to be supplied in bi-prism form. Which eye should be supplied in bi-prism form and how much prism would be removed by slab-off?

A R 2.4Δ   B L 2.4Δ   C L 3.2Δ   D R 3.2Δ   E L 4.0Δ

23 How can a horizontal prismatic effect of 2Δ base in be obtained at a near visual point that lies 2mm inwards from the distance optical centre, for the prescription R −3.00/−2.00 × 90 Add +2.50, which is to be dispensed as a 35 flat-top bifocal? (Ignore all vertical prismatic effect at the NVP)

A order an inset of 6mm
B order an inset of 4mm
C order an inset of 2mm
D order an inset of 8mm
E order a cemented prism segment design with 2Δ base in added to the segment

24 The prescription DV −4.00/+2.00 × 90, NV −2.00/+2.25 × 90 is to be dispensed as a cemented bifocal with the segment on the concave surface, using an 8.00D contact surface. What is the power of the concave surface of the segment?

A −6.00/−0.25 × 90   B −6.00/+0.25 × 90
C −6.00/+0.25 × 180   D −5.75/+0.25 × 90
E −5.75/+0.25 × 180

Chapter 11

1 A trifocal lens has an intermediate addition of +1.50 and a near addition of +2.50. What is the IP/NP ratio for the lens?

A 67%   B 60%   C 57%   D 55%   E 50%

2 A myope whose total amplitude of accommodation is +1.50D is prescribed a near addition of +2.00 for close work at 33.3cm. The subject is a violinist and requires a continuous clear range of vision from the near point out to 75cm, at which distance the music score is placed, often in conditions of poor illumination. What intermediate addition would serve the purpose?

A +1.00   B +1.50   C +1.37   D +1.25   E +1.12

3 A fused trifocal lens is constructed from glasses of 1.53, 1.61 and 1.69. What percentage of the reading addition is the intermediate addition?

A 40%   B 45%   C 50%   D 55%   E 60%

4 A fused trifocal lens with a near addition of +3.00 is constructed from glasses of 1.52 for the main lens, 1.60 for the intermediate portion and 1.64 for the near portion. What is the addition of the intermediate portion?

A +2.00   B +1.75   C +1.62   D +1.37   E +1.25

5 A concentric downcurve trifocal is made to the prescription +2.00 Add +2.50 for near, with a 60% IP/NP ratio, the segment diameters being 38 and 22 with the IP segment top lying 2mm below the distance optical centre. What is the vertical prismatic effect at a point 4mm below the segment tops in each of the intermediate and near portions?

A IP 0.5Δ base down, NP 0.5Δ base down
B IP 1.05Δ base up, NP 1.05Δ base up
C IP 1.05Δ base up, NP 1.05Δ base down
D IP 1.05Δ base down, NP 1.05Δ base down
E IP 1.05Δ base down, NP 1.05Δ base up

6 What is the jump exerted by the segments in Question 5?

A IP 2.85Δ base down, NP 2.75Δ base down
B IP 2.85Δ base down, NP 1.1Δ base down
C IP 2.75Δ base down, NP 2.85Δ base down
D IP 1.1Δ base down, NP 2.75Δ base down
E IP 1.1Δ base down, NP 2.85Δ base down

Chapter 12

1 What jump is exerted by the progressive power lens +1.50 add +2.50?

A 2.5   B 1.5   C 1.0   D none   E 4.0

2 An oblate ellipsoid is used to model the tangential meridian of the progression zone for a +6.00D base Add +2.50 progressive power lens made in a plastics material of refractive index 1.60. What p-value is necessary to provide this addition over a progression length of 14mm?

A +7.0   B +8.2   C +9.3   D +10.4   E +11.6

3 A progressive power lens with addition +2.50D has a progression zone 12mm in length. Assuming a linear power law through the progression, what addition would you expect the wearer to obtain 8mm below the start of the progression?

A +1.25D   B +1.33D   C +1.50D   D +1.67D   E +1.75D

4 Why is it important to take monocular CD measurements when fitting progressive power lenses?

A to ensure that the optical centres coincide with the distance reference points
B to ensure during convergence and depression that the visual axes remain in the centre of the progression corridors
C to ensure that there is no prismatic effect at the distance reference points
D to ensure that there is no horizontal prismatic effect at the distance reference points
E to ensure that there is no vertical prismatic effect at the distance reference points

5 If a standard thinning prism is applied to a progressive power lens with prescription plano Add +1.50, how much prism would you expect to find at the distance reference point of the lens?

A none   B 1.0Δ base up
C 1.0Δ base down   D 2.0Δ base up
E 2.0Δ base down

6 On verification of a progressive power uncut, the power at the distance reference point that lies 4mm above the geometrical centre of the uncut is found to be +5.00DS and it is noted that the prismatic effect at the point is 4Δ base down. What thinning prism has been incorporated in the lens?

A 1.0Δ base down   B 1.5Δ base down
C 2.0Δ base down   D 2.5Δ base down
E 3.0Δ base down

7 Which of the following subjects may have trouble adapting to a new pair of progressive power lenses?

A a young presbyope who needs a correction for distance and a near add of +1.00
B an experienced wearer whose add has increased from +1.50D to +2.00D
C someone whose lifestyle, work or hobby does not require wide intermediate or near portions on the lenses
D someone who has worn bifocal lenses for many years
E subjects who do not want dividing lines on their lenses

8 How can you tell which eye a progressive power lens is intended for by inspection of its engraved markings?

A the add is engraved under the right-hand circle
B the add is engraved under the left-hand circle
C the add is engraved under the temporal circle
D the add is engraved under the nasal circle
E it is impossible to tell

9 What power lenses would you order for a subject whose prescription is BE +2.50 for distance, Add +2.00 for near and for whom you have dispensed a pair of Essilor *Interview* lenses?

A +2.50   B +2.00   C +3.50   D +4.00   E +4.50

10 A subject whose distance prescription is BE +2.50 has a total amplitude of accommodation of +1.50D and has been prescribed an add of +2.00 for near vision at 33.3cm. What power lenses would you order in this case if you dispense a pair of Essilor *Interview* lenses?

A +2.50   B +2.00   C +3.50   D +4.00   E +4.50

11 A subject whose distance prescription is BE –3.50 has a total amplitude of accommodation of +1.50D and has been prescribed an add of +2.00 for near vision at 33.3cm. What power lenses would you order in this case if you dispense a pair of Rodenstock *Cosmolit P* progressive lenses?

A you cannot select this design since the power is outside the range
B –2.00
C –1.50
D –1.00
E +2.00

12 On verification of a Zeiss *Gradal RD* lens the power at the painted circle is found to be –1.50/–1.00 × 90. What is the distance prescription for this subject?

A –2.00/–1.00 × 90   B –1.75/–1.00 × 90
C –1.50/–1.00 × 90   D –1.25/–1.00 × 90
E –2.50/–1.00 × 90

13 You decide to dispense *Access* lenses to a subject whose prescription is +2.00 Add +1.75. What prescription would you order?

A +1.25   B +1.75   C +2.00   D +2.50   E +3.75

14 What would be the power in the intermediate viewing area of the correctly ordered *Access* lens described in Question 13?

A plano   B +0.75   C +2.00   D +2.50   E +3.75

15 A new progressive lens design has an isocylinder plot for the power plano Add 2.00, which indicates that the areas on the lens in which the astigmatism exceeds 0.25D are confined entirely to zones below the 180 meridian of the lens. How would you classify this design?

A as a soft design
B as a hard design
C as a design that is soft in the near portion
D as a design that should prove comfortable to wear by a subject with a low near addition
E as a design that is likely to prove suitable for an architect viewing large-scale plans

16 What feature is peculiar to the Zeiss *Gradal Top* and the Rodenstock *Multigressiv* designs that is not shared by progressive power lenses from other sources?

A both are available in aspheric form
B both have the correcting cylinder combined with the progressive surface
C both have atoroidal surfaces when the lens is astigmatic
D both have the progressive surface on the front of the lens
E both have the progressive surface on the back of the lens

Chapter 13

1 What is the size of the annular scotoma of a +14.00D spectacle lens edged 40mm in diameter and mounted 25mm in front of the eye's centre of rotation?

A 11.8°   B 11.6°   C 11.4°   D 11.2°   E 11.0°

2 When the eye turns to view through off-axis zones of a correctly centred point-focal aspheric lens, the distance from the eye to the back surface of the lens increases. The result is that:

A the oblique vertex sphere powers of the lens increase
B the oblique vertex sphere powers of the lens decrease
C the mean oblique power of the lens increases
D the lens is no longer point-focal
E there is no change from the paraxial power

3 Why are errors caused by near vision effectivity more significant with aspheric lenses?

A the image quality is better with an aspheric lens
B the lens is thinner
C the lens is thicker
D the mean oblique image vergence becomes greater than the paraxial value for L'_2
E the mean oblique image vergence becomes less than the paraxial value for L'_2

4 During refraction, best visual acuity is obtained for distance with an equi-convex trial lens of power +12.00 that has been adjusted before the eye so that the pantoscopic angle is 10° and the optical centre has been lowered by 5mm to compensate for the angle. Assuming no change in vertex distance, what power final lens will best duplicate the effect of the trial lens?

A +12.25/+0.50 × 180   B +12.25/+0.50 × 90
C +12.00/+0.25 × 90   D +12.00/+0.25 × 180
E +12.00

5 A subject is corrected for near vision at 33.3cm by a +13.00D plano-convex trial lens that has an axial thickness of 9mm and is designed to be worn with the curved surface facing the eye. The final lens for near that is dispensed has a +15.00D front curve and an axial thickness of 9mm. Assuming the refractive index of each lens is 1.5, what are the NVEEs of the trial lens and the final lens?

A 0.00 and +0.50   B 0.00 and −0.50
C +0.05 and −0.50   D −0.05 and +0.50
E −0.05 and −0.50

6 What power lens must be ordered for near vision for the situation described in Question 5 if the final lens is to have the same paraxial effect as the trial lens?

A +12.50   B +12.75   C +13.00   D +13.25   E +13.50

Chapter 14

1 What is the most significant difference between the old BS 2092 and the more recent EN Standards on safety lenses?

A the recommendations for low-energy impact
B the recommendations for high-energy impact
C the recommendations for the diameter of the steel ball used in the test
D the recommendations for the weight of the steel ball used in the test
E the recommendations for lens retention during the test

2 Which of the following activities has been shown to give rise to most eye injuries?

A accidents in the home   B adult sport
C farm working   D industrial accidents
E assault

3 Which of the following occupations has been shown to give rise to most ocular injury from foreign bodies?

A metalworker   B sheet metalworker
C electrician   D welder
E press/machine tool operator

4 Which of the following safety lenses is least likely to give rise to sharp splinters when fractured?

A laminated lens
B heat-toughened lens
C polycarbonate
D CR39
E chemically toughened lens

5 Which of the following best retains the safety aspects of polycarbonate lenses?

A leaving the lens a little overlarge and mounting in a metal rim
B leaving the lens a little overlarge and mounting in a plastics frame
C glazing the lens normally to a metal rim
D glazing the lens normally to a plastics frame
E glazing the lens loosely to a plastics frame

6 Taking all the risk factors into account, which of the following materials is the safest for use as a spectacle lens material?

A uncoated polycarbonate
B coated polycarbonate
C CR39
D mid-index plastics
E chemically toughened glass

Chapter 15

1 A −5.00D lens is made in glass of refractive index 1.6 with a +4.00D front curve and axial thickness of 1.2mm. What is the shape factor for the lens?

A 3%   B 2%   C 1%   D 0.3%   E 0.1%

2 If the lens described in Question 1 is mounted 15mm in front of the eye's entrance pupil, what is its power factor?

A +4.00   B −5.00   C −4%   D −5%   E −7%

3 What is the equivalent power of a spectacle magnifier whose nominal magnification is 4×?

A +1.00   B +4.00   C +16.00   D +20.00   E +25.00

4 An afocal Galilean telescopic unit is made up from thin +15.00D and –27.00D trial lenses. What is the separation of the lenses and what magnification is achieved?

A d=66.7mm, M=1.5×   B d=40mm, M=1.5×
C d=29.63mm, M=1.5×   D d=29.63mm, M=1.8×
E d=40mm, M=1.8×

5 An afocal telescopic unit has a magnification of 2× when used for near vision at 25cm from the objective lens. If the device is adapted for use at distance by the addition of a –4.00D cap over the objective, what magnification would be obtained for distance vision?

A 2.0×   B 1.9×   C 1.8×   D 1.7×   E 1.6×

6 The specification –1.00/–3.75×180 for DV and +1.50/–4.00×180 for NV is to be dispensed as solid visible bifocals with a –7.00DS segment surface. What is the power of the DP surface?

A –9.00×180/–9.00×90   B –9.25×180/–9.50×90
C –9.25×90/–9.50×180   D –9.50×90/–9.75×180
E –9.50×180/–9.75×90

Chapter 16

1 Which of the following sports has legislation concerning personal eye protection?

A table tennis
B badminton
C cricket
D hockey
E squash

2 A spectacle lens made in CR39 has a power in air of –4.50. What power would it have when totally immersed in water?

A –13.50   B –4.50   C –2.00   D –1.50   E –1.25

3 A spectacle lens, made in plastics material of refractive index 1.666, has surface powers in air of +6.00 and –8.00. What power will this lens have when mounted in a swimming goggle and worn under water (assume the refractive index of the water to be 1.333)?

A –7.00   B –6.00   C –5.00   D –4.00   E –2.00

4 A +4.00D lens is mounted 27mm in front of the eye's centre of rotation and decentred 4mm downwards in order to compensate for a lens pantoscopic tilt of 8°. Through what angle, expressed in prism dioptres, will the eye rotate in order to view a distant object?

A 1.8Δ   B 1.7Δ   C 1.6Δ   D 1.5Δ   E 1.4Δ

5 A subject whose prescription is BE +2.00D is to be dispensed a pair of wrap-round sports spectacles with dihedral angles of 13.5° for each lens which is to be compensated for by outward decentration. If the lenses are mounted 25mm in front of the eye's centres of rotation, what decentration would be specified for each lens?

A BE 10mm out   B BE 9mm out
C BE 8mm out   D BE 7mm out
E BE 6mm out

6 What ocular rotation would be required by each eye for the prescription described in Question 5 in order for the subject to view an object lying directly ahead?

A 1.2Δ inwards   B 1.3Δ inwards
C 1.4Δ inwards   D 1.5Δ inwards
E 1.6Δ inwards

Chapter 17

1 How much prism must be incorporated in the specification R –2.00/–2.00×90 to shift the optical centre 5mm inwards?

A 1Δ base in   B 1Δ base out
C 2Δ base in   D 2Δ base out
E 2Δ base down

2 How much prism must be incorporated in the specification R +2.00/–2.00×45 to shift the optical centre 5mm inwards?

A 0.71Δ base in   B 0.71Δ base up at 45
C 0.71Δ base down at 45   D 0.71Δ base up at 135
E 0.71Δ base down at 135

3 A spherical generator with a tool of diameter 85mm and cutting head radius of 2mm is used to produce a convex surface of power +6.00D on CR39 material of refractive index 1.498. Through what angle must the generator head rotate?

A 30.00°   B 31.65°   C 32.00°   D 32.65°   E 33.00°

4 A tyre-form toroidal surface ground on a material of refractive index 1.50 has a power of +8.00 DC/+12.00 DC. What is the sagittal power of the base curve at a point 20mm above the vertex of the surface?

A +7.54   B +7.64   C +7.74   D +7.84   E +7.94

5 What is the sag of a paraboloidal surface of power +6.00D worked on a material of refractive index 1.50 at a point 15mm above and 20mm out from the vertex of the surface?

A 3.0mm   B 3.25mm   C 3.5mm   D 3.75mm   E 4.0mm

6 Which of the following methods has not yet been applied to the production of aspherical surfaces on spectacle lenses?

A shaping the surface by pressing
B shaping the surface by heat and pressure
C eroding the surface by removing material with an ion beam.
D forming the surface by heat and sagging (slumping)
E shaping the surface by grinding and polishing

Chapter 18

1 A fused bifocal with segment on the +4.00D convex surface has a depression curve of power –6.00D and is made using glasses, main lens n=1.55, segment n=1.66. What is the reading addition of the lens?

A +1.50   B +1.75   C +2.00   D +2.25   E +2.50

2 A fused bifocal with segment on the –8.00D concave surface has a depression curve of power –16.00D and is made using glasses, main lens n=1.52, segment n=1.65. What is the reading addition of the lens?

A +1.00   B +1.25   C +1.50   D +1.75   E +2.00

3 Under which of the following conditions is it easiest to control the final diameter of a fused bifocal segment when working the segment side of the lens?

A when the Add is high
B when the DP curve is high and the Add is high
C when the DP curve is high and the Add is low
D when the DP curve is low and the Add is high
E when the DP curve is low and the Add is low

4 What is the prescription of a solid bifocal lens with surface powers F_1 +2.50, DP curve −6.75 and NP curve −4.50?

A +4.25 Add +2.25   B −2.25 Add +2.75
C +2.25 Add +2.75   D −2.00 Add +2.25
E −4.25 Add +2.25

5 In the production of a solid bifocal surface, which operation normally follows DP roughing?

A DP smoothing   B NP roughing
C NP smoothing   D DP polishing
E NP polishing

6 A solid-prism segment bifocal made in spectacle crown glass has a difference between its minimum and maximum depths of ridge of 1.29mm. How much prism has been incorporated in the segment?

A 2.25   B 2.00   C 1.75   D 1.50   E 1.25

Answers to multiple choice questions

Chapter 1

1 **C** 23.7°
2 **B** 3.07cm
3 **D** 90cm
4 **E** 4.9Δ
5 **B** 3.0Δ
6 **A** 2.25Δ
7 **E** −7.00D
8 **D** +10.00
9 **C** 20cm behind the lens
10 **C** +8.00
11 **D** +7.44
12 **E** +13.00
13 **A** −5.25
14 **E** −12.50
15 **C** −11.50
16 **B** +3.50
17 **A** 1.6mm
18 **D** +1.00/+2.00 × 170

Chapter 2

1 **B** 0.12Δ (TCA = P/V = 0.8 × 6/40)
2 **A** OAE +0.14, MOP +4.83, MOE −0.17
3 **C** OAE −0.75, MOE −0.62
4 **D** +14.25 and +12.25
5 **E** +1.50 base meniscus
6 both C and E describe the lens form correctly but C is the preferred answer
7 **C** CVF = 0.70 reflectance = 7.4%
8 **D** transmission = 89.4%
9 **D** a little lighter
10 **E** 28mm
11 **B** −7.75
12 **A** 1.75

Chapter 3

1 **D** compare this answer with definition 01 113 given in BS 3521 Part 1: 1991
2 **E** segment drop refers to the position of the distance optical centre in relation to the segment top; no information is given about the distance optical centre in the question
3 **C** you should reduce your measurement of the PD by 0.5mm
4 **C** inter CD = 64mm
5 **E** order geometrical insets R 3.0 in, L 2.7 in
6 both B and D are correct; however, B is preferred since it is better to stipulate vertical decentration from the HCL (or the actual *standard optical centre position* if it is located elsewhere) rather than the lower horizontal tangent to the lens periphery; see, for example, the definition given earlier in the text

7 **D** 2.4Δ base down and 1.5Δ base in
8 **C** 2.6Δ base down and 1.5Δ base in
9 **E** 2Δ base in
10 **E** 58 − to avoid 1.2Δ of vertical differential prism
11 **B** iso-V-prism zone is a band 10mm wide along 180
12 **A** 11.5mm wide lying along 30

Chapter 4

1 **D** parabola
2 **D** hyperboloid with vertex radius 50 mm
3 **E** the astigmatism of an aspherical surface can neutralize the astigmatism of oblique incidence
4 **A** 6.3mm
5 **B** 5.8mm
6 **C** +4.00
7 **D** they are flatter and use an aspherical surface
8 **B** it is about the same as the performance of lenses made with spherical surfaces
9 **C** a low-power aspheric lens has about the same distortion as a best-form lens with spherical surfaces
10 **D** +5.00D
11 **A** 1.74mm
12 **E** the atoroidal surface of the *Hypal* does not include the cylindrical correction
13 **D** 32.5/30.5
14 **E** decentre lenses 4 in each eye from the box centre and apply a reverse dihedral angle of 4° to each lens
15 **C** by asking for the lens to be decentred 3mm out after the prism has been surfaced
16 **C** because the decentration will shift the pole of the surface from the visual axis
17 **A** 8.4Δ and 7.35Δ
18 **B** +262.11mm

Chapter 5

1 **C** the ghost image must be superimposed upon the refracted image
2 **E** 4.8%
3 **A** 0.33%
4 **D** 4.00D
5 **C** +2.50
6 **B** 37.8mm
7 **D** 11.6%
8 **C** 82.4%
9 **B** 1.249
10 **A** 101.4nm

11 **E** to enable the amplitude condition to be satisfied
12 **E** to ensure that the mean free path of the molecules of coating material is 1 metre

Chapter 6

1 **D** can be reformed after heating
2 **E** hard coating, MAR, single-layer anti-reflection, hydrophobic coating
3 **C** interference patterns become visible on the surface when the lens is anti-reflection coated
4 **C** they have a high wetting angle
5 **A** because the dirt shows more
6 **E** 90%

Chapter 7

1 **C** BS 169 and BS 379
2 **A** at the blue end of the visible spectrum
3 **E** 0.19
4 **D** infrared radiation
5 **B** 64%
6 **E** D_{65}
7 **B** light/dark
8 **B** reversible whereas in the latter it is fatiguing
9 **C** silver bromide and silver iodide
10 **C** 1500nm
11 **A** 8%
12 **D** 0.8
13 **B** 20.6%
14 **E** 0.1 τ_V
15 **E** 50 000 lux (±3000)

Chapter 8

1 **D** +3.00 and −11.00
2 **C** 84°
3 **B** (i) 1.3mm, (ii) 1.6mm, (iii) 2.0mm
4 **D** 6.4mm
5 **C** 4.1mm
6 **E** 7.9mm
7 **D** 7.0mm
8 **A** 4.9mm
9 **C** +4.75DC
10 **B** 4mm
11 **E** bonded lenticular
12 **E** at the cornea and the back surface of the lens

Chapter 9

1 **C** +5.75
2 **D** −4.00
3 **E** +11.00

4 **B** 74°
5 **D** 6.4mm
6 **A** 2.5mm
7 **D** 4.4mm
8 **C** 2.9mm
9 **D** 120°
10 **B** 45mm
11 **E** +8.00 made in 1.60 glass and edged 40mm round
12 **A** −1.00D

Chapter 10

1 **D** +2.50
2 **D** +4.00 Add +1.75
3 **D** 2 below the horizontal centre line
4 **C** 1.25Δ base down
5 **A** nil
6 **B** 0.6Δ base down
7 **D** +6.25 Add +2.25
8 **A** +1.75
9 **D** +2.48
10 **C** +1.97
11 **B** +2.37
12 **E** old +3.00 new +3.25
13 **E** 24 × 2 × 3 segment drop 3
14 **C** extra-deep 45 solid
15 **D** 1.7Δ base down and 1.2Δ base in
16 **E** 0.6Δ base down
17 **A** 2.1Δ base down R eye
18 **B** −0.06Δ
19 **D** 38
20 **D** 38
21 **E** 3.5Δ base up at 103
22 **C** L 3.2Δ
23 **A** order an inset of 6mm
24 **B** −6.00/+0.25 × 90

Chapter 11

1 **B** 60%
2 **D** +1.25
3 **C** 50%
4 **A** +2.00
5 **E** IP 1.05Δ base down, NP 1.05Δ base up
6 **B** IP 2.85Δ base down, NP 1.1Δ base down

Chapter 12

1 **D** none
2 **E** +11.6
3 **D** +1.67D
4 **B** to ensure during convergence and depression that the visual axes remain in the centre of the progression corridors
5 **C** 1.0Δ base down
6 **C** 2Δ base down
7 **D** someone who has worn bifocal lenses for many years
8 **C** the add is engraved under the temporal circle
9 **E** +4.50
10 **E** +4.50
11 **B** −2.00
12 **A** −2.00/−1.00 × 90
13 **E** +3.75
14 **D** +2.50
15 **B** as a hard design
16 **C** both have atoroidal surfaces when the lens is astigmatic

Chapter 13

1 **D** 11.2°
2 **B** the oblique vertex sphere powers of the lens decrease
3 **E** the mean oblique image vergence becomes less than the paraxial value for L'_2
4 **A** +12.25/+0.50 × 180
5 **C** +0.05 and −0.50
6 **E** +13.50

Chapter 14

1 **B** the recommendations for high-energy impact
2 **D** industrial accidents
3 **E** press/machine tool operators
4 **C** polycarbonate
5 **E** glazing the lens loosely to a plastics frame
6 **A** uncoated polycarbonate

Chapter 15

1 **D** 0.3%
2 **E** −7%
3 **C** +16.00
4 **D** d = 29.63mm, M = 1.8×
5 **A** 2×
6 **B** −9.25 × 180/−9.50 × 90

Chapter 16

1 **E** squash
2 **D** −1.50
3 **C** −5.00
4 **A** 1.8Δ
5 **E** BE 6mm out
6 **B** 1.3Δ inwards

Chapter 17

1 **D** 2Δ base out
2 **B** 0.71Δ base up at 45
3 **A** 30°
4 **B** +7.64
5 **D** 3.75mm
6 **C** eroding the surface by removing material with an ion beam

Chapter 18

1 **C** +2.00
2 **E** +2.00
3 **D** when the DP curve is low and the add is high
4 **E** −4.25 Add +2.25
5 **B** NP roughing
6 **A** 2.25Δ

Index

Minimum system requirements

Windows

Windows 2000 or higher
1.4Ghz processor
128 MB RAM
4x CD-ROM drive
VGA Monitor supporting 800x600 at millions of colours

Note:
Some of the content in this product is available in PPT format. You need Microsoft PowerPoint 2003, or an equivalent product, to view this content. In absence of this, use PowerPoint Viewer located in the root folder of the CD (under Microsoft folder). This is for Windows only.
Some of the content in this product is available in XLS format. You need Microsoft Excel, or an equivalent product, to view this content.

Mac

Apple G4 Macintosh
Mac OS 10 or later
128 MB RAM
4x CD-ROM drive
VGA Monitor supporting 800x600 at millions of colours

Note:
Some of the content in this product is available in PPT format. You need Microsoft PowerPoint 2003, or an equivalent product, to view this content.
Some of the content in this product is available in XLS format. You need Microsoft Excel, or an equivalent product, to view this content.

instructions

Windows
If your system does not support Autorun, navigate to your CD drive and double click on 'Jalie.exe' to begin. Alternatively, click Start, Run and type 'D: Jalie.exe ' to begin. If D: is not your CD drive, substitute D: with the appropriate drive letter.

Mac
If the CD does not autorun, open the CD icon that appears on the desktop and select ' Jalie' to begin.

Technical Support
Technical support for this product is available between 7.30 a.m. and 7.00 p.m. CST, Monday through Friday. Before calling, be sure that your computer meets the minimum system requirements to run this software.
Inside the United States and Canada, call 1-800-692-9010.
Inside the United Kingdom, call 00-800-692-90100.
Outside North America, call +1-314-872-8370.
You may also fax your questions to +1-314-997-5080,
or contact Technical Support through e-mail: technical.support@elsevier.com.

ELSEVIER CD-ROM LICENCE AGREEMENT